# Practical Perinatal Care: The Baby Under 1000 grams

# Practical Perinatal Care:
# The Baby Under 1000 grams

**Gill Levitt** BSc DCH MRCP MRCPCH
Consultant Paediatrician
Department of Haematology and Oncology
Great Ormond Street Hospital for Children NHS Trust
London

**David Harvey** MBBS FRCP FRCPCH
Professor of Paediatrics and Neonatal Medicine
Imperial College School of Medicine
Hammersmith Hospital
London

**Richard Cooke** MD FRCP FRCPCH
Professor of Paediatric Medicine
Department of Child Health
University of Liverpool
Liverpool

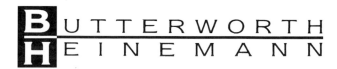

**B**UTTERWORTH
**H**EINEMANN

OXFORD   AUCKLAND   BOSTON   JOHANNESBURG   MELBOURNE   NEW DELHI

Butterworth–Heinemann
Linacre House, Jordan Hill, Oxford OX2 8DP
225 Wildwood Avenue, Woburn, MA 01801-2041
A division of Reed Educational and Professional Publishing Ltd

A member of the Reed Elsevier plc group

First published 1999

**British Library Cataloguing in Publication Data**
A catalogue record for this book is available from the British Library

**Library of Congress Cataloguing in Publication Data**
A catalogue record for this book is available from the Library of Congress

ISBN 0 7506 1717 9

Composition by Scribe Design, Gillingham, Kent
Printed and bound in Great Britain by The Bath Press, Somerset

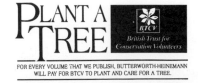

PLANT A TREE

BTCV
British Trust for
Conservation Volunteers

FOR EVERY VOLUME THAT WE PUBLISH, BUTTERWORTH-HEINEMANN
WILL PAY FOR BTCV TO PLANT AND CARE FOR A TREE.

# Contents

# Preface

The idea for the first edition of this book arose from a conference of neonatal specialists held at Maidstone, Kent in 1984. It was at a time when the survival of infants born weighing less than 1000 grams was becoming more the rule than the exception. Apparently new problems such as periventricular leukomalacia and metabolic bone disease were becoming more prominent, and disorders such as retinopathy of prematurity, thought to be conquered, were reappearing. Neonatal care for those at the limits of viability seemed the ultimate challenge for the nascent speciality of universal neonatal intensive care.

Fifteen years on, a great deal of progress has been made. The likelihood of survival at a birthweight below 1000 grams has improved several-fold, and the quality of that survival has not deteriorated. New technologies for respiratory care, nutritional support and neuroimaging have contributed to these improvements and to our understanding of the origins of residual morbidity. Careful follow-up studies have focused more than ever before on this extensively studied group, and in a cost conscious age, the financial wisdom of providing care for these children has been questioned.

In the age of the Internet and electronic data transfer, many people consider that the textbook, even when multi-authored, has had its day. However, this medium remains highly favoured amongst staff in training, and those at the workface of neonatal care as a rapid source of practical reference, experience and as a starting point for further enquiry. This volume with its authors drawn from most of the UK's major neonatal centres, provides an authoritative guide to the challenges surrounding the care of the extremely preterm infant into the next millennium.

# List of contributors

**Elizabeth Bryan** MD FRCP FRCPCH
*Honorary Consultant Paediatrician and Director of the Multiple Births Foundation, Queen Charlotte's and Chelsea Hospital, Hammersmith Hospitals NHS Trust; Reader in Paediatrics, Imperial College School of Medicine at Hammersmith Hospital, London, UK*

**Ashley Buckner**
*Research Fellow, Ninewells Hospital and Medical School, Dundee, UK*

**Geoffrey Chamberlain** MD FRCS FRCOG FACOG
*Emeritus Professor of Obstetrics and Gynaecology, Singleton Hospital, Swansea, UK*

**David Clark** BM FRCS FRCO DO
*Consultant Ophthalmologist, Aintree Hospitals NHS Trust, Liverpool, UK*

**Richard Cooke** MD FRCP FRCPCH
*Professor of Paediatric Medicine, Institute of Child Health, Royal Liverpool Children's NHS Trust, Alder Hey, Liverpool; Clinical Director, Neonatal Services, Liverpool Women's Hospital, Liverpool, UK*

**Malcolm Coulthard** MSc MBBS FRCP MRCPCH
*Consultant Paediatric Nephrologist, Children's Kidney Unit, The Royal Victoria Infirmary, Newcastle upon Tyne, UK*

**Lilly Dubowitz** MD FRCP FRCPCH
*Honorary Consultant Paediatrician, The Hammersmith Hospitals NHS Trust; Senior Lecturer, Department of Paediatrics and Neonatal Medicine, Imperial College School of Medicine at Hammersmith Hospital, London, UK*

**Murdo Elder** DSc MD FRCS FRCOG
*Professor of Obstetrics and Gynaecology, Chairman of the Division of Paediatrics, Obstetrics and Gynaecology, Imperial College School of Medicine at Hammersmith Hospital, London, UK*

**Janet Eyre** BSc MBChB DPhil FRCP
*Professor of Paediatric Neuroscience and Consultant Paediatric Neurologist, University of Newcastle, Newcastle upon Tyne, UK*

**Janice Fearne** BDS FDS RCS(Eng) PhD
*Consultant in Paediatric Dentistry, The Royal Hospitals NHS Trust Dental Institute, London, UK*

**Anne Greenough** MD FRCP FRCPCH DCH
*Clinical Director of the Department of Child Health, and Honorary Consultant Paediatrician, King's College Hospital; Professor of Clinical Respiratory Physiology, Department of Child Health, King's College School of Medicine and Dentistry, London, UK*

**Michael Hall** MBChB DCH FRCP FRCPCH
*Consultant Paediatrician and Neonatologist, Princess Anne Hospital; Honorary Senior Lecturer in Child Health, University of Southampton, Southampton University Hospital NHS Trust, Southampton, UK*

**Henry Halliday** MD FRCPE FRCP FRCPCH DCH D(Obst)RCOG
*Consultant Neonatologist, Royal Maternity Hospital, Belfast; Honorary Professor of Child Health, The Queen's University of Belfast, UK*

**David Harvey** MBBS FRCP FRCPCH
*Professor of Paediatrics and Neonatal Medicine, Imperial College School of Medicine at Hammersmith Hospital; Honorary Consultant Paediatrician, Queen Charlotte's and Chelsea Hospital, The Hammersmith Hospitals NHS Trust, London, UK*

**Barbara Holland** MBBCh BAO DCH FRCP FRCPCH
*Consultant Neonatal Paediatrician, The Queen Mother's Hospital, Royal Hospital for Sick Children, Glasgow, UK*

**Robert Irontron** BM BCh DPhil FRCP FRCPCH
*Consultant Neonatal Paediatrician, Princess Anne Hospital, Southampton University Hospital NHS Trust, Southampton, UK*

**Jean Keeling** MBBS FRCPath FRCP(Edin) FRCPCH
*Consultant Paediatric Pathologist and Head of Department, Edinburgh Sick Children's NHS Trust; Honorary Senior Lecturer in Pathology, University of Edinburgh, Edinburgh, UK*

**Ronnie Lamont** BSc MD FRCOG
*Consultant in Obstetrics and Gynaecology, Northwick Park and St Marks NHS Trust, Harrow, UK; Honorary Senior Lecturer, Division of Paediatrics, Obstetrics and Gynaecology, Imperial College School of Medicine, Hammersmith Hospital, London, UK*

**Elizabeth Letsky** MBBS FRCPath FRCOG FRCPCH
*Consultant Perinatal Haematologist and Honorary Senior Lecturer, Queen Charlotte's and Chelsea Hospital, Hammersmith Hospitals NHS Trust, London, UK*

**Neil McIntosh** MBBS BSc FRCP FRCPE FRCPCH DSc(Med)
*Professor of Child Life and Health, and Head of Department, Edinburgh Sick Children's NHS Trust and University of Edinburgh, Edinburgh, UK*

**Ann Maloy** RGN RM ENB402
*Neonatal Services Manager, Hammersmith Hospitals NHS Trust, Queen Charlotte's and Chelsea Hospital, London, UK*

**Eugenio Mercuri** MD PhD
*Lecturer in Paediatric Neurology, Imperial College School of Medicine at Hammersmith Hospital, London, UK*

**Gary Mires** MD MRCOG
*Senior Lecturer in Obstetrics and Gynaecology, Ninewells Hospital and Medical School, Dundee, UK*

**Sally Mitton** MD MRCP
*Senior Lecturer and Consultant in Paediatric Gastroenterology and Nutrition, St George's Hospital Medical School, London, UK*

**Neena Modi** MBChB MD FRCP FRCPCH
*Senior Lecturer and Consultant in Neonatal Paediatrics, Imperial College School of Medicine at Hammersmith Hospital, London, UK*

**Richard Mupanemunda** BSc BM MRCP FRCPCH
*Consultant in Neonatal Medicine, Princess of Wales Maternity Unit, Birmingham Heartlands Hospital NHS Trust, Birmingham, UK*

**Gareth Parry** BSc MSc
*Research Fellow in Statistics, Medical Care Research Unit, University of Sheffield, Sheffield, UK*

**Naren Patel**
*Professor of Obstetrics and Gynaecology, Department of Reproductive Medicine, Ninewells Hospital and Medical School, Dundee, UK*

**Janet Rennie** MA MD FRCP FRCPCH DCH
*Consultant and Honorary Senior Lecturer in Neonatal Medicine, Department of Child Health, King's College Hospital, London, UK*

**Martin Richards** MA PhD
*Professor of Family Research and Director of the Centre for Family Research, University of Cambridge, Cambridge, UK*

**N.R.C. Roberton** MA MB FRCP
*Former Consultant Paediatrician, Rosie Maternity Hospital, Cambridge, UK*

**Irene Roberts** MD FRCP FRCPath DRCOG
*Senior Lecturer in Haematology, Imperial College School of Medicine at Hammersmith Hospital; Honorary Consultant Paediatric Haematologist, Hammersmith Hospitals NHS Trust, London, UK*

**Peter Rolfe** BSc PhD CEng MIEEE FIPEM FIEE
*Director of Science and Technology, Oxford Bioengineering Ltd; Director of WHO Collaborating Centre; Visiting Professor, Department of Informatica, Systemistica and Telematica, Genoa University, Italy*

**Nicholas Rutter** MD FRCP FRCPCH
*Professor of Paediatric Medicine and Honorary Consultant Paediatrician, Queens Medical Centre, Nottingham, UK*

**Ben Shaw** MBChB MD FRCP FRCPCH
*Consultant in Neonatal and Respiratory Paediatrics, Liverpool Women's Hospital and Royal Liverpool Children's NHS Trust, Alder Hey, Liverpool, UK*

**Ann Stewart** MRCP FRCPCH
*Honorary Senior Lecturer, Department of Paediatrics, University College London Medical School and Department of Psychological Medicine, Institute of Psychiatry, King's College, London, UK*

**William Tarnow-Mordi** BA MBChB MRCP FRCPCH
*Reader in Neonatal Medicine and Perinatal Epidemiology, Ninewells Hospital and Medical School, Dundee, UK*

**Charles Wardrop** MBChB FRCPE
*Senior Lecturer and Honorary Consultant in Haematology, University of Wales College of Medicine, Cardiff, UK*

**Andrew Whitelaw** MD FRCPCH
*Professor of Neonatal Medicine, University of Bristol, Neonatal Intensive Care Unit, Southmead Hospital, Bristol, UK*

**James Wilkinson** MB ChB FRCP FRACP FACC FRCPCH
*Director of Cardiology, Royal Children's Hospital, Melbourne; Honorary Cardiologist, Royal Melbourne Hospital, Melbourne; Honorary Cardiologist, Monash Medical Centre, Melbourne; Honorary Cardiologist, Geelong Hospital, Geelong, Australia*

**Anthony Williams** BSc MBBS DPhil FRCP FRCPCH
*Senior Lecturer and Consultant in Neonatal Paediatrics, Department of Child Health, St George's Hospital Medical School, London, UK*

**Victor Yu** MD MSc FRACP FRCP FRCPCH DCH
*Professor of Neonatology, Monash University; Director of Neonatal Intensive Care, Monash Medical Centre, Clayton, Victoria, Australia*

# Glossary of abbreviations

| | |
|---|---|
| ABR | auditory brainstem response |
| AC | abdominal circumference |
| ADH | antidiuretic hormone |
| AER | active expiratory reflex |
| AGA | appropriate for gestational age |
| AITP | autoimmune thrombocytopenia |
| ANP | atrial natriuretic peptide |
| APACHE | (Chapter 28) |
| APCR | activated protein C resistance |
| ATP | adenosine triphosphate |
| AVP | arginine vasopressin |
| BBB | blood–brain barrier |
| BCG | Bacille Calmette Guerin vaccine |
| BMC | bone mineral content |
| BP | blood pressure |
| BPD | biparietal diameter |
| BPD | bronchopulmonary dysplasia |
| BV | blood volume |
| CBF | cerebral blood flow |
| CBV | cerebral blood volume |
| CI | confidence interval |
| CLP | chronic lung disease of prematurity |
| CMV | cytomegalovirus |
| CPAP | continuous positive airways pressure |
| CRIB | clinical risk index for babies |
| CSF | cerebrospinal fluid |
| CT | computerized tomography |
| CVP | central venous pressure |
| CVS | chorionic villus sampling |
| DEXA | dual energy X-ray absorptiometry |
| DIC | disseminated intravascular coagulation |
| DPG | diphosphoglycerate |
| DPPC | dipalmitoylphosphatidyl choline |
| ECF | extracellular fluid |
| ECG | electrocardiogram |
| ECMO | extracorporeal membrane oxygenation |
| EEG | electroencephalogram |
| ELBW | extremely low birth weight (<1000 g) |
| EMG | electromyelogram |
| EPO | erythropoietin |
| ERR | event rate ratio |
| ETT | endotracheal tube |
| FG | Foley gauge |
| $F_{IO_2}$ | fraction of inspired oxygen concentration |
| FL | femur length |
| FRC | functional residual capacity |
| GA | gestational age |
| GABA | gamma amino butyric acid |
| GAGA | gamma amino glutaric acid |
| GFR | glomerular filtration rate |
| GLH | germinal layer haemorrhage |
| GLH/IVH | germinal layer/intraventricular haemorrhage |
| GMH/PVH | germinal layer/periventricular haemorrhage |
| Gunn rats | rats with error of bilirubin metabolism leading to kernicterus |
| GVHD | graft-versus-host disease |
| HbA | adult haemoglobin |
| HbF | fetal haemoglobin |
| HC | head circumference |
| HCT | haematocrit |
| HDN | haemorrhagic disease of the newborn |

| | | | |
|---|---|---|---|
| HELLP | haemolysis, elevated liver enzymes and low platelet count | PEEP | positive end expiratory pressure |
| HFJV | high frequency jet ventilation | PG | phosphatidyl glycerol |
| HFO | high frequency oscillation | PGA | postgestational age |
| HFPPV | high frequency positive pressure ventilation (>60 breaths min$^{-1}$) | PHVD | posthaemorrhagic ventricular dilation |
| HIV | human immunodeficiency virus | PI | phosphatidyl inositol |
| HMWK | high molecular weight kininogen | PIE | pulmonary interstitial emphysema |
| HPA$^1$ | human platelet antigen 1 | PIP | peak inspiratory pressure |
| i.m. | intramuscular | PK | prekallikrein |
| i.v. | intravascular | PG | phosphatidyl glycerol |
| ICP | intracranial pressure | PMA | post menstrual age |
| IgA | immunoglobulin A | $Po_2$ | partial pressure of oxygen |
| IgB | immunoglobulin B | PRISM | paediatric risk of mortality |
| IgM | immunoglobulin M | PROM | preterm rupture of the membranes |
| IMV | intermittent mandatory ventilation | PT | prothrombin time |
| IPL | intraparenchymal echodense lesion | PTT | partial thromboplastin time |
| IPPV | intermittent positive pressure ventilation | PTV | patient-triggered ventilation |
| | | PUFA | polyunsaturated fatty acids |
| IQ | intelligence quotient | PVC | poly(vinyl chloride) |
| ITP | idiopathic thrombocytopenia | PVH | periventricular haemorrhage |
| IUGR | intrauterine growth retardation | PVL | periventricular leucomalacia |
| IVH | intraventricular haemorrhage | QALY | quality-adjusted life years |
| IWL | insensible water loss | RAAS | renin–angiotensin–aldosterone system |
| L/S ratio | lecithin/sphingomyelin ratio | RCT | randomized controlled trial |
| LBW | low birth weight (<2500 g) | RCV | red-cell volume |
| MAP | mean airways pressure | RDEP | respiratory distress of extreme prematurity |
| MAP | mean arterial pressure | | |
| MRS | magnetic resonance spectroscopy | RDS | respiratory distress syndrome |
| | | ROP | retinopathy of prematurity |
| NEC | necrotizing enterocolitis | RR | relative ratio |
| NICHD | National Institute of Child Health and Human Development (USA) | $Sao_2$ | oxygen saturation |
| | | SCBU | special care baby unit |
| | | SD | standard deviation |
| | | SGA | small for gestational age |
| NICU | neonatal intensive care unit | SHO | Senior House Officer |
| NIRS | near infrared spectroscopy | SIDS | Sudden Infant Death Syndrome |
| OFC | occipitofrontal head circumference | SLE | systemic lupus erythematosus |
| | | SNAP | score for acute neonatal physiology |
| OPCS | Office of Population Censuses and Surveys | TAR | (Table 14.3) |
| OR | odds ratio | $tcPco_2$ | transcutaneous partial pressure for carbon dioxide |
| $Paco_2$ | partial pressure of arterial carbon dioxide | | |
| | | $tcPo_2$ | transcutaneous partial pressure for oxygen |
| PAL | pulmonary air leak | | |
| $Pao_2$ | partial pressure of arterial oxygen | TEWL | transepidermal water loss |
| | | TI | inflation time |
| PCA | postconceptional age | TLC | total lung capacity |
| $Pco_2$ | partial pressure of carbon dioxide | tc $Pco_2$ | transcutaneous partial pressure for carbon dioxide |
| PCV | packed cell volume | tc $Po_2$ | transcutaneous partial pressure for oxygen |
| PDA | patent ductus arteriosus | | |

| | | | |
|---|---|---|---|
| TNF | tumour necrosis factor | VLBW | very low birth weight (<1500 g) |
| tPA | tissue plasminogen activator | VOTN | Vermont–Oxford Trials |
| TRH | thyrotrophin-releasing hormone | | Network |
| TT | thrombin time | VPS | ventriculoperitoneal shunt |
| TTP | (Table 14.3) | VSD | ventricular septal defect |
| VEP | visual evoked potential | VWF | von Willebrand factor |

# 1

# Aetiology and incidence

**Gary Mires and Naren Patel**

Any attempt to define the incidence of babies born weighing less than 1000 g (ELBW) is fraught with problems. The commonly quoted figure of just under 1% [1] only relates to live or stillbirths after 28 weeks of gestation, and is inherently biased to exclude stillbirths or babies born dead earlier than this gestation (late abortions). In an attempt to discover obstetric factors leading to delivery of livebirths of less than 1000 g, one must look at late abortions at less than 28 weeks' gestation. The survivors at birth are only a minority of the pregnancies that have come to grief.

The majority of ELBW infants are small because of extreme prematurity (less than 28 weeks' gestation) but some are small-for-dates at a later gestation. Much of the published data deal with birth weight alone and it is understandable why this is so. Weight is easily established, length of gestation is much more difficult to assess retrospectively. It has been long recognized that a woman's recall of the date of her last menstrual period is poor; about one fifth of UK women surveyed in 1970 were unable to provide reliable enough dates to calculate length of gestation [2] and this has been confirmed by other workers [3]. Paediatric scoring systems for assessing gestational age are difficult to perform on these infants as they are designed for longer gestations. Unless reliable ultrasound data are available from earlier in the pregnancy, it is not always possible to estimate gestational age. Since we cannot predict which women will produce a baby weighing less than 1000 g, all women in

an obstetric population would have to have an ultrasound measurement of crown–rump length (at 7–11 weeks' gestation) or biparietal diameter (at 14–20 weeks' gestation) for us to know the gestational age at birth.

Preterm birth is defined as delivery occurring before 37 completed weeks of gestation. Few studies have addressed the aetiologic factors relating specifically to very preterm delivery. Walker and Patel [4] reported a retrospective study of infants born at 20–28 weeks' gestation, and identified uncomplicated spontaneous preterm labour as the most frequent precipitating cause (47%), with antepartum haemorrhage (15%) and preterm rupture of the membranes (PROM) (14%) also being significant precedents. The factors that lead to the delivery of these ELBW infants are likely to be the same as those causing late abortions in midtrimester and later preterm delivery.

Despite primary prevention programmes, preterm birth rates have remained virtually unchanged in developed countries over the past decade [5], and the prevention of preterm delivery remains one of the major modern obstetric challenges. This chapter considers current thoughts on aetiological factors associated with preterm delivery.

## Spontaneous preterm labour

### Uncomplicated preterm labour

Despite recent advances in knowledge about prostaglandins and other locally acting agents involved in parturition, we still do not know why the human uterus starts to contract at term, and we know even less about causes of preterm labour. In studies which have considered factors associated with delivery at <37 weeks [6,7] uncomplicated spontaneous preterm labour, that is labour without other recognizable aetiologic factors, accounts for approximately one in five deliveries. Lettieri *et al.* [8], however, argue that an exhaustive evaluation plan can identify possible pathological precipitating causes in the majority (96%) of 'idiopathic' preterm labours that result in preterm delivery.

A number of possible associations with uncomplicated preterm labour have been investigated, and are discussed below.

### Psychosocial stress

Several studies have been performed to determine the influence, if any, of psychological stress on the incidence of preterm delivery, but the reports are conflicting.

Standardized questionnaires have been designed to measure perceived levels of anxiety and depression along with a record of recent life events. Some of these earlier studies were performed in retrospect – interviewers visited the women after a preterm delivery [9]. This was a major criticism of their method, since women who have had an adverse outcome tend to seek a cause and this tendency has been recognized in other retrospective studies [10]. Perhaps the best example of this, is a study by Stott [11], which showed that mothers who had delivered a child with Down's syndrome had experienced more 'shocks' during that pregnancy than mothers with normal children. It was two years later that the first report linking Down's syndrome and chromosomal abnormality appeared!

Poor socioeconomic status has been shown to be associated with preterm labour [5]. Unmarried women and teenagers are also known to be at increased risk of uncomplicated spontaneous preterm labour [12], as are women with increased maternal stress [13]. Using a modified Life Events Inventory these workers identified that single teenagers would experience more stressful life events than married women, and this may explain the association. Newton and Hunt [14] demonstrated a significant association between the experience of major life events in pregnancy and preterm delivery. However, in a more recent prospective study no significant association was identified between life events and preterm delivery when a similar inventory was applied [15]. The mechanism by which psychosocial stress may play a role in precipitating labour is unknown. More recently, a reappraisal of the 1958 British Perinatal Mortality Survey [16] failed to confirm that sociodemographic factors including employment status and social class have a substantial impact on the risk of preterm birth. It did, however, demonstrate that low maternal age (<20 years) was significantly predictive of preterm birth, and concluded that preventative measures aimed at social demographic adversity are unlikely to reduce preterm birth rates [17].

### Physical activity

The contribution, if any, of physical activity and employment in increasing the risk of preterm labour has not been conclusively determined, but it seems that whereas strenuous activity and lifting are not important risk factors, prolonged standing may have an influence on the incidence of preterm labour [18].

### Drug use

Of increasing importance in today's society are certain maternal behavioural activities, and in particular drug use in pregnancy. Ney *et al.* [19] reported a positive urine toxicology screen in 17% of women with suspected preterm labour compared to 3% in uncomplicated term patients. Similar findings had previously been reported by MacGregor *et al.* [20].

### Smoking

Smoking has been shown to increase the risk of preterm birth by 40% compared with non-smokers, particularly in women with a high caffeine intake. The effect was dose related, with women smoking 6–10 cigarettes per day having a threefold increase in risk, and women smoking >10, a fivefold increase in risk of preterm birth compared with non-smokers for the same caffeine intake [21].

## Complicated preterm delivery

### Bleeding in pregnancy

Threatened abortion seems to predispose to an increased risk of preterm birth. In a study of threatened abortion, in which the bleeding settled and the pregnancy appeared to progress satisfactorily, the incidence of preterm labour was 16.5% compared with 6.5% in all booked cases [22].

Placenta praevia, placental abruption and non-specific antepartum haemorrhage are all associated with preterm delivery [6,7]. Approximately 1% of deliveries are complicated by placental abruption, and 60% of these will result in preterm birth [23]. Some studies have reported antepartum haemorrhage as the highest risk factor for preterm delivery [24].

### Premature rupture of the membranes

Spontaneous rupture of the membranes precedes the onset of labour in a high percentage of preterm deliveries [6,7]. In the study by Walker and Patel [4] of pregnancies ending spontaneously between 20 and 28 weeks, spontaneous PROM was the principal precipitating obstetric factor in 14% of cases. The mechanism whereby the amniotic membranes rupture prematurely in some women is not entirely clear. Tension in the intact membranes appears to increase as full term approaches, but there is a significant decrease in the elasticity of the membranes which rupture spontaneously before the onset of labour [25]. The epithelial surfaces of amnion and chorion are hydrophobic and it has been demonstrated that in women with spontaneous PROM the surface energy is significantly higher than in controls. This probably results in impaired mechanical resistance. One interesting suggestion was that this phenomenon may be regulated by the deposition of surfactant from the amniotic fluid [26].

### Infection

Infection, either clinical or subclinical, is considered to play a role in a significant proportion of cases of preterm labour and delivery. Lamont *et al.* [27] highlighted the association between abnormal colonization of the genital tract and preterm labour, and associated chorioamnionitis in preterm deliveries. Chorioamnionitis has been estimated to account for up to 25% of preterm deliveries [28].

Several studies have attempted to identify a specific cervical infection which might weaken membranes and make spontaneous PROM more likely. An association has been found between spontaneous PROM and infection of amniotic fluid with bacteria which produce high phospholipase $A_2$ activity [29,30]. However, this association was also found in premature labour where the membranes were intact, so the mechanism may be increased uterine activity rather than weakening of the membranes.

Specific infections such as syphilis and gonorrhoea are associated with an increased risk of preterm delivery, but the role of organisms such as *Ureaplasma urealyticum*, *Chlamydia trachomatis* and *Mycoplasma hominis* is less well established. McDonald *et al.* [31] demonstrated a twofold risk of preterm birth, and a threefold risk of PROM in women with second trimester evidence of carriage of *Ureaplasma urealyticum*. Ngassa and Egbe [32] demonstrated that a positive Chlamydial swab taken between 28 and 34 weeks increased the risk of preterm delivery. Results from randomized trials, however, have failed to demonstrate a reduction in preterm delivery or PROM rate by treating antenatally diagnosed *Mycoplasma hominis* or *Ureaplasma urealyticum*, but did give an increased birth weight [33,34]. Similarly, in a randomized trial of metronidazole in women with bacterial vaginosis flora by McDonald *et al.* (1997), no significant reduction in preterm birth rate was observed. However, in a subset analysis of women in the study who had had a previous preterm delivery, a reduced risk was noted in the treatment arm [39].

Studies into genital tract colonization with group B streptococci have again provided conflicting results, although there is a more consistent association with PROM [36,37]. Women with group B streptococci in their *urine* seem to have a significantly increased risk of PROM and delivery [38,39], and the treatment of asymptomatic bacteriuria in pregnancy is associated with a reduction in the incidence of preterm labour [40]. McKenzie *et al.* [41], however, failed to confirm this association, but demonstrated that the risk of preterm delivery was doubled in the presence of urinary antibodies to E. coli and group B streptococci. Urinary antibodies appear to be a marker for underlying genital tract infection.

Several randomized trials have been performed relating to the use of antibiotics in threatened preterm labour with intact membranes. Crowley has undertaken a meta-analysis of eight such trials [42]. The conclusion from this analysis was there was no evidence to support their use in this clinical situation. However, in a similar analysis of 13 trials where membrane rupture had occurred, antibiotic use was associated with a delay in delivery and reduced maternal and neonatal infection. However, this benefit has not been reflected in a demonstrable effect on perinatal mortality or long-term morbidity [43].

### Cervical incompetence

The incidence of true cervical incompetence is probably between 1 and 2% [44]. It is difficult to be so sure since the condition is often overdiagnosed, and whilst the number of cerclage operations may well reflect the frequency of diagnosis, this is not necessarily the true incidence. Cervical incompetence has been estimated to be the principal precipitating cause in up to one fifth of late miscarriages [44]. The classical picture is of late miscarriage resulting in the birth of a live fetus following a short painless labour not preceded by significant bleeding. Cervical incompetence is thus a loose term which describes the failure of the cervix to fulfil its role in the second trimester of pregnancy as a sphincter for the uterus. Much effort has been made to determine the causes.

The first report of abortion due to cervical incompetence was published by Gream [45] and he campaigned against the then-fashionable practice of surgically dividing or forcefully dilating the cervix for treatment of adolescent dysmenorrhoea. It seems to have taken more than a century for this practice to be abandoned but iatrogenic damage still occurs.

The dilated incompetent cervix can expose the fetal membranes to the vaginal microflora and secretions, predisposing to both PROM and chorioamnionitis. Rupture of the membranes can be a complication of an attempt to manage an incompetent cervix with cervical cerclage. The presence of suture material can act as a nidus for infection and subsequent PROM or preterm labour.

Cone biopsy of the cervix has also been implicated, with subsequent cervical incompetence being related to the volume of the tissue excised [46]. The introduction of colposcopy has significantly reduced the need for cone biopsy in most centres. Uterine abnormalities [47] and *in utero* exposure to diethylstilboestrol [48] have also been implicated. It is interesting to note that whilst dilatating an unripened cervix with blunt Hegar dilators beyond 10 mm has been shown to cause rupture [49], the increased incidence of second trimester induced abortions in the last 15 years does not seem to have resulted in increased risk of spontaneous abortion in subsequent pregnancies [50]. This is almost certainly due to the improved techniques available.

### Multiple pregnancy

It has long been recognized that multiple pregnancy is associated with a high risk of preterm labour, and contributes significantly to the number of ELBW babies admitted to special baby care units. The Scottish Office Review of Twin Pregnancies 1986–1990 [51] demonstrated that 11% of twins were born before 32 weeks' gestation compared to 1% of singletons, and overall 47% of twins had been born by the end of the 36th week compared to 6% of singletons. Quite why multiple pregnancies should feature as such a significant underlying cause in the gestational age group is not entirely clear. While it may be true that many multiple pregnancies deliver before term because the uterus is very distended and simply cannot accommodate any more volume, this cannot satisfactorily explain the high incidence of spontaneous labour at less than 28 weeks when a twin pregnancy does not yet distend the uterus as much as a 36 week singleton gestation. Some more subtle factor may be at work. In addition to increased total fetal weight, there is also a much greater placental size and oestrogen levels are much higher. It may be that this alters myometrial activity and predisposes to earlier onset of spontaneous labour. The rate of uterine distension may also be an aetiological factor.

### Fetal abnormality

Early detection of fetal abnormality is now an important part of antenatal care in the UK.

Apart from specific investigations for groups at particular risk, e.g. amniocentesis and chorionic villus sampling (CVS), many UK centres now perform whole-population screening for specific abnormalities, e.g. serum α-fetoprotein to detect neural tube defects and abdominal wall defects, and biochemical Down's risk assessment. These biochemical tests need to be interpreted in conjunction with accurate gestational data obtained by a 'booking' scan, and in addition, many centres now routinely offer a second trimester fetal anomaly ultrasound scan.

Fetal abnormalities are associated with preterm delivery [6,8], and in particular it could be anticipated that those abnormalities associated with the development of polyhydramnios, e.g. anencephaly, would be at greater risk. As antenatal detection of fetal abnormalities becomes more effective, fetal abnormality as a cause of preterm delivery should become a less common cause of birth weight less than 1000 g. Randomized trials are, however, required to assess to efficacy of anomaly scanning.

## Fetal growth

Fetal growth has been extensively investigated by many centres with access to good ultrasound facilities but most studies have concentrated on detection of poor fetal growth late in the third trimester. This is partly because some authors feel that the small for gestational age fetus (SGA) only becomes manifest after 30 weeks gestation [52]. This hypothesis is not universally accepted [53]. Another reason why the emphasis has been placed on investigation later in pregnancy is the knowledge that intervention at less than 30 weeks gestation is fraught with hazard for the fetus and the feeling that there is little point in detecting poor growth until the fetus is sufficiently mature to have a good chance of survival if delivered. Because of this there is a lack of data on ELBW babies, and it is not possible to be certain what role poor fetal growth plays in these deliveries. A recent paper by Hediger *et al.* [54], however, demonstrated that at 32 weeks' gestation all fetuses later delivered preterm had significantly smaller head circumference (HC), biparietal diameter (BPD), abdominal circumference (AC) and femur

length (FL) than fetuses later delivered at term. Further stratification by cause of preterm delivery for fetuses later delivered for medical or obstetric indications identified that only AC was decreased and that the HC–AC ratio was elevated suggesting asymmetric growth retardation. This suggests that in this group growth failure is occurring later in pregnancy. Those neonates born after unsuccessful treated PROM or preterm labour were symmetrically smaller in all measurements. This implies an overall slowing of growth in these fetuses that may originate early in pregnancy. The findings of this study do therefore suggest that fetal growth may play a role in preterm labour, but this requires further investigation.

## Biochemical and immunological factors

The investigation of biochemical influences in the aetiology of preterm labour is in its infancy. Studies have, however, suggested an association between raised serum relaxin concentrations and preterm delivery [55], and also reduced concentrations of the naturally occurring phospholipase $A_2$ inhibitor gravidin in women giving birth preterm [56]. A positive test for fetal fibronectin, a protein found in amniotic fluid, placental tissue and the extracellular substance of the decidua basalis, has also been found to give a positive predictive value of approaching 50% for delivery before 37 weeks, based on samples taken weekly from 24 weeks' gestation in women considered to be at risk of preterm delivery [57]. However, Chien *et al.* (1997) in an overview including nine studies to determine the accuracy with which cervicovaginal fetal fibronectin predicts preterm delivery concluded that the technique has limited accuracy in predicting such an outcome [58].

Immunological factors including the identification of antiphospholipid antibodies (antinuclear, lupus anticoagulant and anticardiolipin) have also been associated with miscarriage and preterm delivery, and in the study by Lettieri *et al.* [8], antiphospholipid antibodies were present in 30% of cases labelled as 'idiopathic' preterm labour. It is clear, however, that the immunochemical characterization of preterm labour still requires further investigation.

> ## Practical points
>
> 1. ELBW infants can be small as a result of extreme prematurity or small for dates at a later gestation.
> 2. The most common causes of birth at 20–28 weeks are spontaneous preterm labour, antepartum haemorrhage and preterm rupture of the membranes.
> 3. The pathophysiology of spontaneous preterm labour remains unclear.
> 4. Infection plays a significant role in preterm delivery.
> 5. Multiple pregnancies remain a group at particular risk of preterm delivery.
> 6. The role of associated factors such as fetal growth and biochemical/ immunological parameters in preterm delivery require further investigation.

# References

1. National Centre for Health Statistics (1984) *Health, United States*, Public Health Service, Washington DC
2. Chamberlain, G., Philipp, E., Howlett, B. and Masters, K. (1970) *British Births Survey*, Vol. 1, Heinemann Medical, London, pp. 8–54
3. Hall, M.H., Carr-Hill, R.A., Fraser, C., Campbell, D. and Samphier, M.L. (1985) The extent and antecedents of uncertain gestation. *Br. J. Obstet. Gynaecol.*, **92**, 445–451
4. Walker, E.M. and Patel, N.B. (1987) Mortality and morbidity in infants born between 20 and 28 weeks gestation. *Br. J. Obstet. Gynaecol.*, **94**, 670–674
5. Lumley, J. (1993) The epidemiology of pre term birth. In Preterm labour and delivery (G.E. Rice and S.P. Brennecke eds). *Baillieres Clin. Obst. Gynaecol.*, **7** (3), 477–498
6. Schneider, H., Naiem, A., Malek, A. and Hanggi, W. (1994) Etiologic classification of premature deliveries and its significance for prevention. *Geburtshilfe Frauenheilkd.*, **54**, 12–19
7. Connon, A.F. (1994) Assessment of key aetiologic factors associated with preterm birth and perinatal mortality. *Aust. N. Z. J. Obstet. Gynaecol.*, **32**, 200–203
8. Lettieri, L., Vintzileos, A.M., Rodis, J.F., Albini, S.M. and Salafia, C.M. (1993) Does ideopathic preterm labor resulting in preterm birth exist? *Am. J. Obstet. Gynecol.*, **168**, 1480–1485
9. Newton, R.W., Webster, P.A.C., Binu, P.S., Maskrey, N. and Philips, A.B. (1979) Psycho-social stress in pregnancy and its relation to the onset of premature labour. *Br. Med. J.*, **ii**, 411
10. Brown, G.W. and Harris, T. (1978) *Social Origins of Depression*, Tavistock, London
11. Stott, D.H. (1958) Some psycho-somatic aspects of casualty in reproduction. *J. Psychosom. Res.*, **3**, 42
12. White D.R., Hall, M.H. and Campbell, D.M. (1986) The aetiology of preterm labour. *Br. J. Obstet. Gynaecol.*, **93**, 733–738
13. Newton, R.W., Webster, P.A., Binn, P.S., Maskey, N. and Phillips, A.B. (1979) Psychosocial stress in pregnancy and its relation to the onset of preterm labour. *Br. Med. J.*, **ii**, 411–413
14. Newton, R.W. and Hunt, L.P. (1984) Psychosocial stress in pregnancy and its relation to low birth weight *Br. Med. J.*, **288**, 1191–1194
15. Honnor, M.J., Zubrick, S.R. and Stanley, F.J. (1994) The role of life events in different categories of preterm birth in a group of women with previous poor pregnancy outcome. *Eur. J. Epidemiol.*, **10**, 181–188
16. Fedrick, J. and Anderson, A.B.M. (1976) Factors associated with spontaneous preterm birth. *Br. J. Obstet. Gynecol.*, **83**, 342–350
17. Wildscutt, H.I.J., Nas, T. and Golding, J. (1997) Are sociodemographic factors predictive of preterm birth? A reappraisal of the 1958 British Perinatal Mortality Survey. **104**, 57–63
18. Colie, C.F. (1993) Preterm labour and delivery in working women. *Semin. Perinatol.*, **17**, 37–44
19. Ney, J.A., Dooley, S.L., Keith, L.G., Chasnoff, I.J. and Socol, M.L. (1990) The prevalence of substance abuse in patients with suspected preterm labour. *Am. J. Obstet. Gynecol.*, **162**, 1562–1567
20. MacGregor, S.N., Keith, L.G. and Chasnoff, I.J. (1987) Cocaine use during pregnancy: adverse perinatal outcome. *Am. J. Obstet. Gynecol.*, **157**, 686–690
21. Wisborg, K., Henriksen, T.B., Hedegaard, M., Secher, N.J. (1997) Smoking during pregnancy and pre term birth. *Br. J. Obstet. Gynecol.*, **157**, 686–690
22. Turnbull, E.P.N. and Walker, J. (1956) The outcome of pregnancy complicated by threatened abortion. *J. Obstet. Gynaecol. Br. Emp.*, **63**, 553
23. Blair, R.G. (1973) Abruption of the placenta: a review of 189 cases occuring between 1965 and 1969. *J. Obstet. Gynaecol. Br. Comnwlth.*, **80**, 242–245
24. Bakketeig, L.S. and Hoffman, H.J. (1981) Epidemiology of preterm birth: results from a longitudinal study of births in Norway. In *Preterm Labour* (M.G. Elder and L.H. Hendricks eds), Butterworths, London
25. Parry-Jones, E. and Priya, S. (1976) A study of the elasticity and tension of fetal membranes and the relation of the area of the gestational sac to the area of the uterine cavity. *Br. J. Obstet. Gynaecol.*, **83**, 205
26. Hills, B.A. and Cotton, D.B. (1984) Premature rupture of membranes and surface energy. Possible role of surfactant. *Am. J. Obstet. Gynaecol.*, **149**, 896
27. Lamont, R.L., Taylor Robinson, D. and Newman, M. (1986) Spontaneous early preterm labour associated with abnormal genital bacterial colonisation. *Br. J. Obstet. Gynaecol.*, **93**, 804

28. Guziac, D.S. and Winn, K. (1985) The association of chorioamnionitis and preterm delivery. *Obstet. Gynecol.*, **65**, 11

29. Bejar, R., Curbelo, V., Davis, C. and Gluck, L. (1981) Premature labour, II. Sources of phospholipase. *Obstet. Gynecol.*, **57**, 479

30. Curbelo, V., Bejar, R., Benirschke, K. and Gluck, L. (1981) Prostaglandin precursors in human placental membranes. *Obstet. Gynecol.*, **57**, 473

31. McDonald, H.M., O'Loughlin, J.A., Jolley, P. *et al.* (1992) Prenatal microbiological risk factors associated with preterm birth. *Br. J. Obstet. Gynaecol.*, **99**, 190–196

32. Ngassa, P.C. and Egbe, J.A. (1994) Maternal genital chlamydia trachomatis infection and the risk of preterm labour. *Int. J. Gynecol. Obstet.*, **47**, 241–246

33. McCormack, W.M., Rosner, B., Lee, Y. *et al.* (1987) Effect on birthweight of erythromycin treatment of pregnant women. *Obstet. Gynecol.*, **69**, 202–207

34. Eschenbach, D.A., Nugent, R.P., Rao, A.V. *et al.* (1991) A randomised, placebo controlled trial of erythromycin for the treatment of *Ureaplasma urealyticum* to prevent premature delivery. *Am. J. Obstet. Gynecol.*, **164**, 734–742

35. McDonald, H.M., O'Loughlin, J.A., Vigneswaran *et al.* (1997) Impact of metronidazole therapy on preterm birth in women with bacterial vaginosis flora (Gardnerella vaginalis): a randomised, placebo controlled trial. *Br. J. Obstet. Gynecol.*, **104**, 1391–1397

36. Regan, J.A., Choa, S. and James, L.S. (1981) Premature rupture of membranes, preterm delivery and group B streptococcal colonisation of mothers. *Am. J. Obstet. Gynecol.*, **141**, 184–186

37. Bobitt, J.R., Damato, J.D. and Sakakini, J. Jr (1985) Perinatal complications in group B streptococcal carriers: a longitudinal study of prenatal patients. *Am. J. Obstet. Gynecol.*, **151**, 711–717

38. Moller, M., Thomsen, A.C., Borch, K. *et al.* (1984) Rupture of fetal membranes and premature delivery associated with group B streptococci in urine of pregnant women. *Lancet*, **ii**, 586

39. White, C.P., Wilkins, E.G.L., Roberts, C. *et al.* (1984) Premature delivery and group B streptococcal bacteriuria. *Lancet*, **ii**, 586

40. Romero, R., Sibai, B., Caritis, S. *et al.* (1993) Antibiotic treatment of preterm labour with intact membranes: a multicenter, randomised, double blind, placebo controlled trial. *Am. J. Obstet. Gynecol.*, **169**, 764–774

41. McKenzie, H., Donnet, M.L., Howie, P.W. *et al.* (1994) Risk of preterm delivery in pregnant women with group B streptococcal urinary infections or urinary antibodies to group B streptococcal and E coli antigens. *Br. J. Obstet. Gynaecol.*, **101**, 107–113

42. Crowley, P. (1995) Antibiotics in preterm labour with intact membranes. In: *The Cochrane Collaboration; Issue 2*, Update Software, Oxford

43. Crowley, P. (1995) Antibiotics for preterm prelabour rupture of membranes. In: *The Cochrane Collaboration; Issue 2*, Update Software, Oxford

44. McDonald, I.A. (1980) Cervical cerclage. *Clin. Obstet. Gynecol.*, **7**, 461–479

45. Gream, G.T. (1865) Dilation or division of the cervix uteri. *Lancet*, **i**, 381

46. Leiman, G., Harrison, N.A. and Rubin, A. (1980) Pregnancy following conisation of the cervix and complication related to cone size. *Am J Obstet. Gynecol.*, **136**, 14–18

47. Craig, C.J.T. (1974) Congenital abnormalities of the uterus and fetal wastage. *Obstet. Gynecol. Surv.*, **29**, 612–614

48. Quinlan, R.W. and Cruz, A.C. (1980) Reproductive failure and cervical incompetence in women exposed to diethyl stilbestrol. *S. Afr. Med. J.*, **73**, 89

49. Liu, D.T.Y., Black, M., Meldner, D.A., Melville, M.A.H. and Cameron, S. (1975) Dilation of the parous non-pregnant cervix. *Br. J. Obstet. Gynaecol.*, **82**, 246–251

50. Chung, C.S., Smith, R.G., Steinhoff, P.G. and Ming-Pi, Mi (1982) Induced abortion and spontaneous fetal loss in subsequent pregnancies. *Am. J. Public Health*, **72**, 548–554

51. Report on Maternal and Perinatal Death in Scotland 1986–1990. Scottish Office Home and Health Department

52. Beischer, N.A., Albell, D.A. and Drew, J.H. (1984) Intrauterine growth retardation. *Prog. Obstet. Gynaecol.*, **4**, 83

53. Geirsson, R.T. and Persson, P. (1984) Diagnosis of intrauterine growth retardation using ultrasound. *Clin. Obstet. Gynecol.*, **11**, 457–480

54. Hediger, M.L., Scholl, T.O., Miller, L.W. and Fischer R.L. (1995) Fetal growth and the etiology of preterm delivery. *Obstet. Gynecol.*, **85**, 175–182

55. Peterson, L.K., Skajaa, K. and Uldbjerg, N. (1992) Serum relaxin as a potential marker for preterm labour. *Br. J. Obstet. Gynaecol.*, **99**, 292–295

56. Wilson, T. (1993) Minireview: Gravidin: an endogenous inhibitor of phospholipase A2. *Gen. Pharmacol.*, **24**, 1311–1318

57. Nageotte, M.P., Casal, D. and Seneyi, A.E. (1994) Fetal fibronectin in patients at increased risk for premature birth. *Am. J. Obstet. Gynecol.*, **170**, 20–25

58. Chien, P.F.W., Khan, K.S., Ogston, S., Owen, P. (1997) The diagnostic accuracy of cervico-vaginal fetal fibronectin in predicting pre term delivery: an overview. *Br. J. Obstet. Gynecol.*, **104**, 436–444

# 2

# Antenatal care of the very small baby

**Geoffrey Chamberlain**

In England and Wales in 1990, the National Statistics Office reported that among babies born with a birth weight under 1000 g, the still-birth rate was 280 per 1000 total births, the neonatal death rate 390 per 1000 live births and the perinatal mortality rate was 515 per thousand total births [1]. These rates in the UK had been static until the mid-1970s but each had been reducing since then (Fig. 2.1). Neonatal deaths have improved at a sharper rate than still births since 1980, associated with the expansion of improvement in neonatal care. There are some who

allege that by saving very small babies we are providing problems for society later on. In a recent follow-up in N.W. Region, the disability rate among survivors at 10 years was 68%. Most of this was blindness following retinopathy [2]. A wider picture is seen from birthweight and gestational specific data (Figs 2.2 and 2.3).

By far the most common associated cause of death in babies with a birth weight under 1000 g is respiratory distress syndrome (about 40%), and the next largest is congenital abnormalities (about 15%).

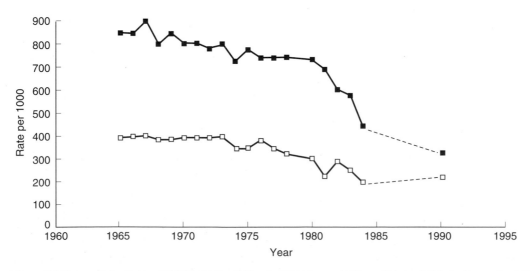

**Figure 2.1** Neonatal deaths per 1000 live births (■) and stillbirths per 1000 total births (□) in babies under 1000 g birth weight in England and Wales (1960–95)

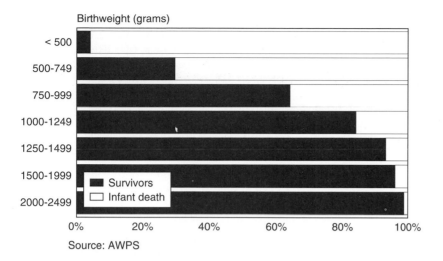

**Figure 2.2** Birth weight specific infant survival to 1 year. Cumulative data 1993–5. (Acknowledgements to the All Wales Perinatal Survey Annual Report (1996))

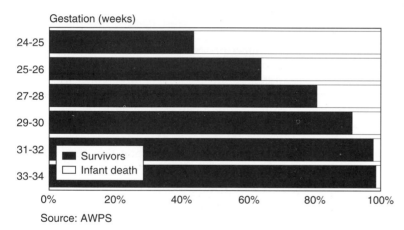

**Figure 2.3** Gestation specific infant survival to 1 year. Cumulative data 1993–5. (Acknowledgements to the All Wales Perinatal Survey Annual Report (1996))

## Management

In all branches of medicine the best management of any condition is to prevent it, then no one has to deal with so many and such severe primary or secondary problems that might arise. This may seem a counsel of perfection but it applies very much in the obstetric field of ELBW infants. Antenatal care as currently practised serves many functions but the one that particular concerns this chapter is the prevention of very early preterm labour.

### Background

During the course of antenatal care, women at higher risk of preterm labour should be identified and special attention paid to them. For example, the woman who has had a previous preterm labour has at least twice the risk of another preterm delivery.

The three major components of perinatal epidemiology are age, parity and socioeconomic class. Very little data are collected on babies born below 1000 g birth weight so the relevant effects are not easily seen. Surrogates are the data on babies born under 1500 g which mirror but exaggerate the changes seen in the under 1000 g group. The younger and older aged mothers are at increased risk of having ELBW babies. A similar phenomenon is seen with parity; the lowest incidence is with para 1 whilst those having their first or third baby or subsequent have an increased incidence.

The socioeconomic class influence on those born under 1500 g follows the national trends of the problems which go with social deprivation but numbers are too few to show a strong trend.

Any association seen in this area seems to be a feature of the mother's body size rather than the simple categorization of their partner's occupation. Cigarette smokers have a much greater increased risk as have women bearing multiple pregnancies. Such women should be advised about their increased risks of preterm labour and warned of the signs of onset of such a labour. If their work is physically heavy they should be advised to try to reduce that effort, for fatiguing and boring jobs have been shown to double the risk of preterm labour [3] although this has been refuted in other studies [4]. Such guidance is not always possible to follow in a society such as ours, where employment is at a premium, but if it could be arranged that a woman works less hard this may well postpone the onset of a very preterm labour. Work has many components, not the least of which is getting to work. Travelling to and from work in unpleasant circumstances for an hour each day can be as stressful as all the other features of work itself [5].

### Fetal growth

During the antenatal period most obstetricians try to estimate the growth of the fetus. Clinical estimation is not good enough by itself; Paul, Koh and Monfared [6] showed long ago that most clinicians underestimate the size of babies weighing under 1500 g. In the UK almost 95% of women have an ultrasound reading of fetal size before the 20th week of pregnancy and some have a repeat of this later on. The first estimation confirms the dates of pregnancy assessed from the last menstrual period and enables a precise measure of fetal growth to be obtained by placing the baby on the correct part of the birth weight and gestational age chart.

When a woman who has had early ultrasound runs into problems later in pregnancy, a repeat ultrasound estimation of the fetal head circumference and abdominal circumference can give a very good measure of the estimated fetal weight. This is extremely useful in guiding obstetricians and neonatologists about delivery. Altman and Chitty [7] have derived a series of charts from which the fetal size can be calculated from the biparietal diameter and the abdominal circumference. These should be available in all labour wards; obstetricians at registrar or a more senior level should be capable of using an ultrasound machine to make scans and so estimate fetal weight from such measurements. However, in the ELBW baby there is still a lack of sufficient data to make valid charts of estimated birth weight and so errors of prediction are more likely. A fuller ultrasound scan should be performed by a more experienced ultrasonographer if time allows and labour does not follow immediately on admission. Some then use charts associating fetal measurements with probably fetal size [8].

### Cervical incompetence

Once of the major reasons for early preterm labour among ELBW babies is cervical incompetence. This concept has grown up in the last 40 years; it owes acceptance in the obstetrical world to its simplistic nature. The diagnosis of this condition would ideally be made before pregnancy when a woman who has had a previous midtrimester abortion or an early preterm labour should be investigated. She may be found to have a cervix which will accept an 8 mm dilator in the outpatient department without any anaesthesia. She may require X-ray or ultrasound investigations to show the incompetence of the cervix. These are relatively crude but show up the worst cases.

In pregnancy, X-ray investigations like these cannot be performed; one starts with the history of previous midtrimester abortion or early preterm labour which gives rise to suspicion. Ultrasound visualization of the cervix in early midpregnancy is rewarding, provided a machine of sufficient resolution is used and the ultrasonographer is experienced. Varma, Patel and Pillai [9] first showed that accurate and reproducible readings could be made of the length of the canal and its diameter at the internal os; such measurements provided an objective method of diagnosing an incomplete cervix and also helped to avoid unnecessary cerclage operations which might have been performed on history alone.

Treatment is simple and consists of putting in a non-absorbable suture at about the level of the internal cervical os to stop the cervix dilating. Shirodkar was the pioneer in this, although most people follow the technique of McDonald [10]. Unfortunately this simple operation has its complications. Stimulation of the myometrium to produce an abortion, and septicaemia have been reported. Because of these doubts, the Medical Research Council and

Royal College of Obstetrics and Gynaecology performed a multicentre randomized controlled trial of cervical suture. The results indicate that there may be some prevention of the very early preterm birth of babies to mothers who had a late midtrimester abortion in a previous pregnancy. This applies also to women who have had previous deliveries at 24–28 weeks of gestation [9].

The cervical suture is best inserted before it is needed, usually at 14 weeks of gestation, having allowed time for spontaneous abortions due to chromosomal abnormalities to have taken place. If the suture succeeds, pregnancy will proceed well past the time relevant to this chapter and the suture can be removed at about 37 weeks' gestation.

## Tocolysis

The manipulation of uterine contractions has been the wish of many in obstetrics. For the last 80 years sympathomimetics have been the predominant drugs for the control of myometrial contractions. In the 1960s intravenous alcohol had a brief phase of popularity and spasmolytics such as isoxsuprine were tried. Whilst our knowledge of smooth muscle physiology of the uterus has increased greatly, the mechanisms responsible for starting the onset of contractions are still unknown and so the use of sympathomimetics is slightly illogical. They do not act against the factors that cause preterm labour, only against the uterine contractions once started.

In very early preterm labour, it is difficult for anyone – mother or doctor – to make the diagnosis. The differences between Braxton Hicks contractions of pregnancy and early labour contractions do not exist as well in practice as they seem to in the text books; it takes the passage of time with a competent observer watching and assessing the myometrial contractions to make the differential diagnosis. A tocograph helps, and assessment of cervical dilation finally allows Braxton Hicks contractions to be ruled out. In consequence, studies of tocolytic agents are bedevilled by the problems of deciding which women to enter into the study. The well-known placebo effect is important here. If one cares for a patient and looks after her properly, 25–50% of women will go out of labour even if given placebo therapy [12].

In essence there is little evidence that the use of betamimetics has improved fetal outcome. Certainly labour has been postponed by hours and days but the ultimate measurement of the fetal condition by perinatal mortality or morbidity has not been greatly improved. A *British Medical Journal* leading article over ten years ago said: 'On balance and in terms of fetal outcome, the use of drugs to inhibit labour is usually unnecessary, frequently ineffective and occasionally harmful' [13]. It is very hard to find truly randomized studies; to set these up is difficult for very few women present in the appropriate gestational stage who fulfil all the criteria and are willing to be randomized. A meta-analysis published in 1995 did not show any long-term beneficial effect of betamimetics in truly randomized controlled studies – either from perinatal mortality or morbidity rates (Table 2.1).

These agents have their side-effects on the mother with an unpleasant tachycardia and, more seriously, pulmonary oedema. The only statistically helpful effect was a significant reduction in the numbers of deliveries within 14 hours in the betamimetic treated group. This allowed an interval for action either to transfer the mother to a tertiary referral centre or to give steroids to help mature the neonatal respiratory tract. The use of such betamimetic agents has now decreased in the UK and they are used mostly to cover first aid situations to postpone labour to allow the use of steroids to help maturation of the fetal lungs (see Chapter 4).

### *In utero* transfer

If the woman is at risk of going into very early preterm labour, she should be delivered at the place where the best paediatric care is available. If it is thought that the fetus is under 1000 g, this should be at a tertiary referral centre with expert neonatal help. The best incubator in which to transfer a baby of this size is the mother's uterus. This can be done after consultation between the peripheral and central units

At the recipient unit the doctor concerned should be of senior registrar or consultant level and should deal directly on the telephone with a consultant or registrar of the donor unit. It should firstly be established that the woman is not likely to give birth during the course of transfer. Hence it is unusual to accept women

**Table 2.1    Effect of betamimetic tocolytics in preterm labour on perinatal death (from Chalmers *et al.* 1989 with thanks)**

| Study | EXPT | | CTRL | | Odds ratio | Graph of odds ratios and confidence intervals |
|---|---|---|---|---|---|---|
| | *n* | *(%)* | *n* | *(%)* | *(95% CI)* | 0.01  0.1  0.5  1  2  10  100 |
| Christensen *et al.* (1980) | 1/14 | (7.14) | 0/16 | (0.00) | 8.52 (0.17–99.99) | |
| Spellacy *et al.* (1979) | 1/15 | (6.67) | 4/15 | (26.67) | 0.25 (0.04–1.64) | |
| Barden (unpub) | 1/12 | (8.33) | 0/13 | (0.00) | 8.03 (0.16–99.99) | |
| Hobel (unpub) | 2/17 | (11.76) | 0/16 | (0.00) | 7.42 (0.44–99.99) | |
| Cotton *et al.* (1984) | 1/19 | (5.26) | 4/19 | (21.05) | 0.26 (0.04–1.67) | |
| Howard *et al.* (1982) | 1/16 | (6.25) | 1/21 | (4.76) | 1.33 (0.08–22.65) | |
| Ingemarsson (1976) | 0/15 | (0.00) | 0/15 | (0.00) | 1.00 (1.00–1.00) | |
| Larsen *et al.* (1986) | 1/49 | (2.04) | 2/50 | (4.00) | 0.52 (0.05–5.09) | |
| Calder and Patel (1985) | 0/37 | (0.00) | 1/39 | (2.56) | 0.14 (0.00–7.19) | |
| Scommegna (unpub) | 0/16 | (0.00) | 1/17 | (5.88) | 0.14 (0.00–7.25) | |
| Mariona (unpub) | 1/4 | (25.00) | 1/5 | (20.00) | 1.29 (0.07–25.50) | |
| Wesselius-De Casparis *et al.* (1971) | 2/33 | (6.06) | 1/30 | (3.33) | 1.81 (0.18–18.08) | |
| Leveno *et al.* (1986) | 2/56 | (3.57) | 3/55 | (5.45) | 0.65 (0.11–3.87) | |
| Larsen *et al.* (1980) | 11/131 | (8.40) | 2/45 | (4.44) | 1.78 (0.49–6.46) | |
| Adam (1966) | 9/28 | (32.14) | 7/24 | (29.17) | 1.15 (0.36–3.69) | |
| Typical odds ratio (95% confidence interval) | | | | | 0.95 (0.55–1.67) | |

with a cervix over 4 cm dilated. Another contraindication is vaginal bleeding which might imply the presence of placenta praevia. The senior registrar or consultant in the recipient unit should then check with his paediatric opposite number that there are staffed cots available within the neonatal intensive care unit and should know whether there are any expected problems from their own obstetrical unit that might need these cots.

After this, and only then, acceptance is given and arrangements for escorted transport made. There is a further problem in the UK of transfer across regions. In the old South West Thames Region recently, of the women accepted for *in utero* transfer at the tertiary referral NICU in St. George's Hospital, 30% came from out of the region implying some deficiency in the provision of care for the ELBW baby in the London area, as the different regions have insufficient facilities for modern neonatal care.

The major features in deciding whether to use *in utero* transfer are the condition of the fetus and the maturity. This should have been estimated by ultrasound in the peripheral unit. The presentation might sway transfer for, if it is a breech presentation, it is more than likely that operative delivery will be required. The site of the placenta should be known.

It is very important to know where the family lives and their whereabouts, and to ensure that they are fully consulted before the woman leaves the donor centre. Much ill will has been engendered in the past when people have been transferred from one hospital to another without their family being fully informed of the reasons.

When the woman arrives at the recipient centre, the possibility of maturation of the lungs and postponement of labour must be considered again if these factors have not been fully worked out at the donor centre. At the stage of gestation appropriate for an under 1000 g baby it is unlikely that the lecithin–sphingomyelin ratio will be useful, as the results are not helpful at this very early stage of gestation and probably will not cause any change in the management of the case. If a test is not going to influence any clinical action taken there is little point in doing it. It may be performed in special cases and a phospholipid glycerol level may also be obtained by cross electrophoresis. Howie and Liggins [14] were the first to show that betamethasone has a maximal effect in reducing respiratory distress syndrome when given for 48 hours at a gestational age of between 32 and 34 weeks. It is probable that between 28 and 30 weeks a singleton baby (especially if female) would benefit from steroids given *in utero* to a greater extent than the disadvantages the therapy entails [15]. This means the postponement of delivery for about 48 hours, hence the use of betamimetics to aid this. The efficacy and problems of the use of steroids are discussed in Chapters 3 and 5.

## Conclusions

More babies under 1000 g estimated birth weight are presenting in our labour wards each year. The obstetrician, in conjunction with the paediatrician, must consider the best way of managing these cases. Background information of reported uterine contractions may warn of impending early preterm labour. The place of suturing of the cervix is at present less certain than it seemed ten years ago. The reduction of respiratory problems after appropriately timed steroids given to the mother is now accepted practice.

The features of the pregnancy should be reviewed and women at high risk for delivery of very small babies should be offered accommodation in or close to obstetrical units that can look after them. If a woman goes into labour with such a small baby, she should be transferred in labour to a unit where intensive neonatal care will be of the highest standards.

**Practical points**

1. Clinical estimates of probable birth weight are very inexact: ultrasound gives a better answer, especially if the first reading is early in pregnancy.
2. Try to prevent preterm birth: this gives the best result of any treatment.
3. If the birth of a very preterm baby is expected, ensure it is in the best place, i.e. arrange *in utero* transfer to a tertiary referral unit.
4. Give steroids to the mother to help mature fetal surfactant secretion and so reduce risks of respiratory distress syndrome.
5. If delivery is inevitable, have a senior obstetrician and neonatal paediatrician in the labour ward.
6. Ensure delivery is by the best route allowing for maturity and presentation of fetus, i.e. use Caesarean section judiciously.

## References

1. OPCS (1993) *Perinatal and Infant Mortality Statistics.* DHJ3, no 25, HMSO, London
2. Emsley, H.C., Wardle, S.P., Sims, D.G. *et al.* (1998) Increased survival and deteriorating developmental outcome in 23- to 25-week-old gestation infants, 1990–4 compared with 1984–9. *Arch. Dis. Child. Fetal Neonatal Ed.*, **78**, F99–F104
3. Peoples-Sleps M.D., Siegel, E., Suchindran, C.M. *et al.* (1991) Maternal employment in pregnancy: effects on birth weight. *Am. J. Pub. Health*, **81**, 1007–1012
4. Klebanoff, M., Shiono, P. and Carey, J. (1990) The effect of physical activity in pregnancy on preterm delivery and birth weight. *Am. J. Obstet. Gynaec.*, **163**, 1450–1456
5. Rodrigues-Escudero, R., Belanstegreguria, A. and Gutierrez-Martinez, S. (1980) Perinatal complications of work in pregnancy. *An. Esp. Pediatr.*, **13**, 465–476
6. Paul, R., Koh, K. and Monfared, A. (1979) Obstetric factors influencing outcome in infants weighing from 1001 to 1500 g. *Am. J. Obstet. Gynecol.*, **133**, 503–508
7. Altman D. and Chitty L., (1994) Charts of fetal size. *Br. J. Obstet. Gynaecol.*, **101**, 29–43
8. Jeanty, J. and Romero, R. (1984) *Obstetrical Ultrasound*, McGraw Hill, New York, pp. 163–166
9. Varma, T., Patel, R. and Pillai, U. (1987) Ultrasonic assessment of the cervix in at-risk patients. *Int. J. Obstet.*, **25**, 25–34

10. McDonald, I. (1957) Suture of the cervix for inevitable miscarriage. *J. Obstet. Gynaecol. Br. Comnwlth*, **64**, 346

11. Quinn, M. (1993) Final report of the MRC/RCOG randomised controlled trial of cervical cerclage. *Br. J. Obstet. Gynaecol.*, **100**, 1154–5

12. Ingemarsson, I. (1984) Pharmacology of tocolytic agents. *Clin. Obstet. Gynecol.*, **11**, 337–351

13. Anon (1981) Drug treatment of premature labour. *Br. Med. J.*, **283**, 395–396

14. Howie, R. and Liggins, G.C. (1977) Clinical trial of antepartum betamethasone therapy. In *Preterm Labour* (A. Anderson, R. Beard, J.M. Brudenell and P.M. Dunn, eds.), Royal College of Obstetricians and Gynaecologysts, London, pp. 281–289

15. Crowley, P. (1998) Corticosteroids prior to preterm labour. The Cochrane Database of Systematic Reviews, issue 1, Oxford: Update Software

# 3

# Mode of delivery

**Ronnie Lamont and Murdo Elder**

The decision about the route of delivery of the extremely low birth weight (ELBW) fetus estimated to weigh less than 1000 g will be influenced by a number of factors:

(1) Many women who present in preterm labour have a past history of fetal or neonatal loss and this may persuade the obstetrician to choose an operative delivery.

(2) Those babies who are estimated to weigh less than 1000 g because of severe intra-uterine growth retardation (IUGR) may be considered to have insufficient reserves to withstand a full labour and vaginal delivery.

(3) Where elective delivery is planned at an early gestation for conditions such as severe IUGR, pregnancy-induced hypertension or antepartum haemorrhage, the state of the cervix may be so unfavourable that successful induction of labour and vaginal delivery would be improbable or impossible.

(4) Unless vaginal delivery is imminent, cardiotocographic evidence of intrapartum asphyxia will require delivery by Caesarean section if the fetus is estimated to weigh more than 750 g and neonatal intensive facilities are available.

(5) Most progressing spontaneous preterm labours are of relatively short duration but if it is felt that labour is becoming prolonged, or if there is evidence of intra-uterine infection, most obstetricians would expedite delivery by Caesarean section.

While these factors raise little controversy, the choice of a particular route of delivery continues to cause much argument.

## Considerations for vaginal delivery

Cord complications such as compression or prolapse are more common with breech birth. The lower limbs and trunk of the small fetus presenting by the breech may be delivered through an incompletely dilated cervix and this may lead to entrapment of the fetal head. Abdominal visceral injuries are more common when the soft abdomen of a breech, rather than the bony pelvis, has been compressed during manipulation at birth, and intracranial haemorrhage is more common after a vaginal breech delivery either as a result of trauma or intrapartum asphyxia. While these risks of vaginal breech delivery apply to breech presentation at all gestations, the lower the birth weight, the higher the risk.

For vertex presentations, high intrauterine pressures during the expulsive phase of the second stage of labour may cause excessive head compression. With delivery of the tiny fetus, the increased size of the maternal pelvis relative to the size of the fetus may result in a compound presentation. It can be worrying to see a scalp electrode disappear into the vagina with each maternal expulsive effort, as one realizes that the tiny fetus is gradually folding up into the vagina so that an arm or shoulder will soon appear at the introitus.

## Considerations for Caesarean section

Caesarean section carries a ten-fold risk of maternal mortality and morbidity over vaginal delivery. In the most recent triennium (1991–1993) of the *Confidential Enquiry into Maternal Deaths*, there were 76 maternal deaths associated directly with Caesarean section. Although, due to deficient data, it was not possible to calculate a rate of maternal death, it was likely to have been approximately 0.3/1000 as in the previous triennium.

Lethal congenital malformations (especially if these are associated with excess or deficiency of the liquor volume) are associated with an increased incidence of preterm delivery. It is estimated that up to 13% of preterm infants presenting by the breech have congenital malformations [1]. If appropriate steps are not taken to exclude such malformations where possible, up to 50% of Caesarean sections may be performed unnecessarily because of cardiotocographic evidence of intrapartum asphyxia in such instances [2].

Caesarean section below 30 weeks' gestation is a technically difficult procedure because of the poorly formed lower segment and, as with vaginal delivery, the fetus presenting by the breech may suffer head entrapment. This may require extension of the uterine excision into the upper segment.

Idiopathic respiratory distress syndrome (RDS) is more common after Caesarean section, though this may only apply to elective Caesarean sections where there has been no labour to stimulate release of endogenous fetal cortisol. It is less likely to occur in cases of IUGR where the fetus has been stressed for some time.

## Delivery of the very low birth weight (VLBW) infant (<1500 g)

### Breech

Using pooled data from 11 studies, Crowley and Hawkins [3] showed that preterm infants presenting by the breech and born vaginally suffered twice the mortality rate of comparable infants born by Caesarean section. However, when the figures were presented as birth weight specific perinatal mortality rates, Caesarean section only showed a reduction in mortality for those infants presenting by the breech who had a birth weight of 1000 g and 1500 g. Since that time, other review articles [4,5] have confirmed the findings of Crowley and Hawkins.

The results of this policy of Caesarean section for infants presenting by the breech who were estimated to have a birth weight between 1000 g and 1500 g have been published [2]. Survival of such infants with a birth weight of below 1500 g was 100% for those delivered by Caesarean section compared to 63% for those delivered by the breech vaginally.

The rate of periventricular haemorrhage (PVH) in the same group of infants was 21% for breech presentation babies under 1500 g delivered by Caesarean section compared to 59% for infants delivered vaginally.

### Vertex

Studies which give recommendations for the best route of delivery for the VLBW infant presenting by the vertex are far fewer than those for the preterm infant presenting by the breech. For those vertex presentations above 34 weeks' gestation, in an otherwise uncomplicated labour, most obstetricians would agree that the vaginal route is the better mode of delivery.

For infants weighing between 800 and 1350 g, Haesslein and Goodlin [6] showed an improvement in survival for infants delivered by Caesarean section. Westgren *et al.* [7] recorded that for infants weighing less than 1500 g, delivery by Caesarean section resulted in a reduced incidence of subsequent IVH over those infants delivered vaginally by the vertex. In a carefully matched study of infants weighing less than 2000 g, Westgren *et al.* [8] showed that at follow up 18–24 months later, infants delivered vaginally by the vertex had a higher incidence of psychomotor retardation over infants delivered by Caesarean section.

In an observational study, Lamont [9] recorded the outcome for 309 infants presenting by the vertex who were delivered before 34 weeks' gestation as a result of spontaneous preterm labour. Those infants who were delivered by Caesarean section before 30 weeks' (and who had a birth weight of less than

1500 g) had a higher survival rate and a lower rate of IVH compared to infants delivered vaginally. This was in spite of the fact that the Caesarean section was only performed for vertex presentations when there were some intrapartum complications such as haemorrhage, infection or cardiotocographic evidence of intrapartum asphyxia.

## Delivery of the infant weighing less than 1000 g (ELBW)

The data pertaining to the optimum mode of delivery for the ELBW infant are very difficult to obtain. A literature search for English language papers in the last 15 years concerned with the mode of delivery of the ELBW revealed about 80 publications.

### Breech

Only 11 papers gave adequate statistics from which conclusions could be drawn. The mortality of the infant weighing less than 1000 g presenting by the breech was calculated according to whether the delivery was vaginal or by Caesarean section. These studies and their results are shown in Table 3.1.

Using the figures in Table 3.1 in combination, the mortality rate for infants presenting by the breech was 73% for vaginal deliveries compared to 47% for infants delivered by Caesarean section ($P$ <0.001).

Four studies of infants presenting by the breech quoted data for infants of 700 g (or 750 g)–1000 g [10–13]. When only these infants were considered (Table 3.2), the overall mortality for these infants was 67% for those delivered vaginally compared to 39% for those delivered by Caesarean section ($P$ <0.02).

In only three studies was it possible to quantify the rate of PVH among infants presenting by the breech. Morales and Koerten [14] detected PVH in 22 of 24 infants (92%) with birth weight of 500–1000 g who were delivered vaginally, compared to 26 of 32 infants (81%) for infants with similar birth weights who were delivered by Caesarean section. Main et al. [11] detected PVH in 17 of 34 infants (50%) weighing 750–999 g delivered vaginally compared to six of ten infants (60%) delivered by Caesarean section. Malloy et al. [13] found PVH in ten of 23 infants (43%) with birth weights of 501–1000 g who were delivered vaginally compared to 21 of 43 infants (49%) for infants of similar birth weights delivered by Caesarean section.

### Vertex

Only five studies quoted adequate statistics for calculation of the mortality rate for infants weighing less than 1000 g and presenting by the vertex. These studies and the results are shown in Table 3.3.

For infants with a birth weight of 500–1000 g presenting by the vertex (Table 3.3) the trend

**Table 3.1** Hospital mortality rates of infants presenting by the breech according to mode of delivery

| Authors | Birth weight range (g) | Caesarean section | | Vaginal delivery | |
|---|---|---|---|---|---|
| | | *n* | *Deaths* | *n* | *Deaths* |
| Yu et al. [15] | 501–1000 | 3 | 1 | 28 | 16 |
| Doyle et al. [10] | 500–999 | 10 | 3 | 49 | 33 |
| Morales & Koerten [14] | 500–1000 | 32 | 18 | 24 | 16 |
| Bowes et al. [16][a] | 501–1000 | 5 | 3 | 34 | 29 |
| Effer et al. [17][b] | 500–999 | 25 | 11 | 23 | 14 |
| Worthington et al. [12] | 500–999 | 10 | 2 | 18 | 13 |
| Mann & Gallant [18] | 500–1000 | 5 | 4 | 29 | 27 |
| Main et al. [11] | 750–999 | 15 | 9 | 52 | 45 |
| Nissell et al. [1] | <1000 | 0 | 0 | 16 | 16 |
| Yang et al. [19] | <1000 | 1 | 0 | 2 | 1 |
| Malloy et al. [13][a] | 501–750 | 43 | 26 | 66 | 49 |
| Malloy et al. [13][b] | 751–1000 | 74 | 28 | 30 | 13 |
| Total (%) | | 223 | 105 (47)[c] | 371 | 272 (73)[c] |

[a]Stillbirth plus neonatal deaths
[b]Neonatal mortality
[c]$P$ <0.001

**Table 3.2.    Hospital mortality rates for infants of 750–1000 g according to presentation and mode of delivery**

| Authors | Presentation | Caesarean section | | Vaginal delivery | |
|---|---|---|---|---|---|
| | | n | Deaths | n | Deaths |
| Doyle *et al.* [10][a] | Breech | 8 | 2 | 40 | 26 |
| Worthington *et al.* [12] | Breech | 8 | 2 | 8 | 3 |
| Main *et al.* [11] | Breech | 15 | 9 | 52 | 45 |
| Malloy *et al.* [13] | Breech | 74 | 28 | 30 | 13 |
| Breech total (%) | | 105 | 41 (39)[b] | 130 | 87 (67)[b] |
| Worthington *et al.* [12] | Vertex | 12 | 4 | 36 | 12 |
| Main *et al.* [11] | Vertex | 9 | 5 | 132 | 73 |
| Vertex total (%) | | 21 | 9 (43) | 168 | 85 (51) |

[a]700–999 g
[b]$P < 0.01$

**Table 3.3.    Hospital mortality rates of infants presenting by the vertex according to mode of delivery**

| Authors | Birth weight range (g) | Caesarean section | | Vaginal delivery | |
|---|---|---|---|---|---|
| | | n | Deaths | n | Deaths |
| Yu *et al.* [15] | 501–1000 | 21 | 8 | 42 | 21 |
| Main *et al.* [11] | 500–1000 | 9 | 5 | 132 | 73 |
| Morales & Koerten [14] | 500–1000 | 26 | 9 | 88 | 32 |
| Worthington *et al.* [12] | 500–999 | 6 | 2 | 49 | 26 |
| Yang *et al.* [19] | <1000 | 0 | 0 | 9 | 5 |
| Total (%) | | 62 | 24 (39) | 320 | 157 (49) |

was the same as for infants presenting by the breech (Table 3.1). Vaginal delivery was associated with a mortality rate of 49% compared with 39% for delivery by Caesarean section (Table 3.3). Two of these studies quoted mortality rates in the birth weight band of 750–1000 g [11,12]. In this birth weight range, the mortality rate for vertex presentations delivered vaginally was 51% compared to 43% for those infants delivered by Caesarean section (Table 3.2).

The incidence of PVH among babies presenting by the vertex and weighing 500–1000 g was 59 of 88 infants (67%) delivered vaginally compared to 16 of 26 infants (62%) delivered by Caesarean section [14].

## Long-term follow up

There was only one report of survival at follow up for infants weighing 501–1000 g, depending on the presentation at birth and the mode of delivery. The survival at two years for vertex presentations with a birth weight of 501–1000 g was 11 of 13 (85%) delivered by Caesarean section compared to 17 of 21 (81%) compar-

able infants delivered vaginally. The survival at 2 years for breech presentations with a birth weight of 501–1000 g was one of two (50%) delivered by Caesarean section compared to 8 of 12 (67%) of comparable infants delivered vaginally [15].

Data relating to handicap at long-term follow up could not be found which quoted figures for the baby weighing less than 1000 g and which also analysed the data with respect to presentation and mode of delivery.

## Intrapartum management

The importance of ultrasound cannot be over-emphasized for a woman admitted in preterm labour when the birth weight is thought to be less than 1000 g. The scan will give an estimate of birth weight, may detect congenital malformations and will identify presentation of the fetus and position of the placenta, all of which are essential if the optimal mode of delivery is to be chosen.

To reduce the dangers of head compression of the infant presenting by the vertex, many will advocate leaving the membranes intact. The membranes then act as the presenting part and spread the rise of intrauterine pressure that occurs during a contraction evenly over the liquor and fetus. This also reduces the incidence of cord prolapse. If external monitoring is unsatisfactory, it may be necessary to rupture the membranes and apply a fetal scalp electrode to monitor the fetal heart rate.

The transition of the fetus with its immature hindbrain from intrauterine to extrauterine life will be helped if it is not depressed by central analgesics. Epidural analgesia is therefore the preferred method of analgesia rather than the use of opiates. The use of forceps for delivery of the VLBW baby to protect the fetal head from compression at delivery has been advocated. Not only are forceps too big for the tiny baby, but there is no evidence that the use of prophylactic forceps is beneficial [16]. Instead, we would advocate an adequate episiotomy to reduce the perineal resistance to delivery of the fetal head and an experienced midwife to conduct the delivery.

The use of Caesarean section has been advocated by Haesslein and Goodlin [6]. As a universal policy, this seems unnecessary. Westgren *et al.* [7] found that a T-extension to the transverse lower segment uterine incision was needed in only three of the 43 cases. The delivery of the preterm infant by Caesarean section should be carried out by the most experienced member of the obstetric staff available and the decision about the uterine incision should depend on the findings at the time of operation rather than by a routine policy in advance. Irrespective of the decision, some difficulty in delivering a tiny baby through thick myometrium may be encountered. In practice, the operation is not always as easy for the infant as one might expect.

## Standardization

As increased attention is given to the infant weighing less than 1000 g, better standardization is required, as the data have to be compared and accumulated. The LBW baby and VLBW baby are well defined birth weight groups. The nomenclature for the baby weighing less than 1000 g varies from 'tiny newborn' to 'extremely low birth weight (ELBW)'. The latter would therefore seem more appropriate

and should be adopted for standardization. There is a great difference in survival rates between babies weighing 500–749 g and babies of 750–1000 g. It would therefore seem appropriate not to consider the group with birth weights of less than 1000 g as a whole, but rather to group these babies into 250 g bands of 500–749 g and 750–999 g.

Many studies including those reviewed in this chapter quote birth weight ranges of 500–999 g or 501–1000 g or 500–1000 g. This may seem unimportant but for a busy regional referral centre the difference of one gram can result in a number of infants each year being allocated to higher or lower birth weight bands which might adversely or favourably affect figures.

## Conclusion

For the ELBW baby presenting by the vertex, there is evidence that Caesarean section may result in a decrease in neonatal mortality and morbidity [9]. For the vertex presentation below 1000 g, there also appears to be a trend towards improved survival following Caesarean section (Table 3.3). The evidence, however, is not strong enough to recommend a policy of elective Caesarean section for all preterm infants presenting by the vertex.

Despite the limitations of the studies with regard to the VLBW infant presenting by the breech, a policy of Caesarean section for infants estimated to weigh 1000–1500 g appears to be vindicated [5].

From Table 3.2, mortality rates following Caesarean section (39%) for infants of 750–1000 g presenting by the breech, were significantly less than for such infants delivered vaginally (67%) ($P < 0.01$). It would appear that with improved neonatal intensive care and hence improved survival for infants of 750–1000 g, the policy of Caesarean section for infants presenting by the breech should be extended to cover infants with an estimated birth weight of 750–1500 g.

Finally, the views of the mother must not be ignored. Despite a poor prognosis, some women will request a Caesarean section because they feel it gives their baby an increased chance of survival, however tiny. Conversely, others may be totally against surgery for various reasons and these views must be respected, provided the woman has been fully informed of the situation.

## Practical points

1. The decision with respect to the mode of delivery will be multifactorial.
2. Nearly 50% of babies with severe congenital malformations delivered before 34 weeks' gestation were undiagnosed and so were erroneously delivered by Caesarean section because of intrapartum complications.
3. While some advocate Caesarean section for delivery of the preterm infant presenting cephalically, this is not widely recommended. However, those babies presenting cephalically who were delivered by Caesarean section because of complications and who should have fared worse than those delivered vaginally, had a lower morbidity and mortality.
4. Delivery of the preterm infant presenting by the breech should be by Caesarean section when the estimated birth weight lies between 1000 and 1500 g corresponding to a gestational age of approximately 28–34 weeks.
5. Most of the perinatal mortality associated with preterm breech presentation is associated with footling presentation, so those obstetricians who wish to use Caesarean sections sparingly may wish to accept this high risk group for Caesarean section.
6. The final decision with respect to the mode of delivery should be with the informed consent of the parents after a full discussion of the advantages and disadvantages of the chosen route.

# References

1. Nissell, H., Bistoletti, P. and Palme, C. (1981) Preterm breech delivery: early and late complications. *Acta Obstet. Gynecol. Scand.*, **60**, 363–366
2. Lamont, R.F., Dunlop, P.D.M.D., Crowley, P. and Elder, M.G. (1983) Spontaneous preterm labour and delivery under 34 weeks gestation. *Br. Med. J.*, **286**, 454–457
3. Crowley, P. and Hawkins, D.F. (1980) Preterm breech delivery – the caesarean section debate. *J. Obstet. Gynecol.*, **1**, 2–6
4. Howie, P.W. and Patel, N.B. (1984) Obstetric management of preterm labour. *Clin. Obstet. Gynecol.*, **11**, 373–390
5. Steel, S.A. and Pearce, J.M. (1986) Delivery of the very low birthweight baby. *Br. J. Hosp. Med.*, **36**, 328–334
6. Haesslein, H.C. and Goodlin, R.C. (1979) Delivery of the tiny newborn. *Am. J. Obstet. Gynecol.*, **134**, 192–198
7. Westgren, M., Ingermarsson, I., Ahlstrom, H., Lindroth, M. and Svenningsen, M.W. (1982) Delivery and long-term outcome of very low birthweight infants. *Acta. Obstet. Gynecol. Scand.*, **61**, 25–30
8. Westgren, M., Dolfin, R., Halperin, M. *et al.* (1985) 1. Mode of delivery in the low birthweight fetus: delivery by caesarean section independent of fetal lie versus vaginal delivery in vertex presentation. *Acta. Obstet. Gynecol. Scand.*, **64**, 51–57
9. Lamont, R.F. (1985) Factors influencing the route of delivery of the preterm infant. In *Proceedings of the Thirteenth Study Group of the Royal College of Obstetricians and Gynaecologists* (R.W. Beard and F. Sharp, eds.) Royal College of Obstetrics and Gynaecology, London, pp. 263–271
10. Doyle, L.W., Rickards, A.L., Ford, G.W., Pepperell, R.J. and Kitchen, W. (1985) Outcome for the very low birthweight (500–1499 g) singleton breech: benefit of caesarean section. *Aust. N.Z. J. Obstet. Gynaecol.*, **25**, 259–265
11. Main, D.M., Main, E.K. and Maurer M.M. (1983) Caesarean section versus vaginal delivery for the breech fetus weighing less than 1500 grams. *Am. J. Obstet. Gynecol.*, **146**, 580–584
12. Worthington, D., Davis, L.E., Grausz, J.P. and Sobocinski, K. (1983) Factors influencing survival and morbidity with very low birthweight delivery. *Obstet. Gynecol.*, **62**, 550–555
13. Malloy, M.H., Onstad, L., Wright, E., National Institute of Child Health and Human Development Neonatal Research Network (1991) The effect of caesarean delivery on birth outcome in very low birthweight infants. *Obstet. Gynecol.*, **77**, 498–503
14. Morales, W.J. and Koerten, J. (1986) Obstetric management and intraventricular haemorrhage in very low birthweight infants. *Obstet. Gynecol.*, **68**, 35–40
15. Yu, V.Y.H., Bajuk, B., Cutting, D., Orgill, A.A. and Astbury, J. (1984) Effect of mode of delivery on outcome in very low birthweight infants. *Br. J. Obstet. Gynaecol.*, **91**, 633–639
16. Bowes, W.A. (1977) Results of the intensive perinatal management of very low birth weight infants. In *Preterm Labour* (Anderson, A., *et al.* eds). Royal College of Obstetrics and Gynaecology, London, pp 331–335
17. Effer, S.B., Saigal, S., Raud, C. *et al.* (1983) Effect of delivery method on outcomes in the very low birthweight breech infant: is the improved survival related to caesarean section or other perinatal case manoeuvres? *Am. J. Gynecol.*, **145**, 123–128
18. Mann, L.I. and Gallant, J.M. (1979) Modern management of the breech delivery. *Am. J. Obstet. Gynecol.*, **134**, 611–614
19. Yang, Y.C., Jou, T.J., Wu, C.H., Wang, K.G., Lan, C.C. and Shen, E.Y. (1990) The obstetric management in very low birthweight infants. *Asia-Oceania J. Obstet. Gynecol.*, **16**, 339–335

# 4

# Resuscitation

## N.R.C. Roberton

Intubation and intermittent positive pressure ventilation (IPPV) should be used routinely to resuscitate all extremely low birth weight (ELBW) neonates and should be started as soon as the infant reaches the resuscitation trolley. The only possible exceptions to this rule are:

(1) Previable infants of less than 400–500 g birth weight and less than 22–23 weeks' gestation. The decision not to resuscitate, an ethical one, should only be taken by an experienced neonatologist [1], after weighing the baby (which can be done virtually instantaneously on modern electronic scales), and after pre-delivery discussion with the parents and their obstetrician about the problems and prognosis of a very immature infant. It is not fair to leave a junior paediatrician in the early stages of his neonatal training to make snap decisions of this nature in the middle of the night.
(2) A baby, usually small for gestational age, who by the time it arrives on the resuscitation trolley is pink, vigorous, howling, waving arms and legs about, and clearly in excellent condition.

The justification for this aggressive management is based on five major lines of evidence:

(1) The high incidence of low Apgar scores in ELBW neonates which may not necessarily mean severe biochemical asphyxia, but undoubtedly identify an at-risk infant who will rapidly develop the biochemical features of severe asphyxia if not resuscitated promptly.
(2) The literature suggesting that if an ELBW infant is spared hypoxia, hypercapnia, hypotension and acidaemia in the first few hours of life it is much less likely to develop complications of prematurity such as respiratory distress syndrome (RDS), germinal layer/periventricular haemorrhage (GMH/PVH), periventricular leucomalacia (PVL), and subsequent neurological handicap.
(3) The association between active resuscitation at birth and improved neonatal outcome.
(4) The deficiencies in methods of neonatal resuscitation other than intubation and IPPV.
(5) Practical advantages inherent in active resuscitation.

Recently a 'softly-softly' approach has been recommended from Denmark [2], in which only nasal CPAP is given, even to babies weighing <1000 g in the labour ward. Their data, however, suggest that this results in a higher mortality from RDS, particularly in those that go on to require IPPV [3] and this approach has not been validated in an adequate prospective controlled trial.

## High incidence of low Apgar scores in ELBW infants

The traditional method of assessing the severity of asphyxia at birth is the Apgar score and

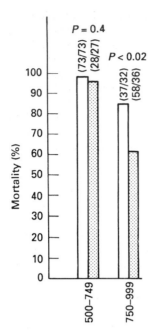

**Figure 4.1** Neonatal mortality in asphyxiated infants (white bars) and unasphyxiated infants (shaded bars). Asphyxia is defined as those babies needing IPPV for >1 min after delivery. Figures in parentheses show absolute number of babies/number surviving. *P* values compare outcome in asphyxiated and non-asphyxiated groups. From McDonald *et al.* [4], with permission

it is well recognized that the score is lower, the more premature the baby [4,5]. Furthermore, it is clear that those with low Apgar scores are less likely to survive [4,6] (Figure 4.1) though the low Apgar score is a poor predictor of neurological outcome [7]. What is not clear, however, is whether the reduced survival is due to asphyxia, or whether the poor Apgar score is a measure of more complex depression of vital functions caused by something other than the acid–base changes of asphyxia.

The most accurate and physiologically acceptable way of assessing the presence of asphyxia at birth is to measure the blood gases in a segment of umbilical artery double-clamped immediately after delivery [8]. Even this is less than perfect, since adequate interpretation of cord blood gas values requires some assessment of the mother's acid–base status [9]. Furthermore, cord blood gas analysis may give a falsely optimistic indication of the likely incidence of early neonatal problems. The neonate may have suffered severe asphyxia, for example early in the second stage of

labour, from which it has recovered from the acid–base point of view by the time of delivery, but may nevertheless have suffered serious myocardial, pulmonary or neurological damage which will cause symptomatic disease in the 3–4 hours after delivery. There are, unfortunately, relatively few studies measuring umbilical cord blood gases in preterm babies, and even fewer in those under 1000 g at birth. Luthy *et al.* [10] show a correlation between cord blood pH and gestation but most studies do not [11–13]. A low pH is, however, a marker of increased morbidity and mortality in these studies as, of course, is a low Apgar [4,11–13]. As with term babies [14] the data suggest that the Apgar score is a poor indicator of asphyxia and acidaemia, and that a low score correlates very much better with gestation [5,11,15]. One of the problems with recent studies of this sort is that with modern perinatal care, intrapartum acidaemia even in preterm infants is so rare that it is difficult to establish statistically significant correlates for the few babies with intrapartum acidaemia [10]. However, Goldenberg *et al.* [11] showed that although many preterm babies can have a low Apgar score without asphyxia, those that are asphyxiated (pH <7.25) are much more likely to have a low Apgar score with its attendant risk of a higher neonatal mortality.

The low one-minute Apgar score in the ELBW infant does not, therefore, necessarily mean asphyxia in the strict biochemical sense of the term, but the neonate with a low score clearly has a problem whether or not it is asphyxia since it is more likely to die than the baby with a good Apgar score (Figure 4.1). Furthermore, if a baby with a 'non-asphyxial' low Apgar score is not promptly and adequately resuscitated, then hypoxia and asphyxia will be added rapidly to all the other pre-existing problems, and this should clearly be avoided at all costs.

## Perinatal asphyxia and subsequent morbidity

### Respiratory distress syndrome (RDS)

There is a large literature relating perinatal and intrapartum asphyxia, assessed either by Apgar score or cord blood gas analysis, to subsequent RDS [16–18].

*In utero* only 10% of the cardiac output goes to the lungs, but during fetal asphyxia lung perfusion may fall to even lower levels, which may cause ischaemic damage to pulmonary capillaries. Fetal resuscitation is then followed by pulmonary hyperperfusion [19] and a leak of protein rich pulmonary oedema onto the alveolar surface where it inhibits the action of surfactant [20, see below]. If this type of prenatal damage has occurred, the infant's fate is sealed before birth, and it is very likely to develop severe surfactant-deficient RDS. There is every reason, nevertheless, to try to minimize these prenatal effects, and to reverse any intrapartum asphyxia as quickly as possible after delivery by prompt and vigorous resuscitation.

However, the single most important justification for active resuscitation of ELBW babies is to prevent asphyxia developing in the first few minutes of life in small, puny, previously biochemically stable babies who, even in the best of all possible worlds, have great difficulty establishing adequate alveolar ventilation after birth. Common sense dictates, as with any seriously ill patient, that it is important for the physician to establish control as soon as possible over such vital functions as ventilation, oxygenation and perfusion. More specifically in the ELBW infant at high risk from RDS, every effort must be made to avoid early neonatal events which are likely to increase the severity and complications of the disease. In theory at least there are five ways in which this can be done, all involving prompt vigorous resuscitation:

(1)  Preventing postnatal hypoxic damage to lung capillaries leading to pulmonary oedema and RDS.
(2)  Preventing decreased surfactant synthesis in the presence of acidaemia and hypoxia.
(3)  Ensuring effective surfactant release from the type II pneumonocytes.
(4)  Rapidly establishing normal blood gases and normal pulmonary perfusion.
(5)  Avoiding and correcting systemic hypotension: postnatal hypotension is important in the aetiology not only of RDS but also of GMH/PVH and PVL.

### Hypoxic capillary damage and RDS

In both fetal and neonatal animals hypoxaemia can cause pulmonary oedema. In part this is due to an increase in filtration pressure in the microcirculation and in part it is due to hypoxic ischaemic damage to the capillary and alveolar lining cells [20–22]. The resultant pulmonary oedema causes the surfactant-producing cells to slough off and die, and this is an early histological feature of fatal cases of RDS [23]. However, it is now recognized that the most damaging effect of asphyxia and pulmonary oedema on the preterm lung is that the protein which leaks through the capillary walls [24] inhibits surfactant activity [25,26]. It is interesting that this leak can be inhibited by antenatal treatment with steroids [27] and this may be one of the beneficial effects of this form of treatment. Furthermore, the immediate institution of IPPV after delivery may prevent the deleterious effects of asphyxia on the preterm lung [28].

Every effort should therefore be made in the first 10–20 minutes after delivery to prevent asphyxia. This means using IPPV to establish immediate ventilation.

### Surfactant synthesis and pH (see also Chapter 5)

Merritt and Farrell [29] (in monkey lung tissue slices) showed that dipalmitoyl phosphatidyl choline synthesis was pH sensitive and a fall in the pH of the tissue culture supernatant to just 7.20 was associated with reduced synthesis (Figure 4.2). This has a clear clinical message: the further the pH in a preterm neonate is below 7.20, the less likely it is to synthesize an adequate amount of surfactant. At resuscitation, therefore, every endeavour must be made to get the pH above 7.20 as quickly as possible, in part by ventilation and blowing off $CO_2$. Every effort should also be made to avert metabolic acidaemia (lactic acidaemia) by preventing hypoxia, anaemia, hypotension and hypoperfusion (Figure 4.3). Although asymptomatic term neonates who have suffered intrapartum asphyxia may be left safely postnatally to correct spontaneously a metabolic acidaemia of 10–20 mmol l$^{-1}$ [30], there is no point in speculatively leaving an ELBW infant with a base deficit of more than 10 mmol l$^{-1}$ in the hope that it might correct spontaneously. The ability of sick low birth weight babies to correct metabolic acidaemia is reduced [31] and the data relating infusions of base to neonatal GMH/PVH are extremely

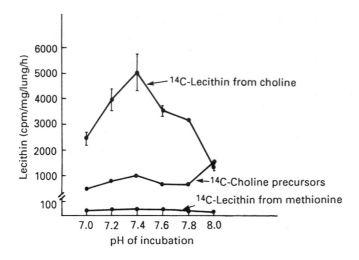

**Figure 4.2** Rate of incorporation of $^{14}C$ into lecithin in monkey lung slices. From Merritt and Farrell [29], with permission

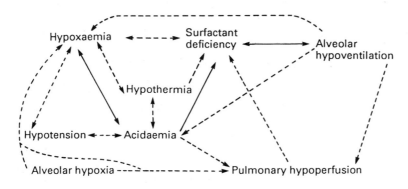

**Figure 4.3** Inter-relationships of factors affecting surfactant production in ill neonates. Solid arrows indicate major effects. From Roberton [84], with permission

unimpressive since they deal with inappropriate rates and volumes of bicarbonate given to infants, many of whose cerebral haemorrhages were not of the periventricular variety [32,33].

Clearly in neonatal resuscitation the priority must be to prevent those conditions which predispose to acidaemia; however if the base deficit is more than 10 mmol$^{-1}$ in an ELBW infant in the first 3–60 min of life, it should be corrected with infusions of base given no faster than 0.5–1.0 mmol kg$^{-1}$ min$^{-1}$ [34,35].

### Surfactant release

Surfactant release at birth is a complex combination of mobilization of intracellular reserves, pharmacologically mediated release of surfactant and adequate physical expansion of the neonate's lungs [36,37]. Infants of less than 1000 g have stiffer lungs with a higher airways resistance than full term infants [38,39]. In addition, they have a very compliant chest wall [40] which may cave in, even during the feeble respiratory efforts generated by their weak muscles [41]. Furthermore, these muscles fatigue easily [42] and their activity is often compromised by hypoxia and acidaemia [43]. Hypoxia in its own right is a respiratory depressant in ELBW infants [44]. The result is that the ELBW infant has considerable difficulty in expanding the fluid-filled surfactant-deficient lungs at birth [45], and has even greater problems maintaining a functional residual capacity [46].

There is, therefore, a potential vicious circle being created (Figure 4.3). Poor ventilation leads to poor surfactant release, resulting in hypoxia, hypercapnia, acidaemia and thus weaker muscles further compromising surfactant release. The most effective way of preventing this cycle is to ventilate the baby from birth, maximizing the release of whatever surfactant stores they possess and reversing all the adverse changes (Figure 4.3).

An important factor to remember when ventilating such babies is that *over*-ventilation does reduce surfactant levels unless a small amount of positive end expiratory pressure (PEEP) is added [47].

## Pulmonary perfusion and ventilation

The major cause of hypoxia in RDS is ventilation–perfusion imbalance in the diseased lungs [48,49]. There is also some right-to-left shunting through the patent ductus [50] and foramen ovale [51]. These true shunts are bigger in the presence of pulmonary hypertension which may be present in many neonates with severe RDS [52,53]. Many factors are involved in reducing pulmonary artery pressure after birth. There seems to be a rapid reduction in response to ventilation, a fall in $Pa\text{CO}_2$ and a rise in $Pa\text{O}_2$ [54,55] and a slower one due to interaction of vasodilator and vasoconstrictor agents. Vasodilator prostaglandins, nitric oxide and bradykinin increase, and endothelin I levels fall [56–59].

## Hypotension

Hypotension, one of the cardinal features of terminal apnoea [60], is well recognized in asphyxiated babies, particularly those with myocardial injury [61]. It is also likely to develop in neonates who are hypoxic and acidaemic, and is virtually inevitable in neonates who have bled or have become anaemic for some other reason. Hypotension can damage many body systems in the neonate causing renal failure and necrotizing enterocolitis. In preterm neonates hypotension at birth has been reported to be associated with an increased incidence of RDS, and in particular an increased mortality from it [17,62]. It is also of crucial importance in the aetiology of PVH. Its role in PVL is less clear.

Resuscitation by preventing hypoxia and acidaemia is likely to minimize the incidence of hypotension. In addition it is essential to measure the blood pressure (BP) in all ELBW infants within the first 30–60 min after birth, and if the blood pressure is low (systolic BP <40 mmHg: mean BP <30 mmHg) to correct it promptly. The blind use of albumen in such babies is to be deprecated [63,64] and care has to be taken even in those who are hypotensive to differentiate those who are volume depleted (and would benefit from early albumen infusion) from those who have myocardial pump failure in whom albumen could be detrimental and who require inotrope infusions [65].

## Periventricular haemorrhage (PVH) and leucomalacia (PVL)

It is now widely accepted in the aetiology of GMH/PVH that brain hypoperfusion and ischaemia secondary to hypotension are most important aetiological factors. In addition, periventricular venous infarction and torrential blood flow through areas already damaged by ischaemia may play a role in specific situations [66,67]. The use of antenatal steroids reduces the incidence of GMH/PVH by at least 50% [68].

The aetiology of PVL is less clear. Hypotension may still be important [69], but other factors such as perinatal sepsis and neonatal hypocapnia are also frequently found [70]. The overall incidence of GMH/PVH now seems to be falling, but PVL occurs in 5–10% of ELBW neonates [70]. The fate of some babies as regards developing GMH/PVH may be more or less sealed before they are delivered. Careful cranial ultrasound studies show that many GMH/PVH appear shortly after delivery [71,72] supporting this view, as does the fact that some epidemiological studies show an association between vaginal delivery and prenatal asphyxia and an increased incidence of GMH/PVH [11,73–76]. Nevertheless, in such babies resuscitation will prevent any further damage to the periventricular vasculature that might be caused by postnatal asphyxia.

Once the baby is delivered there is a clear association between the development of a PVH and RDS [77] in particular the incidence of RDS complicated by a pneumothorax [78]. Therefore, minimizing RDS in the ways outlined above, and in particular resuscitation and early correction of hypotension to avoid cerebral hypoperfusion and ischaemia, is likely to decrease the incidence of GMH/PVH.

## Other acute neonatal illness

Birth asphyxia in term babies can damage many other body systems, causing renal failure, necrotizing enterocolitis, bleeding disorders, especially disseminated intravascular coagulation, and adrenal haemorrhage [79]. It is not unreasonable to assume that these illnesses may also be sequelae of intrapartum asphyxia in ELBW neonates and their incidence in such infants can be minimized by preventing postnatal asphyxia and hypotension.

## Long-term neurological sequelae

Prevention of postnatal asphyxia and reduction in the incidence of RDS, PVL and GMH/PVH is likely to reduce the incidence of neurological sequelae causing handicap.

## Studies on the effect of early intervention

Two attempts have been made to evaluate active resuscitation methods. Robson and Hey [80] compared consecutive periods in Newcastle when the resuscitation of infants weighing 1000–2000 g was passive or active. In the period with active resuscitation the babies were in better condition when admitted to the neonatal unit, and there was a statistically significant decrease of 20% in the mortality from RDS. Drew [81] prospectively randomized infants weighing 500–1500 g to elective resuscitation by intubation and ventilation or resuscitation by bag and mask and IPPV only when clinically indicated. He showed a very clear reduction in the morbidity and mortality in actively resuscitated infants. The overall mortality fell from 49% in the control group to 23% in the actively treated group ($P < 0.01$) and from 86% to 59% when the analysis was limited to ELBW babies ($P < 0.05$).

## Why intubation?

It is hoped that the reader is now convinced that active resuscitation is indicated immediately after delivery in all ELBW infants. The next step is to justify why resuscitation should be carried out by intubation and positive pressure ventilation. This is based on studies on term infants since no comparable studies have, as yet, been done on preterm ones.

When using a bag and mask to resuscitate a term baby who has never breathed after deliv-

**Table 4.1   Expiratory volume achieved with first three breaths using bag and mask ventilation or endotracheal tubes. All babies were ventilated at pressures of approximately 30 cmH$_2$O. The expiratory volume gives a close estimate of the tidal exchange [82]**

|  | Expiratory volume (ml) | | |
|---|---|---|---|
|  | *Breath 1* | *Breath 2* | *Breath 3* |
| Bag and mask | 3.0 | 4.7 | 3.9 |
| ETT and IPPV | 14.3 | 10.5 | 17.0 |

ery, it is a common clinical experience to find that, despite dramatic hissing and squelching noises as the gas escapes over the baby's face from under the mask, the chest does not move and air cannot be heard to enter the lungs.

Milner, Vyas and Hopkin [82] showed that unless the physical assault on the baby is sufficient to provoke him to gasp or breathe on his own, useful tidal exchange does not take place during bag and mask ventilation (Table 4.1).

In the ELBW infant who has surfactant-deficient lungs with their inherent inability to establish a functional residual capacity (FRC), these data suggest that a bag and mask ventilation is unlikely to be of any benefit.

Even with endotracheal intubation and IPPV in term babies, the tidal volume achieved for a given inflation pressure is much smaller than that which occurs with an identical pressure change during a spontaneous inhalation. The FRC is also slow to form during IPPV even down an endotracheal tube unless the inspiratory time is 3–5 s during the first few inflations [83].

### Practical advantages

There are certain basic technical advantages which accrue when resuscitation is carried out by intubation and positive pressure ventilation down an endotracheal tube:

(1)   Laryngoscopy is required and this allows the paediatrician to clear extraneous material out of the airway in a precise and accurate way, rather than blindly thrusting a suction catheter down the back of the baby's throat.

(2)   The period between resuscitation in the labour ward and stabilizing the ELBW neonate in an incubator in the neonatal intensive care unit (NICU) is often the

**Table 4.2** Tidal exchange and FRC established in term neonates taking a first spontaneous breath, and in the first inflation of those resuscitated with a 1 second and 2–5-second inflation time down on endotracheal tube. Mean values are given with range in parentheses [83]

| | Spontaneous breath | 1-second inflation of IPPV | 2- to 5-second inflation of IPPV |
|---|---|---|---|
| Inspiratory/inflation pressure (cmH₂O) | 33   (6.1–103) | 30 | 30 |
| Tidal exchange (ml) | 40.3 (2.7–90) | 18.6 (0–62.5) | 33.6 (16.9–70) |
| FRC (ml) | 18.7 (2.7–40) | 7.5 (0–15.5) | 15.9 (11.7–23.2) |

most hazardous 20–30 min of the ELBW neonate's existence [84]. Control of care during this period and the transportation involved does become considerably easier if the baby is intubated. The incidence of the hypoxia, hypercapnia, acidaemia and hypotension which is so damaging to ELBW neonates in the first 60–90 min of life can thus be reduced to the absolute minimum.

(3) A study in which the decision to intubate ELBW infants at birth was left to clinical judgement found that the majority were intubated anyway [4] (Figure 4.1), and delay in intubation has been shown to increase morbidity and mortality [81].

(4) In routine clinical practice the majority of ELBW neonates end up on IPPV anyway because of recurrent apnoea or surfactant deficient RDS; since they are going to be intubated anyway, they might as well be intubated at birth to establish immediate control of their respiratory function and minimize the adverse sequelae outlined above.

(5) The evidence is now very strong [85] that prophylactic surfactant is preferable to rescue therapy in babies of less than 30 weeks' gestation. The surfactant should therefore be given as an integral part of resuscitating ELBW babies.

The fact that laryngoscoping and intubating ELBW infants does require considerable skill should not be used as an excuse for relying on bag and mask ventilation which is a dangerously inadequate form of resuscitation. Rather it should motivate those responsible for the care of such fragile patients and their mothers to ensure that the birth takes place in a unit with adequate neonatal facilities.

It has been suggested that over-vigorous neonatal resuscitation leads to an increase in chronic lung disease of prematurity [86]. It is difficult to understand how 20–30 minutes of IPPV can do harm if and when it is withdrawn quickly as soon as it is clear that the baby is stable, well oxygenated and adequately ventilated. Both this and the Scandinavian 'softly, softly' approach alluded to earlier [2,3] have not been adequately evaluated in ELBW babies in an era when prenatal steroids and postnatal surfactant should be the norm. I believe in active management of the first hour with IPPV and rapid stabilization of the 'milieu interieur'.

## Technique of resuscitation

Much of what goes on when resuscitating newborn babies is common to those of all birth weights, for example taking the perinatal history, providing appropriate equipment and drugs, and many of the techniques which are used [79]. In this section only those aspects of resuscitation which are specific to the ELBW baby will be considered.

### Location and personnel

Infants weighing less than 1000 g should all be delivered in a level 3 NICU, but if in an emergency one needs to be delivered elsewhere, the most experienced paediatrician available must be present for resuscitation. Ideally a second person should be in the labour ward or immediately available should any complication arise.

### Temperature control

In a conventional labour ward at 21°C (70°F) the naked, wet ELBW infant loses heat about ten times faster than they can generate it, and as a result the body temperature may fall by

0.25–0.3°C min$^{-1}$. The room in which the resuscitation takes place should, therefore, be as warm as possible, windows and doors should be shut and air conditioning turned off in an attempt to minimize convective and evaporate heat loss. To minimize radiant and conductive heat loss the radiant heater on the resuscitation trolley should be full on and warm towels should be available in which the baby can be wrapped as soon as it is delivered, and with which it can be dried.

### Laryngoscope and endotracheal tubes (ETT)

In general, straight-bladed laryngoscopes should be used. A common mistake is to use those with a ⊂ or L cross-section. Particularly in the small mouth of the ELBW infant the cross-section of the laryngoscope blade should be C-shaped and large enough to pass the ETT through it and still visualize the laryngeal entrance. Although 2.5 mm ETTs have a much higher internal resistance than 3.0 mm ones, in most circumstances they will have to be used since the 3.0 mm tube will not pass through the vocal cords. For routine purposes a shouldered Cole's oral ETT should be used. Compared with nasal ETTs these are much easier to insert. Pushing the ETT too far into one or other division of the bronchial tree resulting in poor ventilation and increasing the risk of pneumothorax is also much less likely to occur with a shouldered tube. Furthermore, since they are quicker and easier to insert the adverse physiological changes which take place during intubation [87] are likely to be minimized.

Although it is often suggested that nasal ETTs cause fewer complications when used for long-term IPPV, and they are extensively used in neonates, the evidence on which this belief is based is far from convincing [88] and it is certainly absent where short-term intubation is concerned.

### Inflation pressures and gas composition

Inflation pressures of 30 cmH$_2$O are likely to expand the lungs of most newborn babies [83]. Ideally the inflation time should be at least 1 s, and initially nearer 3 s, in an endeavour to establish an FRC as soon as possible; the ventilation rate will therefore be slow, no more than 30–40 min$^{-1}$.

Self-inflating bags are frequently used for ventilation during neonatal resuscitation, but there is much to be said for using a simple Y-connector attached to a blow-off valve since this allows for greater control of the duration of each inflation.

The practical and financial realities are such that, although 40–60% oxygen is theoretically preferable to pure oxygen for resuscitation, it is rarely used.

### Drug administration

It is doubtful if blind drug therapy should ever be given to an ELBW infant in the labour ward. Those drugs that might be considered include:

(1) *Naloxone.* If the mother received an opiate during the 6 h before delivery and the baby makes no spontaneous respiratory effort, naloxone can be given. However, from what has been said it will be clear that the intention is to artificially ventilate the baby in any case, and there is therefore no urgency about giving an opiate antagonist to reverse apnoea. Never waste time by giving naloxone to the apnoeic baby before intubation and establishing artificial ventilation.

(2) *Sodium bicarbonate.* Given the impossibility of assessing the severity of acidaemia clinically, this drug should not be used in the labour ward without measuring the neonate's blood gases. If a cord blood gas analysis has not been done, this can usually wait until the baby is transferred to the NICU. Bicarbonate should only be considered if there is persisting bradycardia (<60 min$^{-1}$) in the absence of some technical errors in the resuscitation, or in the case of a stillbirth when 5–10 mEq may be given intravenously over 1–2 min.

(3) *Glucose.* This should never be given unless hypoglycaemia is confirmed by Dextrostix or BM stix.

(4) *Adrenaline.* This is of benefit in the baby with extreme bradycardia or asystole. Give one or two doses of 0.25 ml 1:1000 adrenaline intratracheally [89]. If this does not work, give the same dose intracardiac.

(5) *Other drugs.* No other drugs should be considered for the neonate during routine resuscitation. In the event of a

**Table 4.3  The causes of poor response to resuscitation at birth**

*Malformations*
Upper respiratory tract:
  Choanal atresia
  Pierre–Robin syndrome
  Laryngeal and tracheal malformations
    atresia
    webs
    luminal tumours
    clefts
Lung:
  Pulmonary hypoplasia
    Potter's syndrome
    prolonged membrane rupture
    idiopathic
  Pleural effusions; hydrops
  Congenital cystic adenomatoid malformation
  Congenital lobar emphysema
  Pulmonary lymphangiectasia
Extrapulmonary:
  Diaphragmatic hernia
  Diaphragmatic eventration
  Intrathoracic space-occupying tumours
  Gross abdominal distension splinting the diaphragm
    tumours
    hepatosplenomegaly
    ascites ± hydrops
    dilated renal tract
  Small chest
    asphyxiating thoracic dystrophy
    thanatophoric dwarfism
*Pulmonary disease*
Severe RDS
Congenital pneumonia (esp. Group B streptococcus)
Pneumothorax

cardiac arrest appropriate dosages of calcium gluconate, atropine and sympathomimetic drugs may be given in addition to bicarbonate. However, the outcome for full cardiopulmonary resuscitation in ELBW babies could at best be described as poor [90–92]. Whether it is justified, therefore, to initiate external cardiac massage, IPPV, and the use of cardio-resuscitative drugs in the delivery suite in the asystolic neonate weighing <750–800 g is doubtful, and if done it should not continue for more than 10 minutes at the most in the absence of a return of cardiac output.

# The ELBW infant who does not respond to resuscitation

Despite carrying out the procedures outlined above the baby may remain cyanosed and often bradycardic at 5 min of age. The commonest cause for this is some technical error in the resuscitation procedure, and it is therefore essential to check as quickly as possible whether:

(1)  the endotracheal tube is in the wrong place, either in the oesophagus, or down one main stem bronchus, or even in some more distant part of the bronchial tree;
(2)  an adequate inflation pressure (usually set to $30 \, cmH_2O$) is being applied. The blow-off valve on the resuscitation trolley may become inadvertently set at a low pressure;
(3)  the oxygen has been disconnected.

As soon as these errors are recognized and remedied, the infant will rapidly pink-up and become vigorous and active. The other causes of poor response to resuscitation are listed in Table 4.3 and are usually easy to diagnose clinically or by chest X-ray.

---

**Practical points**

(1)  With extremely low birth weight babies if in doubt resuscitate. If they are pre-viable it is much easier and safer to withdraw care later than to start care after 15–20 minutes if a putative fetus fails to die quickly.
(2)  Unless the baby is pink, screaming and trying to crawl off the resuscitaire, intubate for resuscitation using a 2.5 mm endotracheal tube in babies weighing <750 g and a 3.0 mm tube in those weighing 750–1000 g.
(3)  give prophylactic surfactant down the endotracheal tube to all these babies.
(4)  For babies who do not respond to IPPV via the ETT, a technical error, commonly too small an ETT, or the ETT in the wrong place is the most likely diagnosis.
(5)  Do not give drugs including bicarbonate unless there is a clear indication, e.g. a base deficit >10 mmol l⁻¹ or Narcan unless opiates have been used in the latter stages of labour.
(6)  Keep the baby warm at all times. A drop in body temperature of 2°C during resuscitation is likely to at least double the mortality.

# References

1. Campbell, A.G.M. (1999) Ethical problems in neo-natal care. In *Textbook of Neonatology*, 3rd edn, (J.M. Rennie and N.R.C. Roberton, eds), Churchill Livingstone, London and Edinburgh, pp. 1345–1350.

2. Kamper, J., Wulft, K., Larsen, C. and Lindequist, S. (1993) Early treatment with nasal continuous positive airway pressure in very low-birth-weight infants. *Acta Paediatr. Scand.*, **82**, 193–197

3. Roberton, N.R.C. (1993) Does CPAP work when it really matters? *Acta Paediatr. Scand.*, **82**, 206–207

4. McDonald, H.M., Mulligan, J.C., Allen, A.C. and Taylor, P.M. (1980) Neonatal asphyxia. I. Relationship of obstetric and neonatal complications to neonatal mortality in 28,405 consecutive deliveries. *J. Pediatr.*, **96**, 898–902

5. Catlin, E.A., Carpenter, M.W., Brann, B.S. *et al.* (1986) The Apgar score revisited: influence of gestational age. *J. Pediatr.*, **109**, 865–868

6. Rehnke, M., Carter, R.L., Hardt, N.S., Eyler, F.D., Cruz, A.C. and Resnick, M.B. (1987) The relationship of Apgar scores, gestational age and birthweight to survival of low-birthweight infants. *Am. J. Perinatol.*, **4**, 121–124

7. Nelson, K.B. and Ellenberg, J.H. (1981) Apgar scores as predictors of chronic neurologic disability. *Pediatrics*, **68**, 36–44

8. Wible, J.L., Petrie, B.H., Koons, A. and Perez, A. (1982) The clinical use of umbilical cord acid base determinations in perinatal surveillance and management. *Clin. Perinatol.*, **9**, 387–397

9. Dijxhoorn, M.J., Visser, G.H.A., Huisjes, H.J., Fidler, V. and Touwen, B.C.L. (1985) The relation between umbilical pH values and neonatal neurological morbidity in full-term appropriate for dates infants. *Early Hum. Dev.*, **11**, 32–42

10. Luthy, D.A., Shy, K.K., Strickland, D. *et al.* (1987) State of infants at birth and risk for adverse neonatal events and long term sequelae. A study in low birthweight infants. *Am. J. Obstet, Gynecol.*, **157**, 676–679

11. Goldenberg R.L., Huddleston, J.F. and Nelson, K.G. (1984) Apgar scores and umbilical arterial pH in preterm newborn infants. *Am. J. Obstet. Gynecol.*, **149**, 651–654

12. Stark, C.F., Gibbs, R.S. and Freedman, W.L. (1990) Comparison of umbilical artery pH and 5 minute Apgar score in the low birthweight and very low birthweight infant. *Am. J. Obstet. Gynecol.*, **163**, 818–823

13. Hibbard, J.U., Hibbard, M.C. and Whalen, M.P. (1991) Umbilical cord blood gases and mortality and morbidity in the very low birth weigh infant. *Obstet. Gynecol.*, **78**, 768–773

14. Sykes, G.S., Molloy, P.M., Johnson, P. *et al.* (1982) Do Apgar scores indicate asphyxia? *Lancet*, **i**, 494–497

15. Perkins, R.P. and Papile, L.A. (1985) The very low birthweight infant: incidence and significance of low Apgar scores, "asphyxia" and morbidity. *Am. J. Perinatol.*, **2**, 108–113

16. Jones, M.D., Burd, L.J., Bowes, W.A., Battaglia, F.C. and Lubchenko, L.O. (1975) Failure of association of premature rupture of membranes with respiratory distress syndrome. *N. Engl. J. Med.*, **292**, 1253–1257

17. Linderkamp, O., Versmold, H.T., Fendel, H., Riegel, K.P. and Betke, K. (1978) Association of neonatal respiratory distress with birth asphyxia and deficiency of red cell mass in premature infants. *Eur. J. Pediatr.*, **129**, 167–173

18. Thibeault, D.W., Hall, F.K., Sheehan, M.B. and Hall, R.T. (1984) Postasphyxial lung disease in newborn infants with severe perinatal acidosis. *Am. J. Obstet. Gynecol.*, **150**, 393–399

19. Dawes, G.S. and Mott, J.C. (1962) The vascular tone of the fetal lung. *J. Physiol.*, **164**, 465–477

20. Davis, J.A. and Stafford, A. (1964) Respiratory distress in newborn rabbits. *Biol. Neonate*, **7**, 129–140

21. Adamson, T.M., Boyd, R.D.H., Hill, J.R., Normand, I.C.S., Reynolds, E.O.R. and Strang, L.B. (1970) Effect of asphyxia due to umbilical cord occlusion in the foetal lamb on leakage of liquid from the circulation and permeability of lung capillaries to albumin. *J. Physiol.*, **207**, 493–505

22. Hansen, T.I., Hazinski, T.A. and Bland, R.D. (1984) Effects of asphyxia on lung fluid balance in fetal lambs. *J. Clin. Invest.*, **74**, 370–376

23. Gandy, G.M., Jacobson, W. and Gairdner, D. (1970) Hyaline membrane disease, I. Cellular changes. *Arch. Dis. Childh.*, **45**, 289–310

24. Jeffries, A.L., Coates, G. and O'Brodovich H. (1984) Pulmonary epithelial permeability in hyaline membrane disease. *N. Engl. J. Med.*, **311**, 1075–1080

25. Ikegami, M., Jacobs, H. and Jobe, A. (1983) Surfactant function in respiratory distress syndrome. *J. Pediatr.*, **102**, 443–447

26. Kobayashi, T., Nitta, K., Ganzuka, M., Inui, S., Grossman, G. and Robertson, B. (1991) Inactivation of exogenous surfactant by pulmonary edema fluid. *Pediatr. Res.*, **29**, 353–356

27. Ikegami, M., Berry, D., Elkady, T., Pettenazzo, A., Seidner, S. and Jobe, A. (1987) Corticosteroids and surfactant change lung function and protein leaks in the lungs of ventilated premature rabbits. *J. Clin. Invest.*, **79**, 1371–1378

28. Berry, D., Jove, A., Ikegami, M., Seidner, S., Pettenazzo, A. and Elkady, T. (1988) Pulmonary effects of acute prenatal asphyxia in ventilated premature lambs. *J. Appl. Physiol.*, **65**, 26–33

29. Merritt, T.A. and Farrell, P.M. (1976) Diminished pulmonary lecithin synthesis in acidosis. Experimental findings as related to respiratory distress syndrome. *Pediatrics*, **57**, 32–40

30. Spencer, J.A.D., Robson, S.C. and Farkas, A. (1993) Spontaneous recovery after severe metabolic acidaemia at birth. *Early Hum. Dev.*, **32**, 103–111

31. Allen, A.C. and Usher, R.H. (1971) Renal acid excretion in infants with respiratory distress syndrome. *Pediatr. Res.*, **5**, 345–355

32. Simmons, M.A., Adcock, E.Q., Bard, H. and

Battaglia, F.C. (1974) Hypernatremia and intracranial hemorrhage in neonates. *N. Engl. J. Med.*, **291**, 6–10

33. Wigglesworth, J.S., Keith, J.H., Girling, D.J. and Slade, S.A. (1975) Hyaline membrane disease, alkali and intraventricular haemorrhage. *Arch. Dis. Childh.*, **51**, 755–762

34. Baum, J.D. and Roberton, N.R.C. (1975) Immediate effects of alkaline infusion in infants with respiratory distress syndrome. *J. Pediatr.*, **87**, 255–261

35. Fanconi, S., Burger, R., Ghelfi, D., Uehlinger, J. and Arbenz, U. (1993) Haemodynamic effects of sodium bicarbonate in critically ill neonates. *Intens. Care Med.*, **19**, 65–69

36. Jobe, A. (1988) The role of surfactant in neonatal adaptation. *Semin. Perinatol.*, **12**, 113–123

37. Chander, A. and Fisher, A.B. (1990) Regulation of lung surfactant secretion. *Am. J. Physiol.*, **258**, L241–L253

38. Greenspan, J.S., Abbasi, S. and Bhutani, V.K. (1988) Sequential changes in pulmonary mechanics in the very low birth weight (≤1000 grams) infant. *J. Pediatr.*, **113**, 732–737

39. Abbasi, S. and Bhutani, V. (1990) Pulmonary mechanics and energetics of normal, non-ventilated low birthweight infants. *Pediatr. Pulmonol.*, **8**, 89–95

40. Stocks, J. (1977) The functional growth and development of the lung during the first year of life. *Early Hum. Dev.*, **1**, 285–309

41. Keens, T.G., Bryan, A.C., Levison, H. and Ianuzzo, C.D. (1978) Developmental pattern of muscle fibre types in human ventilatory muscles. *J. Appl. Physiol.*, **44**, 909–913

42. Muller, N., Gulston, G., Cade, D., Witton, J., Froese, A.B. and Bryan, M.H. (1979) Diaphragmatic muscle fatigue in the newborn. *J. Appl. Physiol.*, **46**, 688–695

43. Watchko, J.F., LaFramboise, W.A., Standaert, T.A. and Woodrum, D.E. (1986) Diaphragmatic function during hypoxemia: neonatal and developmental aspects. *J. Appl. Physiol.*, **60**, 1599–1604

44. Alvaro, R., Alvarez, J., Kwiatkowski, K., Cates, D. and Rigatto, W. (1992) Small preterm infants (≤1500 g) have only a sustained decrease in ventilation in response to hypoxia. *Pediatr. Res.*, **32**, 403–406

45. Scarpelli, E.M., Clutario, B.C. and Traver, D. (1979) Failure of immature lungs to produce foam and retain air at birth. *Pediatr. Res.*, **13**, 1285–1289

46. Scarpelli, E.M. (1984) Perinatal lung mechanics and the first breath. *Lung*, **162**, 61–71

47. Wyszogrodski, I., Kyei-Aboagye, K., Tauesch, H.W. and Avery, M.E. (1975) Surfactant inactivation by hyperventilation, conservation by end-expiratory pressure. *J. Appl. Physiol.*, **38**, 461–466

48. Strang, L.B. and McLeish, M.H. (1961) Ventilatory failure and right to left shunt in newborn infants with respiratory distress. *Pediatrics*, **28**, 17–27

49. Warley, M.A. and Gairdner, D. (1962) Respiratory distress syndrome of the newborn – principles of treatment. *Arch. Dis. Childh.*, **37**, 455–465

50. Roberton, N.R.C. and Dahlenburg, G.W. (1969) Ductus arteriosus shunts in respiratory distress syndrome. *Pediatr. Res.*, **3**, 149–159

51. Stahlman, M. (1964) Treatment of cardiovascular disorders of the newborn. *Pediatr. Clin. N. Am.*, **11**, 363–400

52. Evans, N.J. and Archer, L.N.J. (1991) Doppler assessment of pulmonary artery pressure and extrapulmonary shunting in the acute phase of hyaline membrane disease. *Arch. Dis. Childh.*, **66**, 6–11

53. Skinner, J.R., Boys, R.J., Hunter, S. and Hey, E.N. (1992) Pulmonary and systematic arterial pressure in hyaline membrane disease. *Arch. Dis. Childh.*, **67**, 366–373

54. Cassin, S., Dawes, G.S., Mott, J.C., Ross, B.B. and Strang, L.B. (1964) The vascular resistance of the foetal and newly ventilated lungs of the lamb. *J. Physiol.*, **171**, 61–79

55. Teitel, D.F., Iwamoto, H.S. and Rudolph, A.M. (1990) Changes in pulmonary circulation during birth related events. *Pediatr. Res.*, **27**, 372–378

56. Cassin, S. (1987) Role of prostaglandins, thromboxanes and leucotrienes in the control of the pulmonary circulation in the fetus and newborn. *Semin. Perinatol.*, **11**, 53–63

57. Velvis, H., Moore, P. and Heymann, M.A. (1991) Prostaglandin inhibition prevents the fall in pulmonary vascular resistance as a result of rhythmic distension of the lungs of fetal lambs. *Pediatr. Res.*, **30**, 62–68

58. Ziegler, J.W., Ivy, D.D., Kinsella, J.P. and Abman, S.H. (1995) The role of nitric oxide, endothelin and prostaglandins in the transition of the pulmonary circulation. *Clin. Perinatol.*, **22**, 387–403

59. Greenough, A. (1999) Neonatal pulmonary physiology. In *Textbook of Neonatology* 3rd edn (J.M. Rennie and N.R.C. Roberton, eds) Churchill Livingstone, Edinburgh, pp. 455–480

60. Dawes, G.S., Hibbard, E. and Windle, W.F. (1964) The effect of alkali and glucose infusion on permanent brain damage in rhesus monkeys asphyxiated at birth. *J. Pediatr.*, **65**, 801–806

61. Cabal, L.A., Devaskar, U., Siassi, B., Hodgman, J.E. and Emmanouilides, G. (1980) Cardiogenic shock associated with perinatal asphyxia in preterm infants. *J. Pediatr.*, **961**, 705–710

62. Phibbs, R.H., Clements, J.A., Creary, R.G. *et al.* (1976) Lung maturity, intrauterine growth, neonatal asphyxia and shock and the risk of hyaline membrane disease. *Pediatr. Res.*, **10**, 466 (Abstract)

63. Bland, R.D., Clarke, T.L., Harden, L.B. *et al.* (1973) Early albumen infusion to infants at risk for respiratory distress. *Arch. Dis. Childh.*, **48**, 800–805

64. Roberton, N.R.C. (1997) Use of albumin in neonatal resuscitation. *Eur. J. Pediatr.*, **156**, 428–431

65. Gill, A.B. and Weindling, M. (1993) Randomized controlled trial of plasma protein fraction versus dopamine in hypotensive very low birthweight infants. *Arch. Dis. Childh.*, **69**, 284–287

66. Pape, K.E. (1989) Etiology and pathogenesis of intra-

ventricular haemorrhage in newborns. *Pediatrics*, **84**, 382–385

67. Volpe, J.J. (1989) Intraventricular haemorrhage in the premature infant – current concepts I & II. *Ann. Neurol.*, **25**, 3–11 and 109–116

68. Crowley, P.A. (1995) Antenatal corticosteroid therapy: A meta-analysis of the randomised trials 1972–1994. *Am. J. Obstet. Gynecol.*, **173**, 322–335

69. Volpe, J.J. (1997) Brain injury in the premature infant: Neuropathology, clinical aspects, pathogenesis and prevention. *Clin. Perinatol.*, **24**, 567–587

70. de Vries, L.S. and Rennie, J.M. (1999) Preterm brain injury. In *Textbook of Neonatology* 3rd edn (J.M. Rennie and N.R.C. Roberton, eds), Churchill Livingstone, Edinburgh and London, 1252–1270

71. Ment, L.P., Duncan, C.C., Ehrencranz, R.A. *et al.* (1984) Intraventricular hemorrhage in the preterm neonate: timing and cerebral blood flow changes. *J. Pediatr.*, **104**, 410–425

72. McDonald, M.M., Koops, B.L., Johnson, M.L. *et al.* (1984) Timing and antecedents of intracranial hemorrhage in the newborn. *Pediatrics*, **74**, 32–36

73. Bada, H.S., Korones, S.B., Anderson, G.D., Magill, H.L. and Wong, S.P. (1984) Obstetric factors and relative risk of neonatal germinal layer intraventricular hemorrhage. *Am. J. Obstet. Gynecol.*, **148**, 798–804

74. Meidell, R., Martinelli, P. and Pettet, G. (1985) Perinatal factors associated with early onset intracranial hemorrhage in premature infants. *Am. J. Dis. Child.*, **139**, 160–163

75. Westgren, L.M., Malcus, P. and Svenningsen, N.W. (1986) Intrauterine asphyxia and long term outcome in preterm fetuses. *Obstet. Gynecol.*, **67**, 512–516

76. Szymonowicz, W., Yu, V.Y.H. and Wilson, F.E. (1984) Antecedents of periventricular haemorrhage in infants weighing 1250 g or less at birth. *Arch. Dis. Childh.*, **59**, 13–17

77. Dykes, F.D., Lazzara, A., Ahmann, P., Blumenstein, B., Schwartz, J. and Brann, A.W. (1980) Intraventricular hemorrhage. A prospective evaluation of etiopathogenesis. *Pediatrics*, **66**, 42–49

78. Lipscombe, A.P., Thorburn, R.J., Reynolds, E.O.R. *et al.* (1981) Pneumothorax and cerebral haemorrhage in preterm infants. *Lancet*, **i**, 414–416

79. Roberton, N.R.C. (1999) Resuscitation. In *Textbook of Neonatology* 3rd edn (J.M. Rennie and N.R.C.

Roberton, eds), Churchill Livingstone, Edinburgh and London, 241–267

80. Robson, E. and Hey, E. (1982) Resuscitation of preterm babies at birth reduces the risk of death from hyaline membrane disease. *Arch. Dis. Childh*, **57**, 184–186

81. Drew, J.H. (1982) Immediate intubation at birth for very-low-birthweight infants. *Am. J. Dis. Child.*, **136**, 207–210

82. Milner, A.D., Vyas, H. and Hopkin, I.E. (1984) Efficacy of face mask resuscitation at birth. *Br. Med. J.*, **289**, 1563–1565

83. Milner, A.D. and Vyas, H. (1985) Resuscitation of the newborn. In *Neonatal and Paediatric Respiratory Medicine* (eds A.D. Milner and R.J. Martin), Butterworths, London, pp. 1–16

84. Roberton, N.R.C. (1993) *A Manual of Neonatal Intensive Care*, 3rd edn, Edward Arnold, London, Chapters 17 and 18

85. Morley, C.J. (1997) Systematic review of prophylactic versus rescue surfactant. *Arch. Dis. Childh.*, **77**, 70–75

86. Poets, C.F., and Sens, B. (1996) Changes in intubation rates and outcome of very low birthweight infants: a population based study. *Pediatrics*, **98**, 24–27

87. Kelly, M.A. and Finer, N.N. (1984) Nasotracheal intubation in the neonate: physiologic responses and affects of atropine and pancuronium. *J. Pediatr.*, **105**, 303–309

88. McMillan, D.D., Rademaker, A.W., Buchan, K.A., Reid, A., Machin, G. and Sauve, R.S. (1986) Benefits of oral tracheal and nasotracheal intubation in neonates requiring ventilatory assistance. *Pediatrics*, **77**, 39–44

89. Schwab, K.O. and Stockhausen, H.B. (1994) Plasma catecholamines after endotracheal administration of adrenaline during postnatal resuscitation. *Arch. Dis. Childh.*, **70**, 213–217

90. Lantos, J.D., Miles, S.H., Silverstein, M.D. and Stocking, C.B. (1988) Survival after cardiopulmonary resuscitation in babies of very low birth weight. *N. Engl. J. Med.*, **318**, 91–95

91. Davis, D.J. (1993) How aggressive should delivery room cardiopulmonary resuscitation be for extremely low birth weight neonates. *Pediatrics*, **92**, 447–450

92. Sood, S. and Giacoia, G.P. (1992) Cardiopulmonary resuscitation in very low birthweight infants. *Am. J. Perinatol.*, **9**, 130–133

# 5

# Prevention and management of respiratory distress syndrome

## Henry Halliday

Respiratory failure in the extremely low birth weight infant is not always due to surfactant deficiency (the respiratory distress syndrome, RDS). Although biochemical immaturity of the lungs is undoubtedly important, poor pulmonary anatomical development and immaturity in other organ systems have roles to play in the aetiology of respiratory distress. Furthermore, it is often difficult to distinguish between RDS and congenital pneumonia, although the latter may also be associated with surfactant deficiency. There have been relatively few clinical trials focusing specifically on the baby of less than 1000 g and therefore much of the information given in this chapter has been extrapolated from physiological, biochemical and clinical studies of larger preterm babies.

## Incidence

Whilst the incidence of babies born with a weight of less than 1000 g is about 0.4% of all births the incidence of RDS in these babies is not clearly established. A review of a consecutive series of 100 babies weighing less than 1000 g who were managed in the neonatal unit of the Royal Maternity Hospital, Belfast in 1992–93, shows that 82% needed mechanical ventilation. Although 55% of mothers were given betamethasone about half of the babies needed to be intubated at birth and 50% were given surfactant to treat severe RDS. Mechan-

ical ventilation was needed in 20% some time after birth because of apnoea or infection. 10% of those with early respiratory failure had congenital pneumonia. Eight babies had severe congenital anomalies (three chromosomal, one hydrops, one complex congenital heart disease, one Russell–Silver dwarf, one multiple limb deformities and one pulmonary hypoplasia) and seven of these died. Excluding these babies with abnormalities, overall survival was 71%. Survival in babies born elsewhere was 50% which was poorer than that of babies born in the regional hospital at 76%. Hack *et al.* [1] have reported outcomes for very immature babies in seven centres in a US Neonatal Network born in 1988. Survival was 34% at <751 g birth weight (range between centres 20–55%), and 66% at 751–1000 g (range 42–75%). Of these babies 67% had RDS and the need for both oxygen and ventilatory support at 28 days increased with decreasing birth weight. Of babies less than 751 g, 79% needed oxygen for 28 days (range 67–100%) compared to 45% of those of 751–1000 g (range 20–68%). The requirement for mechanical ventilation of more than 27 days was 68% in infants <751 g and 29% at birth weight 751–1000 g. This study demonstrated the importance of inter-centre variation of neonatal outcomes [1]. Two quite recent studies have looked at outcomes of very premature infants according to gestational age [2,3]. These single centre studies show clearly how outcome improves from 23 to 27 weeks of gestation with survival increasing from 16% [2] to 89% [3].

# Development of the lung

About 26–28 weeks the terminal air sacs or alveoli appear as outpouchings of the bronchioles. At about the same time the capillary network proliferates close to the developing airway to facilitate gas exchange. Before 26–28 weeks gas exchange must take place across terminal bronchioles into the developing capillary network [4]. The number of alveoli increases linearly from 28 weeks to term when about 120 million are present [5]. In the very preterm baby, low alveolar numbers probably contribute to respiratory dysfunction. Airway maturation may be important in the development of pulmonary interstitial emphysema. The airways of the very preterm baby are characterized by progressive deformability with positive pressure ventilation, and structural disruption with loss of elasticity occurs on repetitive deformation [6]. This susceptibility of the airways of the very immature baby to injury probably contributes to the development of bronchopulmonary dysplasia. Both mechanical and humoral factors influence growth of the fetal lung but the former are probably more important.

Biochemical maturation of the lung, on the other hand, relies more on humoral control mechanisms than mechanical factors [7]. Lamellar bodies which store surfactant appear at about 22–24 weeks' gestation; glucocorticoids increase their numbers and also stimulate surfactant production [8]. Thyroid hormones also stimulate surfactant synthesis and this effect is synergistic with that of glucocorticoids. Thyrotropin-releasing hormone which crosses the placenta [8], may also have effects on the structural maturation of the lung.

Surfactant is a complex mixture of phospholipids, neutral lipids and apoproteins; the main components are dipalmitoylphosphatidyl choline (DPPC), phosphatidyl glycerol (PG) and the four surfactant associated apoproteins A to D [9]. Surfactant is needed to maintain alveolar stability during expiration which prevents atelectasis. Immature infants have both a quantitative and qualitative deficiency of surfactant which predispose to the development of RDS. In addition, capillary leakage will allow inhibitors from the plasma to reach the alveoli and inactivate any surfactant that may be present [10]. Hypoxia, acidosis and hypothermia will reduce surfactant synthesis

which is necessary to replenish surfactant that is lost from the system and cannot be recycled.

The pulmonary antioxidant enzyme system (superoxide dismutase, catalase and glutathione peroxidase) develops in parallel to the surfactant system [11]. Deficiency of both surfactant and antioxidant defences explains why the very preterm infant is at great risk of developing chronic lung disease such as bronchopulmonary dysplasia.

In addition to humoral and mechanical factors, maternal diet may play an important role in the development of biochemical maturity in the lung. The babies of women with anorexia nervosa appear to have a high incidence of RDS. Palmitic acid [12] and inositol [13] supplements to the maternal diet may reduce the incidence of RDS in their babies.

Before birth the lungs are filled with fluid, but during labour fluid secretion by alveolar epithelial cells ceases and fluid is absorbed. This effect is due to catecholamine release, but in preterm animals labour has much less effect on lung fluid secretion and reabsorption than in mature animals [14]. Delay in resorption of lung fluid will interfere with the establishment of alveolar volume and increase surface tension within the lung [15]. Elective delivery before the onset of labour will further increase the risk of RDS, perhaps by exaggerating this failure to reduce lung liquid secretion.

After birth the lungs of the very immature baby are prone to develop oedema especially during mechanical ventilation [16]. Protein in this pulmonary oedema fluid will inactivate surfactant [10,17] and these problems increase as gestational age decreases [16,17]. In preterm rabbits, maternal treatment with corticosteroids or thyrotrophin-releasing hormone (TRH) decreases protein leaks following delivery [18]. The effect of surfactant replacement on neonatal lung pathology has been extensively reviewed [19].

# Development of other organs

Apart from the lung, immaturity of the heart, cardiovascular system, and the central nervous system may be important in adding to the respiratory problems. After birth, pulmonary vascular resistance falls more slowly in the very immature baby and the ductus arteriosus is more likely to remain patent [20], because of

**Table 5.1** Antecedents of preterm birth and its outcome

| Antecedent | Distribution (%) | | Survival (%) | |
|---|---|---|---|---|
| | ≤1500 g[a] | ≤1000 g | ≤1500 g[a] | ≤1000 g |
| Spontaneous labour | 30 | 42 | 68 | 62 (69) |
| Premature rupture of membranes | 20 | 16 | 80 | 69 (75) |
| Emergency delivery | 25 | 22 | 65 | 59 (73) |
| Elective delivery | 25 | 20 | 90 | 80 (80) |
| Totals | 100 | 100 | 75 | 66 (71) |

Figures in parentheses refer to corrected survival after excluding deaths from congenital anomalies.
[a]From [23–25].

reduced circular smooth muscle content, blunted response to hypoxia and raised prostaglandin levels. Right-to-left shunting of blood may soon give way to large left-to-right shunts which flood the lungs with fluid, reducing compliance and increasing respiratory distress. This problem may be increased after surfactant treatment [21].

Immaturity of the central nervous system [22] and indeed of the chest wall may lead to hypoventilation or apnoea. These will lead to hypoxia, acidosis, bradycardia and reduced lung volume; assisted ventilation is often needed even though the baby does not have severe RDS.

# Prevention of respiratory problems

A great advance in perinatal medicine would be an understanding of what triggers preterm labour leading to preterm birth, especially of babies under 1000 g. Once the mechanisms of preterm birth have been elucidated it should be possible to target preventive measures at the causes. Antecedents of preterm birth can be divided into four approximately equal groups (Table 5.1) [23–25]. There is some evidence that factors associated with preterm birth (<37 weeks) differ from those antecedents of very preterm birth (<30 weeks) [26]. Cervical cerclage is a generally low yield procedure but if used selectively in women with a previous midtrimester loss it will prevent one preterm labour for every 25–30 cerclages performed [27].

Preterm rupture of the membranes probably reduces the risk of RDS but the risk of congenital pneumonia may increase. Pre-eclampsia does not decrease the risk of RDS and in fact may increase it as elective delivery by

Caesarean section prior to the onset of labour is frequently necessary [28].

# Promotion of fetal lung maturity

Three drugs used to induce maturity of the fetal lungs have been studied: corticosteroids, thyrotropin releasing hormone and ambroxol [29,30].

## Corticosteroids

Twelve randomized controlled trials have assessed the efficacy of antenatal corticosteroids in preventing RDS [29–31]. Antenatal treatment with a total of 24 mg betamethasone or 24 mg dexamethasone or 2 g hydrocortisone, is associated with a significant reduction in the risk of RDS of the order of 40–60%. The benefit appears to apply to babies born at all the gestational ages at which RDS may occur [32,33] and is independent of gender. The reduction in the risk of RDS is accompanied by decreases in periventricular haemorrhage and necrotizing enterocolitis and this in turn results in an approximately 40% reduction in the odds of death. These benefits are obtained without any detectable increase in the risk of maternal, fetal or neonatal infection, even in the presence of prolonged rupture of the membranes. One study has looked specifically at babies weighing 600–1000 g born in 1983–86 [33]. Control of labour was attempted with intravenous ritodrine in all mothers of 5 cm cervical dilatation or less and if control was obtained betamethasone was given 30 minutes later. Mortality, the incidence of respiratory distress syndrome and the need for mechanical ventilation were all reduced in the 33 babies born after 24 hours of betamethasone compared to the 53 born earlier than this [33].

## Thyrotropin-releasing hormone

TRH has been used in conjunction with corticosteroids in three studies [34–36] with promising results. In one trial there was an important reduction in the need for artificial ventilation and in the incidence of bronchopulmonary dysplasia [35]. In another trial of 103 babies of less than 1500 g birth weight [36], betamethasone plus TRH (4 doses of 400 µg 8 hourly) did not reduce the incidence of RDS but did decrease the risk of bronchopulmonary dysplasia (oxygen need at 28 days; RR 0.40, 95% CI 0.26–0.80, $P$ <0.05). TRH may have important effects on lung development in addition to those on the surfactant system of the lung. However, a recent large multicentre trial from Australia (ACTOBAT) showed that following maternal TRH and corticosteroid treatment the infants were more likely to develop RDS and need ventilation [37]. At follow-up TRH treated babies had an increased risk of motor delay and sensory impairment (38). Administration of TRH to mothers at risk of preterm labour can no longer be recommended.

## Ambroxol

Antenatal ambroxol (bromhexine metabolite VIII) in a dose of 1 g day$^{-1}$ intravenously over 5 days has been shown to reduce the incidence of RDS in babies of less than 36 weeks' gestation [39]. However, the main disadvantage of ambroxol therapy appears to be that five days are needed to complete the course of treatment. Further trials are warranted with this drug and evidence of beneficial effects on very preterm babies is presently lacking.

# Management of preterm labour

Acidosis, hypothermia, trauma and drugs can all adversely affect the very preterm baby and increase the risk of respiratory distress. Obstetric management is designed to prevent these complications [40] and to present the ELBW baby to the paediatrician in the best possible condition. Promotion of fetal lung maturity [29] and prolongation of pregnancy should be major goals of the obstetrician. The use of antibiotics to reduce the risk of preterm delivery is controversial [41] and a multicentre trial is presently being undertaken to explore their use (ORACLE, overview of the role of antibiotics in curtailing labour and early delivery).

Since infection and especially chorioamnionitis is associated with preterm labour, cultures of the genital tract should be taken and antibiotics begun if there are maternal signs of infection or if group B streptococci have been isolated [42]. In labour, if it has been decided that the fetus is viable, attempts should be made to avoid asphyxia and acidosis by careful monitoring [40]. Analgesia should be used sparingly and an epidural may be preferred. For breech presentations consideration of Caesarean section should be given, especially if there is evidence of fetal distress [43]. The place of delivery is important and improved outcomes are obtained with maternal transfer to regional perinatal centres prior to the birth of very preterm babies [44,45].

# Surfactant treatment

Surfactant treatment to prevent or modify the natural history of RDS has now become a reality. Although surfactant deficiency [46] is the major cause of RDS in preterm babies, it is not the only factor which is involved in the pathogenesis of respiratory failure in the very immature baby [47]. In the 1970s several animal studies showed that surfactant replacement improved lung function in immature rabbits [48], lambs [49] and monkeys [50]. In the preterm lamb the magnitude and duration of the response to surfactant depend upon the gestational age of the animal [51]. Lambs treated with 50 mg of natural sheep surfactant at 128 days' gestational age have a sustained improvement in arterial oxygen tension if they receive additional small doses of surfactant. However, lambs at 120 days, although they initially respond to surfactant, develop recurrent respiratory failure despite supplemental surfactant doses [51]. Similar findings have been reported by Maeta *et al.* in lambs and baboons [52]. All of these studies used natural surfactants containing phospholipids and surfactant apoproteins.

In the early 1980s the first studies on babies treated with natural [53] and synthetic [54] surfactants took place. Since then over 30 randomized controlled trials have demonstrated that surfactant prophylaxis or treat-

**Table 5.2   Surfactant preparations in clinical use**

| Name | Composition and concentration | Dose (mg/kg) | No. of doses | Prophylaxis or treatment | Dose volume (ml kg$^{-1}$) |
|---|---|---|---|---|---|
| **Synthetic** | | | | | |
| ALEC (Pumactant®) Britannia | DPPC: PG 7 : 3 100 mg ml$^{-1}$ | 100 | 4 | P | 2 |
| Colfosceril palmitate (Exosurf®) Burroughs Wellcome | DPPC 13.5 Hexadecanol 1.5 Tyloxapol 1.0 13.5 mg ml$^{-1}$ | 67.5 | 2–4 | P, T | 5 |
| **Natural** | | | | | |
| Surfactant TA (Surfacten®) Tokyo Tanabe | Bovine mince plus DPPC, tripalmitin and triacylglycerol 30 mg ml$^{-1}$ | 120 | 3 | P, T | 4 |
| Beractant (Survanta®) Abbott | Bovine mince plus DPPC, tripalmitin and triacyclglycerol 25 mg ml$^{-1}$ | 100 | 4 | P, T | 4 |
| Bovactant (Alveofact®) Boehringer–Ingelheim | Bovine lavage 41.7 mg ml$^{-1}$ | 50 | 4 | P | 1.2 |
| Calf lung surfactant extract (CLSE, Infasurf®) Forrest | Calf lung lavage 25–30 mg ml$^{-1}$ | 90–100 | 3 | P, T | 3–4 |
| Porcine lung surfactant extract (Curosurf®) Chiesi | Porcine mince 80 mg ml$^{-1}$ | 100–200 | 3 | P, T | 1.25–2.5 |

ment reduces neonatal mortality by about 40% and pneumothorax by a half [55,56]. These trials enrolled babies of various gestational ages and many were more than 1000 g birth weight. Some trials excluded babies of birth weight below 750 g. The types of surfactant used in these trials are shown in Table 5.2.

There have been only a few trials that have been designed to study babies under 750 g [57–61]. Two of these trials have used protein-free, synthetic surfactants [57,58] and three bovine-derived surfactants [59–61]. Three studies were of prophylaxis [57–59], one of rescue treatment [60] and one compared prophylaxis and rescue [61]. A meta-analysis of the three prophylaxis studies shows that surfactant therapy in babies <750 g or ≤27 weeks' gestation is associated with a reduction in the odds of neonatal mortality of about 40% (Table 5.3). The risk of intraventricular

haemorrhage is not significantly increased, but there is a trend that needs to be studied further. The one trial of treatment of established RDS in babies of 600–750 g did not show a significant reduction in neonatal mortality [60] (Table 5.3). This is in keeping with the findings of the study comparing prophylaxis and rescue treatment which showed an improved survival (64/85 (75%) versus 39/72 (54%); $P$ <0.01) in babies < 26 weeks' gestation treated prophylactically [61]. There is new evidence from meta-analyses of randomized trials showing that prophylaxis with natural surfactant in babies ≤31 weeks' gestation is superior to rescue treatment [62,63].

It is generally agreed that infants of less than 28 weeks' gestation should be given surfactant in the labour ward, especially if their mothers have not received a full course of prenatal steroids [66] or if the babies need to be

**Table 5.3  Effect of surfactant therapy on neonatal mortality and periventricular haemorrhage in babies ≤750 g or ≤27 weeks**

|  | *Treated* | *Control* | *Odds ratio* | *95% CI* |
|---|---|---|---|---|
| **Prophylaxis** | | | | |
| Neonatal mortality | | | | |
| ALEC [57] | 13/43 | 15/32 | 0.49 | 0.17–1.41 |
| Exosurf® [58] | 51/106 | 60/109 | 0.76 | 0.43–1.34 |
| Survanta® [59] | 5/26 | 14/28 | 0.24 | 0.06–0.93 |
| Typical estimate | | | 0.59 | 0.37–09.93 |
| Periventricular haemorrhage | | | | |
| ALEC [57] | 14/42 | 10/31 | 1.05 | 0.35–3.17 |
| Exosurf® [58] | 45/106 | 39/109 | 1.32 | 0.74–2.38 |
| Survanta® [59] | 7/26 | 7/28 | 1.11 | 0.28–4.40 |
| Typical estimate | | | 1.23 | 0.77–1.98 |
| **Treatment** | | | | |
| Neonatal mortality | | | | |
| Survanta® [60] | 35/81 | 36/76 | 0.85 | 0.43–1.67 |

95% CI = 95% confidence interval

intubated for resuscitation [63]. Follow-up studies of extremely immature infants of gestational age 23–26 weeks [65] did suggest a significant improvement in survival during the post-surfactant era. Indeed, Ferrara *et al.* [65] suggested that the impact was greater at 23–24 weeks gestation than at 25–26 weeks.

In keeping with animal studies [51,52] there is evidence that babies weighing 750–1000 g have a sustained response in only 50% of cases, response with relapse in about 25% and a transient or no response in about 25% [47]. It has been suggested that this is evidence that surfactant deficiency is not the only cause of respiratory failure in very preterm babies. Support for this comes from the improved clinical response to surfactant treatment seen both in animals [14] and infants [66] whose mothers had been treated with corticosteroids.

The combination of antenatal corticosteroid treatment and prophylactic surfactant seems to be the optimal and most cost-effective combination [67] for the very immature baby.

### Early or prophylactic surfactant

This can now be advocated for all babies of gestational age <31 weeks (estimated fetal weight <1250 g). If rapid pulmonary function testing [68] is available the paediatrician can be more selective in treating only those babies with an immature lung profile. There is a difference between true prophylaxis, which is the administration of surfactant in the delivery room prior to the first breath, and early treatment which involves the instillation of surfactant within the first 30–60 minutes after birth. Early treatment may be given in the neonatal intensive care unit after stabilization of the baby. Both natural and synthetic surfactants have been used in prophylaxis.

After intubation of the trachea, surfactant may be given slowly (e.g. Exosurf) or rapidly by bolus (e.g. Survanta and Curosurf) (Table 5.2). Both types of surfactant appear efficacious when compared with controls but comparative trials suggest that matural surfactants are associated with a reduced risk of pneumothorax and a trend towards lower mortality [69,70]. It has been suggested that protein-free surfactants (Exosurf or ALEC) may be useful for prophylaxis before the lungs have been injured by ventilation and fluid leaks, whereas natural surfactants (Survanta, Curosurf or Infasurf) may be best for treatment of established RDS when a rapid response is needed [71]. It has been further suggested that the dose of surfactant needed for prophylaxis might be less than that needed for rescue treatment as inactivation by inhibitors should be less [71]. At least 50 mg phospholipids $kg^{-1}$ is needed for prophylaxis and 100 mg $kg^{-1}$ for rescue treatment. Multiple doses may be needed for babies who relapse and this is more likely when a lower initial dose is administered.

The combination of prenatal corticosteroids and prophylactic surfactant therapy is the most cost-effective because it produces the greatest number of survivors and the lowest number of intensive and high dependency care days in hospital [67]. Not all babies can be treated prophylactically however, and inevitably rescue treatment will be needed for babies who are >30 weeks' gestation or who are born in hospitals where surfactant is not available [72].

## Late surfactant treatment

Once RDS has developed and treatment with oxygen, continuous positive airway pressure or mechanical ventilation has been initiated, the very preterm baby is at grave risk of pulmonary air leaks and subsequently bronchopulmonary dysplasia [73]. Late surfactant treatment of the baby <1000 g therefore represents a sub-optimal situation. Indeed, Kendig *et al.* showed improved survival rates for babies <26 weeks' gestation treated prophylactically compared to late [61].

Several factors have been shown to affect the response to surfactant treatment and these include the severity of RDS, pre-existing asphyxia or acidosis, gestational age, male gender, age at treatment, and hospital allocation [74–77]. The response pattern is an important determinant of outcome [76,77]. Most babies showing rapid and sustained responses to treatment will survive but about 40% of those showing poor response or relapse will die [77]. A high peak arterial oxygen tension within 30 minutes of treatment may be associated with an increased incidence of grade I–II intraventricular haemorrhage but a sustained good response at 24 hours is associated with a lower incidence of grade III–IV haemorrhage [76]. Babies with a good response may have a higher incidence of patent ductus arteriosus [76].

Haemodynamic effects of surfactant administration have been described but their pathogenesis remains uncertain. Changes in blood pressure and cerebral blood flow velocities have been reported in some studies with both natural [78,79] and synthetic [80] surfactants but not in others [81,82]. It is not known if these effects occur in babies <1000 g or if they are significant. Cerebral blood flow has been measured by near-infrared spectroscopy [83–85] and Xenon[133] clearance [83,84] in babies treated with the natural surfactant, Curosurf. These studies show that there are no significant changes in cerebral blood flow after

surfactant administration and in particular no evidence of cerebral ischaemia despite a modest decrease in blood pressure [84].

Cerebral oxygenation and cerebral blood volume have also been measured by near-infrared spectroscopy [83–85] and in general there is a large increase in the former and a small rise in the latter which is equivalent to a 2 kPa increase in arterial carbon dioxide tension. These changes are probably related to changes in carbon dioxide tension and are not associated with any increased risk of intraventricular haemorrhage [83,85]. Transient suppression of the EEG occurs after surfactant administration and it is seen with both natural and synthetic preparations [86,89]. The effect is variable and the cause is unexplained. There is no correlation between EEG changes, hypotension and risk of intraventricular haemorrhage [83].

More research is needed into the acute effects of surfactant therapy especially in the very preterm baby. There have been very few studies comparing different methods of instilling surfactant although animal studies suggest that natural surfactants are less effective if given slowly. This is probably due to less effective distribution of surfactants in the lung during slow instillation.

## Ventilator settings after surfactant

There is very little published information on this subject and none referring to the baby <1000 g. Synthetic surfactants generally have a slower onset of action in both human [88,89] and animal studies [90,91] and this means that the clinician can gradually lower inspired oxygen concentrations after administration provided that continuous blood gas monitoring is available.

Lowering of ventilator pressures can also take place gradually after analysis of arterial blood gases. For natural surfactants the response in animals [90,91,92] and babies [76,89,93–95] is generally rapid so that it is vital to reduce ventilator settings within minutes in responding babies. Inspired oxygen concentration should be lowered first to reduce the peak arterial oxygen tension level [76]. It is usually possible to reduce the inspiratory time (for example from 0.5 s to 0.4 or 0.3 s) and keep the respirator rate high (about 60 $min^{-1}$) by increasing the expiratory time. Peak inspiratory pressure can be lowered soon afterwards using chest wall movement and carbon dioxide tension from blood gas analysis as guidelines [73]. Whatever type of surfactant is used for late treatment, it is important to monitor the infant carefully for his or her response. Surfactant treatment should be given in Neonatal Intensive Care Units with adequate staffing and equipment levels. Modification of the severity of RDS will reduce the incidence of pulmonary air leaks but does not significantly alter the risks of intraventricular haemorrhage and chronic lung disease.

### Poor response to surfactant treatment

This can be caused by various factors, for example, incorrect primary diagnosis, inadequate dosage or administration of surfactant, or interference from other intensive care practices [96]. Examples of incorrect diagnosis are pulmonary hypoplasia which may be associated with very prolonged rupture of the membranes [97], persistent fetal circulation [74], shock and asphyxia and congenital pneumonia [98]. The presence of a large shunt through a patent ductus arteriosus has been associated with a transient surfactant response or relapse sometime later [75,99].

Administration of 60 mg human surfactant $kg^{-1}$ transiently improves respiratory failure but relapses mean that re-treatment is needed [100]. Two studies have shown that 100–120 mg surfactant $kg^{-1}$ is better than 50–60 mg $kg^{-1}$ with improved oxygenation [101,102] and a reduced incidence of bronchopulmonary dysplasia [101]. A high initial surfactant dose probably decreases the number of infants who do not respond [96] and reduces the need for re-treatment [103]. Although animal studies do not suggest harmful effects from accumulation of repeated administrations of surfactant [104], clinical trials point to a failure to further improve long-term outcome by continuing to re-treat beyond two [105] or three [103] doses. A study of the turnover of artificial surfactant in preterm babies also suggested that two doses gave improved tracheal phospholipid profiles that lasted for up to one week [106]. Some babies may require very high doses of surfactant, so that the dose regimen should be flexible and tailored to meet the needs of the individual baby [96]. About 100 mg $kg^{-1}$ seems to be needed for the first dose and re-treatment criteria have been suggested for babies who relapse and need more than 30–40% oxygen [107].

The quality of exogenous surfactant is also likely to influence the response [108]. The method of administration may also affect the response to surfactant, but nebulization is hampered by reduced bioavailability [109]. In one small clinical trial up to eight times the usual dose of surfactant needed to be administered by a nebulizer to obtain a significant clinical effect [110]. More research is needed to determine the optimal method of administering surfactant to all babies and especially those <1000 g.

Treatment practices in the neonatal intensive care unit can also affect the clinical response [96]. These include excessive fluid intake, low circulating blood volume and high ventilator pressures. Using a logistic regression analysis, Hallman [111] and Merritt *et al.* [112] found that high fluid intake significantly contributed to a poor outcome after surfactant treatment. Blood volume depletion, on the other hand, from blood sampling or inadequate use of colloid infusions is also associated with a poor outcome [112]. In these babies surfactant treatment may lead to hypotension and increased pulmonary vascular resistance.

Mechanical ventilation has been discussed above. It is important to note that appropriate ventilation and surfactant treatment increase functional residual capacity (FRC) [95], and decrease lung oedema. This should allow a substantial decrease in airway pressures. Excessive ventilation pressures after surfactant treatment can acutely increase pulmonary vascular resistance, decrease pulmonary perfusion and lead to an apparently poor response [96].

## Other post-natal drug treatments

These include administration of ambroxol [113,114], inositol [115–117] and corticosteroids [118,119]. Each of these drugs can be given antenatally to the mother; this has already been discussed.

### Ambroxol

Preliminary results from two trials have demonstrated benefits of postnatal ambroxol administered intravenously (up to 30 mg $kg^{-1}$ $day^{-1}$ for 5 days) from soon after birth to preterm babies at high risk of developing RDS [113,114]. Ambroxol-treated infants needed less oxygen and appeared to recover more quickly. Treated babies also had lower incidences of BPD, PVH and acquired pneumonia [114]. Pulmonary air leaks and PDA were not reduced by ambroxol. Further trials of ambroxol perhaps in conjunction with surfactant treatment are probably warranted. Evidence of a beneficial effect in babies <1000 g is so far lacking.

## Inositol

Myo-inositol (inositol) is a regulator of pulmonary surfactant synthesis and increases phosphatidyl-inositol and decreases phosphatidyl glycerol in surfactant [115]. It also potentiates the steroid-induced acceleration of fetal lung maturation [120]. Hallman *et al.* in three published trials [115–117] administered inositol for 5 to 10 days to babies <2000 g who needed ventilation for RDS [115] or were at risk of developing RDS because of immature lung profiles [116,117]. Inositol supplementation decreased the incidence of bronchopulmonary dysplasia or death by a similar amount. In one study the improved neonatal survival without BPD was evident only in the babies who did not receive surfactant; but the incidence of retinopathy of prematurity was also reduced by inositol supplementation [117]. More trials are needed before inositol can be recommended for babies <1000 g.

## Corticosteroids

Post-natal steroids have been used at various times in the neonatal period in babies with early or established chronic lung disease (see Chapter 7).

A number of randomized controlled trials have studied the early post-natal use of corticosteroids [121,122]. Yeh *et al.* [121] found improvement in respiratory distress and pulmonary compliance so that extubation by 14 days was more successful in the steroid treated group. Although neither chronic lung disease nor mortality were significantly improved their combination was decreased [121]. Sanders *et al.* [122] gave 0.5 mg kg$^{-1}$ of dexamethasone at 12–18 hours of age and repeated 12 hours later and compared the outcome with a saline placebo in babies of <30

weeks gestation [122]. The steroid treated group required shorter stays in hospital but longer term benefits, although suggested, were not proven. These encouraging results, together with evidence that babies who develop bronchopulmonary dysplasia have early adrenal insufficiency [123] suggest a need for further trials of steroid treatment. Such a trial comparing early and late treatment with either dexamethasone or inhaled budesonide is currently being undertaken (OSECT, open study of early corticosteroid treatment). Systemic reviews of postnatal corticosteroid treatment suggests that treatment at 7–14 days of age may be the most effective, reducing the incidence of chronic lung disease [124] but significant adverse effects probably occur.

## Complications of RDS

These may be categorised as acute: pneumothorax, pulmonary interstitial emphysema, periventricular haemorrhage, patent ductus arteriosus and pulmonary haemorrhage; or chronic: bronchopulmonary dysplasia, retinopathy of prematurity and neurodevelopmental sequelae. Meta-analysis of all surfactant trials [55,56,125] and of those enrolling babies of ≤ 750 g or ≤ 27 weeks [126] (Table 5.3) show a significant reduction in the odds of neonatal mortality of about 40%. Similar meta-analyses have been performed for many of the complications of RDS listed above.

## Pneumothorax

The incidence of pneumothorax in babies enrolled as controls in the prophylaxis surfactant trials ranged from 11% to 54%, compared to 20–80% for babies treated in rescue trials [55,56,127]. The higher rate in babies with established RDS is to be expected as these babies all have severe disease but up to half of those babies treated prophylactically may not have developed RDS if left untreated. The effect of surfactant treatment is to significantly lower the incidence of pneumothorax by over 60% for prophylaxis with natural surfactant, about 30% for prophylaxis with synthetic surfactant, about 60% for rescue with natural surfactant and 40% for rescue with synthetic surfactant [55,56,71] (Table 5.4). The effect of

**Table 5.4  Typical estimates of event rate ratios and 95% confidence intervals for the effects of surfactants on the complications of RDS**

| | Event rate ratio | 95% CI | Event rate ratio | 95% CI |
|---|---|---|---|---|
| | *Natural surfactant* | | *Synthetic surfactant* | |
| **Prophylaxis** | | | | |
| Neonatal death | 0.66 | 0.49–0.88 | 0.74 | 0.62–0.88 |
| Pneumothorax | 0.36 | 0.26–0.49 | 0.68 | 0.51–0.92 |
| Pulmonary interstitial emphysema | 0.23 | 0.12–0.46 | 0.75 | 0.54–1.05 |
| Periventricular haemorrhage | 0.94 | 0.75–1.17 | 0.90 | 0.74–1.10 |
| Severe PVH | 0.97 | 0.69–1.35 | — | — |
| Patent ductus arteriosus | 1.09 | 0.93–1.27 | 1.12 | 1.01–1.25 |
| Bronchopulmonary dysplasia | 0.75 | 0.61–0.92 | 1.01 | 0.79–1.29 |
| BPD or death at 28 days | 0.72 | 0.61–0.83 | 0.87 | 0.75–1.01 |
| **Treatment** | | | | |
| Neonatal death | 0.68 | 0.57–0.80 | 0.67 | 0.54–0.83 |
| Pneumothorax | 0.43 | 0.35–0.52 | 0.60 | 0.50–0.72 |
| Pulmonary interstitial emphysema | 0.38 | 0.26–0.57 | 0.54 | 0.45–0.64 |
| Periventricular haemorrhage | 0.90 | 0.76–1.08 | 0.87 | 0.73–1.03 |
| Severe PVH | 0.98 | 0.75–1.27 | — | — |
| Patent ductus arteriosus | 1.07 | 0.93–1.22 | 0.86 | 0.76–0.94 |
| Bronchopulmonary dysplasia | 0.94 | 0.72–1.22 | 0.68 | 0.48–0.95 |
| BPD or death at 28 days | 0.76 | 0.65–0.90 | 0.65 | 0.55–0.78 |

Data in table derived from reviews in *Effective Care of the Newborn Infant* (J.C. Sinclair and M.B. Bracken, eds) (see refs [55,56]).
95% CI = 95% confidence interval

reduction of pneumothorax appears greater for natural than synthetic surfactants and this is in keeping with the findings from comparative trials [69,70]. Prophylaxis is also associated with a greater reduction in incidence of pneumothorax than rescue treatment [61,62].

## Pulmonary interstitial emphysema

The incidence of PIE in control babies in the surfactant trials ranges from 26% to 48% in prophylaxis studies and 22% to 73% in rescue studies [56]. In randomized controlled trials natural surfactant prophylaxis at birth and later treatment both reduce the incidence of PIE by about 70%. Synthetic surfactant, however, does not reduce the incidence of PIE when given prophylactically and the reduction with rescue therapy is about 45% [56] (Table 5.4).

## Periventricular haemorrhage

The incidence of PVH in control babies in the surfactant trials ranges from 14% to 72% in prophylaxis studies and 18–65% in rescue trials [55,127,128]. As these ranges are similar the severity of RDS may not be the only factor determining the incidence of PVH [129]. In the trials using natural surfactants the incidences of severe PVH (Papile III or IV) [130] have

been reported. These are 0–40% for prophylaxis trials and 14–50% in rescue trials [55]. These figures may not represent the true incidence for these groups of babies, as some trials excluded babies with severe PVH [88,93]. Surfactant treatment has been associated with both a decrease [128,131–133] and an increase [134] in the incidence of PVH. The trial of Horbar *et al.* with Survanta also found an increase in the relative risk of severe PVH (2.50, 95% CI, 1.21–5.16) but can be considered to be unique as overviews show that the effect of surfactant on PVH is of an insignificant reduction [55,129] (Table 5.4). It has been argued that because only 25% of both prophylaxis and rescue trials of surfactant administration demonstrated a reduction in the incidence of PVH, the contribution of RDS to the occurrence of intracranial haemorrhage is likely to be small [129]. Indeed no surfactant trial has yet shown a reduction in severe PVH (grade III/IV) in treated babies although one trial has demonstrated that early treatment of babies in <40% oxygen reduces the risk of PVH compared to waiting until oxygen requirements are >60% [135]. For babies ≤750 g or ≤27 weeks the risk of PVH is insignificantly increased (Table 5.3) in those treated prophylactically compared to controls. Further studies of prophylaxis in babies <1000 g are warranted

**Table 5.5**   **Incidence of pulmonary haemorrhage and patent ductus arteriosus in surfactant trials**

| Surfactant | Prophylaxis or treatment | Birth weight (g) | n | Pulmonary haemorrhage | | Patent ductus arteriosus | |
|---|---|---|---|---|---|---|---|
| | | | | Treated (%) | Control (%) | Treated (%) | Control (%) |
| Exosurf | T | 700–1350 | 419 | 1.5 | 2.8 | 57 | 66 |
| Exosurf | P | 700–1100 | 446 | 3.6 | 1.4 | 54 | 50 |
| Exosurf | P | 700–1350 | 385 | 3.1 | 1.6 | 70 | 66 |
| Exosurf | P, T | 700–1350 | 178 | 1.0 | 0 | 48 | 39 |
| Exosurf | P | 500–699 | 215 | 11.3 | 1.8 | 54 | 48 |
| Survanta | P | 600–1250 | 430 | 3.4 | 4.6 | 46 | 38 |
| Survanta | T | 600–1750 | 798 | 7.1 | 5.4 | 51 | 56 |
| Surfactant-TA | T | 750–1750 | 100 | 6.0 | 7.0 | 46 | 37 |
| Human | P | 24–29 weeks | 60 | 6.4 | 10.3 | 74 | 83 |
| | | | | Single dose (%) | Multiple dose (%) | Single dose (%) | Multiple dose (%) |
| Curosurf | T | 700–2000 | 357 | 2.3 | 1.8 | 52 | 57 |

and the risk of PVH and long-term outcome need to be examined more fully.

## Patent ductus arteriosus

This has been shown to be increased in animal studies; and in the first non-randomized trial of Fujiwara *et al.* [53] nine of ten treated babies developed a significant PDA. In the surfactant trials untreated infants had incidences of PDA ranging from 14% to 83% for prophylaxis and 23–83% for rescue treatment. Meta-analysis suggests that use of natural surfactants insignificantly increases the risk of PDA but that synthetic surfactants have a paradoxical effect depending upon their method of use [55] (Table 5.4). For prophylactic synthetic surfactant there is a slight increase in the risk of PDA and for rescue treatment a modest decrease in the risk of PDA [55] (Table 5.4). These differences are not easy to explain but there appears to be an increased risk of PDA in very immature babies treated with synthetic surfactants and perhaps also male infants [58]. An association between PDA and pulmonary haemorrhage has been made for babies of <700 g [58,136] and early use of intravenous indomethacin has been advocated for these babies at risk [58].

## Pulmonary haemorrhage

This has not always been recorded as an adverse outcome in the randomized controlled trials of surfactant replacement. Furthermore, there has been little agreement on what constitutes this complication with opinions ranging from blood-stained fluid in the aspirate from endotracheal tube suctioning [58] to massive pulmonary haemorrhage with significant clinical deterioration and a need for increased mechanical ventilation [136]. The incidence in autopsy material is much higher than the rate diagnosed clinically before death [136]. Table 5.5 shows the incidence of pulmonary haemorrhage and patent ductus arteriosus in various trials of synthetic and natural surfactants. Although most of the trials enrolled babies of over 1000 g birth weight the incidence of pulmonary haemorrhage ranged from 0 to 10.3% in control infants and 1.0–11.3% in treated babies (Table 5.5). There is no convincing evidence that surfactant treatment increases the risk of pulmonary haemorrhage but the highest incidence was found in babies of 500–699 g birth weight who were treated prophylactically with Exosurf [58]. This is in keeping with the results of a recent meta-analysis which showed that the risk of pulmonary haemorrhage was increased about threefold in babies treated with prophylactic synthetic surfactant [137].

Recently it has been shown that further doses of surfactant can safely and beneficially be given to babies who have developed pulmonary haemorrhage after previous doses of surfactants [138].

## Bronchopulmonary dysplasia

The incidence of BPD in control babies in the prophylaxis surfactant trials ranged from 0 to 69% and from 0 to 46% in rescue trials [55]. Prophylactic natural surfactant treatment is associated with a modest decrease in the incidence of BPD (RR 0.75, 95% CI 0.61–0.92), but there is no effect with synthetic surfactant [55]. For rescue treatment the opposite is true, with synthetic surfactant there is a reduction in risk of BPD [RR 0.65, 95% CI 0.55, 0.78] which is not found with natural surfactants [55]. This is difficult to explain as studies have shown the appearance of bronchiolar necrotic lesions within a short time of the onset of breathing in animals with surfactant deficient lungs and this is prevented by giving prophylactic natural surfactant [139]. Perhaps the effect of barotrauma in the aetiology of BPD has been over-stated and the role of oxygen toxicity is of more importance.

## Retinopathy of prematurity

ROP is an important cause of blindness among VLBW babies. Due to improved survival rates, in part due to routine surfactant therapy and the hyperoxaemia that can follow treatment, the risk of ROP might be expected to increase. Two studies have looked at the effect of surfactant on the incidence of ROP [140,141]. Repka *et al.* [140] found that calf lung surfactant extract increased survival from 63% to 79% when given at birth to babies of ≤1000 g. Surfactant-treated babies also had a significantly lower incidence of acute ROP (64% vs 85%) and of threshold disease (stage 3 plus or greater), 3.4% compared to 10%. This surfactant-associated reduction in ROP was independent of gestational age, race or gender [140]. Tubman *et al.* [141] found that 36% of babies <1000 g treated with rescue Curosurf had acute ROP but only 2% had Stage 3 plus disease or greater. These incidence figures are lower than those expected for non-surfactant treated babies <1000 g. Recently, it has been shown that in addition to gestational age, the size and quality of the hospital is an important factor in determining the risk of both mortality and severe ROP in very preterm babies [142].

## Neurodevelopmental sequelae

This subject is covered more fully in Chapter 18. During the past 20 years neonatal survival of babies <1000 g has progressively improved and the number of able-bodied survivors has also increased. However, the population of disabled survivors has generally remained constant. A recent study has demonstrated a fall in the rate of major impairment during the 1980s which was attributed to a reduced rate of blindness but also to improved control of physiological status immediately after birth [143]. Prediction of abnormal long-term outcome is now possible using cerebral ultrasound scanning [144] and this should facilitate appropriate early intervention. In addition to immaturity, factors such as smallness for gestational age, neonatal signs of cerebral depression and low social class are significant predictors of neurodevelopmental problems at age 9 years [145].

Neonatal follow-up examinations are also important predictors of outcome. For babies <1000 g, who at 2 years have no major handicaps, there is a higher risk for intellectual and emotional problems at 5 years than controls of normal birth weight [146].

In surfactant-treated babies there have been at least 10 reported studies of long-term outcome [71,147]. Rates of neurological handicap are not increased by use of surfactants despite the increased survival of immature babies and between 70% and 85% of survivors are apparently normal at 2 years [71,147]. Of the 15% to 30% of babies with handicaps less than half are major.

Pulmonary function has been assessed in relatively few surfactant-treated babies beyond the neonatal period. The incidence of respiratory symptoms and hospital re-admissions of infants treated at birth with surfactant has been reported to be similar to those of controls [148–155]. Pulmonary function testing at about one year of age shows some decrease in dynamic compliance and increase in airways resistance in both surfactant-treated and control babies [149,156].

## Conclusions

Prevention of the respiratory distress syndrome is a realistic goal in many potential

**Practical points**

1. Prevention is better than cure. Prevention of preterm labour is problematic but prevention of RDS with antenatal corticosteroids is effective and probably underused. When delivery is likely from 23 or 24 weeks' gestation antenatal corticosteroids should be given.
2. Perinatal care, the cooperation of obstetrician and paediatrician is vital to ensure the best possible outcome for the very immature baby. The most experienced personnel available should manage delivery and resuscitation. The smaller the baby, the more experienced the doctor should be. During resuscitation the baby must not get cold. Effective radiant warmers are needed.
3. Early respiratory support is helpful using either nasal CPAP or mechanical ventilation if the baby shows any signs of respiratory distress.
4. Surfactant is best given early. There is a case for routine prophylaxis of babies between 23 and 27 weeks' gestation and of very early treatment, after stabilization and radiographic investigation in babies with RDS at other gestations. The best results with surfactant at low gestational ages are obtained in large regional centres where careful monitoring of the response and quick reaction to changing situations are more likely to be available.
5. Problems outside the lungs must be considered. Maintenance of blood pressure, prevention of IVH, fluid and electrolyte balance, temperature control and early nutritional support especially by the enteral route are all important. Good nursing care is also vital for keeping a balance between necessary intervention and minimal handling.
6. Keep the baby's parents informed and find out what their views are.

preterm deliveries. Promotion of fetal lung maturity with maternal corticosteroid therapy should be the rule in all high-risk situations. Treatment of the preterm baby with surfactant is a recognition of the failure to prevent RDS. Surfactant may be given as a true prophylaxis (in the delivery room) to babies of ≤28 weeks' gestation and to those >29 weeks when they need endotracheal intubation. For other babies early treatment within the first 2 hours should be the rule for those showing clinical and radiological signs of RDS. Both synthetic and natural surfactants may be used but the decision about which surfactant should be given will depend upon the timing of treatment and relative costs. In the future, third generation, genetically engineered surfactants may replace the currently available preparations [157].

# References

1. Hack, M., Horbar, J.D., Malloy, M.H., Tyson, J.E. and Wright, L. (1991) Very low birth weight outcomes of the National Institute of Child Health and Human Development Neonatal Network. *Pediatrics*, **87**, 587–597
2. Synnes, A.E., Ling, E.W.Y., Whitfield, H.F. *et al.* (1994) Perinatal outcomes of a large cohort of extremely low gestational age infants (twenty-three to twenty-eight completed weeks of gestation). *J. Pediatr.*, **125**, 952–960
3. Katy, V.C. and Bose, E.L. (1993) Improving survival of the very premature infant. *J. Perinatol.*, **13**, 261–265
4. Avery, M.E., Fletcher, B.D. and Wilkins, R.G. (1981) Lung development. In *The Lung and its Disorders in the Newborn Infant*. 4th edn, WB Saunders, Philadelphia, pp. 3–22
5. Hislop, A.A., Wigglesworth, J.S. and Desai, R. (1986) Alveolar development in the human fetus and infant. *Early Hum. Dev.*, **13**, 1–11
6. Bhutani, V.K. and Shaffer, T.H. (1982) Time-dependent tracheal deformation in fetal, neonatal and adult rabbits. *Pediatr. Res.*, **16**, 830–833
7. Liggins, G.C. and Kitterman, J.A. (1981) Development of the fetal lung. In *The Fetus and Independent Life*. Ciba Foundation Symposium 86, Pitman, London, pp. 308–335
8. Ballard, P.L. (1984) Combined hormonal treatment and lung maturation. *Semin. Perinatol.*, **8**, 283–292
9. Notter, R.H. (1984) Surface chemistry of pulmonary surfactant: the role of individual components. In *Pulmonary Surfactant* (B. Robertson, L.M.G. van Golde and J.J. Batenburg, eds), Elsevier, Amsterdam, pp. 17–65
10. Holm, B.A., Enhorning, G. and Notter, R.H. (1988) A biophysical mechanism by which plasma proteins inhibit lung surfactant activity. *Chem. Phys. Lipids*, **49**, 49–55

11. Frank, L. and Sosenko, I.R.S. (1987) Prenatal development of lung antioxidant enzymes in four species. *J. Pediatrics*, **110**, 1066–1110
12. Nelson, G.H. and McPherson, J.C. (1985) Respiratory distress syndrome in various cultures and a possible role of diet. In *Pulmonary Development: Transition from Intrauterine to Extrauterine Life* (G.H. Nelson, ed.), Marcel Dekker, New York, pp. 159–178
13. Hallman, M. (1987) Myo-inositol and the perinatal development of surfactant. In *Physiology of the Fetal and Neonatal Lung* (D.V. Walters, L.B. Strang and F. Geubelle, eds), MTP Press, Lancaster, pp. 197–208
14. Walters, D.V. and Ramsden, C.V. (1987) The secretion and absorption of fetal lung liquid. In *Physiology of the Fetal and Neonatal Lung* (D.V. Walters, L.B. Strang and F. Geubelle, eds), MTP Press, Lancaster, pp. 61–75
15. Guyton, A.C., Moffett, D.S. and Adair, T.H. (1984) Role of alveolar surface tension is transepithelial movement of fluid. In *Pulmonary Surfactant* (B. Robertson, L.M.G. van Golde and J.J. Batenburg, eds), Elsevier, Amsterdam, pp. 171–186
16. Ikegami, M., Jobe, A.H., Seidner, S. and Yamada, T. (1989) Gestational effects of corticosteroids and surfactant in ventilated rabbits. *Pediatr. Res.*, **25**, 32–37
17. Ikegami, M., Jobe, A., Jacobs, H. and Lam, R. (1984) A protein from airways of premature lambs that inhibits surfactant function. *J. Appl. Physiol.*, **57**, 1134–1142
18. Ikegami, M., Jobe, A.H., Pettenazzo, A., Seidner, S.R., Berry, D.D. and Ruffini, L. (1987) Effects of maternal treatment with corticosteroids, $T_3$, TRH, and their combinations on lung function of ventilated preterm rabbits with and without surfactant treatments. *Am. Rev. Respir. Dis.*, **136**, 892–898
19. Robertson, B. (1995) Surfactant replacement and neonatal lung pathology. *Perspect. Pediatr. Pathol.*, **18**, 5–13.
20. Halliday, H.L. (1988) Neonatal patent ductus arteriosus. *Pediatr. Rev. Commun.*, **3**, 1–17
21. Clyman, R.I., Jobe, A., Heymann, M. *et al.* (1982) Increased shunt through the patent ductus arteriosus after surfactant replacement therapy. *J. Pediatr.*, **100**, 101–107
22. Rigatto, H. (1984) Control of ventilation in the newborn. *Ann. Rev. Physiol.*, **46**, 661–674
23. Halliday, H.L. (1988) Care of preterm babies in the first hour. *Care Crit. Ill.*, **4**, 7–12
24. Wariyar, U., Richmond, S. and Hey, E. (1989) Pregnancy outcome at 24–31 weeks' gestation: mortality. *Arch. Dis. Childh.*, **64**, 670–677
25. Halliday, H.L. (1992) Management of the very low birthweight neonate. *Curr. Obstet. Gynecol.*, **2**, 207–211
26. Macfarlane, A., Cole, S., Johnson, A. and Botting, B. (1988) Epidemiology of birth before 28 weeks of gestation. *Br. Med. Bull.*, **44**, 861–893
27. MRC/RCOG Working Party on Cervical Cerclage (1988) Interim report of the Medical Research Council/Royal College of Obstetricians and Gynaecologists multicentre randomized trial of cervical cerclage. *Br. J. Obstet. Gynaecol.*, **95**, 437–445
28. Tubman, T.R.J., Rollins, M.D., Patterson, C.C. and Halliday, H.L. (1991) Increased incidence of respiratory distress syndrome in babies of hypertensive mothers. *Arch. Dis. Childh.*, **66**, 52–54
29. Crowley, P. (1989) Promoting pulmonary maturity. In *Effective Care in Pregnancy and Childbirth* (I. Chalmers, M. Enkin and M.J.N.C. Keirse, eds), Oxford University Press, Oxford, pp. 746–764
30. Halliday, H.L. (1993) Current views on the use of surfactant. *Contemp. Rev. Obstet. Gynaecol.*, **5**, 65–70
31. Crowley, P., Chalmers, I. and Keirse, M.J.N.C. (1990) The effects of corticosteroid administration before preterm delivery: an overview of the evidence from controlled trials. *Br. J. Obstet. Gynaecol.*, **97**, 11–15
32. Doyle, L.W., Kitchen, W.H., Ford, G.W., Rickards, A.L., Lissenden, J.V. and Ryan, M.M. (1986) Effects of antenatal steroid therapy on mortality and morbidity in very low birthweight infants. *J. Pediatr.*, **108**, 287–292
33. Papageorgiou, A.N., Doray, J.L., Ardila, R. and Kunos, I. (1989) Reduction of mortality, morbidity and respiratory distress syndrome in infants weighing less than 1000 grams by treatment with betamethasone and ritodrine. *Pediatrics*, **83**, 493–497
34. Liggins, G.C., Knight, D.B., Wealthall, S. and Howie, R.N. (1988) A randomised, double-blind trial of antepartum TRH and steroids in the prevention of neonatal respiratory disease. In *Clinical Reproductive Medicine. The Liggins' Years*, Auckland, New Zealand
35. Morales, W.J., O'Brien, W.F., Angel, J.L., Knuppel, R.A. and Sawai, S. (1989) Fetal lung maturation: the combined use of corticosteroids and thyrotropin-releasing hormone. *Obstet. Gynecol.*, **73**, 111–116
36. Ballard, R.A., Ballard, P.L., Creasy, R.K. *et al.* (1992) Respiratory distress in very-low-birthweight infants after prenatal thyrotropin-releasing hormone and glucocorticoid. TRH Study Group. *Lancet*, **339**, 510–515
37. ACTOBAT Study Group (1995) Australian collaborative trial of antenatal thyrotropin releasing hormone (ACTOBAT) for prevention of neonatal respiratory distress. *Lancet*, **345**, 877–882
38. Crowther, C.A., Hiller, J.E., Haslam, R.R. *et al.* (1997) Australian collaborative trial of antenatal thyrotropin releasing hormone: adverse effects at 12 month follow up. ACTOBAT Study Group. *Pediatrics*, **99**, 311–317
39. Wauer, R.R., Schmalisch, G., Menzel, K. *et al.* (1982) The antenatal use of Ambroxol (bromhexine metabolite VIII) to prevent hyaline membrane disease: a controlled double-blind study. *Biol. Res. Pregn. Perinatol.*, **3**, 84–91
40. Maresh, M. (1992) The obstetric management of preterm labour. *Curr. Obstet. Gynecol.*, **2**, 199–206
41. Morales, W.J., Angel, J.C., O'Brien, W.T. *et al.* (1988). A randomized study of antibiotic therapy in idiopathic preterm labour. *Obstet. Gynecol.*, **72**, 829–833.

42. Boyer, D.M. and Gotoff, S.P. (1986) Prevention of early onset neonatal group B streptococcal disease with selective intrapartum chemoprophylaxis. *N. Engl. J. Med.*, **314**, 1665–1669

43. Bowes, W.A. (1990) Cesarean section versus vaginal delivery: the obstetrician's perspective. In *The Micropremie: the next frontier* (R.M. Cowett, W.W. Hay, eds). Report of the Ninety-ninth Ross Conference on Pediatric Research. Ross Laboratories, pp. 4–13, Columbus, Ohio

44. Roper, H.P., Chiswick, M.L. and Sims, D.G. (1988) Referrals to a regional neonatal intensive care unit. *Arch. Dis. Childh.*, **63**, 403–407

45. Sidhu, H., Heasley, R.N., Patterson, C.C., Halliday, H.L. and Thompson, W. (1989) Short term outcome in babies refused perinatal intensive care. *Br. Med. J.*, **299**, 647–649

46. Avery, M.E. and Mead, J. (1959) Surface properties in relation to atelectasis and hyaline membrane disease. *Am. J. Dis. Child.*, **97**, 517–523

47. Jobe, A.H. (1990) The respiratory distress syndrome. Is it all surfactant deficiency? In *The Micropremie: The Next Frontier* (R.M. Cowett and W.W. Hay, eds). Report of the Ninety-ninth Ross Conference on Pediatric Research. Ross Laboratories, pp. 21–28, Columbus, Ohio

48. Enhorning, G. and Robertson, B. (1973) Lung expansion in the premature rabbit fetus after tracheal deposition of surfactant. *Pediatrics*, **50**, 58–66

49. Adams, F.H., Tower, B., Osher, A., Ikegami, M., Fujiwara, T. and Nozaki, M. (1978) Effects of tracheal instillation of natural surfactant in premature lambs. *Pediatr. Res.*, **12**, 841–848

50. Enhorning, G., Hill, D., Sherwood, G., Cutz, E., Robertson, B. and Bryan, C. (1978) Improved ventilation of prematurely delivered primates following tracheal deposition of surfactant. *Am. J. Obstet. Gynecol.*, **132**, 529–536

51. Walther, F.J., Blanco, C.E., Houdjik, M. and Bevers, E.M. (1985) Single versus repetitive doses of natural surfactant as treatment of respiratory distress syndrome in premature lambs. *Pediatr. Res.*, **19**, 224–227

52. Maeta, H., Vidyasagar, D., Raju, T., Bhat, R. and Matsuda, H. (1988) Response to bovine surfactant (surfactant TA) in two different HMD models (lambs and baboons). *Eur. J. Pediatr.*, **147**, 162–167

53. Fujiwara, T., Chida, S., Watabe, Y., Maeta, H., Morita, T. and Abe, T. (1980) Artificial surfactant therapy in hyaline membrane disease. *Lancet* **i**, 55–59

54. Morley, C.J., Bangham, A.D., Miller, N. and Davis, J.A. (1981) Dry artificial surfactant and its effect on very premature babies. *Lancet*, **i**, 64–68

55. Soll, R.F. and McQueen, M.C. (1992) Respiratory distress syndrome. In *Effective Care of the Newborn Infant* (J.C. Sinclair and M.D. Bracken, eds), Oxford University Press, Oxford, pp. 325–358

56. Halliday, H.L. (1992) Other acute lung disorders. In *Effective Care of the Newborn Infant* (J.C. Sinclair and M.B. Bracken, eds), Oxford University Press, Oxford, pp. 359–384

57. Ten Centre Study Group (1987) Ten centre trial of artificial surfactant (artificial lung expanding compound) in very premature babies. *Br. Med. J.*, **294**, 991–996

58. Stevenson, D., Walther, F., Long, W. *et al.* (1992) Controlled trial of a single dose of synthetic surfactant at birth in premature infants weighing 500–699 grams. *J. Pediatr.*, **120**, S3–S12

59. Ferrara, T.B., Hoekstra, R.E., Couser, T.R.J. *et al.* (1991) Effects of surfactant therapy on outcome of infants with birth weight of 600 to 750 grams. *J. Pediatr.*, **119**, 455–457

60. Leichty, E.A., Donovan, E., Porohit, D. *et al.* (1991) Reduction of neonatal mortality after multiple doses of bovine surfactant in low birth weight neonates with respiratory distress syndrome. *Pediatrics*, **88**, 19–28

61. Kendig, J.W., Notter, R.H., Cox, C. *et al.* (1991) A comparison of surfactant as immediate prophylaxis and as rescue therapy in neonates of less than 30 weeks' gestation. *N. Engl. J. Med.*, **324**, 865–871

62. Soll, R.F. and Morley, C.J. (1998) Prophylactic surfactant vs treatment with surfactant (Cochrane Review) In: *The Cochrane Library, Issue 2.* Oxford: Update Software

63. Morley, C.J. (1997) Systemic review of prophylactic vs rescue surfactant. *Arch. Dis. Childh.*, **77**, F70–F74

64. Halliday, H.L. (1997) Prophylactic surfactant. In: *Advances in Perinatal Medicine* (Cochburn, ed), Parthenon Publishing Group, London, pp. 360–370

65. Ferrara, T.B., Hoekstra, R.E., Couser, R.J. *et al.* (1994) Survival and follow-up of infants born at 23 to 26 weeks of gestational age. Effects of surfactant therapy. *J. Pediatr.*, **124**, 119–124

66. Farrell, E.E., Siver, R.K., Kimberlin, L.V., Wolf, E.S. and Dusik, J.M. (1989) Impact of antenatal dexamethasone administration on respiratory distress syndrome in surfactant-treated infants. *Am. J. Obstet. Gynecol.*, **161**, 628–633

67. Egberts, J. (1992) Estimated costs of different treatments of the respiratory distress syndrome in a large cohort of preterm infants of less than 30 weeks of gestation. *Biol. Neonate*, **61** (Suppl 1), 59–65

68. Chida, S., Fujiwara, T., Takahashi, A., Kanehama, S. and Kanedko, J. (1991) Precision and reliability of stable microbubble test as a predictor of respiratory distress syndrome. *Acta Paediatr. Jpn.*, **33**, 15–19

69. Halliday, H.L. (1996) Natural vs synthetic surfactants in neonatal respiratory distress syndrome. *Drugs,* **51**, 226–237

70. Soll, R.F. (1998) Natural surfactant extract vs synthetic surfactant in the treatment of established respiratory distress syndrome. (Cochrane Review) In: *The Cochrane Library*, Issue 2. Oxford: Update Software, Update quarterly.

71. Halliday, H.L. (1991) Surfactant replacement. In *Neonatal and Perinatal Medicine 1991 Yearbook* (M.H. Klaus and A.A. Fanaroff, eds), London, Yearbook Medical Publishers, pp. 13–21

72. Martin, G.I. and Sindel, B.D. (1992). Neonatal management of the very low birth weight infant: the use of surfactant. *Clin. Perinatol.*, **19**, 461–468

73. Speer, C.P. and Halliday, H.L. (1994) Surfactant therapy in the newborn. *Curr. Pediatr.*, **4**, 5–9

74. Charon, A., Tauesch, H.W., Fitzgibbon, C., Smith, G.B., Treves, S.T. and Phelps, D.S. (1989) Factors associated with surfactant treatment response in infants with severe respiratory distress syndrome. *Pediatrics*, **83**, 348–354

75. Fujiwara, T., Konishi, M., Chida, S. and Maeta, H. (1988) Factors affecting the response to a post-natal single dose of a reconstituted bovine surfactant (Surfactant-TA). In *Surfactant Replacement Therapy in Neonatal and Adult Respiratory Distress Syndrome* (B. Lachmann, ed.), Springer Verlag, Berlin, pp. 91–107

76. Collaborative European Multicenter Study Group (1991) Factors influencing the clinical response to surfactant replacement therapy in babies with severe respiratory distress syndrome. *Eur. J. Pediatr.*, **150**, 433–439

77. Segerer, H., Stevens, P., Schadow, B. *et al.* (1991) Surfactant administration in ventilated very low birth weight infants: factors related to response types. *Pediatr. Res.*, **30**, 591–596

78. Cowan, F., Whitelaw, A., Wertheim, D. and Silverman, M. (1991) Cerebral blood flow velocity changes after rapid administration of surfactant. *Arch. Dis. Childh.*, **66**, 1105–1109

79. van Bel, F., de Winter, P.J., Wijnands, H.B., van de Bor, M. and Egberts, J. (1992) Cerebral and aortic blood flow velocity patterns in preterm infants receiving prophylactic surfactant treatment. *Acta Paediatr.*, **81**, 504–510

80. van de Bor, M., Ma, E.J. and Walther, F.J. (1991) Cerebral blood flow velocity after surfactant instillation in preterm infants. *J. Pediatr.*, **118**, 285–287

81. McCord, F.B., Halliday, H.L., McClure, G. and Reid, M. McC. (1989) Changes in pulmonary and cerebral blood flow after surfactant treatment for severe respiratory distress syndrome. In *Surfactant Replacement Therapy in Neonatal and Adult Respiratory Distress Syndrome* (B. Lachmann, ed.), Springer-Verlag, Berlin, pp. 195–200

82. Jorch, G., Rabe, H., Garbe, M., Michel, E. and Gortner, L. (1989) Acute and protracted effects of intratracheal surfactant application on internal carotid blood flow velocity, blood pressure and carbon dioxide tension in very low birth weight infants. *Eur. J. Pediatr.*, **148**, 770–773

83. Skov, L., Bell, A. and Greisen, G. (1992) Surfactant administration and the cerebral circulation. *Biol. Neonate*, **61** (Suppl 1), 31–36

84. Skov, L., Hellstrom-Westas, L., Jacobsen, T., Greisen, G. and Svenningsen, N.W. (1992) Acute changes in cerebral oxygenation and cerebral blood volume in preterm infants during surfactant treatment. *Neuropediatrics*, **23**, 126–130

85. Edwards, A.D., McCormick, D.C., Roth, C.E. *et al.* (1992) Cerebral hemodynamic effects of treatment with modified natural surfactant investigated by near infrared spectroscopy. *Pediatr. Res.*, **32**, 532–536

86. Segerer, H., van Gelder, W., Angenent, F.W.M. *et al.* (1993) Pulmonary distribution and efficacy of exogenous surfactant in lung-lavaged rabbits are influenced by the instillation technique. *Pediatr. Res.*, **34**, 490–501

87. Ueda, T., Ikegami, M., Rider, E.D. and Jobe, A.H. (1994) Distribution of surfactant and ventilation in surfactant-treated preterm lambs. *J. Appl. Physiol.*, **76**, 45–55

88. Phibbs, R.H., Ballard, R.A., Clements, J.A. *et al.* (1991) Initial clinical trial of Exosurf, a protein-free synthetic surfactant, for prophylaxis and early treatment of hyaline membrane disease. *Pediatrics*, **88**, 1–9

89. Horbar, J.D., Wright, L.L., Soll, R.F. *et al.* (1993) A multicenter randomized trial comparing two surfactants for the treatment of neonatal respiratory distress syndrome. *J. Pediatr.*, **123**, 757–766

90. Cummings, J.J., Holm, B.A., Hudak, M.L. *et al.* (1992) A controlled clinical comparison of four different surfactant preparations in surfactant-deficient preterm lambs. *Am. Rev. Respir. Dis.*, **145**, 999–1004

91. Corcoran, J.D., Berggren, P., Sun, B., Halliday, H.L., Robertson, B. and Curstedt, T. (1994) Comparison of surface properties and physiological effects of a synthetic and a natural surfactant in preterm rabbits. *Arch. Dis. Childh.*, **71**, F165–F169

92. Vilstrup, C., Gommers, J.A., Bos, B., Lachmann, B., Werner, O. and Larsson, A. (1992) Natural surfactant instilled in premature lambs increases lung volume and improves ventilation homogeneity within five minutes. *Pediatr. Res.*, **32**, 595–599

93. Collaborative European Multicenter Study Group (1988) Surfactant replacement therapy for severe neonatal respiratory distress syndrome: an international randomized clinical trial. *Pediatrics*, **82**, 683–691

94. Halliday, H.L., McCord, F.B., McClure, B.G. and Reid, M.McC. (1989) Acute effects of instillation of surfactant in severe respiratory distress syndrome. *Arch. Dis. Childh.*, **64**, 13–16

95. Svenningsen, N.W., Bjorklund, L., Vilstrup, C. and Werner, O. (1992) Lung mechanics (FRC and static pressure-volume diagram) after endotracheal surfactant instillation: preliminary observations. *Biol. Neonate*, **61** (Suppl. 1), 44–47

96. Hallman, M., Merritt, T.A., Berry, C. *et al.* (1991) Who doesn't respond to surfactant therapy? In *Hot Topic '91 in Neonatology* (J.F. Lucey, ed.), Ross Laboratories, Columbus, Ohio, pp. 148–156

97. Tubman, T.R.J. and Halliday, H.L. (1990) Surfactant treatment for respiratory distress following prolonged rupture of membranes. *Eur. J. Pediatr.*, **149**, 727–729

98. Auten, R.L., Notter, R.H., Kendig, J.W., Davis, J.M. and Shapiro, D.L. (1991) Surfactant treatment of full-term newborns with respiratory failure. *Pediatrics*, **87**, 101–107

99. Heldt, G., Pesonen, E. and Merritt, T.A. (1989) Closure of the ductus arteriosus and mechanics of breathing in preterm infants after surfactant replacement therapy. *Pediatr. Res.*, **25**, 305–310

100. Hallman, M., Merritt, T.A., Pohjavuori, M. and Gluck, L. (1986) Effect of surfactant substitution on lung effluent phospholipids in respiratory distress syndrome: evaluation of surfactant phospholipid turnover, pool-size and the relationship to severity of respirator failure. *Pediatr. Res.*, **20**, 1228–1235

101. Konishi, M., Fujiwara, T., Naito, T. *et al.* (1988) Surfactant replacement therapy in neonatal respiratory distress syndrome. A multicenter randomised trial: comparison of high-versus low-dose of surfactant-TA. *Eur. J. Pediatr.*, **147**, 20–25

102. Gortner, L. (1992) Natural surfactant in neonatal respiratory distress syndrome, a 1992 update. *J. Perinatol Med.*, **20**, 409–418

103. Halliday, H.L., Tarnow-Mordi, W.O., Corcoran, J.D., Patterson, C.C. and the Collaborative European Multicentre Study Group (1994). A multicentre randomised trial comparing high and low doses surfactant regimens for the treatment of respiratory distress syndrome (The Curosurf 4 Trial). *Arch. Dis. Childh.*, **69**, 276–280

104. Pettenazzo, A., Jobe, A.H., Ikegami, M., Rider, E., Seidner, S.E. and Yanada, T. (1990) Cumulative effects of repeated surfactant treatments in the rabbit. *Exp. Lung Res.*, **16**, 131–143

105. The OSIRIS Collaborative Group (1992) Early versus delayed neonatal administration of a synthetic surfactant – The judgement of OSIRIS. *Lancet*, **340**, 1363–1369

106. Ashton, M.R., Postle, A.D., Hall, M.A., Austen, N.C., Smith, D.E. and Normand, I.C. (1992) Turnover of exogenous artificial surfactant. *Arch. Dis. Childh.*, **67**, 383–387

107. Halliday, H.L. (1997) Surfactant theory in neonates. *Paediatric and Perinatal Drug Therapy*, **1**, 30–40

108. Ikegami, M., Agate, Y., Elkady, T. *et al.* (1987) Comparison of four surfactants: *in vitro* surface properties and responses of preterm lambs to treatment at birth. *Pediatrics*, **79**, 38–46

109. Lewis, J., Ikegami, M., Tabor, B. and Jobe, A. (1990) Physiological response to nebulized surfactants administered to premature lambs. *Pediatr. Res.*, **27**, 310A

110. Samgstad, O.D., Halliday, H.L., Robertson, B. and Speer, C.P. (1993) Replacement therapy with porcine natural surfactant – current status and future challenges. *Biol. Neonate*, **64**, 269–278

111. Hallman, M. (1989) The severity of respiratory distress syndrome during the first two neonatal days in relationship to fluid intake. *Acta. Pediatr. Scand.*, **360** (Suppl), 93–100

112. Merritt, T.A., Hallman, M., Berry, C. *et al.* (1991) A randomized placebo-controlled trial of human surfactant at birth versus rescue administration in very low birthweight infants with lung immaturity. *J. Pediatr.*, **118**, 581–594

113. Wauer, R.R. (1983) Medical treatment of neonatal hyaline membrane disease using bromhexine, ambroxol and CDP-choline. In *Pulmonary Surfactant System* (E.V. Cosmi and E.M. Scarpelli, eds), Elsevier, Amsterdam, pp. 173–189

114. Wauer, R.R., Schmalsch, G., Bohme, B. and Arand, J. (1990) Ambroxol therapy of hyaline membrane disease – preliminary results of a double-blind study. In *Research in Perinatal Medicine 2* (E.L. Grauel, L. Stern, I. Syllm-Rapoport and R.R. Wauer, eds), Verlag Gesundheit GmbH, Berlin, pp. 259–268

115. Hallman, M., Jarvenpaa, A.-L. and Pohjavuori, M. (1986) Respiratory distress syndrome and inositol supplementation in preterm infants. *Arch. Dis. Childh.*, **61**, 1076–1083

116. Hallman, M., Pohjavuori, M. and Bry, K. (1990) Inositol supplementation in respiratory distress syndrome. *Lung*, **168** (Suppl), 877–882

117. Hallman, M., Bry, K., Hoppu, K., Lappi, M. and Pohjavuori, M. (1992) Inositol supplementation in premature infants with respiratory distress syndrome. *N. Engl. J. Med.*, **326**, 1233–1239

118. Avery, G.B., Fletcher, A.B., Kaplan, M. and Bruono, D.S. (1985) Controlled trial of dexamethasone in respirator-dependent infants with bronchopulmonary dysplasia. *Pediatrics*, **75**, 106–111

119. Collaborative Dexamethasone Trial Group (1991) Dexamethasone therapy in neonatal chronic lung disease: an international placebo-controlled trial. *Pediatrics*, **88**, 421–427

120. Hallman, M. (1984) Effect of extracellular myo-inositol on surfactant phospholipid synthesis in the fetal rabbit lung. *Biochim. Biophys. Acta*, **795**, 67–68

121. Yeh, T.F., Torre, J.A., Rastogi, A., Aneybuno, M. and Pildes, R.S. (1990) Early post-natal dexamethasone therapy in premature infants with severe respiratory distress syndrome: a double-blind controlled study. *J. Pediatr.*, **117**, 273–282

122. Sanders, R.J., Cox, C., Phelps, D.L. and Sinkin, R.A. (1994) Two doses of early intravenous dexamethasone for the prevention of bronchopulmonary dysplasia in babies with respiratory distress syndrome. *Pediatr. Res.*, **36**, 122–128

123. Watterberg, K.L. and Scott, S.M. (1995) Evidence of early adrenal insufficiency in babies who develop bronchopulmonary dysplasia. *Pediatrics*, **95**, 120–125

124. Halliday, H.L. (1998) Postnatal corticosteroids for prevention of chronic lung disease in the preterm infantL moderately early treatment (7–14 days). (Cochrane Review) In: *The Cochrane Library*, Issue, 3, Oxford: Update Software

125. Soll, R.F. (1992) 1. Prophylactic administration of any surfactant. 2. Synthetic surfactant treatment of RDS. 3. Natural surfactant treatment of RDS. In *Oxford Database of Perinatal Trials*, Version 1.3, Disk Issue 7, Records 5664, 5252, 5206

126. Halliday, H.L. and Tarnow-Mordi, W.O. (1993) Surfactant replacement therapy – time for thought. *Arch. Dis. Childh.*, **68**, 619

127. Halliday, H.L. (1989) Clinical experience with exogenous natural surfactant. *Dev. Pharmacol. Ther.*, **13**, 173–181

128. McCord, F.B., Curstedt, T., Halliday, H.L., McClure, B.G., Reid, M.McC. and Robertson, B. (1988) Surfactant treatment and incidence of intraventricular haemorrhage in severe respiratory distress syndrome. *Arch. Dis. Childh.*, **63**, 10–16

129. Leviton, A., Van Marter, L. and Kuban, K.C.K. (1989) Respiratory distress syndrome and intracranial hemorrhage: cause or association. Inferences from surfactant clinical trials. *Pediatrics*, **84**, 915–922

130. Papile, L.A., Burstein, J., Burstein, R. and Koffler, H. (1978) Incidence and evolution of subopendynal and intraventricular hemorrhage: a study of infants with birth weights less than 1500 gram. *J. Pediatr.*, **92**, 429–534

131. Enhorning, G., Shennan, A., Possmayer, F. *et al.* (1985) Prevention of neonatal respiratory distress syndrome by tracheal instillation of surfactant: a randomized clinical trial. *Pediatrics*, **76**, 145–153

132. Fujiwara, T., Konishi, M., Chida, S. *et al.* (1990) Surfactant replacement therapy with a single postventilatory dose of a reconstituted bovine surfactant in preterm neonates with respiratory distress syndrome: final analysis of a multicenter, double-blind, randomized trial and comparison with similar trials. *Pediatrics.*, **86**, 753–764

133. Morley, C.J., Greenough, A., Miller, N. *et al.* (1988) Randomized trial of artificial surfactant (ALEC) given at birth to babies from 23 to 34 weeks' gestation. *Early Hum. Dev.*, **17**, 41–54

134. Horbar, J.D., Soll, R.F., Schachinger, M. *et al.* (1990) A European multicentre randomized controlled trial of single dose surfactant therapy for idiopathic respiratory distress syndrome. *Eur. J. Pediatr.*, **149**, 416–423

135. Bevilacqua, G., Halliday, H.L., Parmigiani, S., Robertson, B. on behalf of the Collaborative European Multicentre Study Group (1993) Randomized multicentre trial of treatment with porcine natural surfactant for moderately severe neonatal respiratory distress syndrome. *J. Perinat. Med.*, **21**, 5, 329–40

136. van Houten, J., Long, W., Mullett, M. *et al.* (1992) Pulmonary hemorrhage in premature infants after treatment with synthetic surfactant: an autopsy evaluation. *J. Pediatr.*, **120**, S40–S44

137. Raju, T.N.K. and Langenberg, P. (1993) Pulmonary hemorrhage and exogenous surfactant therapy: A meta-analysis. *J. Pediatr.*, **123**, 603–610

138. Pandit, P.B., Dunn, M.S. and Colucci, E.Z. (1995) Surfactant therapy in neonates with respiratory deterioration due to pulmonary hemorrhage. *Pediatrics*, **95**, 32–36

139. Nilsson, R., Grossmann, G. and Robertson, B. (1978) Lung surfactant and the pathogenesis of neonatal bronchiolar lesions induced by artificial ventilation. *Pediatr. Res.*, **12**, 249–255

140. Repka, M.X., Hudak, M.L., Parsa, C.F. and Tielsch, J.M. (1992) Calf lung surfactant extract prophylaxis and retinopathy of prematurity. *Ophthalmology*, **99**, 531–536

141. Tubman, T.R.J., Rankin, S.J., Halliday, H.L., Johnston, S.S. (1992) Surfactant replacement therapy and the prevalence of acute retinopathy of prematurity. *Biol. Neonate*, **61**, (Suppl 1), 54–58

142. Darlow, B.A., Harwood, L.J., Clemett, R.S. (1992) Retinopathy of prematurity: risk factors in a prospective population-based study. *Paed. Perinat. Epidemiol.*, **6**, 62–80

143. Perlman, M., Claris, O., Hao, Y. *et al.* (1995) Secular changes in the outcomes to eighteen to twenty-four months of age of extremely low birth weight infants, with adjustment for changes in risk factors and severity of illness. *J. Pediatr.*, **126**, 75–87

144. Stewart, A.L., Reynolds, E.O.R., Hope, P.L. *et al.* (1987) Probability of neurodevelopmental disorders estimated from ultrasound appearance of brain in very preterm infants. *Dev. Med. Child. Neurol.*, **29**, 3–11

145. Lindahl, E., Michelsson, K., Helenns, M. and Parre, M. (1988) Neonatal risk factors and later neurodevelopmental disturbances. *Dev. Med. Child. Neurol.*, **30**, 571–589

146. Szatmari, P., Saigal, S., Rosenbaum, P. *et al.* (1990) Psychiatric disorders at five years among children with birthweights <1000 g: a regional perspective. *Dev. Med. Child. Neurol.*, **32**, 954–962

147. Halliday, H.L. (1993) Follow-up data from babies treated with surfactant. In *Surfactant in Clinical Practice* (G. Bevilacqua, S. Parmigiani and B. Robertson, eds), Harwood, Chur, pp. 149–156

148. Kitchen, W.H., Ford, G.W., Doyle, L.W., Rickards, A.L. and Kelly, E.A. (1990) Health and hospital readmissions of very low birth weight and normal birth weight children. *Am. J. Dis. Child.*, **144**, 213–218

149. Walti, H., Boule, M., Moriette, G. and Relier, J.-P. (1992) Pulmonary functional outcome at one year of age in infants treated with natural porcine surfactant at birth. *Biol. Neonate*, **61**, (Suppl 1), 48–53

150. Halliday, H.L., McClure, G. and Reid, M.McC. (1986) Growth and developmental two years after artificial surfactant replacement at birth. *Early Hum. Dev.*, **13**, 323–327

151. Vaucher, Y.E., Merritt, T.A., Hallman, M. *et al.* (1988) Neurodevelopmental and respiratory outcome in early childhood after human surfactant treatment. *Am. J. Dis. Child.*, **142**, 927–930

152. Dunn, M.S., Shennan, A.T., Hoskins, E.M., Lennox, K. and Enhorning, G. (1988) Two-year follow-up of infants of enrolled in a randomized trial of surfactant replacement therapy for prevention of neonatal respiratory distress syndrome. *Pediatrics*, **82**, 543–547

153. Wale, J., Taeusch, H.W., Soll, R.F. and McCormick, M.C. (1990) Health and developmental outcomes of a surfactant controlled trial: follow-up at 2 years. *Pediatrics*, **85**, 1103–1107

154. Morley, C.J. and Morley, R. (1990) Follow-up of premature babies treated with artificial surfactant (ALEC). *Arch. Dis. Child.*, **65**, 667–669

155. Collaborative European Multicentre Study Group (1992) A 2-year follow-up of babies enrolled in a European multicentre trial of porcine surfactant replacement for severe neonatal respiratory distress syndrome. *Eur. J. Pediatr.*, **151**, 372–376

156. Heldt, G.P., Rosas, F., Merritt, T.A. *et al.* (1989) Pulmonary function of infants treated with human surfactant: assessment at 9 months. *Pediatr. Res.*, **25**, 366A

157. Yao, L.-J., Richardson, C., Ford, C. *et al.* (1990) Expression of mature pulmonary surfactant-associated protein B (SP-B) in *Escherichia coli* using truncated human SP-B c DNAs. *Biochem. Cell. Biol.*, **68**, 559–566

# 6

# Ventilation and pulmonary air leak

**Anne Greenough**

The extremely low birthweight (ELBW) infant will usually be resuscitated at birth by endotracheal intubation and manual inflation of the lungs. Indeed, many centres have a gestational age or birth weight cut-off below which their infants are routinely intubated at birth. Only infants who establish vigorous respiration by 2 minutes of age with a heart rate greater than 100 beats $min^{-1}$ escape intubation. ELBW infants will then remain intubated and ventilated for transfer and on admission to the neonatal unit. In one series [1] 168 of 175 extremely preterm (gestational age ≤28 weeks) infants were ventilated from birth. Once on the neonatal unit the indications for ventilation include recurrent apnoea or worsening respiratory distress and are similar to criteria used in larger infants [2], although earlier intervention is usually practised [1].

## Diagnosis

The majority of ELBW infants are ventilated because of respiratory distress syndrome (RDS) or respiratory distress of extreme prematurity (RDEP). Although in one series this diagnosis only accounted for 55% of ventilated ELBW infants [3], in another over 90% of ventilated infants fell into those diagnostic categories [1]. RDEP is diagnosed in infants of less than 24 weeks of gestational age who develop respiratory distress within 4 hours of birth, with a symmetrical ground glass appear-

ance on the chest radiograph and no infectious agent being isolated in the first 48 hours of life. Other diagnoses include pulmonary hypoplasia, septicaemia, congenital pneumonia, apnoea, transient tachypnoea of the newborn [1] and respiratory depression due to birth asphyxia [3].

## Ventilation techniques

### Conventional ventilation

Conventional ventilators are used at rates between 30 and 150 breaths $min^{-1}$. Amongst the present population of ventilated babies, rates in excess of 60 breaths $min^{-1}$ (high frequency positive pressure ventilation (HFPPV) improve oxygenation and carbon dioxide elimination [4]. This advantageous effect, however, is only seen amongst non-paralysed infants and it has become clear that increasing ventilator rate in such babies alters their respiratory interactions [5]. Infants who are actively expiring against positive pressure inflation delivered at a rate of 30 breaths $min^{-1}$, at faster rates tend to breathe synchronously, an interaction which increases tidal volume and hence $CO_2$ elimination. This interaction is most likely to be provoked when the ventilator rate is close to the infant's spontaneous respiratory rate [6]. It is not necessary to match exactly the ELBW infant's own respiratory rate [7], but a ventilator rate faster than the infant's rate measured during a very short period of disconnection from the ventilator should be used [8]. ELBW infants of less than 28 weeks of gestation have a very rapid respiratory rate in the first 48 hours of life and are therefore most likely to benefit from HFPPV. Ventilator performance, however, is an important determinant of the success of this form of ventilation [9]. Inadvertent positive end expiratory pressure (PEEP) is produced if rate is increased in ventilators which do not incorporate an assisted expiratory valve, this reduces delivered volume and hence may cause carbon dioxide retention. Fast rates have not been proven to improve gas exchange in paralysed infants. Indeed, in that group gas trapping can be produced, but this is less likely in immature ELBW infants [10]. Increasing ventilator rates from 30 to 60 breaths $min^{-1}$ significantly improves carbon dioxide elimination, but not oxygenation, in infants, ventilated beyond the first week of life. Raising the ventilator rate above 60 breaths $min^{-1}$, however, did not further improve blood gases, even though the study group include seven ELBW infants [11]. After the first week of life relatively few infants, when being fully ventilated, show any spontaneous respiratory activity [12] and thus it is not unexpected that such infants' results resemble those of paralysed babies [4].

Addition of PEEP during mechanical ventilation increases mean airway pressure, improves oxygenation [13,14] and conserves surfactant [15]. PEEP levels of 10 $cmH_2O$ have been recommended [16], but the relevant data were collected from infants with severe RDS and birthweight >1000 g. In recent studies which have included ELBW infants with acute respiratory distress, high levels of PEEP have resulted in alveolar overdistension with reduced compliance and carbon dioxide retention [17] without improving oxygenation [18]. In chronic respiratory failure, however, a different picture emerges. Amongst 14 ELBW ventilated infants studied at a median postnatal age of 15 days, increasing the PEEP level to 6 $cmH_2O$ significantly improved oxygenation without resulting in carbon dioxide retention [18]. The majority of infants ventilated beyond the first week of life suffer from Type I chronic lung disease [19] and their chest radiographs show evidence of areas of collapse. These underexpanded areas of lung will be recruited by increasing PEEP without causing overdistension and carbon dioxide retention.

## Patient triggered ventilation

It is not always possible to tune the ventilator to the baby's own respiratory efforts, thereby inducing synchrony. An alternative method has been to use the baby's respiratory efforts to trigger the ventilator. This approach, patient-triggered ventilation (PTV), has only recently become available for use in neonates [20]. During PTV, the peak inspiratory pressure (PIP), PEEP and inspired oxygen, are set by the operator, but the rate is controlled by the baby's respiratory efforts, unless synchronous intermittent mandatory ventilation is used. A number of ventilator manufacturers have modified their conventional neonatal ventilator to be patient-triggered and there are now available purpose-built patient-triggered ventilators. These machines incorporate a variety of triggering devices to detect the infant's respiratory efforts. Changes in airway pressure [21], airway gas flow [22] and abdominal movement [20] are used as trigger signals. Although successful in the short term, oesophageal pressure triggering devices have not proved suitable for long-term use, as the continued presence of a balloon in the oesophagus stimulates peristalsis which interferes with the detection of the infant's respiratory efforts [23]. The performance of the triggering device is an important determinant of the success of PTV. The triggering device must have a high sensitivity and thus detect the maximum number of the infant's respiratory effort. The trigger delay, the time from the onset of inspiration to the commencement of positive pressure inflation, must be as short as possible to ensure that inflation occurs early in inspiration and does not continue into expiration. If the trigger delay is very long, the only method of preventing inflation extending into expiration and stimulating an adverse respiratory intervention, is to shorten inflation time to such an extent that the delivered volume is reduced [24]. The trigger delay consists of two components, the time needed for the baby's respiratory efforts to reach the critical trigger level, which is dependent on the pattern of breathing adopted by the baby, and the response time or system delay of the ventilator. Ideally, the system's delay time should not exceed 10% of the total inflation time; a systems delay of 36 ms permits a maximum ventilator rate of 83 breaths $min^{-1}$ [25]. In infants with both acute

[26] and chronic lung disease of prematurity (CLP) [27] comparison of the abdominal movement sensor (MR10 pneumatic capsule) and an airway pressure triggering device revealed the latter to be more sensitive and to have significantly shorter trigger delays, a median of 200 ms compared to 300–550 ms with the pneumatic capsule. The commercial systems now available function better as preliminary studies indicate that, for example, the Draeger Baby Log [28] and SLE 2000 [21] have trigger delays of less than 100 ms in preterm babies with RDS.

Unfortunately PTV is frequently unsuccessful in immature ELBW infants [29], even when one of the commercially available systems with a short trigger delay is used [30]. Very immature infants rapidly develop a metabolic acidosis; their respiratory efforts are irregular and often of insufficient magnitude to consistently trigger the ventilator. PTV has also been attempted in immature infants who require ventilation beyond the second week of life due to CLP, but again, rarely provided a satisfactory alternative to conventional ventilation [31]. It is possible to predict in which infants PTV will be unsuccessful in the long term [32]. Failure of PTV is likely to occur in infants whose oxygenation does not increase after one hour on PTV, compared to a similar period on conventional ventilation. A further indicator of failure is a slow triggering rate when related to the infant's gestational age [29], and an asynchronous respiratory interaction [32]. Despite recent developments in PTV and improvements in performance, PTV still remains relatively unsuccessful in very immature infants. This is, in part, due to the nature of their respiratory efforts, that is those with a weak Hering Breuer reflex tend to fail on long-term PTV [33].

### High frequency jet ventilation

During high frequency jet ventilation (HFJV) frequencies of up to 400 min$^{-1}$ are used. Very little data exist on long-term results and complications and, indeed, ethical considerations have meant that this technique has often been restricted to critically ill children whose respiratory failure has been unresponsive to more conventional therapy. In such infants, HFJV has resulted in temporary improvements in oxygenation [34,35] but there has

been a high incidence of tracheal lesions if HFJV is maintained for more than 8 hours [36,37]. In infants with a birth weight of 1000–2000 g, a randomized trial failed to demonstrate that early intervention with HFJV prevented or substantially reduced the mortality or morbidity rates associated with assisted ventilation [38]. At our current level of knowledge, this technique should probably be reserved for the preoperative management of infants with diaphragmatic hernia who have severe respiratory failure [39,40]. It is also useful as a short-term measure for infants with severe pulmonary interstitial emphysema (PIE); PIE resolving within 24 hours or at least showed signs of improvement in 46% of ELBW patients supported by HFJV compared to only 33% of ELBW infants on conventional ventilation [41]. There was, however, no difference between the two groups in their long-term outcome, that is in the incidence of CLP, periventricular haemorrhage (PVH), patent ductus arteriosus (PDA) or new airleaks.

### High frequency oscillation

During high frequency oscillation (HFO) frequencies of up to 40 Hz may be used, although 10–15 Hz is most commonly employed [42–44]. This technique has provided useful improvements in oxygenation in infants with severe respiratory failure and appears to have only minimal side-effects [45], although there is some evidence to suggest that HFO may increase the occurrence of serious intraventricular haemorrhage (IVH) and periventricular leucomalacia [42]. Randomized studies have given conflicting results as to whether HFO reduces the incidence of CLP [42,43]. Both studies included ELBW infants: 372 in the first [42] and 24 in the second [43]; unfortunately the method of presentation of the results precludes the possibility of determining the outcome of this selected group. It is likely to be some years before the necessary physiological studies and clinical trials have defined the place of this ventilation technique in clinical management of the ELBW infant. Our own clinical experience suggests amongst infants with severe RDS, HFO is likely to be less successful in infants of less than 28 weeks' gestation compared to those of greater maturity [46].

## Extracorporeal membrane oxygenation

This technique provides a method of gas exchange in critically ill infants [47], while avoiding continuance of damaging patterns of mechanical ventilation. Unfortunately, this technique is not suitable for infants less than 1000 g as, in babies prior to 35 weeks' gestation use of ECMO has been associated with a high incidence of PVH [48]. As this complication is related to the need for heparinization during the procedure, the introduction of heparin-bonded circuits may make ECMO more widely applicable.

## Extubation

Few randomized studies have focused on improving the efficiency and speed of weaning from mechanical ventilation and no data are available from trials which have exclusively considered infants of less than 1000 g in birth weight. Limitation of inspiratory time to <0.5 s which, in preterm infants of all birth weights has been demonstrated to significantly shorten weaning [49], would seem logical in ELBW infants as such infants have a short spontaneous inspiratory time. In contrast, a randomized study of weaning comparing PTV to conventional ventilation did not produce encouraging results for the ELBW infant. Although in the trial overall, the duration of weaning by PTV was a median of 30 hours (range 3–186) and significantly shorter than by conventional ventilation which was a median of 61 hours (range 15–262), the three ELBW infants less than 28 weeks of gestation did not tolerate weaning by the PTV [50].

During recovery from RDS, first inflating pressures are reduced and then ventilator rate is steadily decreased until 5 breaths min⁻¹ is reached. At that stage policies differ as to whether it is appropriate to extubate from intermittent mandatory ventilation (IMV) or to place the infant temporarily on endotracheal continuous positive airways pressure (CPAP). It is certainly advisable to avoid a long period on endotracheal CPAP which has been shown to be associated with a higher incidence of extubation complications [51]. Of 22 infants with birth weight less than 1250 g extubation was successful, that is unassociated with apnoea or respiratory acidosis, in all 13 patients extubated

directly from IMV compared to in only seven of 14 infants extubated after 6 hours of endotracheal CPAP. The high failure rate in the latter group was postulated to be due to the increased work of breathing consequent upon the high airways resistance of the narrow endotracheal tubes used to ventilate ELBW infants [51]. Once extubated, infants may be nursed on nasal CPAP or in a headbox. The application of nasal CPAP has theoretical advantages; it can improve functional residual capacity, decreasing the likelihood of postextubation atelectasis and preventing apnoea by improving chest wall stability. It has, however, disadvantages in that the nasal catheter may traumatize the nostrils, increase the infant's agitation and, unless frequently changed, block resulting in hypoxia. It would seem likely that nasal CPAP would be most useful for extubation of infants with acute RDS, this however has not been demonstrated to be the case [52]. A recent randomized study [52] has shown that there is no advantage of either method in infants with acute or chronic respiratory distress. Approximately one-third of patients required re-intubation within 48 hours of extubation regardless of which extubation method was used. The study population consisted of preterm infants of birth weight less than 1880 g, but the majority of the 60 with CLP were ELBW. Physiotherapy prior to extubation has been shown in a retrospective and prospective controlled study [53] to reduce postextubation atelectasis, unfortunately the trial only recruited infants with birth weight greater than 1000 g.

A number of agents have been used to assist weaning. Theophylline appears useful in infants less than 30 days of age [54,55] but no study has concentrated exclusively on ELBW infants. Dexamethasone has been investigated in both non-randomized [56,57] and randomized [58,59] studies. This therapy certain shortens the duration of weaning [58,59] and if given for 6 weeks [60] appears to improve the long-term outcome. Those studies involved infants of birth weight less than 1000 g but it is not possible, because of the manner of presentation of the results, to determine if the effectiveness of the therapy was influenced by birth weight. A recent study has suggested that very early, at less than 48 hours of age, administration of dexamethasone may enhance weaning [61]. Dexamethasone therapy, unfortunately, has numerous side-effects. Perhaps the most well documented is that of hypertension, which can result in serious morbidity [62], the effect of elevation of blood pressure is independent of the postnatal age at administration [63].

# Outcome of ventilation

## Mortality

Mortality is significantly increased in infants of birthweight ≤1000 g ($P = 0.006$). In one series which included 6676 inborn neonates with birth weight less than 1250 g, the 28-day survival rate of infants with birth weight 500–599 g was 30% compared with 91.3% for neonates of 1200–1250 g. Multivariate analysis has demonstrated, however, that gestational age is a more important determinant of survival than birth weight; predictors of survival in order of descending significance were: gestational age, birth weight, sex, race, single birth and small for gestational age status [64]. Mortality of ventilated infants is inversely related to their gestational age, the survival rate of infants of 27 and 28 weeks' gestation being significantly greater than that of ≤24 weeks ($P = 0.003$). The overall mortality of ventilated infants of <29 week gestation infants is 59%, but is higher amongst those born small-for-dates who have only a 25% survival rate [1]. The survival of extremely premature infants documented in 1992 [1] compares favourably with earlier studies which reported mortality rates of 55% in 1976–1980 [65]; 48% in 1980–1984 [66]; and 44% in 1981–1985 [65]. These data suggest that survival rates of even very immature infants are increasingly slowly with time.

## Periventricular haemorrhage (PVH)

Amongst infants of less than 29 weeks of gestational age the occurrence of PVH or the effect of PVH on mortality does not appear to correlate with gestational age or with birth weight: 43% of extremely preterm infants with RDS or RDEP develop PVH of varying severity [1].

## Chronic lung disease

Approximately 37% of extremely preterm ventilated infants are chronically oxygen-dependent at 28 days, CLP. Many of these infants are still oxygen-dependent at a postconceptional age of 36 weeks; the majority (22 of 27) of one series [1] who were so affected had a birth weight less than 1000 g.

## Patent ductus arteriosus

Of ventilated infants (<29 weeks of gestation), 38% developed a PDA; relatively few, however, required surgical ligation [1]. Previous reports have demonstrated that the incidence of PDA amongst infants with birth weight less than 1000 g is 77% [67] and 81% [68]. The low incidence in the most recent series [1] may be explained by a policy of fluid restriction in the acute stage of RDS or differences in the methods of diagnosing PDA in the recent [1] and previous studies [67,68]. Administration of exogenous surfactant to infants of birth weight of less than 1000 g may increase PDA [69].

# Pulmonary air leak

A large series of 230 infants with birth weight of 500–999 g from an eight-year period (1977–1984) reported a pneumothorax incidence of 41% [70], which is very similar to the 36% incidence amongst 59 infants reported from Cambridge between 1980 and 1983 [2]. Pneumothorax developed in 21% of ELBW infants ventilated during a twelve-month period (1985–1986) at King's College Hospital [71] and (at the same institution) in 20% of ventilated infants of less than 29 weeks of gestation during 1985–1988 [1]. The most common form of pulmonary air leak (PAL) amongst ELBW infants is pulmonary interstitial emphysema (PIE), the incidence varying from 14 to 35% [68,70,71] whereas pneumothorax occurs in 11–20% [70,72]. Other forms of PAL – pneumomediastinum, pneumopericardium – are relatively uncommon (less than 3%) as in other birth weight groups [70].

It is well recognized that PIE is much more common in the ELBW infant, with an obvious inverse relationship between the incidence of PIE and birth weight [70,72]. This is explained by the high connective tissue content of the immature lung [73]. In other species, such as the cow, which have a high interstitial tissue content, the lung is more susceptible to widespread PIE [74]. Unfortunately this is worsened by a high interstitial water content, as is found in RDS, which impedes the flow of gas into the perivascular spaces: this then blocks the formation of a pneumomediastinum which is necessary to decompress the interstitial emphysema [75]. The effect of maturity on the likelihood of a pneumothorax is a much more open question [76,77]. Thibeault *et al.* [77] demonstrated a significant difference in the type of PAL according to maturity, with the highest incidence of pneumothorax in term infants and PIE increasingly common with decreasing gestational age. Alder and Wyszogroski [78] also reported a similar association of increased pneumothorax with increased maturity and this was confirmed by evidence from a subsequent animal study [79]. The lungs of rabbit fetuses were inflated after death and the inflating pressures necessary to rupture the lung were found to be significantly higher in the more immature animals. This finding was explained by the lower resistance of the lung at term to rupture due to the reduction in both elastic and surface forces within the lung with increasing maturity. In contrast, however, Madansky *et al.* found that the incidence of all forms of PAL increased with decreasing gestational age [76]. Three recent clinical studies have shown a very poor relationship between the incidence of pneumothorax and birth weight [2,70,80].

Mortality and morbidity in ELBW infants with PAL is greatly increased; 47% of infants with PIE and all infants with pneumothorax dying in one series [70] and 53% dying in another [2]. Mortality associated with PAL decreases with increasing birth weight: 53% with birth weight <1000 g, 33% with birth weight <1500 g and only 8% with birth weight of 1500–2000 g [2]. There is a similar relationship with gestational age; mortality in infants with pneumothorax being 50% in infants of gestational age 27–28 weeks, 92% in those 25–26 weeks and 100% in those less than 25 weeks. Low birth weight infants without air leak have significantly higher survival rates [70]. Although survival amongst ELBW infants without PAL has improved, this is not the case if only infants with PAL are considered [70]. This stresses the need for improvements in both the treatment and, more importantly, the prevention of PAL. The association of PAL and PVH is well known [81,82]. Among 36 ELBW infants ventilated at King's College Hospital in 1986, all eight infants who developed PAL either died and/or developed an IVH, these complications developed in only 13 of the 28 infants without PAL (*P* <0.02). The other important sequel of PAL is an increased incidence of CLP [79]. Escobedo and Gonzalez [83] reported that 58% of ELBW infants with CLP had had at least one pneumothorax and Bhat and Zikos-Labropoulou [84] that 35% had had air leak syndrome. Amongst 16 of 107 ELBW infants with bronchopulmonary dysplasia (BPD) reported by Yu *et al.* [85], PIE was a significant perinatal association (*P* <0.0005). CLP was commoner amongst infants with PAL, their median duration of ventilation was 34 days (range 2–115 days) and median duration of treatment with oxygen was 49 days (range 6–243 days) [85].

**Aetiology**

From studies of preterm infants, including ELBW babies, four main factors have been incriminated. An association between high peak inspiratory pressure (PIP) and PAL was first reported by Oh and Stern [86] and confirmed by Greenough, Dixon and Roberton [80]. Attempts to ventilate at lower peak pressures in one study did not result in a reduction in the incidence of PAL [87], but PIP was documented only just before the air leak and this may not have been a true representation of the PIP used throughout the period of ventilation. Equally important, if PIP is reduced without other compensatory manoeuvres to maintain mean airway pressure (MAP), some estimation must be made of the probably increased infant's respiratory effort, as the latter is known to be associated with the development of PAL [88]. High PIP has been demonstrated recently to be associated with an increased mortality rate in infants with a birth weight of <750 g [89]. Of infants who required a peak pressure of >18 cmH$_2$O at 48 hours or >16 H$_2$O at 72 hours, seven of 10 (90%) subsequently died of respiratory failure. Using these data the authors constructed a 95th centile for PIP requirements during the first 72 hours of life. In a separate series they demonstrated that 80% of infants whose PIP remained below the 95th centile (or were not ventilated) survived compared with 92% mortality in the infants whose PIP requirements crossed the 95th centile.

In one study the introduction of PEEP during IPPV was associated with an increased incidence of both pneumothorax and BPD

[90], but this study was neither randomized nor did it compare two simultaneous time periods.

In a retrospective study comparing ventilator settings of infants with and without air leaks, Primak [91] found that although MAP was higher amongst infants developing PAL, only differences in inspiratory time, TI, between the two groups reached statistical significance. Two physiological studies have confirmed an association between TI and PAL [5,92]. Both have shown that 'active expiration' (a respiratory pattern significantly associated with PAL [88]) can be reduced in some infants by increasing ventilator rate or reducing TI alone. The duration of the positive pressure inflation plateau is significantly longer in infants who actively expire [93].

The association of 'fighting the ventilator' and the development of PAL has long been recognized [94]. Until recently the nature of such respiratory efforts could not be determined and it had been postulated that the most likely mechanism for alveolar rupture during artificial ventilation would be simultaneous inspiratory effects with inflation as this would generate the largest transpulmonary pressure swings [95]. However, a detailed study of infants' respiratory efforts during ventilation demonstrated that the development of PAL was related to expiratory rather than inspiratory efforts during positive pressure inflation [88]. Infants who developed PAL had shown, prior to its development, a consistent respiratory interaction, expiratory efforts during positive pressure inflation and the flow of gas into their lungs was either reduced or in some cases even reversed compared to that which occurred during passive positive pressure inflation. The pattern was designated the 'active expiratory reflex (AER)'. The reflex occurred in infants with the stiffest lungs and was not related to gestational age or birth weight [93,96]. AER occurs in ELBW infants, in one series 12 of 33 infants <28 weeks' gestation were actively expiring during the period of ventilator inflation. The expiratory reflex was provoked if the start of positive pressure inflation occurred during a respiratory window (±0.2 s) around end-inspiration [96]. Using a square wave pressure waveform such a combination would generate the largest transpulmonary pressure swings. The active expiratory reflex which follows inflation of the lungs at end-inspiration may be responsible for

the development of PAL or it may simply be a very reliable marker [97], and hence predictor, of infants at high risk of developing this important condition. Active expiration in those studies [93,96,97] was diagnosed by use of a pneumotachograph to measure tidal flow and an oesophageal balloon to detect spontaneous respiratory activity. In addition the signals were recorded simultaneously with measurement of changes in airway pressure. Unfortunately that equipment is not available on all neonatal units. Two studies, however, have suggested it is possible to detect 'fighting the ventilator' by clinical observation [98,99], particularly if the infant is studied at a series of rates and the infant's response is interpreted in association with the effect of the change in ventilator rate on oxygenation [98]. The reliability of such observations exclusively in the ELBW infant has not been investigated, but neither has the observation that greater than a 10% variation in the coefficient of variation of the beat-to-beat variability of the undamped arterial blood pressure trace [100] is diagnostic of fighting the ventilator.

## Prevention

Two preventative measures have been extensively employed to try to reduce the incidence of PAL: high frequency positive pressure ventilation (HFPPV) and muscle relaxants.

### *HFPPV*

HFPPV using conventional ventilators has been associated with a reduced incidence of PAL in three studies [80,101,102]. In the study of Heicher, Kasting and Richards [102], rates of 60 breaths min$^{-1}$ and a TI of 0.5 s was associated with approximately half the incidence of PAL. In a recently reported multi-centre randomized study, similar ventilator settings when compared with slower rates (30–40 breaths min$^{-1}$ and a longer TI) were associated with a significant reduction in PAL [103]. Even amongst infants with PIE, HFPPV reduces the incidence of pneumothorax [80], although PIE actually worsens on fast rates as, in the absence of a pneumothorax or pneumomediastinum the PIE cannot decompress. The association of a lower incidence of PAL and fast rates may be due to a number of mechanisms. Using certain ventilators, increasing rate increases MAP

[104] and thus PIP could be lowered without impairing oxygenation and barotrauma reduced. Increasing ventilator rates in two physiological studies [5,92] was associated with a reduction in the active expiratory reflex. Spontaneous respiratory rate of low birth weight infants with RDS is inversely related to gestational age [6]. Thus, fast rates (>100 breaths min$^{-1}$) mimic the spontaneous respiratory frequency of ELBW infants and would be likely to induce synchronous respiration, improving oxygenation again enabling ventilation at a lower PIP, as a consequence the likelihood of PAL would be reduced. Indeed, of 21 babies with a gestation less than 28 weeks who all had AER at a ventilator rate of 30 breaths min$^{-1}$ when the rate was increased to 60 breaths min$^{-1}$ six infants breathed synchronously and at 100–120 breaths min$^{-1}$ this figure had risen to 18, with only two showing AER and one an irregular pattern of response [105].

## Muscle relaxants and sedation

Use of muscle relaxants, such as pancuronium, during mechanical ventilation of preterm neonates may be advantageous. Until recently, although this treatment had been associated with a reduction in cerebral blood flow variability [106], mortality [107] and CLP [95], it had not been demonstrated to decrease the incidence of PAL [95,106,107]. However, selective paralysis, that is giving pancuronium only to those infants at high risk of developing air leak, was confirmed in two independent studies [97,99] as an effective method of preventing PAL. Unfortunately in one of the two studies a statistically significant reduction in PAL occurred only in 'more mature' infants [99] and in the second study the only infant who sustained a pneumothorax during paralysis was of 24 weeks gestational age and birth weight <1000 g [97]. More recently the outcome of a group of 37 babies with a gestational age of less than 28 weeks who all had AER in response to ventilator settings of 30 breaths min$^{-1}$ has been reported [103]. Pneumothorax developed in only five of the 22 infants with AER who were paralysed, compared to all 15 who were not paralysed. In contrast, only two of 41 babies who did not show AER and remained nonparalysed went on to develop pneumothoraces. A number of potentially serious problems have been associated with the use of muscle relax-

**Practical points**

1. High frequency positive pressure ventilation (>60 breaths min$^{-1}$) is particularly useful for the infant of birth weight <1000 g as their spontaneous respiratory rate is fast. Care, however, must be taken to use an appropriate ventilator, so that increasing rate does not cause inadvertent positive end expiratory pressure.
2. Except in chronically ventilated infants, positive end expiratory pressure levels should usually be kept low to avoid overdistension and carbon dioxide retention.
3. Despite improvements in patient triggered ventilators, this form of ventilation is not successful in all very immature infants. Failure of improvement in blood gases after 1 hour on patient triggered ventilation, indicates it is unlikely to be successful in the long term.
4. Prolonged periods on endotracheal continuous positive airways pressure increase the incidence of extubation complications.
5. Manoeuvres to avoid high peak inspiratory pressures during ventilation should be used, as high peak inspiratory pressures are significantly associated with mortality and air leak.
6. Pneumothorax is best avoided by increasing ventilator rate to promote synchrony as, although selective use of pancuronium reduces air leak, neuromuscular blocking agents have important side-effects.

ants; hypoventilation [108], blood pressure abnormalities [109,110], and transient hypoxia [98]. These tend to be acute effects after the drug was first administered and no adverse persisting effect on blood pressure was demonstrated in one series [111]. All paralysed infants, however, did show a significant reduction in heart rate variability which persisted during treatment, this phenomena was not present in the control infants [111]. Unfortunately, paralysed infants develop fluid retention despite fluid restriction, in one series [111] being significantly heavier than the control babies from day 3 onwards and above their birth weight by day seven.

Opiate agents have been used in an attempt to inhibit the infant's respiratory drive. Although there is anecdotal evidence that the newborn infant is more sensitive to the respiratory depressant properties of morphine [112], clinical experience does not support this [100]. Even in high doses morphine may not suppress the infant's ventilatory efforts sufficiently to improve synchrony. Potential side-effects include hypotension [113], fits [114] and withdrawal symptoms. Diamorphine has a more rapid onset of action and is more potent than morphine. In a recent study, but in which a minority of infants included were ELBW, use of diamorphine infusion was associated with synchronization of respiratory efforts with positive pressure ventilation in 19 of 20 infants studied [115]. Pharmokinetic studies of synthetic opioids have been performed in preterm infants. These agents are theoretically attractive as they are associated with greater cardiovascular stability, but in preterm infants their clearance is reduced and their elimination half life prolonged when compared with older children and adults [113]. Randomized studies are required to assess which, if any, of these agents will reduce PAL in the ELBW infant.

# References

1. Chan, V., Greenough, A. and Gamsu, H.R. (1992) Neonatal complications of mechanical ventilation in extremely preterm infants. *Eur. J. Pediatr.*, **151**, 693–696
2. Greenough, A. and Roberton, N.R.C. (1985) Morbidity and survival in neonates ventilated for the respiratory distress syndrome. *Br. Med. J.*, **290**, 597–600
3. Yu, V.Y.H. and Hollingsworth, E. (1979) Respiratory failure in infants weighing 1000g or less at birth. *Aust. Paediatr. J.*, **15**, 152–159
4. Greenough, A., Pool, J., Greenall, F., Morley, C.J. and Gamsu, H. (1987) Comparison of different rates of artificial ventilation in preterm neonates with the respiratory distress syndrome. *Acta Pediatr. Scand.*, **76**, 706–712
5. Greenough, A., Morley, C.J. and Pool, J. (1986) Fighting the ventilator – are fast rates an effective alternative to paralysis? *Early Hum. Dev.*, **13**, 189–194
6. Greenough, A., Greenall, F. and Gamsu, H. (1987) Synchronous respiration – which ventilator rate is best? *Acta Pediatr. Scand.*, **76**, 713–718
7. South, M. and Morley, C.J. (1986) Synchronous mechanical ventilation of the neonate. *Arch Dis. Childh.*, **61**, 1190–1195
8. Hird, M.F. and Greenough, A. (1991) Inflation time in mechanical ventilation of preterm neonates. *Eur. J. Pediatr.*, **150**, 440–443
9. Greenough, A. and Greenall, F. (1987) Performance of respirators at fast rates commonly used in neonatal intensive care unit. *Pediatr. Pulmonol.*, **3**, 357–361
10. Hird, M., Greenough, A. and Gamsu, H.R. (1990) Gas trapping during high frequency positive pressure ventilation using conventional ventilators. *Early Hum. Dev.*, **22**, 51–56
11. Chan, V., Greenough, A. and Hird, M.F. (1991) Comparison of different rates of artificial ventilation for preterm infants ventilated beyond the first week of life. *Early Hum. Dev.*, **26**, 177–83
12. Hird, M.F. and Greenough, A. (1991) Spontaneous respiratory effort during mechanical ventilation in infants with and without acute respiratory distress. *Early Hum. Dev.*, **25**, 69–73
13. Boros, S.J. (1979) Variations in inspiratory:expiratory ratio and airway pressure wave form during mechanical ventilation: the significance of mean airway pressure. *J. Pediatr.*, **94**, 114–117
14. Boros, S.J. and Campbell, K. (1980) A comparison of the effects of high frequency–low tidal volume and low frequency–high tidal volume mechanical ventilation. *J. Pediatr.*, **97**, 108–112
15. Wyszogrodski, I., Kyer-Aboagye, K. and Taeusch, H.W. (1975) Surfactant inactivation by hyperventilation, conservation by end expiratory pressure. *J. Appl. Physiol.*, **38**, 461–464
16. Richardson, C.P. and Jung, A.L. (1978) Effects of continuous positive airway pressure on pulmonary function and blood gases of infants with respiratory distress syndrome. *Pediatr. Res.*, **12**, 771–774
17. Field, D., Milner, A.D. and Hopkin, I.E. (1985) Effects of positive end expiratory pressure during ventilation of the preterm infant. *Arch. Dis. Childh.*, **60**, 843–847
18. Greenough, A., Chan, V. and Hird, M.F. (1992) Positive end expiratory pressure in acute and chronic neonatal respiratory distress. *Arch. Dis. Childh.*, **67**, 320–323
19. Hyde, I., English, R.E. and Wilhams, J.A. (1989) The changing pattern of chronic lung disease of prematurity. *Arch. Dis. Childh.*, **64**, 448–451
20. Mehta, A., Callan, K., Wright, B.M. and Stacey, T.E. (1986) Patient triggered ventilation in the newborn. *Lancet*, **ii**, 17–19
21. Greenough, A., Hird, M.F. and Chan, V. (1991) Airway pressure triggered ventilation for preterm neonates. *J. Perinat. Med.*, **19**, 471–476
22. Greenough, A. and Pool, J. (1988) Neonatal patient triggered ventilation. *Arch. Dis. Childh.*, **63**, 394–397
23. Greenough, A. and Greenall, F. (1988) Patient triggered ventilation in premature neonates. *Arch. Dis. Childh.*, **63**, 77–78
24. Upton, C.J., Milner, A.D. and Stokes, G.M. (1990) The effect of changes in inspiratory time on neonatal triggered ventilation. *Eur. J. Pediatr.*, **149**, 668–670

25. Epstein, R.A. (1971) The sensitivities and response times of ventilatory assists. *Anaesthesiology*, **34**, 321–326

26. Hird, M.F. and Greenough, A. (1991) Comparison of triggering systems for neonatal patient triggered ventilation. *Arch. Dis. Childh.*, **66**, 426–428

27. Chan, V. and Greenough, A. (1999) Evaluation of triggering systems for patient triggered ventilation for neonates ventilator dependent beyond 10 days of age. *Eur. J. Pediatr.*, **151**, 842–5

28. Hird, M.F. and Greenough, A. (1991) Patient triggered ventilation using a flow triggered system. *Arch. Dis. Childh.*, **66**, 1140–1143

29. Mitchell, A., Greenough, A. and Hird, M.F. (1989) Limitations of neonatal patient triggered ventilation. *Arch. Dis. Childh.*, **64**, 924–929

30. Hird, M.F. and Greenough, A. (1990) Gestational age: an important influence on the success of patient triggered ventilation. *Clin. Phys. Physiol.*, **11**, 307–312

31. Hird, M.F. and Greenough, A. (1991) Patient triggered ventilation in chronically ventilator-dependent infants. *Eur. J. Pediatr.*, **9**, 1–3

32. Hird, M.F. and Greenough, A. (1990) Causes of failure of neonatal patient triggered ventilation. *Early Hum. Dev.*, **23**, 101–108

33. Chan, V., Greenough, A. and Muramatsu, K. (1994) Influence of lung function and reflex activity on the success of patient triggered ventilation. *Early Hum. Dev.*, **37**, 9–14

34. Carlo, W.A., Chatburn, R.L. and Martin, R.J. (1984) Decrease in airway pressure during high frequency jet ventilation in infants with respiratory distress syndrome. *J. Pediatr.*, **104**, 101–107

35. Pokora, T., Bing, D., Mammel, M. and Boros, S. (1983) Neonatal high frequency jet ventilation. *Pediatrics*, **72**, 27–32

36. Boros, S.J., Mammel, M.C., Lewallen, P.K., Coleman, J.M., Gordon, M.J. and Ophoven, J. (1986) Necrotizing tracheobronchitis: a complication of high frequency ventilation. *J. Pediatr.*, **109**, 95–100

37. Fox, W.W., Spiker, A.R. and Musci, M. (1984) Tracheal secretion impaction during hyperventilation for persistent pulmonary hypertension of the neonate. *Pediatr. Res.*, **18**, 323A

38. Carlo, W.A., Sinner, B., Chatburn, R.L., Robertson, S. and Martin, R.J. (1990) Early randomized intervention with high frequency jet ventilation in respiratory distress syndrome. *J. Pediatr.*, **117**, 65–70

39. Bohn, D.J., Tamura, M. and Bryan, C. (1984) Respiratory failure in congenital diaphragmatic hernia: ventilation by high frequency oscillation. *Pediatr. Res.*, **18**, 387A

40. Karl, S.R., Ballantine, T.V.N. and Schnides, M.T. (1983) High frequency ventilation at rates of 375 to 1800 cycles/minute in 4 neonates with congenital diaphragmatic hernia. *J. Pediatr. Surg.*, **18**, 822–828

41. Keszler, M., Donn, S.M., Bucciarelli, R.L. *et al.* (1991) Multicentre controlled trial comparing high frequency jet ventilation and conventional mechanical ventila-

tion in newborn infants with pulmonary interstitial emphysema. *J. Pediatr.*, **119**, 85–93

42. The HIFI Study Group (1989) High frequency oscillatory ventilation compared with conventional mechanical ventilation in the treatment of respiratory failure in preterm infants. *N. Engl. J. Med.*, **320**, 88–93

43. Clark, R.H., Gerstmann, D.R., Null, D.M. and deLemos, R.A. (1992) Prospective randomized comparison of high frequency oscillatory and conventional ventilation in respiratory distress syndrome. *Pediatrics*, **89**, 5–12

44. Chan, V. and Greenough, A. (1993) Determinants of oxygenation during high frequency oscillation. *Eur. J. Pediatr.*, **152**, 350–3

45. Solimano, A.J., Bryan, A.C. and Jobe, A.H. (1984) High frequency oscillation versus conventional mechanical ventilation: barotrauma, surfactant pools and surface tensions in premature lambs. *Pediatr. Res.*, **18**, 348

46. Chan, V., Greenough, A. and Gamsu, H.R. (1994) High frequency oscillation for preterm infants with severe respiratory failure. *Arch. Dis. Childh.*, **70**, F44–46

47. Bartlett, R.H., Gazzaniga, A.B. and Toomasian, J.M. (1986) Extracorporeal membrane oxygenation (ECMO) in neonatal respiratory failure: 100 cases. *Ann. Surg.*, **204**, 236

48. Nicks, J.J. and Bartlett, R.H. (1988) Extracorporeal membrane oxygenation and other new modes of gas exchange. In *Neonatal Respiratory Failure* (W.A. Carlo and R.L. Chatburn, eds), Yearbook Medical Publishers,

49. Greenough, A., Pool, J. and Gamsu, H. (1989) A randomised controlled trial of two methods of weaning from high frequency positive pressure ventilation. *Arch. Dis. Childh.*, **64**, 834–838

50. Chan, V. and Greenough, A. (1993) Randomised controlled trial of weaning by patient triggered ventilation or conventional ventilation. *Eur. J. Pediatr.*, **152**, 51–54

51. Kim, E.H. and Boutwell, W.C. (1987) Successful direct extubation of very low birthweight infants from low intermittent mandatory ventilation rate. *Pediatrics*, **80**, 409–414

52. Chan, V. and Greenough, A. (1993) Randomized trial of methods of extubation in acute and chronic respiratory distress. *Arch. Dis. Childh.*, **68**, 570–572

53. Finer, N.N., Moriartey, R.R., Boyd, J., Phillips, H.J., Stewart, A.R. and Ulan, O. (1979) Post-extubation atelectasis: a retrospective review and prospective controlled study. *J. Pediatr.*, **94**, 110–113

54. Greenough, A., Elias Jones, A., Pool, J., Morley, C.J. and Davis, J. (1985) The therapeutic actions of theophylline in preterm ventilated infants. *Early Hum. Dev.*, **12**, 15–22

55. Rooklin, A.R., Moomjian, A.S. and Fox, W.W. (1979) Theophylline therapy in bronchopulmonary dysplasia. *J. Pediatr.*, **95**, 882–884

56. Donn, S.M., Faix, R.G. and Banagale, R.C. (1983) Dexamethasone for bronchopulmonary dysplasia. (Letter) *Lancet*, **ii**: 460

57. Pomerance, J.J. and Puri, A.P. (1980) Treatment of neonatal bronchopulmonary dysplasia with steroids. *Pediatr. Res.*, **14**, 649A

58. Avery, G.B., Fletcher, A.B., Kaplan, M. and Brudno, D.S. (1985) Controlled trial of dexamethasone in respirator-dependent infants with BPD. *Pediatrics*, **75**, 106–111

59. Collaborative dexamethasone trial group (1991) Dexamethasone therapy in neonatal chronic lung disease: an international placebo-controlled trial. *Pediatrics*, **88**, 421–427

60. Cummings, J.J., D'Eugenio, D.B. and Gross, S.J. (1989) A controlled trial of dexamethasone in preterm infants at high risk for bronchopulmonary dysplasia. *N. Engl. J. Med.*, **320**, 1505–1510

61. Yeh, T.F., Torre, J.A., Rastogi, A., Anyebuno, M.A. and Pildes, R.S. (1990) Early postnatal dexamethasone therapy in premature infants with severe respiratory distress syndrome: a double-blind controlled trial. *J. Pediatr.*, **117**, 273–282

62. Greenough, A., Emery, E.F. and Gamsu, H.R. (1992) Dexamethasone and hypertension in preterm infants. *Eur. J. Pediatr.*, **152**, 134–135

63. Emery, E.F. and Greenough, A. (1992) Effect of dexamethasone on blood pressure: relationship to postnatal age. *Eur. J. Pediatr.*, **151**, 364–366

64. Phelps, D.L., Brown, D.R., Tung, B. *et al.* (1991) 28-day survival rates of 6676 neonates with birth weights of 1250 grams or less. *Pediatrics*, **87**, 7–17

65. Grogaard, J.B., Lindstrom, D.P., Parker, R.A., Cutley, B. and Stahlman, M.T. (1990) Increased survival rate in very low birth weight infants (1500 grams or less): no association with increased incidence of handicaps. *J. Pediatr.*, **117**, 139–146

66. Brothwood, M., Wolke, D., Gamsu, H. and Cooper, D. (1988) Mortality, morbidity, growth and development of babies weighing 501–1000 grams and 1001–1500 grams at birth. *Acta. Pediatr. Scand.*, **77**, 10–18

67. Siassi, B., Blanco, C., Cabal, L.A. and Coran, A.G. (1976) Incidence and clinical features of patent ductus arteriosus in low birth weight infants: A prospective analysis of 150 consecutively born infants. *Pediatrics*, **57**, 347–351

68. Cassady, G., Crouse, D.T. and Kirklin, J.W. (1989) A randomised controlled trial of very early prophylactic ligation of the ductus arteriosus in babies who weighed 1000 gms or less at birth. *N. Engl. J. Med.*, **320**, 1511–1516

69. Raju, T.N.K., Vidyasagar, D., Bhat, R. *et al.* (1987) Double-blind controlled trial of single dose treatment with bovine surfactant in severe hyaline membrane disease. *Lancet*, **i**, 651–656

70. Yu, V.Y.H., Wong, P.Y., Bajuk, B. and Szymonowicz, W. (1986) Pulmonary air leak in extremely low birth weight infants. *Arch. Dis. Childh.*, **61**, 239–241

71. Greenough, A. (1989) Pulmonary air leak. In *The Baby under 1000 g* (D. Harvey, R.W.I. Cooke and G.A. Levitt, eds), Butterworths, London, pp. 78–85

72. Hart, S.M., McNair, M., Gamsu, H.R. and Price, J.F. (1983) Pulmonary interstitial emphysema in very low birthweight infants. *Arch. Dis. Childh.*, **58**, 612–615

73. Reid, L. and Rubino, L. (1958) The connective tissue septa in the fetal human lung. *Thorax*, **14**, 35

74. Reid, L. (1959) The connective tissue septa in the fetal human lung. *Thorax*, **14**, 3–12

75. Thibeault, D.W. (1978) Pulmonary barotrauma. In *Neonatal Pulmonary Care* (D.W. Thibeault and G.A. Gregory, eds), Addison Wesley, London, pp. 307–317

76. Madansky, D.L., Lawson, E.E., Chernick, V. and Taeusch, H.W. (1979) Pneumothorax and other forms of pulmonary air leak in newborns. *Am. Rev. Respir. Dis.*, **120**, 729–737

77. Thibeault, D.W., Lachman, R.S., Laul, V.R. and Kwong, M.S. (1973) Pulmonary interstitial emphysema, pneumomediastinum and pneumothorax. occurrence in the newborn infant. *Am. J. Dis. Child.*, **126**, 611–614

78. Alder, S.M. and Wyszogroski, I. (1973) Pneumothorax as a function of gestational age: clinical and experimental studies. *J. Pediatr.*, **87**, 771–775

79. Stahlman, M.T., Cheatham, W. and Gray, M.E. (1979) The role of air dissection in bronchopulmonary dysplasia. *J. Pediatr.*, **95**, 878–885

80. Greenough, A., Dixon, A. and Roberton, N.R.C. (1984) Pulmonary interstitial emphysema. *Arch. Dis. Childh.*, **59**, 1046–1051

81. Lipscomb, A.P., Reynolds, E.O.R., Blackwell, R.J. *et al.* (1981) Pneumothorax and cerebral haemorrhage in preterm infants. *Lancet*, **i**, 414–417

82. Hill, A., Periman, J.M. and Volpe, J.J. (1982) Relationship of pneumothorax to occurrence of intraventricular hemorrhage in the premature newborn. *Pediatrics*, **69**, 144–149

83. Escobedo, M.B. and Gonzalez, A. (1986) Bronchopulmonary dysplasia in the tiny infant. *Clin. Perinatol.*, **13**, 315–326

84. Bhat, R. and Zikos-Labropoulou, E. (1986) Resuscitation and respiratory management of infants weighing less than 1000 g. *Clin. Perinatol.*, **13**, 285–297

85. Yu, V.Y.K., Orgill, A.A., Lim, S.B., Bajuk, B. and Astbury, J. (1983) Bronchopulmonary dysplasia in very low birthweight infants. *Aust. Pediatr. J.*, **19**, 233–236

86. Oh, W. and Stern, L. (1977) Diseases of the respiratory system. In *Neonatal and Perinatal Medicine: Diseases of the Fetus and Infant* (R.E. Behrman, ed.) CV Mosby, St Louis, p. 558

87. Tarnow-Mordi, W.O., Narang, A. and Wilkinson, A.R. (1985) Lack of association of barotrauma and airleak in hyaline membrane disease. *Arch. Dis. Childh.*, **60**, 555–559

88. Greenough, A., Morley, C.J. and Davis, J.A. (1983) Interaction of spontaneous respiration and artificial ventilation. *J. Pediatr.*, **103**, 769–773

89. Foote, K.D., Hoon, A.H., Sheps, S., Gunawardene, N.R., Hershler, R. and Pendray, M.R. (1990) Peak inspiratory pressure requirements in infants born weighing less than 750 gms. *Arch. Dis. Childh.*, **65**, 1045–1049

90. Berg, T.J., Pagtakhan, R.D., Reed, M.H., Langston, C. and Chernick, V. (1975) Bronchopulmonary dysplasia and lung rupture in hyaline membrane disease: Influence of continuous distending pressure. *Pediatrics*, **55**, 51–53

91. Primak, R.A. (1983) Factors associated with pulmonary air leak in premature infants receiving mechanical ventilation. *J. Pediatr.*, **102**, 764–769

92. Field, D., Milner, A.D. and Hopkin, I.E. (1985) Manipulation of ventilator settings to reduce expiration against positive pressure inflation. *Arch. Dis. Childh.*, **60**, 1036–1040

93. Greenough, A. (1988) The premature infant's respiratory response to mechanical ventilation. *Ealry Hum. Dev.*, **17**, 1–5

94. Stark, A.R., Bascom, R. and Frantz, I.D. (1979) Muscle relaxation in mechanically ventilated infants. *J. Pediatr.*, **94**, 439–444

95. Pollitzer, M.J., Reynolds, E.O.R., Shaw, D.G. and Thomas, R.M. (1981) Pancuronium during mechanical ventilation speeds recovery of the lungs with hyaline membrane disease. *Lancet*, **i**, 346–348

96. Greenough, A., Morley, C.J. and Johnson, P. (1985) An active expiratory reflex in preterm ventilated infants. In *The Physiological Development of the Foetus and Newborn*. (C.T. Jones and P.W. Nathanielsz, eds). Academic Press, London and Orlando, pp. 259–263

97. Greenough, A., Wood, S., Morley, C.J. and Davis, J.A. (1984) Pancuronium prevents pneumothoraces in ventilated premature infants who actively expire against positive pressure ventilation. *Lancet*, **i**, 1–3

98. Greenough, A. and Greenall, F. (1988) Observation of spontaneous respiratory interaction with artificial ventilation. *Arch. Dis. Childh.*, **63**, 168–171

99. Cooke, R.W.I. and Rennie, J.M. (1984) Pancuronium and pneumothorax. *Lancet*, **i**, 286–287

100. Levene, M.I. and Quinn, M.W. (1992) Use of sedatives and muscle relaxants in newborn babies receiving mechanical ventilation. *Arch. Dis. Childh.*, **67**, 870–873

101. Bland, R.D., Kim, M.H. and Light, M.J. (1980) High frequency ventilation in severe hyaline membrane disease: an alternative therapy. *Crit. Care Med.*, **8**, 275–280

102. Heicher, D.A., Kasting, D.S. and Richards, J.R. (1981) Prospective clinical comparison of two methods of mechanical ventilation of neonates: rapid rate and short inspiratory time versus slow rate and long inspiratory time. *J Pediatr.*, **98**, 957–961

103. Oxford Region Controlled Trial of Artificial Ventilation (OCTAVE) Study Group (1991) Multicentre randomised controlled trial of high against low frequency positive pressure ventilator. *Arch. Dis. Childh.*, **66**, 770–777

104. Boros, S.J., Bing, D.R., Mammel, M.C., Hagen, E. and Gordon, M.J. (1984) Using conventional infant ventilators at unconventional rates. *Pediatrics*, **74**, 487–492

105. Milner, A. and Greenough, A. (1988) Adaptation of the respiratory system. *Br. Med. Bull.*, **4**, 909–918

106. Perlman, J.M., McMenamin, J.B. and Volpe, J.J. (1983) Fluctuating cerebral blood flow velocity in respiratory distress syndrome. *N. Engl. J. Med.*, **309**, 204–209

107. Henry, G.W., Stevens, D.C., Schreier, R.L., Grosfield, J.L. and Ballantine, T.V.N. (1979) Respiratory paralysis to improve oxygenation and mortality in large newborn infants with respiratory distress. *J. Pediatr. Surg.*, **94**, 481–487

108. Bourgeois, J., Beithier, J.C., Cottancin, G., Milan, J.J. and Bethenod, M. (1982) Dangers de la curarisation au cours de la ventilation artificielle chez le nouveau-né. *Pediatrie*, **37**, 101–112

109. Cabal, L.A., Siassi, B., Artal, R., Gonzalez, F., Hodgman, J. and Plajstek, C. (1985) Cardiovascular and catecholamine changes after administration of pancuronium in distressed neonates. *J Pediatr.*, **75**, 284–287

110. Bancalari, E., Gerhardt, T., Feller, R. *et al.* (1980) Muscle relaxation during IPPV in prematures with RDS. *Pediatr. Res.*, **14**, 590

111. Greenough, A., Gamsu, H.R. and Greenall, F. (1989) Investigation of the effects of paralysis by pancuronium on heart rate variability, blood pressure and fluid balance. *Acta Pediatr. Scand.*, **78**, 829–834

112. Way, W.L., Costley, E.C. and Way, E.L. (1965) Respiratory sensitivity of the newborn infant to meperidine and morphine. *Clin. Pharmacol. Ther.*, **6**, 454–461

113. Marlow, N., Weindling, A.M., Van Peer, A. and HeyKants, J. (1990) Alfentanil pharmacokinetics in preterm infants. *Arch. Dis. Childh.*, **65**, 349–351

114. Koren, G., Butt, W., Chinyanga, H., Soldin, S., Tan, Y.K. and Pape, K. (1985) Postoperative morphine infusion in newborn infants' assessment of disposition characteristics and safety. *J. Pediatr.*, **107**, 963–967

115. Elias-Jones, A.C., Barrett, D.A., Rutter, N., Shaw, P.N. and Davis, S.S. (1991) Diamorphine infusion in the preterm neonate. *Arch. Dis. Childh.*, **66**, 1155–1157

# 7

# Chronic lung disease of prematurity

**Ben Shaw**

In 1967 Northway and colleagues described the clinical, radiological and pathological features of bronchopulmonary dysplasia (BPD) [1] which is now the most common chronic lung disease that affects extremely low birth weight infants. Babies with BPD had a prolonged dependency on supplemental oxygen and characteristic chest radiographic changes consisting of diffuse linear densities and areas of hyperlucency. There were associated histological abnormalities of the pulmonary parenchyma, interstitium and related vasculature which were initially attributed to oxygen toxicity and barotrauma (lung injury due to ventilator-generated pressures). It was subsequently suggested that the following be used as diagnostic criteria for BPD: positive pressure ventilation during the first 2 weeks of life for a minimum of 3 days, clinical signs of chronic respiratory disease for more than 28 days of age, requirement for supplemental oxygen for longer than 28 days to maintain $PaO_2$ above 6.7 kPa (50 mmHg) and a chest radiograph showing persistent strands of radiodensity and areas of increased lucency [2,3].

Since the first report of BPD by Northway and colleagues it has become clear that many infants who have received neonatal intensive care, whilst not having the radiological or pathological features originally described, have a prolonged dependency on supplementary oxygen. It is likely, therefore, that the BPD of Northway's patients represents the most severe end of the spectrum of chronic lung disease which occurs as a consequence of neonatal intensive care. Furthermore, many other factors besides barotrauma and oxygen toxicity have now been implicated in the pathogenesis of neonatal chronic lung disease.

## Chronic lung disease

For the purposes of this chapter chronic lung disease of prematurity (CLP) will be defined in broader terms as: *dependency on supplementary oxygen beyond 28 days of postnatal age in an infant who has suffered from a respiratory illness within the first 2 weeks of postnatal life and has a persistent radiographic abnormality of the lung parenchyma at 28 days* [4,5]. Infants fulfilling these criteria may have histological evidence of BPD or other milder forms of lung damage, will not all have required mechanical ventilation and clinical features will be variably present. The simplicity of this definition makes it easier to illustrate the multifactorial aetiology of chronic oxygen dependency and to compare data on infants with CLP between centres.

### Incidence

The incidence of CLP in infants of birth weight <1000 g who have been admitted to the neonatal intensive care unit at Liverpool Maternity Hospital during the years 1985–1990 and have survived to 28 days was 50%. This is comparable with other published incidence figures of between 40 and 70% [5–8].

**Table 7.1.  Factors implicated in the pathogenesis of CLP**

Barotrauma
Oxygen toxicity
Increased lung fluid
Infection
Use of intravenous fat emulsions
Gastro-oesophageal reflux
Genetic factors
Nutritional deficiencies
    Antioxidant enzymes
    Enzyme cofactors
    Vitamins A and E

## Aetiology

The factors which have been implicated in the pathogenesis of CLP are shown in Table 7.1 and will now be discussed.

### Barotrauma

This is the term used to describe damage caused to the airway by pressures generated by the ventilator. High inspiratory and mean airways pressures used to maintain satisfactory blood gas tensions can lead to over-distension and mechanical damage to the small airways. There is evidence that this predisposes to CLP. High inspiratory pressures predispose to pulmonary interstitial emphysema which is strongly associated with CLP [9]. Kraybill *et al.* have suggested that CLP is more common in infants who have a low $Pa\text{CO}_2$ in the first 48 hours secondary to overventilation [8] and a comparative study of different neonatal intensive care units has indicated that the use of muscle relaxants necessitating the use of higher ventilator pressures to counteract passive expiration results in a higher incidence of CLP [5]. Work carried out on animals supports the role of barotrauma in the pathogenesis of CLP and has shown that baboons ventilated conventionally with high peak inspiratory pressures (PIP) have findings on postmortem examination similar to those in CLP whereas those ventilated with a lower PIP do not [10].

### Oxygen toxicity

A high inspired oxygen concentration can cause alveolar damage by inactivating cellular enzymes, damaging DNA and causing lipid peroxidation [11]. There is much newborn animal work demonstrating that even in the absence of other factors which may contribute to lung damage, breathing a high concentration of oxygen *per se* is a potent cause of lung damage [12–14].

### Increase in lung fluid

Lung fluid may increase as a consequence of asphyxial damage and hyaline membrane disease owing to an increase in pulmonary blood vessel permeability and transcapillary pressure and a decrease in osmotic pressure. A persistent ductus arteriosus may result in left-to-right shunting, increased pulmonary blood flow predisposing to pulmonary oedema. Lung fluid may reduce lung compliance resulting in a higher inspiratory pressure and inspired oxygen concentration being required to provide optimal ventilation. Studies have shown the presence of a persistent ductus arteriosus to be related to an increased incidence of CLP [15–17]. Other work has suggested that over-hydration in the early neonatal period may predispose to increased respiratory morbidity later on [18–20].

### Infection and inflammation

Neutrophil migration to the lungs in response to cellular damage or infection may amplify pulmonary damage already present [21]. It has been suggested that the presence of one of the mycoplasma species *Ureaplasma urealyticum* in endotracheal secretions of infants weighing less than 1000 g is associated with an increased incidence of CLP [22]. This has implications for neonatal screening for the organism and possible treatment with erythromycin, although it remains unclear how important this organism is as a lung damaging pathogen.

### Lipids

Two studies have suggested that the early use of intravenous fat emulsion (Intralipid) in total parenteral nutrition is associated with an increase in incidence of CLP [23,24]. However, two other clinical studies showed no increase in CLP [25,26] and some animal work has suggested a *protective* effect on the lung of administering fat emulsion [27]. One randomized trial however has failed to confirm an association of early use in intravenous fat emulsions with an increased risk for CLP [28].

### Gastro-oesophageal reflux

Gastro-oesophageal reflux is common in preterm ventilated infants [29] and this may further contribute to lung damage associated with CLP.

### Genetic factors

There is a higher incidence of HLA-A2 in infants with CLP [30] and some workers have suggested that there is an increased risk of CLP in infants with a family history of asthma [31].

### Nutritional deficiencies

Deficiency of various nutritional factors at birth make ELBW infants more susceptible to developing CLP and inadequate nutrition in the postnatal period may contribute to its severity [32].

Low levels of antioxidant enzymes (superoxide dismutase, catalase, glutathione peroxidase) in the ELBW infant may predispose to the development of CLP [33]. These enzymes prevent lipid peroxidation and cellular damage and have been shown to have a protective effect on the lung when administered to newborn animals although human studies have not been conclusive [34]. Deficiency of antioxidant enzyme cofactors such as copper and selenium may impair enzyme activity thus compounding the situation [35].

Deficiency of vitamin E (also an antioxidant) increases susceptibility to oxygen toxicity and thus CLP, however, studies of vitamin E supplementation in human newborns have demonstrated no protective effect against the development of CLP [36]. Preterm infants are deficient in vitamin A, an antioxidant which also regulates epithelial cell growth and differentiation, levels being lowest in those who develop CLP [37]. In vitamin A deficiency states in animals and humans squamous metaplasia and loss of cilia in the bronchial tree occur; similar pathological findings to those found in CLP [38].

Metabolic bone disease secondary to nutritional deficiencies (calcium and phosphate depletion) produces a compliant rib cage, and possibly fractures, which may impair respiration and compound lung damage.

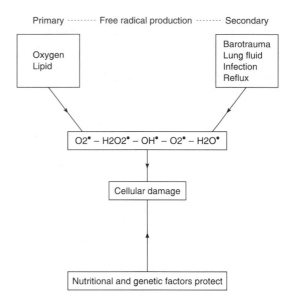

**Figure 7.1** Unifying theory of CLP pathogenesis

It is possible to bring all these factors together in a unifying theory of pulmonary damage based on oxygen free radical production resulting in cellular damage and destruction (Figure 7.1). At the mitochondrial level in the cell the normal process of oxygen reduction produces intermediates (free radicals) in small amounts which are scavenged by superoxide dismutase and catalase. These are hydrogen peroxide ($H_2O_2^\bullet$) superoxide ($O_2^\bullet$) and hydroxyl ($OH^\bullet$). Free radicals have the potential (by donating or abstracting/accepting electrons) to damage cellular components, in particular the phospholipid cell wall [39]. In CLP, free radicals may be increased secondary to hyperoxia fuelling the process of oxygen reduction, barotrauma, increased lung fluid, infection, and gastro-oesophageal reflux. This causes cellular damage with secondary production of free radicals, in addition administration of intravenous fat emulsions contain weak free radicals. Deficiencies of antioxidant enzymes, cofactors and antioxidant vitamins, together with genetic factors, may compound this situation.

## Pathology

Histopathological data is available only from infants who have died as a consequence of CLP and therefore represent the worst end of the clinical spectrum of CLP. Early on in the development of CLP an intra-alveolar exudate forms which may be absorbed to leave a normal lung or a fibrosed alveolar wall, or organized *in situ* so that there is obliteration of the alveolar space [40]. Associated with interstitial fibrosis, distortion of air spaces and enlargement of distal air spaces may occur [41,42]. The latter may be a consequence of overinflation, destruction and failure of alveolar development with alveolar hypoplasia [43,44]. In longer standing severe CLP there may be pulmonary hypertensive lesions, obliterative bronchiolitis and cardiomegaly [45,46]. Delayed mucociliary clearance secondary to large airway damage may compound the picture [47].

## Clinical features

After an initial respiratory insult (usually the requirement for mechanical ventilation, often for hyaline membrane disease) the ELBW baby who has developed CLP remains dependent on supplementary oxygen and hypercapnic. Once weaning from the ventilator has been achieved, which may take weeks, the infant may exhibit persistent tachypnoea, subcostal and intercostal recession and diffuse crackles in the chest on auscultation. There is often a delay in the return to birth weight.

There may be features of hyaline membrane disease or air leak on the chest radiograph initially. These progress to either a diffuse pattern of opacification radiating from the hilar regions (Type 1 CLP; Figure 7.2) or to linear densities interspersed with areas of hyperinflation (type 2 CLP; Figure 7.3) although the chest radiograph may not be easily classified into either type [48]. Type 1 CLP generally has a better outlook in terms of mortality and morbidity [49].

Infants who survive for long enough to fulfil the criteria for the definition of CLP described above, have an approximately 20% mortality in hospital, usually as a consequence of respiratory failure [50] although later unexpected deaths in hospital can occur possibly secondary to pulmonary hypertensive crises or aspiration [51]. Infants who develop overt cor pulmonale seem to have a uniformly bad prognosis.

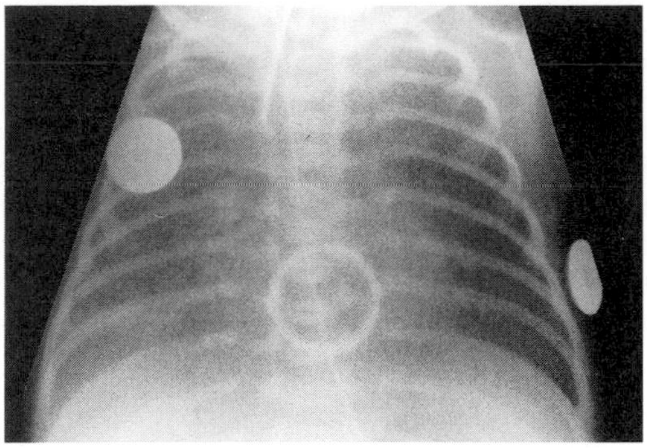

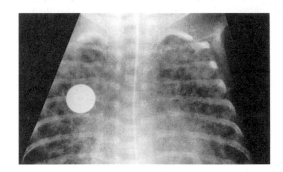

**Figure 7.2** Type 1 chronic lung disease

**Figure 7.3** Type 2 chronic lung disease

## Prevention

Corticosteroids given to the mother antenatally and exogenous surfactant given to the baby via the endotracheal tube early in the neonatal period, have been shown to reduce the mortality from respiratory distress syndrome, although these measures may not result in a reduction in the incidence of CLP [52,53]. It has also been suggested recently that both thyrotrophin-releasing hormone and Inositol given antenatally may reduce the incidence of CLP [54,55] (see Chapter 5).

The severity of CLP may be reduced by minimizing peak airway and mean airway pressures and the inspired oxygen concentration used when treating acute neonatal respiratory disease, although it is not clear what the optimal mechanical ventilator rate should be. Routine use of muscle relaxants for ventilated infants is not associated with a reduction in the incidence of CLP [56].

Avoidance of over-hydration and early treatment of a persistent ductus arteriosus may decrease the likelihood of CLP [15,19]. Recently it has been suggested that administration of vitamin A [57] and the antioxidant superoxide dismutase [34] may be associated with reduction in the incidence of CLP although the former hypothesis has been disputed [57] and further work is needed in both these areas.

## Treatment

To reduce the risk of pulmonary hypertension and to minimize the work of breathing, hypoxia should be prevented in the infant with CLP by keeping oxygen saturations at 93% or above [58]. Oxygen can be administered by headbox or, when the required oxygen concentration is less than 40%, via nasal spectacles or a single nasal cannula. However, care should be taken to avoid hyperoxia in those infants at risk from retinopathy of prematurity (<32 weeks' gestation) although the optimal oxygen saturation in these infants is not known. In the most severe cases (those infants who cannot maintain adequate oxygenation or a satisfactory arterial pH), prolonged periods of mechanical ventilation may be required. In this situation high ventilator pressures should be avoided although an inspiratory time of 0.6 s or more may improve alveolar ventilation [59]. The infant with CLP may develop a compensated respiratory acidosis, and an arterial $P\text{CO}_2$ above the normal range is acceptable in the presence of a normal arterial pH and $P\text{O}_2$; ventilator settings being adjusted according to the latter.

Diuretic therapy with, for example, frusemide and amiloride can improve lung mechanics [60]. It may be useful in the ventilated infant with CLP or when there is a rise in oxygen requirement associated with increased opacification on the chest radiograph due to pulmonary oedema or interstitial fluid [61].

Corticosteroid treatment of infants with CLP will aid in weaning from the ventilator and may reduce the length of oxygen dependency, although no effect on mortality has been shown [62].

Steroids should be used with caution in the ELBW infant as their catabolic effect may impair growth [63,64] and there is a risk of gastric perforation [65]. There is also an increased risk of hypertension and sepsis.

Withdrawal of steroids may cause deterioration. Administration of topical steroids in aerosol form is currently being investigated [66].

Methylxanthines (e.g. aminophylline) may improve lung mechanics in CLP [60] and are used for their central stimulant effect when weaning from the ventilator although there is no clear evidence that they alter the course of CLP [61].

Inhaled bronchodilators given to ventilator-dependent infants may have a beneficial acute effect [67] but a long-term effect on the course of CLP has yet to be demonstrated.

The key to recovery of an infant with CLP is achievement of adequate growth, thus facilitating the growth of new alveoli. If hypoxia can be avoided the addition of an energy supplement, for example with Duocal (Scientific Hospital Supplies) to breast milk or low birth weight formula feeds may provide the extra calories needed for work of breathing or during episodes of infection and may prevent growth impairment. However, there is evidence that infants with CLP have an increased energy expenditure *per se* which may be at the expense of calories required for growth [68], calorie supplementation may therefore not be successful in improving growth velocity.

Correction of anaemia and osteopenia of prematurity may further encourage infants with CLP to thrive.

## Discharge and follow up

Infants who have developed CLP may require supplementary oxygen for several months. Once their inspired oxygen requirement becomes <35–40%, many can be discharged from the neonatal unit with equipment for the administration of oxygen in the home. Factors which affect the decision to discharge a baby who is still requiring oxygen include the presence of other medical problems (such as the need for nasogastric tube feeds), the social circumstances and parental compliance. Before discharge the parents need to be conversant with the use of the various items of equipment such as an oxygen concentrator, oxygen cylinders and tubing for administration of oxygen [69] and may receive training in resuscitation. The child's general practitioner should be fully informed of the situation and contingency plans should be made for readmission to a paediatric ward if the child becomes ill.

Follow-up care of infants with CLP should be by a multidisciplinary approach [70] and should cover the following areas.

### Respiratory

Hypoxia should be prevented to minimize the risk of pulmonary hypertension and cardiac failure and optimize growth. Oxygen may be administered via nasal spectacles, prongs or a single nasal cannula from an oxygen concentrator with a low flow meter attached or, to enable the child to travel, a smaller oxygen cylinder. Pulse oximetry is the most useful way of monitoring oxygen requirements in infants with CLP [71] and in Liverpool supplementary oxygen is prescribed to maintain oxygen saturation consistently at 93% or above.

Recurrent respiratory infections are often viral in origin, although bacterial lower respiratory infections may occur which should be treated with an appropriate antibiotic. Colonization with pseudomonas and other organisms may occur, however there is no proven place for prophylactic antibiotic therapy in infants with CLP. Antiviral therapy may be indicated in specific circumstances, e.g. Ribavirin for bronchiolitis caused by respiratory syncytial virus [72].

The majority of infants develop some degree of airway obstruction usually in the first two years, which may respond to bronchodilators such as ipratropium bromide, salbutamol or terbutaline. Many will be steroid responsive and require regular inhaled or nebulized steroids as well as a short course of oral steroids for acute exacerbations of airways obstruction [73].

It is important to stress to parents the importance of immunization, in particular against pertussis and measles whose respiratory complications are likely to be more severe in infants with CLP.

### Nutrition

Improving somatic growth improves lung growth and may reduce the length of supplementary oxygen requirement [74]. Early involvement of a dietitian for advice regarding calorie intake is important. Calorie supplementation should be considered when weight gain is poor and vitamin supplementation may augment weight gain. Continuing calorie supplementation is often used to promote catch-up growth and maintain growth along the centiles. However, if the infant is hypoxic and expending excess energy on the work of breathing or has an infection then the extra calories provided may be utilized at the expense of growth. As previously mentioned, there is known to be an increased metabolic rate and calorie consumption *per se* in infants who have CLP [68].

As well as providing the correct nutrients it is important to recognize feeding problems in infants with CLP [75]. They may have neuromuscular problems associated with cerebral palsy or be disorganized or difficult feeders in the absence of neurological disability. When oral intake and weight gain are poor, a short period of nasogastric tube feeding either as boluses or continuously overnight may be appropriate. Longer-term feeding via a gastrostomy may be indicated. Infants with CLP may have gastro-oesophageal reflux and recurrent vomiting. If medical treatment (for example with Carobel and Gaviscon) fails, then a Nissen fundoplication may result in dramatic improvement.

### Social

Parents of infants with CLP may feel isolated and overwhelmed by the amount of equipment in their home. The emotional support provided by local neonatal support groups, as well as practical support provided by the social work department in terms of transport, providing a telephone and help claiming disability living and other allowances, is invaluable.

### Others

Infants with CLP may also need to be assessed and treated by the neurodevelopmental team, general and ENT surgeons and ophthalmologists for other associated problems.

## Outcome

There is a significant mortality after discharge from hospital in infants with CLP, usually from a respiratory cause [76]. In the early years there may be frequent hospital admissions as a consequence of respiratory infection and feeding difficulties, although infants gradually improve and grow out of their need for supplementary oxygen.

Of a cohort of 42 infants with CLP who had been followed-up to age 6–10 years in Liverpool, 57% reported wheezing in the previous year and 38% reported increased cough. Other medium-term follow-up studies of survivors of CLP have shown persistent minor abnormalities on the chest radiograph [77], diminished lung function with some degree of airways obstruction (not all of which is reversible), and an increased incidence of airways hyperreactivity [78,79].

## Summary

CLP can now be considered as a multifactorial disease affecting preterm infants who have received neonatal intensive care, particularly those with a birth weight under 1000 g. The majority of infants with CLP survive, and an increasing number are discharged home whilst still requiring supplementary oxygen. This has implications for community care services. Infants with CLP require medium- to long-

term follow up because of the possibility of later respiratory morbidity. The very-long-term consequences of this disease are unknown.

## References

1. Northway, W.H., Rosan, R.C. and Porter, D.Y. (1967) Pulmonary disease following respirator therapy of hyaline membrane disease. *N. Engl. J. Med.*, **276**, 357–368

2. Bureau of Maternal and Child Health and Resources Development. (1989) Guidelines for the care of children with chronic lung disease. *Pediatr. Pulmonol.*, **5**, (Suppl 3), 3–13

3. Bancalari, E., Abdenour, G.E., Feller, R. and Gannon, J. (1979) Bronchopulmonary dysplasia: clinical presentation. *J. Pediatr.*, **95**, 819–823

4. Tooley, W.H. (1979) Epidemiology of bronchopulmonary dysplasia. *J. Pediatr.*, **95**, 851–858

5. Avery, M.E., Tooley, W.H., Keller, J.B. *et al.* (1987) Is chronic lung disease in low birth weight infants preventable? A survey of eight centers. *Pediatrics*, **79**, 26–30

6. Wung, J.-T., Koons, A.H., Driscoll, J.M. Jr. and James, L.S. (1979) Changing incidence of bronchopulmonary dysplasia. *J. Pediatr.*, **95**, 845–847

7. Horbar, J.D., McAuliffe, T.L., Adler, S.M. *et al.* (1988) Variability in 28-day outcomes for very low birth weight infants: an analysis of 11 neonatal intensive care units. *Pediatrics*, **82**, 554–559

8. Kraybill, E.N., Runyan, D.K., Bose, C.L. and Khan, J.H. (1989) Risk factors for chronic lung disease in infants with birth weights of 751 to 1000 grams. *J. Pediatr.*, **115**, 115–120

9. Gaylord, M.S., Thieme, R.E., Woodall, D.L. and Quissell, B.J. (1985) Predicting mortality in low birth weight infants with pulmonary interstitial emphysema. *Pediatrics*, **76**, 219–224

10. Gerstmann, D.R., deLemos, R.A., Coalson, J.J. *et al.* (1988) Influence of ventilatory technique on pulmonary baroinjury in baboons with hyaline membrane disease. *Pediatr. Pulmonol.*, **5**, 82–91

11. Frank, L. (1985) Effects of oxygen on the newborn. *Fed. Proc.*, **44**, 2328–2334

12. Pappas, C.T., Obara, H., Bensch, K.G. and Northway, W.H. Jr. (1983) Effect of prolonged exposure to 80% oxygen on the lung of the newborn mouse. *Lab. Invest.*, **48**, 735–748

13. Delemos, R.A., Coalson, J.J., Gerstmann, D.R., Kuehl, T.J. and Null, D.M. Jr. (1987) Oxygen toxicity in the premature baboon with hyaline membrane disease. *Am. Rev. Respir. Dis.*, **136**, 677–682

14. Davis, J.M., Dickerson, B., Metlay, L. and Penney, D.P. (1991) Differential effects of oxygen and barotrauma on lung injury in the neonatal piglet. *Pediatr. Pulmonol.*, **10**, 157–163

---

**Practical points**

1. Inspiratory and mean airway pressures should be kept to a minimum when ventilating infants in order to reduce the risk of CLP.
2. Overhydration should be avoided in the early neonatal period as this may predispose to CLP.
3. Corticosteroid treatment of infants with CLP will aid in weaning from the ventilator and may reduce the length of oxygen dependency although impaired growth and other side-effects may occur.
4. Once the infant with CLP is stable, has no other medical problems and is receiving an inspired oxygen concentration of 35–40% or less, they can be discharged from the neonatal unit with supplementary oxygen for use in the home.
5. At follow up, many infants with CLP have developed some degree of airways obstruction which will respond to bronchodilators and steroids.

15. Brown, E.R. (1979) Increased risk of bronchopulmonary dysplasia in infants with patent ductus arteriosus. *J. Pediatr.*, **95**, 865–866

16. Dudell, G.G. and Gersory, W.M. (1984) Patent ductus arteriosus in neonates with severe respiratory disease. *J. Pediatr.*, **104**, 915–920

17. Van de Bor, M., Verlooove Vanhorick, S.P., Brand, R. and Ruys, J.H. (1988) Patent ductus arteriosus in a cohort of 1338 preterm infants; a collaborative study. *Paediatr. Perinat. Epidemiol.*, **2**, 328–326

18. Brown, E.R., Stark, A., Sosenko, I., Lawson, E.E. and Avery, M.E. (1978) Bronchopulmonary dysplasia: possible relationship to pulmonary edema. *J. Pediatr.*, **92**, 982–986

19. Van Marter, L.J., Leviton, A., Allred, E.N., Pagano, M. and Kuban, K.C. (1990) Hydration during the first days of life and the risk of bronchopulmonary dysplasia in low birth weight infants. *J. Pediatr.*, **116**, 942–949

20. Van Marter, L.J., Pagano, M., Allred, E.N., Leviton, A. and Kuban, K.C.K. (1992) Rate of bronchopulmonary dysplasia as a function of neonatal intensive care practices. *J. Pediatr.*, **120**, 938–946

21. Ogden, B.E., Murphy, S.A., Saunders, G.C., Pathak, D. and Johnson, J.D. (1984) Neonatal lung neutrophils and elastase/proteinase imbalance. *Am. Rev. Respir. Dis.*, **130**, 817–821

22. Cassell, G.H., Waites, K.B., Crouse, D.T. *et al.* (1988) Association of *Urea plasma urealyticum* infection of the lower respiratory tract with chronic lung disease and death in very-low-birth-weight infants. *Lancet*, **2**, 240–245

23. Cooke, R.W.I. (1991) Factors associated with chronic lung disease in preterm infants. *Arch. Dis. Childh.*, **66**, 776–779

24. Hammerman, C. and Aramburo, M.J. (1988) Decreased lipid intake reduces morbidity in sick premature neonates. *J. Pediatr.*, **113**, 1083–1088

25. Pearlman, M. and Fabrizio, M. (1990) Effect of postnatal lipid nutrition in long-term outcome of children with bronchopulmonary dysplasia. (Abstract) *Am. Rev. Respir. Dis.*, **141**, A158

26. Sosenko, I.R.S., Innis, S.M. and Frank, L. (1991) Intralipid increases lung polyunsaturated fatty acids and protects newborn rats from oxygen toxicity. *Pediatr. Res.*, **30**, 413–417

27. Sosenko, I.R.S., Innis, S.M. and Frank, L. (1991) Intralipid increases lung polyunsaturated fatty acids and protects newborn rats from oxygen toxicity. *Pediatr. Res.*, **30**, 413–417

28. Alwaiah, M.H., Bowden, L., Shaw, B. and Ryan, S.W. (1995) Randomized trial of effect of delayed intravenous lipid administration on chronic lung disease in preterm neonates. *J. Ped. Govt. Nut.,* **22;3**, 303–306

29. Newell, S.J., Booth, I.W., Morgan, M.E.I., Durbin, G.M. and McNeish, A.S. (1989) Gastro-oesophageal reflux in preterm infants. *Arch. Dis. Childh.*, **64**, 780–786

30. Clark, D.A., Pincus, L.G., Oliphant, M. *et al.* (1982) HLA-A2 and chronic lung disease in neonates. *J. Am. Med. Assoc.*, **248**, 1868–1869

31. Nickerson, B.G. and Taussig, L.M. (1980) Family history of asthma in infants with bronchopulmonary dysplasia. *Pediatrics*, **65**, 1140–1144

32. Frank, L. and Sosenko, I.R.S. (1988) Undernutrition as a major contributing factor in the pathogenesis of bronchopulmonary dysplasia. *Am. Rev. Respir. Dis.*, **138**, 725–729

33. Frank, L. and Sosenko, I.R.S. (1987) Development of lung antioxidant enzyme system in late gestation: Possible implications for the prematurely born infant. *J. Pediatr.*, **110**, 9–14

34. Rosenfeld, W., Evans, H., Concepcion, L., Jhaveri, R., Schaeffer, H. and Friedman, A. (1984) Prevention of bronchopulmonary dysplasia by administration of bovine superoxide dismutase in preterm infants with respiratory distress syndrome. *J. Pediatr.*, **105**, 781–785

35. Bancalari, E. and Sosenko, I.R.S. (1990) Pathogenesis and prevention of neonatal chronic lung disease. *Pediatr. Pulmonol.*, **8**, 109–116

36. Sinkin, R.A. and Phelps, D.L. (1987) New strategies for the prevention of bronchopulmonary dysplasia. *Clin. Perinatol.*, **14**, 599–620

37. Shenai, J.P., Chytil, F. and Stahlman, M.T. (1985) Vitamin A status of neonates with bronchopulmonary dysplasia. *Pediatr. Res.*, **19**, 185–188

38. Zachman, R.D. (1989) Retinol (vitamin A) and the neonate: special problems of the human premature infant. *Am. J. Clin. Nutr.*, **50**, 413–424

39. Halliwell, B. (1989) Tell me about free radicals, doctor: a review. *J. R. Soc. Med.*, **82**, 747–752

40. Reid, L. (1979) Bronchopulmonary dysplasia-pathology. *J. Pediatr.*, **95**, 836–841

41. Erickson, A.M., de la Monte, S.M., Moore, G.W. and Hutchins, G.M. (1987) The progression of morphologic changes in bronchopulmonary dysplasia. *Am. J. Pathol.*, **127**, 474–484

42. Van Lierde, S., Cornelis, A., Devlieger, H., Moerman, P., Lauwergus, J. and Eggermont, E. (1991) Different patterns of pulmonary sequelae after hyaline membrane disease; heterogeneity of bronchopulmonary dysplasia? *Biol. Neonate.*, **60**, 152–162

43. Margraf, L.R., Tomashefski, J.F. Jr., Bruce, M.C. and Dalms, B.B. (1991) Morphometric analysis of the lung in bronchopulmonary dysplasia. *Am. Rev. Respir. Dis.*, **143**, 391–400

44. Chambers, H.M. and Van Velzen, D. Ventilator related pathology in the extremely immature lung. *Pathology.*, **21**, 79–83

45. Stocker, J.T. (1986) Pathologic features of long-standing 'healed' bronchopulmonary dysplasia; a study of 28 3–40-month-old infants. *Hum. Pathol.*, **17**, 943–961

46. Anderson, W.R. and Engel, R.R. (1983) Cardiopulmonary sequelae of reparative stages of bronchopulmonary dysplasia. *Arch. Pathol. Lab. Med.*, **107**, 603–608

47. Lee, R.M. and O'Brodovich, H. (1988) Airway epithelial damage in premature infants with respiratory failure. *Am. Rev. Respir. Dis.*, **137**, 450–457

48. Hyde, I., English, R.E. and Williams, J.A. (1989) The

changing pattern of chronic lung disease of prematurity. *Arch. Dis. Childh.*, **64**, 448–451

49. Shaw, N.J., Pilling, D.W., Cooke, R.W.I. and Ashby, D. (1992) The chest radiograph and outcome in chronic lung disease of prematurity. *Pediatric. Rev. Commun.*, **6**, 257–261

50 Shaw, N.J. and Cooke, R.W.I. (1991) Outcome and oxygen dependency in neonatal chronic lung disease. *Pediatr. Rev. Commun.*, **6**, 56

51. Abden, S.H., Burchell, M.F., Schaffer, M.S. and Rosenberg, A.A. (1989) Late sudden unexpected deaths in hospitalized infants with bronchopulmonary dysplasia. *Am. J. Dis. Childh.*, **143**, 815–819

52. Morley, C.J. (1991) Surfactant treatment for premature babies – a review of clinical trials. *Arch. Dis. Childh.*, **66**, 445–450

53. Crowley, P., Chalmers, I. and Keirse, M.J.N.C. (1990) The effects of corticosteroid administration before preterm delivery; an overview of the evidence from controlled clinical trials. *Br. J. Obstet. Gynaecol.*, **97**, 11–25

54. Ballard, R.A., Ballard, P.L., Creasy, R.K. *et al.* (1992) Respiratory disease in very-low-birthweight infants after prenatal thyrotropin-releasing hormone and glucocorticoid. *Lancet*, **339**, 510–515

55. Hallman, M., Bry, K., Hoppu, K., Lappi, M. and Pohjavuori, M. (1992) Inositol supplementation in premature infants with respiratory distress syndrome. *N. Engl. J. Med.*, **326**, 1233–1239

56. Shaw, N.J., Cooke, R.W.I., Gill, A.B., Shaw, N.J. and Saeed, M. (1993) Randomised trial of routine versus selective paralysis during ventilation for neonatal respiratory distress syndrome. *Arch. Dis. Childh.*, **69**, 479–482

57. Shenai, J.P., Kennedy, K.A., Chytil, F. and Stahlman, M.T. (1987) Clinical trial of Vitamin A supplementation in infants susceptible to bronchopulmonary dysplasia. *J. Pediatr.*, **111**, 269–277

58. Mok, J.Y.Q., McLaughlin, J.F., Pintar, M., Hak, R.N.H., Amaro-Galvez, R. and Levison, H. (1986) Transcutaneous monitoring of oxygenation: what is normal? *J. Pediatr.*, **108**, 365–371

59. Goldman, S.L., McCann, E.M., Lloyd, B.W. and Yup, G. (1991) Inspiratory time and pulmonary function in mechanically ventilated babies with chronic lung disease. *Pediatr. Pulmonol.*, **11**, 198–201

60. Kao, L.C., Durand, D.J., Phillips, B.L. and Nickerson, B.G. (1987) Oral theophylline and diuretics improve pulmonary mechanics in infants with bronchopulmonary dysplasia. *J. Pediatr.*, **111**, 439–444

61. Davis, J.M., Sinkin, R.A. and Aranda, J.V. (1990) Drug therapy for bronchopulmonary dysplasia. *Pediatr. Pulmonol.*, **8**, 117–125

62. Anon (1991) Dexamethasone for neonatal chronic lung disease. *Lancet*, **338**, 982–983

63. Brownlee, K.G., Ng, P.C., Henderson, M.J., Smith, M., Green, J.H. and Dear, P.R.F. (1992) Catabolic effect of dexamethasone in the preterm baby. *Arch. Dis. Childh.*, **67**, 1–4

64. Williams, A.F. and Jones, M. (1992) Dexamethasone increases plasma amino acid concentrations in bronchopulmonary dysplasia. *Arch. Dis. Childh.*, **67**, 5–9

65. O'Neil, E.A., Chwals, W.J., O'Shea, M.D. and Turner, C.S. (1992) Dexamethasone treatment during ventilator dependency: possible life threatening gastrointestinal complications. *Arch. Dis. Childh.*, **67**, 10–11

66. Silverman, M. (1994) Chronic lung disease of prematurity: are we too cautious with steroids? *Eur. J. Pediatr.*, **153**, S30–S35

67. Wilkie, R.A. and Bryan, M.H. (1987) Effects of bronchodilators on airway resistance in ventilator-dependent neonates with chronic lung disease. *J. Pediatr.*, **111**, 278–282

68. Kalhan, S.H. and Denne, S.C. (1990) Energy consumption in infants with bronchopulmonary dysplasia. *J. Pediatr.*, **116**, 662–664

69. Angell, C. (1991) Equipment requirements for community based paediatric oxygen treatment. *Arch. Dis. Childh.*, **66**, 755

70. Tansey, S., Doyle, C. and Shaw, N.J. (1995) The role of the Clinical Nurse Specialist in the management of infants with oxygen dependent chronic lung disease. *J. Mater. Child Health,* **3**, 88–92

71. Ramanathan, R., Durand, M. and Larrazabal, C. (1987) Pulse oximetry in very low birth weight infants with acute and chronic lung disease. *Pediatrics*, **79**, 612–617

72. Isaacs, D., Moxon, E.R., Harvey, D. *et al.* (1988) Ribavirin in respiratory syncytial virus infection. *Arch. Dis. Childh.*, **63**, 986–990

73. Fiascone, J.M., Rhodes, T.T., Grandgeorge, S.R. and Knapp, M.A. (1989) Bronchopulmonary dysplasia: a review for the pediatrician. *Curr. Probl. Pediatr.*, **19**, 169–227

74. Markestad, T. and Fitzhardinge, P.M. (1981) Growth and development in children recovering from bronchopulmonary dysplasia. *J. Pediatr.*, **98**, 597–602

75. Sauve, R.S., McMillan, D.D., Mitchell, I. *et al.* (1989) Home oxygen therapy; outcome of infants discharged from NICU on continuous treatment. *Clin. Pediatr.*, **28**, 113–118

76. Sauve, R.S. and Singhal, N. (1985) Long-term morbidity of infants with bronchopulmonary dysplasia. *Pediatrics*, **76**, 725–733

77. Griscom, N.T., Wheeler, W.B., Sweezey, N.B. *et al.* (1989) Bronchopulmonary dysplasia: radiographic appearance in middle childhood. *Radiology.*, **171**, 811–814

78. Northway, W.H. Jr, Moss, R.B., Carlisle, B.K. *et al.* (1990) Late pulmonary sequelae of bronchopulmonary dysplasia. *N. Engl. J. Med.*, **323**, 1793–1799

79. Blayney, M., Kerem, E., Whyte, H. and O'Brodovich, H. (1991) Bronchopulmonary dysplasia: improvement in lung function between 7 and 10 years of age. *J. Pediatr.*, **118**, 201–206

# 8

# Hazards of an immature skin

**Nicholas Rutter**

The skin is an important barrier between man and his environment. It keeps out noxious agents and keeps in the main body constituent: water. If there is extensive skin loss as a result of trauma or disease, death commonly results. In most preterm infants problems due to immaturity of the skin do not occur. Illness and outcome are largely determined by delivery, resuscitation and the development of cerebral, respiratory and bowel complications. Babies born before 30 weeks' gestation, however, especially those below 28 weeks' gestation (who will usually weigh less than 1000 g), suffer from profound immaturity of all the organ systems of the body including the skin. Immaturity of the skin as a barrier leads to major clinical problems of fluid and heat loss, accidental absorption of toxic agents and superficial trauma.

## Structure of the skin

The outer layer of the skin, the epidermis, provides its barrier properties. Epidermal cells are produced in the basal layer, migrate upwards, flatten, become filled with a fibrous protein (keratin) and die. The dead keratinized cell plates are tightly interlocked and overlapping, forming the stratum corneum. It is this layer which resists the escape of water or the entry of toxic agents. Keratinization of the fetal epidermis starts at about 18 weeks when the periderm begins to disappear [1,2]. By about 26 weeks the development of a keratinized stratum corneum involves the whole body surface but the epidermis is only two or three cells thick and a keratinized stratum is barely visible. In the last trimester the epidermis increases in thickness, keratinization becomes more marked and the stratum corneum well defined, so that by term the epidermis resembles that of an adult [3] (Figure 8.1). However, these maturational changes which occur in the last trimester are greatly accelerated if the infant is born prematurely. No matter how immature the infant is at delivery, by two weeks of age the epidermis resembles that of a term infant (Figure 8.2). Thus the epidermis of an infant of 25 weeks' gestation at two weeks of age is similar to that of a term infant, rather than an infant of 27 weeks' gestation.

Birth therefore triggers a rapid acceleration of epidermal maturation, similar to the changes which are seen in adult skin which has been damaged by stripping or by superficial burns. The very immature infant is a water dwelling animal forced prematurely to live on dry land. Presumably the stimulus to the hastened epidermal maturation is exposure to air but the mechanism by which it occurs is unknown. It means, however, that clinical problems associated with an immature skin are only relevant in the early neonatal period.

## Barrier properties of immature skin

### Transepidermal water loss (TEWL)

Water is lost from the skin by two routes: secretion of sweat via the sweat ducts and

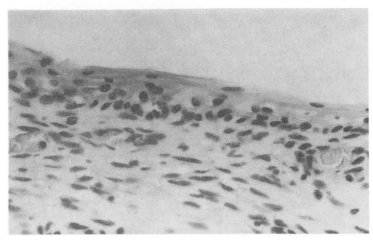

*(a)*

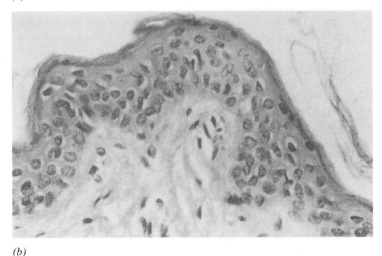

*(b)*

**Figure 8.1** The effect of gestation on maturation of the epidermis. *(a)* Section of abdominal skin of an infant born at 26 weeks' gestation who died shortly after delivery. Note the thin epidermis, 2–3 cells thick, with little formation of a keratinized stratum corneum. *(b)* The abdominal skin of an infant delivered at 40 weeks' gestation who died in intrapartum. There is a well developed epidermis. Magnification × 90. (Reproduced with permission [39])

passive diffusion of water through the epidermis (transepidermal water loss). Babies born before 36 weeks' gestation are unable to sweat in the early neonatal period [4–6] so that all skin water loss is through the epidermis.

### TEWL and the effect of gestational age

Gestational age has a very marked effect on TEWL [7,8] as would be expected from the epidermal histology. Losses rise exponentially before 30 weeks, and can reach values of 100 g m$^2$ h$^{-1}$ in infants of 24 weeks' gestation on the first day or so of life. By 32 weeks' gestation losses are lower, and by term have fallen to about 6 g m$^2$ h (Figure 8.3).

### TEWL and the effect of postnatal age

There is an accelerated fall in TEWL after birth in babies born before 30 weeks' gestation so that by about two weeks of age losses are only a little higher than those of a term infant [7,9–11]. This parallels the acceleration in epidermal maturation (Figure 8.4).

### TEWL and the effect of environmental factors

TEWL is a physical process and not under physiological control. It is determined not only by the effectiveness of the epidermal barrier, but also by environmental factors.

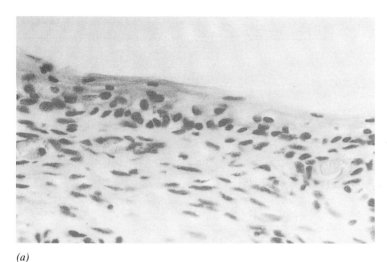

*(a)*

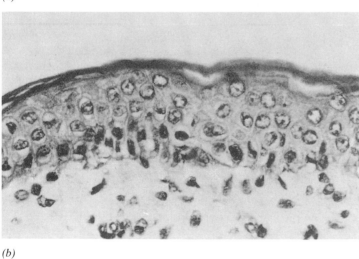

*(b)*

**Figure 8.2** The effect of extra-uterine existence on maturation of the epidermis. *(a)* From an infant born at 26 weeks' gestation who died shortly after delivery (Figure 8.1). *(b)* The abdominal skin of an infant born at 26 weeks' gestation who died at 16 days. The epidermal development is comparable to that of a term infant. Magnification × 90. (Reproduced with permission [39])

**Figure 8.3** The effect of gestation on transepidermal water loss (TEWL). TEWL was measured at three representative skin sites on the first day of life (ambient relative humidity 50%). Redrawn from the data of Hammarlund and Sedin [8]

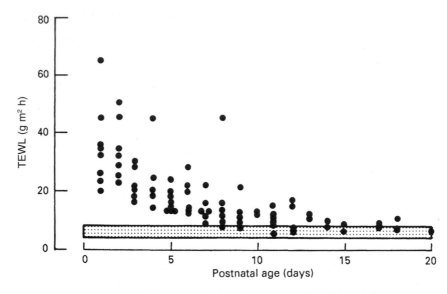

**Figure 8.4** The effect of extrauterine existence on transepidermal water loss (TEWL). Serial measurements were made from the abdominal skin of 17 infants born at 25–29 weeks' gestation. The shaded part represents values of TEWL found in full term infants. Redrawn from the data of Harpin and Rutter [11]

*Temperature*

The temperature of the skin and air is positively related to TEWL [12], although the effect is not great over the narrow range of skin and air temperatures found in a neonatal unit.

*Air speed*

This is positively related to TEWL. When air speed is low, natural convection exists and there is a boundary layer of still air close to the skin. This becomes relatively saturated and reduces TEWL. When air speed is high, the boundary layer is lost and TEWL is higher

[13–15]. These conditions of forced convection are found when infants below 30 weeks' gestation are nursed naked in incubators or under radiant warmers, and therefore exposed to draughty air.

*Humidity*

Ambient humidity is a powerful determinant of TEWL; at low relative humidity TEWL is high, at 100% relative humidity TEWL is abolished. The relationship is linear and the effect more marked in the most immature infants [8,16] (Figure 8.5).

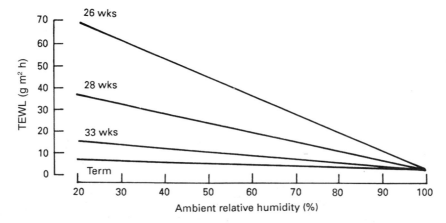

**Figure 8.5** The effect of ambient relative humidity on transepidermal water loss (TEWL). Redrawn and modified from the data of Hammarlund and Sedin [8]

**Table 8.1** Measurements of insensible weight loss in preterm infants of birth weight <1000 g (note that two studies include heavier infants)

| Reference | Weight of infants (g) | Method of nursing | Insensible water loss (mean ± SEM (ml kg⁻¹ 24h⁻¹) |
|-----------|----------------------|-------------------|---------------------------------------------------|
| Fanaroff *et al.* [25] | 700–1250 | Incubator | $84.0 \pm 16.8$ |
| Wu and Hodgman [18] | <1000 | Incubator | $64.8 \pm 4.8$ |
| Bell *et al.* [19] | 790–1310 | Incubator | $38.4 \pm 7.2$ |
|  |  | Radiant warmer | $58.6 \pm 4.8$ |
| Baumgart *et al.* [26] | 660–1000 | Radiant warmer | $127.2 \pm 18.5$ |

*Radiation*

Exposure of the skin to radiant energy increases TEWL. This is important in very immature infants nursed under radiant warmers or phototherapy. Radiant warmers increase TEWL by a factor of 0.5–2.0 [17–19]; phototherapy by 0.4–2.0 [18,20]. The two together have an additive effect [21]. Although part of the increase in TEWL can be explained by the higher skin temperatures, higher air speeds and lower ambient humidity which occur when infants are nursed under radiant warmers, there is an unexplained direct effect of radiant energy [22].

Although it is clear that very immature infants have a high TEWL when measurements are made from local areas of skin, there is disappointingly little information available about the overall water loss from the whole body – the insensible water loss. It is this parameter which would be so useful to know in planning the fluid intake of such an infant. Insensible water loss has been measured directly and indirectly (as insensible weight loss) by many investigators, but most studies have included very few infants under 1000 g birth weight or below 28 weeks' gestation. Furthermore, studies based on measurement of insensible weight loss have probably overestimated water loss because the balances have been affected by temperature changes [23,24]. Table 8.1 summarizes the results of those investigations which include predominantly infants of less than 1000 g.

Insensible water loss in the term infant is approximately 8–11 g m² h⁻¹. This is equivalent to about 11–15 ml k⁻¹ day⁻¹. Depending on environmental conditions, insensible water loss in very immature infants can range from 50 to 150 ml kg⁻¹ day⁻¹. The highest value might be found in an infant of 24 weeks' gestation nursed naked under a radiant warmer and phototherapy lamp in the immediate neonatal period.

Babies with a high TEWL pose problems in the management of fluid balance. Since heat is lost from the evaporation of water they are also difficult to keep warm [22].

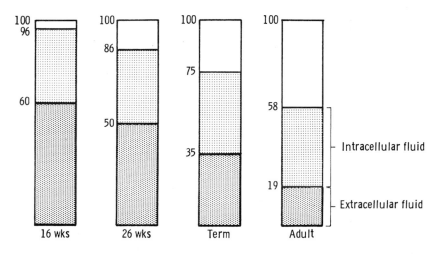

**Figure 8.6** Body water content (intracellular and extracellular) as a percentage of total body weight

## Management of fluid balance

The infant born before 28 weeks' gestation has a higher water content than a term infant (Figure 8.6), entirely due to a higher extracellular fluid volume. This accounts for half the infant's weight. Administration of too much or too little fluid therefore has a more harmful effect than in mature infants. Too much fluid is the more serious. Clinically it may result in a rapid weight gain or failure of the normal weight loss, and appearances of oedema, although the latter is a common finding in very immature infants. It makes respiratory distress worse, with a need for decreasing ventilation and inspired oxygen. Similarly it results in deterioration in infants with chronic lung disease. Patent ductus arteriosus [27] and necrotizing enterocolitis are more common. Too little fluid results in excessive weight loss, clinical dehydration, oliguria, hypernatraemia [28] and reduced excretion of drugs (especially gentamicin).

Since insensible water loss of an immature infant depends on so many factors, it cannot be accurately predicted. Fluid balance is greatly simplified if steps are taken to reduce the high TEWL, whether the infant is nursed in an incubator or under a radiant warmer. Assessment of fluid balance is then made by clinical examination and investigation, allowing fluid needs to be calculated. Body weight is a very useful method of assessment and should be measured as accurately as possible. Daily or even twice daily weighing may be necessary, especially if TEWL is high. Since even the most immature infant has some ability to excrete or conserve water, measurement of the degree of concentration of the blood and urine will be useful (Table 8.2). Plasma sodium levels in the first week of life are particularly helpful in very immature infants: a low sodium reflects fluid overload and a high sodium fluid depletion. After the first week, plasma sodium levels are less useful because they reflect urinary sodium losses rather than the state of hydration.

If TEWL is effectively reduced the fluid requirements of an immature infant will be similar to those of other preterm infants (60 ml kg$^{-1}$ day$^{-1}$ on day 1, increasing by 30 ml kg$^{-1}$ day$^{-1}$ to 150 ml kg$^{-1}$ day$^{-1}$ on day 4). If TEWL is not reduced, fluid requirements in the first few days will be much higher, up to 200 ml kg$^{-1}$ day$^{-1}$. It is better to give too little fluid rather than too much, particularly in the

**Table 8.2    Assessment of fluid needs in immature infants**

**Body weight**
Average percentage weight loss in the first week [29]
   <26 weeks    –  20%
   26–28 weeks  –  15%
Less than 10% weight loss (or no weight loss, or weight gain) suggests too much fluid.
Greater than 20% weight loss suggests too little fluid.

**Blood**
Sodium: normal range, 130–145 mmol l$^{-1}$
Osmolality: normal range, 260–290 mOsmol kg$^{-1}$
Lower levels suggest too much fluid; higher levels suggest too little fluid.

**Urine**
Osmolality: aim to maintain between 150 and 300 mOsmol kg$^{-1}$
Specific gravity: aim to maintain between 1.005 and 1.010

early stages of respiratory distress syndrome [30].

## Temperature control

Each millilitre of water which evaporates from the skin removes 560 calories of heat. The infant below 1000 g is already at a major disadvantage because of his high surface area to weight ratio, so that the heat loss by all channels is high relative to heat production. A high TEWL as well will render the very immature infant susceptible to hypothermia. In the delivery room, for example, body temperature can drop by 1°C every five minutes, in spite of the provision of supplementary heat.

The very immature infant can either be nursed in an incubator or under a radiant warmer. Since the infant is likely to be ill and require intensive care, nursing is easier if the infant is naked. The major advantage of the radiant warmer in this situation is that the infant can be effectively kept warm whilst doctors and nurses have ready access for intubation, placing of intra-arterial and intravenous catheters, etc. Fluid balance, though, is more difficult. Immature infants can be kept warm in an incubator if carefully nursed, but practical procedures are difficult to carry out and cause cold stress.

### Incubators

The very immature infant nursed naked in an incubator can only be kept warm if steps are

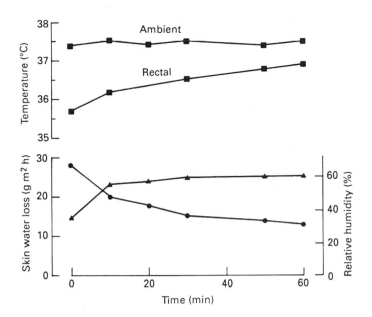

**Figure 8.7** The effect of increasing ambient relative humidity within an incubator. The infant, 26 weeks' gestation and birth weight 960 g, had a persistently low rectal temperature of 35.8°C at 10 hours of age, despite a high incubator air temperature. When humidification is added, relative humidity (▲—▲) increases from 36% to 61%, skin water loss (●—●) falls and rectal temperature rises to normal within an hour. Reproduced with permission [34]

taken to reduce the high TEWL. A high ambient temperature close to 37°C will be necessary. Although TEWL can be reduced using a waterproof covering such as a plastic thermal bubble blanket [31] or topical soft paraffin [32,33], in practice the only effective method is to increase the ambient humidity [8,16]. It is otherwise impossible to avoid hypothermia [34]. It would require an ambient temperature in excess of 39°C to maintain a normal body temperature in a very small and immature infant without the use of humidity. For safety reasons such a temperature is not permitted in the UK.

Some, although not all, current incubators can be very effectively humidified. A relative humidity of 85–90% can be achieved at the highest air temperature setting, a level at which TEWL is greatly reduced (Figure 8.5). The effect of providing a humid environment on temperature control is dramatic [34] (Figure 8.7). When the incubator portholes are opened for access to the infant, relative humidity falls to 50–60%, still higher though than the levels of 25–40% which are found in dry incubators. Although plastic coverings will reduce water loss from the skin by as much as 75% [31], as well as reducing heat loss by convection and radiation, they impair observation of the infant and frequently have to be removed for access. This results in episodes of very high TEWL.

The main worry about incubator humidifica-

tion is a possible increased risk of bacterial infection, particularly as a result of water-borne organisms such as *Pseudomonas aeruginosa*. This can be reduced if the humidifier is drained daily, run dry for a brief spell, then filled with fresh sterile water. Use of humidification should be confined to those infants who need it (infants less than 30 weeks' gestation for the first week of life) and not be extended to all preterm infants nursed in incubators. Another possible hazard of the use of high humidity is overhydration, with an increased incidence of patent ductus arteriosus.

### Radiant warmers

These devices allow very immature infants to have enormous heat losses from evaporation of water and convection without the development of hypothermia. This is achieved by providing a large amount of radiant heat to compensate for the losses. The advantages of visibility and access have been mentioned, but there is a risk of overheating unless obsessional nursing care is practised, and fluid balance is much more difficult than for infants nursed in incubators. It is both possible and desirable to reduce the high TEWL of very immature infants nursed under radiant warmers by use of plastic waterproof coverings [35–37]. Thin polyethylene film is transparent to long wave radiation but impermeable to water and is therefore a suitable material. It can be draped directly over the infant's body but this carries the risk of maceration of the moist skin and increased bacterial colonization. It is best suspended a few centimetres above the infant like a framed tent.

## Absorption of drugs and chemicals

The immature epidermal barrier greatly increases the risk of absorption of topically applied agents in the early neonatal period. Significant absorption can result in systemic toxicity [38]. This was first noted when aniline marker dyes produced methaemoglobinaemia [39–42], but subsequent effects have been confined to the use of topical antiseptics. Hexachlorophene myelinopathy [43–46], iodine-induced goitre [47], alcohol-related skin necrosis [48,49], and neomycin ototoxicity have been described [50]. Any antiseptic agent should be used sparingly and with care. Although the commonly used chlorhexidene is not known to have any toxic effects, it is certainly systemically absorbed [51]. Any water soluble drug or chemical is rapidly absorbed through the skin of immature infants.

A major concern is that since the most immature infants are expected to have a high mortality and morbidity rate, disasters which result from percutaneous absorption of toxic agents will pass unrecognized.

## Gas exchange

Mature epidermis is a barrier to the diffusion of oxygen and carbon dioxide. In the adult only about 1% of respiratory gas exchange occurs across the skin. However, in very immature infants in the early newborn period when the epidermal barrier is weak, appreciable amounts of oxygen can enter the body and carbon dioxide can leave via the skin [52]. The epidermis is about six times more permeable to these gases. It is estimated that if an immature infant is surrounded by oxygen at 95% concentration but continues to breathe air, up to 20% of the resting oxygen requirements and a similar proportion of carbon dioxide excretion can be met percutaneously [53]. Percutaneous oxygen delivery results in an increase in arterial oxygen tension of 5–15 mmHg [54].

## Resistance to trauma

Mature skin is an effective body defence against external trauma: immature skin is not. Adhesive trauma is the most commonly encountered in the newborn intensive care unit, because the skin is such a convenient site for monitoring or for anchoring. Heart rate, breathing, tc$PO_2$ and tc$PCO_2$ and temperature are monitored by probes which are stuck to the skin by adhesive. Intravenous cannulae, arterial lines and chest drains are anchored to the skin by adhesive tape. When the adhesive is removed, the superficial layers of the epidermis are removed with it. This is of no importance if the skin is mature, but in immature infants it causes pain and leaves an area of skin with little or no epidermal covering. TEWL is increased and there is a risk of surface and systemic sepsis. The surface area of a 600 g infant is low in relation to the size of the probes and tape: up to 15% of the skin surface can be subjected to trauma each day. Although skin damage caused by monitoring probes is transient and usually heals completely, scarring occasionally happens [55]. Adhesive tape of adult type can leave an area of roughened irregular skin which looks like the peel of an orange.

Prevention of trauma to the skin can be achieved by limiting use of surface monitoring, reduction in size of the probes and by use of weaker adhesive tape. Karaya gum, used to protect the abdominal skin around surgical stomas, is an effective material for ECG electrodes [56]. It gives good quality traces, but the electrodes can be removed easily and resited on multiple occasions without causing pain or epidermal trauma. Any adhesive tape should be weak and capable of being removed with minimal disturbance to the infant. It is possible to provide an artificial skin to protect the immature skin when it is most vulnerable [57]. A clear semipermeable membrane made of polyurethane (available as the surgical skin dressing 'Opsite' and 'Tegaderm') has been shown to reduce TEWL by 50%. ECG electrodes and temperature probes can be attached to it and give good recordings, although it limits gas diffusion and therefore prevents accurate recording of tc$PO_2$ and tc$PCO_2$. The membrane does not damage the skin when it is removed, nor does it delay the normal maturation of the epidermis [58].

**Practical points**

1. The epidermal barrier is poorly developed and functionally immature in babies below 30 weeks' gestation. There is rapid maturation after birth, which is usually complete by about two weeks of age.
2. The consequences of the immature epidermal barrier are a high transepidermal water loss and susceptibility to percutaneous absorption.
3. A high transepidermal water loss leads to hypothermia and difficulties in fluid balance. Management is simplified if this is reduced. In an incubator this is achieved by the use of high humidity, and under a radiant warmer by the use of polythene drapes.
4. Percutaneous absorption of toxic agents readily occurs. Great care should be taken to avoid putting chemically active agents on the skin in the early newborn period, particularly antiseptics.
5. The physical barrier is weak and susceptible to trauma, especially from adhesive stripping. Probes with weak adhesives only should be used.

# References

1. Holbrook, K.A. (1979) Human epidermal embryogenesis. *Int. J. Dermatol.*, **18**, 329–356
2. Holbrook, K.A. (1982) A histological comparison of infant and adult skin. In *Neonatal Skin* (H.I. Maibach, ed.), Marcel Dekker, New York, pp. 3–31
3. Evans, N.J. and Rutter, N. (1986) Development of the epidermis in the newborn. *Biol. Neonate*, **49**, 74–80
4. Harpin, V.A. and Rutter, N. (1982) Sweating in preterm babies. *J. Pediatr.*, **100**, 614–619
5. Hey, E.N. and Katz, G. (1969) Evaporative water loss in the newborn baby. *J. Physiol.*, **200**, 605–619
6. Foster, K.E., Hey, E.N. and Katz, G. (1969) The response of the sweat glands of the newborn baby to thermal stimuli and to intradermal acetyl choline. *J. Physiol.*, **203**, 13–29
7. Rutter, N. and Hull, D. (1979) Water loss from the skin of term and preterm babies. *Arch. Dis. Childh.*, **54**, 858–868
8. Hammarlund, K. and Sedin, G. (1979) Transepidermal water loss in newborn infants. III. Relation to gestational age. *Acta Paediatr. Scand.*, **68**, 795–801
9. Hammarlund, K., Sedin, G. and Stromberg, B. (1982) Transepidermal water loss in newborn infants. VII. Relation to postnatal age in very preterm and full term appropriate for gestational age infants. *Acta Paediatr. Scand.*, **71**, 360–374
10. Hammarlund, K., Sedin, G. and Stromberg, B. (1983) Transepidermal water loss in the newborn. VIII. Relation to gestational age and postnatal age in appropriate and small for gestational age infants. *Acta Paediatr. Scand.*, **72**, 721–728
11. Harpin, V.A. and Rutter, N. (1983) Barrier properties of the newborn infant's skin. *J. Pediatr.*, **102**, 419–425
12. Grice, K., Sathar, H., Sharratt, M. and Baker, H. (1971) Skin temperature and transepidermal water loss. *J. Invest. Dermatol.*, **57**, 108–110
13. Clark, R.P., Cross, K.W., Goff, M.R. *et al.* (1978) Neonatal natural and forced convection. *J. Physiol.*, **284**, 22–23
14. Stothers, J.K. (1980) The effect of forced convection on neonatal heat loss. *J. Physiol.*, **305**, 778
15. Thompson, M.H., Stothers, J.K. and McLellan, N.J. (1984) Weight and water loss in the neonate in natural and forced convection. *Arch. Dis. Childh.*, **59**, 951–956
16. Sedin, G., Hammarlund, K., Nilsson, G.E., Stromberg, B. and Oberg, P.A. (1985) Measurements of transepidermal water loss in newborn infants. *Clin. Perinatol.*, **12**, 79–99
17. Williams, P.R. and Oh, W. (1974) Effects of radiant warmer on insensible water loss in newborn infants. *Am. J. Dis. Child.*, **128**, 511–514
18. Wu, P.Y.K. and Hodgman, J.E. (1974) Insensible water loss in preterm infants: changes with postnatal development and non-ionizing radiant energy. *Pediatrics*, **54**, 704–712
19. Bell, E.F., Weinstein, M.R. and Oh, W. (1980) Heat balance in premature infants: comparative effects of convectively heated incubator and radiant warmer with and without plastic heat shield. *J. Pediatr.*, **96**, 460–465
20. Oh, W. and Karecki, H. (1972) Phototherapy and insensible water loss in the newborn infant. *Am. J. Dis. Child.*, **124**, 230–232
21. Bell, E.F., Neidich, G.A., Carshore, W.J. and Oh, W. (1979) Combined effect of radiant warmer and phototherapy on insensible water loss in low birthweight infants. *J. Pediatr.*, **94**, 810–813
22. Wheldon, A.C. and Rutter, N. (1982) The heat balance of small babies nursed in incubators and under radiant warmers. *Early Hum. Dev.*, **6**, 131–143
23. Darnall, R.A. (1981) Insensible weight loss measurements in newborn infants: possible over-estimation with the Potter baby scale. *J. Pediatr.*, **99**, 794–797
24. Doyle, L.W. and Sinclair, J.C. (1981) Thermal effect on a Potter baby scale. *Pediatr. Res.*, **15**, 658
25. Fanaroff, A.A., Wald, M., Gruber, H.S. and Klaus, M.H. (1972) Insensible water loss in low birth weight infants. *Pediatrics*, **50**, 236–245
26. Baumgart, S., Engle, W.D., Fox, W.W. and Polin, R.A. (1982) Radiant warmer power and body size as determinants of insensible water loss in the critically ill neonate. *Pediatr. Res.*, **15**, 1495–1499

27. Bell, E.F., Warburton, D. and Stonestreet, B.S. (1980) Effect of fluid administration on the development of symptomatic patent ductus arteriosus and congestive heart failure in premature infants. *N. Engl. J. Med.*, **302**, 598–604

28. Jones, R.W.A., Rochfort, M.J. and Baum, J.D. (1976) Increased insensible water loss in newborn infants nursed under radiant heaters. *Br. Med. J.*, **ii**, 1347–1350

29. Gill, A., Yu, V.Y.H., Bajuk, B. and Astbury, J. (1986) Postnatal growth in infants born before 30 weeks' gestation. *Arch. Dis. Childh.*, **61**, 549–553

30. Costarino, A. and Baumgart, S. (1986) Modern fluid and electrolyte management of the critically ill premature infant. *Pediatr. Clin. N. Am.*, **33**, 153–178

31. Marks, K.H., Friedman, Z. and Maisels, M.J. (1977) A simple device for reducing insensible water loss in low birth weight infants. *Pediatrics*, **60**, 223–226

32. Rutter, N. and Hull, D. (1981) Reduction of skin water loss in the newborn. I. Effect of applying topical agents. *Arch. Dis. Childh.*, **56**, 669–672

33. Brice, J.E.H., Rutter, N. and Hull, D. (1981) Reduction of skin water loss in the newborn. II. Clinical trial of two methods in very low birthweight babies. *Arch. Dis. Childh.*, **56**, 673–675

34. Harpin, V.A. and Rutter, N. (1985) Humidification of incubators. *Arch. Dis. Childh.*, **60**, 219–224

35. Baumgart, S., Engle, W.D., Fox, W.W. and Polin, R.A. (1981) Effect of heat shielding on convection and evaporation and radiant heat transfer in premature infants. *J. Paediatr.*, **99**, 948–956

36. Baumgart, S., Fox, W.W. and Polin, R.A. (1982) Physiologic implications of two different heat shields for infants under radiant warmers. *J. Pediatr.*, **100**, 787–790

37. Baumgart, S. (1984) Reduction of oxygen consumption, insensible water loss, and radiant heat demand with use of a plastic blanket for low birthweight infants under radiant warmers. *Pediatrics*, **75**, 89–99

38. Rutter, N. (1987) Percutaneous drug absorption in the newborn: hazards and used. *Clin. Perinatol.*, **14**, 911–930

39. Rayner, W. (1886) Cyanosis in newly born children caused by aniline marking ink. *Br. Med. J.*, **i**, 294–295

40. Scott, E.P., Prince, G.E. and Rotando, C.C. (1946) Dye poisoning in infancy. *J. Pediatr.*, **28**, 713–718

41. Kagan, B.M., Mirman, B., Calvin, J. and Lundeen, E. (1949) Cyanosis in premature infants due to aniline dye intoxication. *J. Pediatr.*, **34**, 574–578

42. Fisch, R.O., Berglund, E.G., Bridge, A.G., Finley, P.R., Quie, P.G. and Raille, R. (1963) Methemoglobinaemia in a hospital nursery. *J. Am. Med. Assoc.*, **185**, 760–763

43. Curley, A., Hawks, R.G., Kimbrough, R.D., Nathesson, G. and Finberg, L. (1971) Dermal absorption of hexachlorophene in infants. *Lancet*, **ii**, 296–297

44. Kopelman, A.E. (1973) Cutaneous absorption of hexachlorophene in low birth weight infants. *J. Pediatr.*, **82**, 972–975

45. Powell, H., Swarner, O., Gluck, L. and Lampert, P. (1973) Hexachlorophene myelinopathy in premature infants. *J. Pediatr.*, **82**, 976–981

46. Shuman, R.M., Leech, R.W. and Alvord, E.C. (1974) Neurotoxicity of hexachlorophene in the human. *Pediatrics*, **54**, 689–695

47. Chabrolle, J.P. and Rossier, A. (1978) Goitre and hypothyroidism in the newborn after cutaneous absorption of iodine. *Arch. Dis. Childh.*, **53**, 495–498

48. Schick, J.B. and Milstein, J.M. (1981) Burn hazard of isopropyl alcohol in the neonate. *Pediatrics*, **68**, 587–588

49. Harpin, V.A. and Rutter, N. (1982) Percutaneous alcohol absorption and skin necrosis in a preterm infant. *Arch. Dis. Childh.*, **57**, 477–479

50. Morrell, P., Hey, E., Mackee, I.W., Rutter, N. and Lewis, M. (1985) Deafness in a preterm baby associated with topical antibiotic spray containing neomycin. *Lancet*, **i**, 1167–1168

51. Aggett, P.J., Cooper, L.V., Ellis, S.H. and McAinsh, J. (1981) Percutaneous absorption of chlorhexidene in neonatal cord care. *Arch. Dis. Childh.*, **56**, 878–880

52. Evans, N.J. and Rutter, N. (1986) Percutaneous respiration in the newborn infant. *J. Pediatr.*, **108**, 282–286

53. Cartlidge, P.H.T. and Rutter, N. (1987) Percutaneous respiration in the newborn infant. *Biol. Neonate*, **52**, 301–306

54. Cartlidge, P.H.T. and Rutter, N. (1988) Percutaneous oxygen delivery to the preterm infant. *Lancet*, **i**, 315–317

55. Cartlidge P.H.T., Fox, P.E. and Rutter, N. (1990) The scars of newborn intensive care. *Early Hum. Dev.*, **21**, 1–10

56. Cartlidge, P.H.T. and Rutter, N. (1987) Karaya gum electrodes for the preterm infant. *Arch. Dis. Childh.*, **62**, 1281–1282

57. Anon (1989) *Lancet*, **ii**, 1138

58. Knauth, A., Gordin, M., McNelis, W. and Baumgart, S. (1989) Semipermeable polyurethane membrane as an artificial skin for the premature neonate. *Pediatrics*, **83**, 945–950

# 9

# Monitoring

Peter Rolfe

The challenges of monitoring key physiological variables in the ELBW baby are evident immediately after birth during initial assessment and resuscitation. Attaching sensors or electrodes to the highly hydrated, thin baby with fragile skin is really the essence of the problem [1]. Although it was in the mid 1970s that the particular monitoring needs of the small neonate were recognized [2–4], ideal sensors and instruments for the ELBW baby are still not available.

Technological developments continue to take place, and improvements to both invasive and non-invasive approaches are being made steadily. Advances in other fields of science and technology offer new sensing techniques, devices, and computer-based instrumentation, and these may improve monitoring of the ELBW baby.

The improvements in survival of ELBW babies, probably largely due to advances in respiratory support, will only continue if the methods of diagnosis and therapy are thoroughly assessed in an organized prospective manner. Existing and new monitoring systems should be assessed for their impact on outcome; at the same time these monitoring systems can represent the core of an assessment regimen, if carefully planned [5].

## The monitoring strategy

The primary aim of monitoring is, of course, to gather pertinent physiological data to allow effective clinical decision making. In addition, the clinical care of the ELBW baby must contain elements of development, and of research, as new ideas are tried and evaluated and as the successful approaches move into routine clinical practice. A planned monitoring strategy does not only ensure optimum care for an individual baby, but also represents a key component of development and evaluation.

The methods and devices used for monitoring the ELBW baby will inevitably be a sub-set of the monitoring facilities in the NICU [5]. Indeed, this is essential to ensure uniformity as part of the improvements arising from assessment. In practice, this means that monitoring facilities for all babies should be planned as a package, including sensors, electrodes, monitors, displays, and means for data storage and analysis. If sensors are suitable for ELBW babies they will almost certainly be suitable for bigger babies, but particular care is needed with the ELBW baby to avoid skin trauma with externally applied sensors [6]. Therefore the following key points relate to monitoring in general, but they are critical in achieving effective results with all babies.

### Avoiding data gaps

The full potential of monitoring can only be achieved when there is continuity of data collection. Hand-written records, perhaps supplemented by strips of chart recordings, continue to be the norm in most centres, and this is unlikely to be replaced by complete automation of data collection in the forseeable future. Nevertheless, there are simple ways to minimize the likelihood of *data gaps*. The essence of this is to standardize the sequence of manual and automatic data collection, and utilize a graphical representation, probably manually annotated, to depict the key events from birth continuing into the intensive care period.

With the ELBW baby there is a particular need to collect key physiological variables as soon as possible after delivery. In fact, there is an argument to be made for taking advantage of fetal monitoring signals when they are available, and achieving this is just a logistical issue. For example, scalp clip fetal ECG electrodes may remain in place long enough to provide immediate access for heart rate information. However, even with this approach there will be a data gap between the moment of birth and the first monitored events: the first breath; the first heart rate measurement; core temperature at delivery and so on.

The next most frequent break in continuity of data occurs after the initial clinical assessment of the baby, and possible resuscitation, when the baby is transported to the NICU. Portable battery-operated monitors are available and should be part of the standard equipment.

### Ensuring the validity of data

Monitoring of physiological variables, using sensors of any type, makes it essential to validate measurements. This most frequently entails *calibration*, whether this be of the blood gas sensor attached to the baby, or the laboratory instrument used for *in vitro* analysis [7]. Confirmation of each calibration point can then be included in the record system. This then helps with the task of interpreting events when, as is common, monitoring sensors or instruments are found to have drifted out of calibration.

### The role of computers

Both of the first two key points can benefit from a clear policy for the use of computers. This matter is influenced by departmental and hospital policies, although storage of data from clinical monitors can be localized rather than being passed to a hospital information system.

Given the widespread general acceptance and use of computers, it is reasonable to ask how they might simplify and improve monitoring the ELBW baby. There is always a danger of complicating any task simply by using a computer when it is not really necessary; so great caution is needed. Computers are good at several tasks, such as processing signals, statistical analysis, creating data bases, providing clinical decision support, and improving the display of information. However, if used badly computers merely expand data rather than compress them, and thereby add confusion to already complex situations and tasks. It must also be remembered that reliable computer software is expensive to develop and to maintain.

The clinical monitoring instruments now used almost invariably contain their own microcomputers for processing and displaying the signals and some derived variables, but the user need not be aware of the role of the computer here. Nevertheless, there is probably even more need now to question the addition of further computers to such computer-based monitors, unless the case has been considered very carefully.

### Manipulating signals and data

The primary signals from monitors can be manipulated to derive secondary indices, such as long-term heart rate variability, or the trend of $Pa_{O_2}$. Monitoring babies over two or three days generates a huge number of data, and computers can usefully be used to *compress* this quantity by producing indices, rather than merely recording all of primary data [8]. Summaries of key variables over the duration of intensive care can then be generated semi-automatically by a relatively simple program running on an inexpensive PC or similar computer.

### Support for clinical decisions

The field of artificial intelligence was launched upon the medical world with the promise of bringing fundamental changes to diagnosis and therapy [9]. More than two decades later, very little tangible progress has been made in influencing clinical practice. An extension of basic computer processing of monitored signals is to perform automated signal interpretation, both as part of data verification and in an attempt to contribute to clinical decision making.

# Cardiac monitoring

Continuous monitoring of heart rate and breathing are, of course, still the minimum requirements for all ELBW babies. The addition of continuous arterial pressure monitoring is considered essential by some, whilst others are content with intermittent measurements. The combination of heart rate and breathing monitoring has also attracted some attention as the basis of pattern analysis in so-called cardiorespirography. Numerous combinations of sensors have been developed for such monitoring, and in assessing their use for preterm babies certain conclusions may be drawn concerning their use with the very smallest babies.

## ECG and heart rate monitoring

### *Electrodes*

There is no doubt that the initial resuscitation and stabilization of the ELBW baby immediately after delivery is greatly facilitated by the use of an efficient means for heart rate monitoring. This is best achieved by detecting the ECG, which is most likely to give a reliable signal for heart rate monitoring. Many approaches for the attachment of ECG electrodes have been tried, including conventional adhesives, clips, clamps and even needles. Electrodes can be attached by suction [1]. A relatively low negative pressure ($\approx 80$ mmHg) applied in an annular groove around a soft plastic moulding containing a silver/silver chloride electrode has been found to be quite successful, and this level of suction is tolerated by the skin of the ELBW baby for the period of resuscitation. Three of these electrodes may be placed on the resuscitation table and the baby laid directly on them as the wet skin improves the security of the suction attachment.

The evolution of ECG electrodes for longer-term monitoring of tiny babies has been a long and difficult process. The earlier large and rigid electrodes have been replaced by smaller, flexible electrodes, but chemical adhesive attachment is at present an unhappy result. On the

one hand, aggressive adhesives are more likely to keep the electrode in place, but some skin damage seems inevitable, and on the other hand the milder adhesives lead to annoying false alarms due to electrode detachment. In the last 5 years good experience has been gained with electrodes made of natural Karaya gum [10,1]. This has very good skin compatible characteristics, and electrodes are now available from several firms. The moistened gum adheres quite well to even the smallest babies, and the incorporated thin silver film does not require the normal electrode conductive gel or cream. Remoistening of the gum is needed frequently when the baby is nursed under a radiant warmer, but the incidence of skin trauma is very low.

Most cables and leads for connecting electrodes to monitors are still not ideal. The basic arrangement of having a single relatively heavy and robust cable connected to the monitor, with a small connector block at its end for attachment of the three lighter, individual electrode leads, is a sound principle. The cable can generally withstand the harsh treatment to which it is subject in a busy neonatal unit, but the electrode leads still require improvement. Very fine, light, and flexible electrode leads have some advantages for the ELBW baby, but they do frequently become tangled and can then make rapid access to the baby awkward and inconvenient.

Future research on ECG electrodes, leads, cables and associated amplifiers and displays is undoubtedly still needed to produce more reliable heart rate monitoring for the ELBW baby. Ideally, of course, the electrode attachment and contact problem should be eliminated entirely, and there were attempts, some twenty years ago, to use a thin metallized plastic plate on which to place the naked baby and thereby eliminate individual fixed electrode connections. This approach was clearly unencumbering for the baby, but signal reliability was poor, but could perhaps now be improved using modern electronic and computing techniques. An alternative approach for the elimination of electrode contact problems is to take advantage of nasogastric tubes whenever they are in place. Polymer feeding tubes can easily be constructed to incorporate small conductive regions, using wire or ring elements, and very reliable oesophageal ECG monitoring can be achieved.

## Monitoring instruments

Of course, once the problems of electrodes, leads and cables have been completely solved, the selection of an associated ECG and heart rate monitor has no special requirements for the ELBW baby. Nevertheless, the noise and artefact produced by non-ideal electrodes and cables are less likely to be troublesome with the high quality ECG amplifiers found in monitors such as those available from, for example, Hellige, Kontron and Hewlett–Packard.

The electronic systems used in monitors for detecting each cardiac complex are now quite sophisticated and can cope with rather poor signals and high noise levels, and so highly reliable calculation of heart rate is possible. In fetal monitoring, calculation of heart rate variability can have clinical value and there is some evidence that neonatal heart rate variability monitoring may also be useful [11]. Current ECG monitors do have the option for calculation and display of short-term and long-term heart rate variability, and the evaluation of these parameters in the ELBW baby could be helpful.

## Arterial pressure measurement

In many centres it is still common to insert umbilical artery catheters for blood gas and pH measurement, and arterial pressure measurement via the catheter is then useful in its own right, as well as providing an important guide to catheter patency. In very small babies it is of course necessary to use small catheters (eg 4 FG), and the problem of catheter lumen blockage due to thrombus formation can be significant. The phasic arterial pressure waveform can be monitored reliably through small bore catheters by means of modern low volume-displacement pressure transducers, which may be connected either directly to the Luer fitting of the catheter, or at some 60 cm distance attached by saline-filled monometer tubing. Ideally the phasic pressure waveform should be displayed on a monitor screen so that smoothing

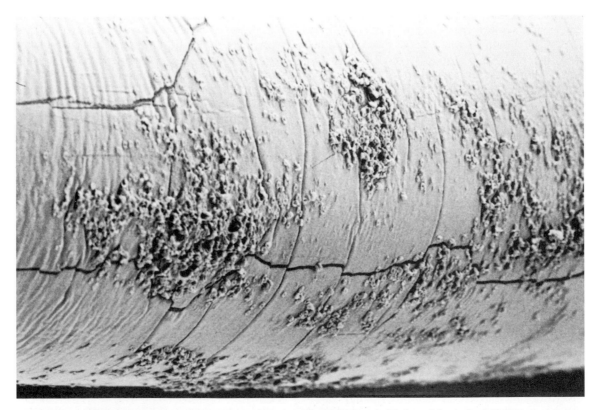

**Figure 9.1** An SEM of an umbilical artery catheter after use. The catheter was fabricated from plasticized poly(vinyl chloride)

and damping of the waveform due to progressive lumen blockage can be easily detected. The Luer fitting transducers have been commercially available for many years [2] and in the last decade single-use disposable transducers have become widely used (eg Gould). The use of conventional blood pressure transducers (eg Hewlett-Packard) was greatly simplified by the introduction of disposable pressure domes, obviating the need for the cumbersome and time-consuming sterilization of the transducer which was necessary in the past. Catheter patency can undoubtedly be improved by continuous infusion through the catheter by means of intra-flow devices or similar. In spite of these precautionary measures arterial catheters must still be regarded as potential hazards through thrombus formation, and improved catheter materials are needed. It is now well established that plasticized poly(vinyl chloride) (PVC) catheters have far worse haemocompatibility characteristics than the more recently introduced material polyurethane (see Figure 9.1). In spite of this PVC catheters continue to be used in many centres.

Non-invasive arterial pressure measurement is clearly desirable. Many systems are now available based on the use of limb encircling cuffs and the so-called oscillometric principle. With this technique mean arterial pressure is first measured from a measurement of the cuff pressure at which cardiac related pulsations in the cuff reach maximum amplitude. Subsequently systolic and diastolic pressures may be obtained. These arterial pressure monitors are now widely used for semicontinuous monitoring. However, the cuff needs to be matched to the size of the baby's limb, otherwise systematic errors will be introduced. Furthermore, repeated automatic inflation of the cuff is not recommended in very small fragile babies with poor peripheral perfusion. A non-invasive technique for continuous arterial pressure measurement has been described, but further research is necessary before this technique is available for routine use [12].

## Respiratory assessment

### Monitoring breathing and detecting apnoea

Reliable, meaningful monitoring of breathing and detection of apnoea are still difficult to achieve in very small babies. The basic problem arises from the difficulties of constructing appropriately small, sensitive, reliable, unencumbering sensors and connecting cables. The choice of methods includes those that measure: impedance, EMG, chest expansion, pressure, movements and air flow.

The improved ECG electrodes mentioned above may also be used for monitoring transthoracic electrical impedance to give a moderately reliable breathing signal. In spite of this electrode improvement, further significant improvements are needed in the impedance monitors themselves to deal with movement artefacts before this method is adequate for the ELBW baby. Although under certain circumstances impedance pneumography can produce signals which correlate well with tidal volume, this is difficult to achieve over extended periods of time. Nevertheless, the basic signal is used for apnoea detection.

A further technique employing abdominal surface electrodes records the diaphragm EMG, and processing of this leads to a signal which has been reported to correlate with tidal volume [13].

Dimensional changes of the chest and abdomen associated with breathing can be recorded with strain gauges, magnetometers, inflatable jackets and inductive straps [3, 5,14,15]. However, none of these methods is ideal for the ELBW baby because of the encumbrance of the necessary straps, bands or coils which must be placed around the chest or abdomen. Changes in curvature of the chest or abdominal wall during breathing can be detected by a small plastic pressure capsule, such as that developed by Wright & Callan [16]. This technique has acceptable performance as an apnoea detector, and can be improved in terms of reliability by using two capsules, one to detect thoracic cage movement and the other abdominal movements.

The conventional lung function approach of recording intra-oesophageal pressure changes can be useful in some very small babies. Ideally, of course, an appropriate latex rubber balloon attached to a flexible plastic catheter should be used to make accurate measurements of intra-oesophageal, and thereby intra-thoracic, pressure changes. However, a liquid filled, open-ended catheter or feeding tube is almost as good for quantitative pressure monitoring, and is adequate for apnoea monitoring in the very small baby. Furthermore, the feeding tube can be further modified to carry small wire contacts to enable either EMG detection or electrical impedance monitoring of breathing via the oesophagus, and this is actually more convenient and more reliable than using surface electrodes on the chest or abdomen.

Apnoea detection without electrodes or other sensors attached directly to the baby first became feasible with the introduction of Lewin's air-filled multi-compartment mattress [17]. That device is still used, although it lacks the sensitivity needed for very small babies. Mattress-type apnoea monitors using the same approach of detecting the weight re-distribution produced by breathing have now been improved by using very sensitive, thin, pressure sensitive pads. These monitors (eg Draeger Medical or Eastwood and Son) perform well with the very small babies, although it is important to position the pad such that cardiac movement during apnoea does not prevent the alarm being activated.

Obstructive apnoea will not be detected by any of the methods mentioned above, since all are indirect and do not sense respired gas flow. Small thermistors or thermocouples can be used to detect nasal gas flow, but this approach is not entirely reliable and cannot easily be used as a clinical routine. Undoubtedly this is an area for further research, and consideration should perhaps be given to improved $CO_2$ sensors or to the use of microphones for detection of gas flow.

Monitoring lung function is something which has not really been achieved as a routine clinical procedure, despite the large amount of work done within clinical research [18]. The difficulties of monitoring lung function in spontaneously breathing babies of course relate to the practical problems of attaching flow and pressure measuring sensors to the airway; single measurements can be made, but continuous monitoring is not feasible. However, in the mechanically ventilated baby there are good opportunities to make continuous long-term measurements of certain key respiratory variables.

## Blood gas and pH measurement

### Invasive methods

The umbilical artery catheter is still widely used to allow arterial sampling for intermittent $Po_2$, $Pco_2$ and pH measurement. Laboratory blood gas analysers which have been introduced over the last 5 years now allow very small volumes of blood to be used, and of course this is important for the small baby. The problems associated with thrombus formation in arterial catheters have already been mentioned above, and at present these put a limitation on the time during which blood gas and pH assessment may be achieved on the basis of arterial sampling. Polyurethane catheters undoubtedly improve this problem, but substantial further research is needed to produce new polymers or surface coatings to achieve long-term haemocompatibility [19]. This is particularly important when it is necessary to resort to the use of radial artery puncture or catheterization.

Indwelling $Po_2$ sensors have promised much over the past 2 decades, but the reality has been disappointing. The first devices to be used in the human neonate gave very exciting indications of abrupt changes and short-term trends in arterial $Po_2$, in spite of the fact that these devices were based on PVC catheters and membranes which are now known to be inferior [20,21,22]. Since those early days more is demanded of the performance of arterial $Po_2$ sensors, in terms of reliability, stability and safety, and it seems clear that there is no suitable commercial device available for use in the ELBW baby. Once again, the key to success will be the utilization of modern polymers to construct 3.5–4.0 FG catheter tip $Po_2$ sensors, together with the incorporation of haemocompatible gas permeable membranes for the active part of the sensor [23].

Fibreoptic catheter oximeters are available for continuous arterial oxygen saturation monitoring (eg Oximetrix). These are available in 4 FG catheters, and the use of polyurethane together with an end sampling eye produces quite good haemocompatible features. The use of oxygen saturation for the control of arterial oxygen levels in the small preterm baby is not entirely satisfactory. The S-shaped oxyhaemoglobin binding curve means that at relatively high levels of oxygenation very small changes in saturation accompany very large changes in oxygen partial pressure. The prevention of hyperoxaemia in terms of oxygen partial pressure is therefore very demanding of precision and accuracy in oxygen saturation measurement. This situation is worsened by a

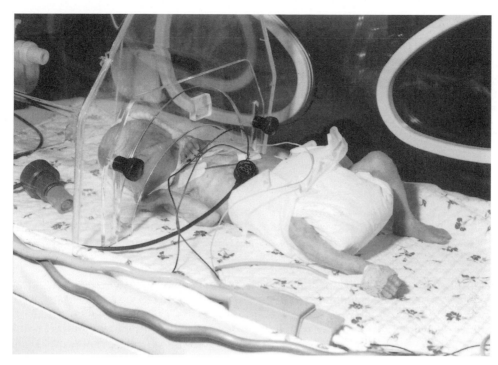

**Figure 9.2** Sensors for monitoring ECG transcutaneous $P_{O_2}$ and $P_{CO_2}$ and oxygen saturation attached to an ELBW baby

significant left shift of the binding curve with fetal haemoglobin. Thus if one's clinical approach is to achieve control of arterial $P_{O_2}$ by $O_2$ saturation monitoring, it is essential, first, to determine the precise position of the oxyhaemoglobin binding curve and, second, to ensure that the precision and accuracy of the oximeter is adequate.

The direct arterial monitoring of $P_{CO_2}$ and pH in the small newborn baby is still not yet feasible as a clinical routine. Catheter tip sensors have been described in the literature [24,25] but as yet these have not been refined sufficiently to overcome the major problems of stability and freedom from thrombogenesis. It is possible that optical sensors based on spectrophotometric and fluorimetric techniques will eventually produce invasive sensors for $P_{O_2}$, $P_{CO_2}$ and pH [26].

### Non-invasive techniques

Non-invasive estimation of arterial $P_{O_2}$ and $P_{CO_2}$, using so-called transcutaneous techniques, can be used to complement intermittent arterial blood sampling (Figure 9.2). The relationships between skin surface and arterial

values of $P_{O_2}$ and $P_{CO_2}$ are, of course, influenced by epidermal thickness and gas permeability, as well as many other factors. In the very small preterm baby this leads to skin surface $P_{O_2}$ values which may be approximately 10% above arterial $P_{O_2}$ in the range 8–12 kPa (60–90 mmHg). Early theoretical work by Thunstrom *et al.* [27] and Lubbers [28], together with more recent clinical results, has emphasized the fact that the relationship between the $P_{O_2}$ at the skin and in an artery is non-linear; the skin surface $P_{O_2}$ is significantly lower than arterial $P_{O_2}$ when it is above 13 kPa. The electrical heating of skin surface gas sensors is critically important, and can be problematical. On the one hand adequate heating of the skin is necessary to induce the maximal vasodilatation which is essential for the $P_{O_2}$ measurement to be essentially independent of moderate fluctuations in cutaneous perfusion. On the other hand the small preterm baby's skin can be very sensitive to the required heating, and this necessitates the sensor being moved to a new site every 1 or 2 hours, depending upon the size of the baby [29]. A skin surface temperature of 42°C is probably optimal in very small babies, but it is

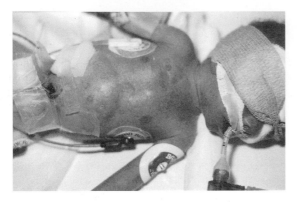

**Figure 9.3** Skin trauma can be caused by heated transcutaneous gas sensors. They should be moved frequently, and skin can be protected by a spray-on dressing [30]

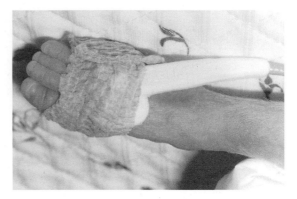

**Figure 9.4** Pulse oximetry optical sensors are still very large when compared with the hand or foot of the ELBW baby

often not appreciated that the sensor temperature which is set on the associated monitor may be as much as 2°C higher than the skin surface temperature achieved beneath the sensor. This temperature gradient between the sensor and the skin surface also varies according to the precise design of the sensor, and will therefore differ from manufacturer to manufacturer. For these reasons it is essential for centres to evaluate the overall performance which is being achieved with the sensors, instrumentation, and protocols being employed. Skin damage produced by transcutaneous sensors can be reduced by using a spray-on dressing [30] (Figure 9.3).

Skin surface $P_{CO_2}$ monitoring is still not used as widely as skin surface $P_{O_2}$ monitoring. Generally the sensor temperature is less critical for $P_{CO_2}$ monitoring, although maximal vasodilatation must still be achieved. Once again it is essential for individual centres to establish their own protocols for this method to produce useful information.

When both skin surface $P_{O_2}$ and $P_{CO_2}$ are to be monitored there is a certain practical advantage in employing a single sensor which combines means for both $P_{O_2}$ and $P_{CO_2}$ measurement. This of course reduces the number of devices which must be attached to the relatively small exposed surface area of the baby, and furthermore it is obviously much less demanding in terms of sensor calibration, membrane changing, and application site rotation. The combined $O_2/CO_2$ transcutaneous sensors are now more reliable and are beginning to be used more widely clinically.

There is now widespread use of pulse oximetry for non-invasive estimation of arterial oxygen saturation. This method, originally developed for use in adults [31] utilizes the pulsatile blood volume change in a digit or palm to calculate, spectrophotometrically, oxygen saturation (Figure 9.4). The method has become popular because it is very much easier to use than conventional transcutaneous gas monitoring. The sensors do not need to be heated, and the optical sensors are very much more stable than the electrochemical sensors for $P_{O_2}$ and $P_{CO_2}$ measurement. However, pulse oximetry should be used with caution in small preterm babies due to the limitations imposed by the shape of the oxyhaemoglobin binding curve at high levels of oxygenation, referred to above. The precision and accuracy of the various commercially available pulse oximeters has not yet been established in detail, and it is therefore not clear at what level of oxygen saturation nominal safety thresholds should be set. Once again there is an urgent need for users to assess the performance and limitations of the means which they employ before basing clinical management on the data derived.

## Monitoring and mechanical ventilation

Since mechanical ventilation represents a critical component of therapy in the ELBW baby it is inevitable that it should be considered within an overall monitoring strategy. Manipulation of the various modes and parameters of mechanical ventilation needs to be recorded alongside key physiological variables, especially blood gas and blood pressure. In this way, then, the mechanical ventilator should be monitored either directly or indirectly. Certainly it is relatively straightforward to monitor pressure and flow waveforms, and then to abstract from these the main descriptors, peak pressure, end expiratory pressure, mean airway pressure, inspired and expired times, for recording and display. Some ventilators now provide output signals for direct monitoring, but if not then use of a blood pressure transducer attached to the endotracheal tube connector, and a small pneumotachograph to record tidal flow, can be employed.

Ventilator monitoring in this way can be extended to allow continuous assessment of lung mechanics [32]. Pressure–volume loops can easily be derived, and derivation of total compliance and airways resistance then performed. Addition of an oesophageal catheter with a pressure transducer then allows more detailed analysis of pulmonary compliance to be performed [33].

# Cerebral monitoring

Hypoxic–ischaemic brain injury remains a major clinical concern. There have been significant research activities since the early 1970s on this major problem, and some interesting new methodologies have emerged, although most of these remain research tools and do not play a major part in routine clinical monitoring. This situation is likely to continue until it becomes firmly established that there is some real benefit to clinical management through the monitoring of one or more of the relevant variables. Beyond the obvious importance of detecting haemorrhage, hydrocephalus etc. using appropriate scanning methods (see Chapter 18) there continues to be interest in the investigation and assessment of cerebral circulation. In this respect the study of intracranial pressure, cerebral blood flow, and cerebral blood volume are relevant.

## Intracranial pressure monitoring

Knowledge of mean arterial pressure and intracranial pressure (ICP) allows the cerebral perfusion pressure to be calculated, and this can be important in deciding whether or not some intervention is required to ensure adequate cerebral perfusion. Invasive and non-invasive techniques have been used in small preterm babies with varying degrees of success. Levene and Evans [34] have evolved an invasive technique for the newborn baby which had originally been developed for adult monitoring by Lundberg [35]. The method involves passing a 16 G intravenous cannula through the lateral margin of the anterior fontanelle into the subarachnoid space. Pressure is then measured via the cannula, either with a miniature Luer fitting pressure transducer or by a conventional blood pressure transducer connected to the cannula by a saline filled manometer tube. Several groups of large infants have been monitored with this invasive technique, and in a small group of babies who had failed to develop regular breathing immediately after birth and who had convulsions and were being mechanically ventilated, maximum pressures ranged from 10 mmHg ($13.6 \text{ cmH}_2\text{O}$) to 48 mmHg ($65.3 \text{ cmH}_2\text{O}$) [34]. Using this method, babies with raised intracranial pressure 8 (above 10 mmHg) ($13.6 \text{ cmH}_2\text{O}$) could be treated with mannitol or dexamethasone [36]. Although when used with great care the invasive technique is an acceptable method for deriving important clinical data, an appropriate non-invasive technique must be preferred in terms of both safety and convenience. Many attempts have been made since the late 1960s to develop satisfactory sensors which may be attached to the anterior fontanelle to derive a reliable estimate of intracranial pressure. The very earliest sensors [37] were relatively large, and were held manually in place over the anterior fontanelle to make single measurements. The principle utilized by these and subsequent non-invasive sensors is that of applanation. With this method, the bulging fontanelle is flattened by the sensor, and in this situation the externally applied pressure exactly balances the intracranial pressure. Continuous non-invasive ICP monitoring became more of a reality when the Ladd miniature sensor became available [38]. This sensor was originally developed for invasive monitoring in adults, but may be fixed to the anterior fontanelle in very small babies. However, the method of fixation is not straightforward and can introduce errors [39], and furthermore the system has a high cost. A small pneumatic sensor was developed [40], and this had the advantage of being low cost, although quantitative performance has not been good [41]. The refinement of a sensor originally developed for non-invasive intravenous pressure in adults has now been found to give good correlations with direct invasive measurements; no errors are associated with attachment, and it is of very low cost [42]. This sensor is small and light, is attached with collodion to the anterior fontanelle, and allows continuous monitoring of pressure for several days if necessary.

## Cerebral blood flow

A knowledge of arterial pressure and of intracranial pressure is useful in making assessments of cerebral perfusion. However, there has long been a desire for a method with which cerebral blood flow (CBF) could be monitored continuously in small newborn babies. It is still the case that no method exists which will allow such continuous monitoring, although for research purposes it is possible to use one or more of a range of methods to obtain some information [43]. Of the available methods, Doppler ultrasound, cranial electrical impedance, and near infra-red spectroscopy (NIRS) are the three which are most likely to allow clinical monitoring to any extent.

It is relatively straightforward to use Doppler ultrasound systems to obtain a qualitative indication of short-term pulsatile changes of arterial or venous blood velocity. Small ultrasound sensors can be positioned to direct a beam of ultrasound at the carotid arteries, the jugular veins, the anterior cerebral arteries, the sagittal sinus, and the middle cerebral artery. In order to derive a quantitative measure of volumetric blood flow (ie ml per 100 g per minute) it is essential to know: the angle between the ultrasound beam and the direction of blood flow; the internal diameter of the blood vessel, including pulsatile changes throughout the cardiac cycle; and the distribution of blood flow across the vessel diameter – the velocity profile. Some of these problems can be overcome when the Doppler ultrasound system is combined with a real-time ultrasound scanner, to produce the so-called Duplex system. In the very small preterm baby it is important to be sure that the resolution of

the Doppler ultrasound system is adequate for the very small blood vessels of interest. The ultrasound scanner allows beam–vessel angle to be determined, as well as enabling individual vessels to be visualized and the depth selectivity of so-called range-gated systems to be adjusted optimally. Nevertheless, in the very small baby lateral and depth resolution of the ultrasound system may be inadequate to separate flow in adjacent vessels. Research and development in this field continues, and improvements to resolution and to the methods of processing the Doppler signals are being made. In the absence of quantitative measures there have been attempts to derive indices from the blood velocity waveforms (eg the pulsatility index), but these must be used with caution [43].

The electrical impedance of the head, measured with four small EEG-type electrodes, is determined by the relative proportions of the main components – the scalp, skull, CSF, brain tissue, and blood. Accumulation of blood in the lateral ventricles will produce a change in the electrical impedance, and this may be detected by an impedance monitor, or may be displayed as a crude image using electrical impedance imaging techniques [44,45]. With each cardiac cycle there is a small reduction in the electrical impedance of the head due to the pulsatile blood volume increase. By means of computer processing techniques this signal can be monitored for several days continuously [46]. The pulsatile impedance signal has been found to exhibit a useful correlation with other non-invasive estimates of CBF, and at present this method is the one which most closely approaches the requirements of a routine clinical monitor although it must be emphasized that it cannot at present provide quantitative measures of CBF.

The technique of *in vivo* NIRS [47] has progressed considerably since it was first developed, and it is described in more detail below. In addition to allowing cerebral oxygenation to be monitored, NIRS can be used to estimate cerebral blood volume (CBV) and possibly CBF (see below).

## Cerebral oxygenation and metabolism

Interest in the investigation of cerebral metabolism in connection with brain haemorrhage

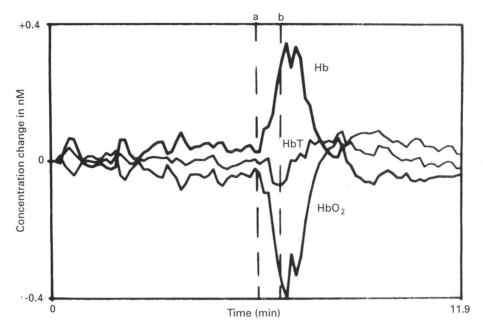

**Figure 9.5** This shows a recording obtained from the head of a baby of 27 weeks' gestation, using near infrared spectroscopy. Heart rate fell from 144 beats min$^{-1}$ at (*a*) to 68 beats min$^{-1}$ at *(b)*. (Reproduced with permission from *Archives of Disease in Childhood* (1991), **66**, 376–380)

and hypoxic-ischaemic brain injury continues. Magnetic resonance spectroscopy (MRS) can provide important information on the relevant phosphorus-linked compounds involved in intracellular metabolic processes [48]. Important studies have been performed in neonates using MRS, but there are considerable practical difficulties in transporting and managing sick babies for this expensive procedure. Since MRS does not allow continuous clinical monitoring the method of *in vivo* NIRS [49] attracted much interest in the mid-1980s as a potential monitoring technique. In the past 5 years substantial progress has been made in establishing the underpinning science of the method, and it is now at the stage where clinical research studies can be performed [50–53].

*In vivo* NIRS relies on the fact that light in the near infrared part of the spectrum (between 750 and 1000 nm) passes through most biological tissues very easily compared to visible light. This means that it is possible to interrogate the neonatal brain by transillumination using specialized monitoring equipment [54–56] (OBC Ltd, Market Drayton, UK). In practice, near infrared light at four wavelengths is fed through a flexible glass fibre to the head, and after passage through the head

the light is collected by a second fibre. There are clear absorption bands for oxyhaemoglobin and deoxyhaemoglobin, and for the key respiratory enzyme cytochrome aa$_3$ [57]. Processing of the absorption at each wavelength then allows estimation of the concentrations of cerebral oxygenated haemoglobin, deoxygenated haemoglobin, total haemoglobin, and possibly oxidized cytochrome aa$_3$.

The recordings of NIRS-derived variables (see Figures 9.5 and 9.6) can give a very good impression of the changes which occur within the brain under a variety of circumstances, such as during apnoea, or with changes in the mode of mechanical ventilation [52,58]. These recordings are semiquantitative, because the absolute values of each variable can not yet be quantified [59]. The calculation of the concentrations of each particular chemical, such as HbO$_2$ or Hb, requires a knowledge of the path length of the light as it passes through the tissue. Since light is significantly scattered in tissues the optical path-length is much greater than the physical path-length, by a factor of around 4.3 [58]. Although an estimate of optical path-length can be made under laboratory conditions it is not yet possible to do this clinically, and until this can be done it will not

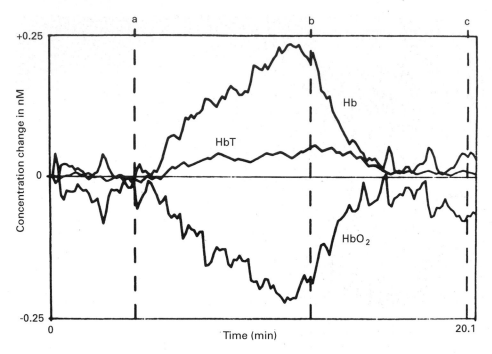

**Figure 9.6** Near infrared spectroscopy recordings from a 30 weeks' gestation baby. Arterial oxygen saturation fell gradually from 94% at *(a)* to 83% at *(b)*. (Reproduced with permission from Archives of Disease in Childhood (1991), **66**, 376–380)

be possible to make continuous quantitative recordings of absolute measurements. Research is underway to develop methods to achieve absolute quantitation, and this is likely to be possible in the near future.

Changes of CBV can be inferred from the calculated concentrations of Hb and $HbO_2$, but it must be assumed that haematocrit remains constant. It has also been reported that $O_2$ may be used as a tracer to calculate single point values of CBF [60]. This involves changing $O_2$ saturation abruptly, as monitored with a rapidly responding pulse oximeter, and then detecting the change of oxyhaemoglobin which occurs in the brain, with CBF then being calculated by means of a Fickian analysis.

The optical fibres and probes used for measurement are still relatively cumbersome for use in the ELBW baby. These are being improved, and already it is possible to apply probes and fibres to the fetal head during labour [61].

It has been conjectured that since cytochrome $aa_3$ is responsible for the utilization of 95% of cellular oxygen in the brain, continuous monitoring of the redox state of this enzyme could possibly provide a more pertinent guide

to oxygen therapy and the general management of very small babies at risk of haemorrhage and hypoxic-ischaemic brain injury [49]. Although there is some evidence that it is possible to detect the redox changes of the enzyme under carefully controlled conditions in animals [62], there is at present no firm evidence that this can be achieved in the human. This controversy is likely to be resolved within the next year or two.

## Multiple sensors

There is clearly an advantage when monitoring the ELBW baby in the use of sensors for measuring more than one variable. This approach means that less space is required on the baby for the devices, and also less time is needed by nursing and clinical staff for sensor attachment and subsequent management. There have already been some attempts to produce multiple sensors, and some are used on a local basis, but most of these have not been produced as commercially available devices.

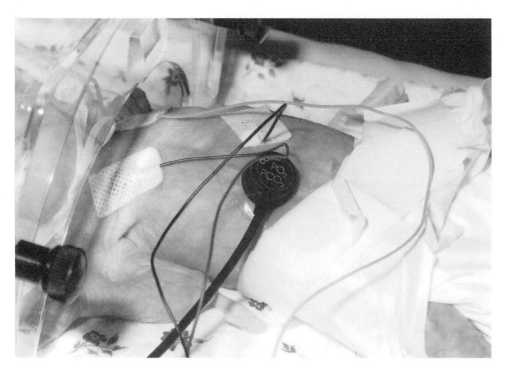

**Figure 9.7** Combined $O_2$/$CO_2$ transcutaneous sensors are now more reliable, but still need to be smaller

A monitoring system which combined sensors within an umbilical artery catheter for measurement of $P\text{a}O_2$, core temperature, systolic and diastolic blood pressure, and heart rate was described and has been used clinically [63]. The multiple sensor consists of a two-lumen catheter, with a $PO_2$ sensor and a thermocouple at its tip, blood pressure being measured through one catheter lumen and heart rate derived from the phasic blood pressure waveform.

Combined $PO_2$ and $PCO_2$ sensors have been produced for both invasive and non-invasive use. For example, a catheter sensor which contained a $PO_2$ electrode and a pH electrode for indirect $PCO_2$ measurement has been described [64], but not extensively used. The combined $O_2$/$CO_2$ transcutaneous sensors are now widely used (Figure 9.7), and are now more convenient in clinical use and are more stable.

In adult intensive care, placement of devices within the oesophagus forms the basis of reliable and convenient monitoring of several physiological variables. As mentioned above, neonatal feeding tubes can be modified to contain ECG electrodes, and these may also be used simultaneously for electrical impedance monitoring of breathing activity. The feeding tube may also contain a thermocouple or thermistor for core temperature monitoring. The lumen of the feeding tube can be used to monitor oesophageal pressure changes associated with breathing. In the adult, it has also proven possible to include ultrasound crystals to measure aortic blood flow.

NIRS has the potential for multiple variable monitoring, for circulatory, blood gas, and metabolic information [52]. The attachment of fibreoptic bundles, one each side of the head, can be combined with a pair of ECG electrodes and a temperature sensor, thus providing a great deal of the information needed for routine monitoring.

## Temperature monitoring

The effective thermal control of the ELBW baby can contribute to improving survival rates. It is helpful to have a complete picture of thermal status from the moment of birth, and, although not ideal, temperature measurement and monitoring can contribute to the creation of such a picture. The actual recording of temperature data from single or continuous measurements can of course be dealt with as described above, but the types and placement of thermometers and sensors is worthwhile considering.

At delivery early measurements of core temperature are useful to detect infection and to assess the likelihood of subsequent hypothermia [65]. Estimation of core temperature from body surface mounted probes can be achieved, as described below, but the method has a long response time and is therefore not suitable for rapid postpartum assessment. It is therefore necessary to use direct rectal measurements, either with a glass thermometer or with an electronic sensor (thermistor or thermocouple). Under controlled environmental conditions the fall in rectal temperature over the first 15 min after birth is a good indication of the baby's ability to respond to thermal stress [66], and so it is useful to make a continuous recording over this period, rather than merely making periodic spot measurements. The interpretation of this period of rectal temperature recording is simplified if there is also a simultaneous recording of the environmental temperature immediately around the baby, since this may well not be stable [67].

If continuous or semicontinuous monitoring of rectal and environmental temperature has been initiated at delivery then the extension of this into longer-term monitoring is straightforward. Monitoring of central and peripheral temperatures, with calculation of temperature difference, is useful during intensive care.

The peripheral temperature is best measured with a loop thermistor sensor taped around the great toe. As with all surface-mounted temperature measurement probes it must be protected from radiant energy emitted by overhead warmers because it will give a falsely high reading. This can be done with silver foil. At the same time the probe should not be covered with a thick layer of insulating tape or other material because the skin surface temperature being measured will begin to rise towards core temperature. A good compromise is to use a perforated double-sided adhesive disc over the sensor, with the connecting cable lightly taped down to the skin a few centimetres away.

Oesophageal, auditory canal, or axillary temperatures may all be used in place of rectal temperature for single or continuous measurements [68]. Of these, axillary measurement is the easiest to measure in small babies, and it lends itself well to continuous monitoring with thermistor or thermocouple sensors attached as described above.

A further method which should be considered for obtaining core temperature measurements non-invasively is the so-called zero temperature gradient technique invented by Fox and Solman in 1971 [69], and further developed by Togawa [68,70]. With this method a skin-mounted temperature sensor is covered by a thermal insulator. This makes the skin temperature rise towards the core temperature. A second sensor is positioned on the surface of the insulator, and this too is then further covered by a small electrical heating coil. The heater increases the temperature of the skin surface further, until there is no gradient between the two temperature sensors: this may take 15–20 minutes after the device has been first applied. At this time both temperature sensors will be recording the core temperature. This method has been evaluated in ELBW babies under special environmental conditions, and good correlation has been found between the zero temperature gradient method and rectal temperature. However, the basic method can only function if ambient temperature is lower than the baby's core temperature and this may not be the case in incubator-nursed babies. To overcome this problem a modification is to include an electronic cooling element in the sensor, but although this approach does work the sensor is rather too large for the ELBW baby: improvements continue to be made.

## Scientific and technical support

Monitoring can only be successful if the equipment is reliable, well-maintained, safe, and properly and regularly calibrated. In discussing the provision of this equipment it is therefore important to plan scientific and technical support. Experience internationally has shown that this is best achieved by having correctly trained *clinical engineers* (technicians and graduates) based within the intensive care unit but professionally integrated within a hospital-based Department of Biomedical Engineering or Medical Physics. First, this arrangement allows these specialized staff to provide rapid service, and this is vital for monitoring equipment including the laboratory blood gas analyser. Second, the arrangement allows these staff to become part of the clinical team, which is important in approaching the problems of working in pressured circumstances. Third, the arrangement ensures that the scientific and technical staff can benefit from their own peer-group review, support, and professional direction. This is now recognized as being essential, to avoid the problems which arise from staff being isolated from their peers. Fourth, the availability of scientific and technical staff as part of the clinical team, linked to the parent scientific department and its facilities, allows refinements and customizing of equipment to be carried out rapidly and at low cost. This is a frequent need in neonatal intensive care.

The costs of health care technology provision increasingly reflect growing pressure, and legislation, to improve standards of safety and quality. The capital costs of neonatal equipment are perhaps well recognized, but the revenue required to operate, maintain and repair equipment to the appropriate standards is not generally appreciated. Considering all medical equipment together it is usual to estimate the revenue requirement as 10% of the replacement value of the equipment. The range is 7–15% depending upon the type of technology and the clinical demands. Intensive care equipment tends to be at the top end of this range, because of the complexity of the equipment and the need for 24-hour cover.

Thus the planning of equipment support, including financial and professional issues, needs to be carried out proactively if the monitoring of the ELBW baby is to be effective.

## Conclusions

The most important difference between monitoring techniques for babies less than and more than 1000 g relates to the sensors required for detecting the variables of interest. Improvements have occurred in recent years, for example in the design of ECG electrodes and their attachment, but significant improvements are still required. The limited surface area available for the attachment of external sensors is a strong motivation for the development of multiple sensors which, in a single device, have means for detecting several variables. The very real problem of attaching any sensor to the skin surface is also an incentive to develop improved biocompatible materials for multiple sensor devices for use in the umbilical artery, in the oesophagus, and attached to the head. Near infrared spectroscopy for cerebral monitoring is now starting to enter the clinical research phase and the results

---

**Practical points**

1. Blood gas and pH assessment and control are central components of the care of the ELBW baby and efficient practical means for combining data from *in vitro* blood analysis, invasive sensors and non-invasive sensors should be established.

2. Attachment of electrodes, optical probes and transcutaneous gas sensors to the skin surface can damage the skin. Use small, lightweight devices having thin very flexible connecting wires. Adhesives can cause allergic reactions as well as fixing the device either too firmly or too loosely; tests should be done locally to develop practices and procedures.

3. Unless monitored data have appropriate precision and accuracy they will not contribute positively to clinical care. Routine procedures need to be established for calibration of all sensors and monitors where quantitative data are presented.

4. Technology for monitoring ELBW babies is still evolving and new, unproven, devices will often need to be used. Protocols for assessing new technologies need to be established prospectively.

5. Practical steps need to be taken to avoid 'data gaps' and achieve continuity of monitored data from the time of delivery, through resuscitation and on into the NICU. Standardization of sensors, probes and monitors, together with agreed policies on the use of manual and automated data records, will be a key to this.

of such research will reveal whether or not NIRS can have a useful role in monitoring the ELBW baby. Successful research and development along these lines must ultimately be followed by effective commercialization in order that the approach may be widely adopted. This continues to be the focus of attention, particularly as monitoring ELBW babies has become more common.

# References

1. Rolfe, P. (1989) Monitoring. In *The Baby Under 1000g* (D. Harvey, R.W.I. Cooke and G. Levitt, eds), Wright, London, pp. 106–119
2. Rolfe, P. (1975) Monitoring in newborn intensive care. *Biomed. Eng.*, **10**, 339–404, 413
3. Rolfe, P. (1976) Monitoring equipment for the neonate. *Br. J. Hosp. Med.*, **1**, 189–205
4. Rolfe, P. (1977) Instruments for the care of ill newborn babies. *Electron. Power*, **23**, 32–39
5. Rolfe, P. (1986) Neonatal critical care monitoring. *J. Med. Eng. Technol.*, **10**, 115–120
6. Boyle, R.J. and Oh, W. (1980) Erythema following transcutaneous oxygen monitoring. *Pediatrics*, **65**, 333–334
7. Veasy, L.G., Clark, J.S., Jung, A.L. *et al.* (1971) A system for computerized automated blood gas analysis; its use in newborn infants with respiratory distress. *Pediatrics*, **48**, 5–17
8. Bristow, C.J. (1980) A microprocessor-based system as an aid to neonatal intensive care. CNAA, M Phil Thesis.
9. Collins, P., Levy, N.M., Boddis, I.R. *et al.* (1979) Apparatus for servo-control of arterial oxygen tension in pre-term infants. *Med. Biol. Eng. Comput.*, **17**, 449
10. Cartlidge, P.H.T. and Rutter, N. (1987) Kuraya gum ECG electrodes for the preterm infant. *Arch. Dis. Childh.*, **62**, 1281–1282
11. Jenkins, J.C., Mitchell, R.H., McClure, B.G., Ritchie, J.W.K. and McCready, P. (1986) The use of a microcomputer for on-line analysis of heart rate variability in newborn infants. In *Neonatal Physiological Measurements* (P. Rolfe, ed.), Butterworths, pp. 49–55.
12. Rolfe, P., Kanjilal, P.P., Murphy, C. and Burton, P.J. (1986) Continuous non-invasive beat-by-beat blood pressure (BP) measurement in the newborn. In *Proceedings of the 3rd International Symposium on Continuous Transcutaneous Monitoring*, Zurich.
13. O'Brien, M.J. *et al.* (1983) Monitoring respiratory activity in infants – a non-intrusive diaphragm EMG technique. In *Non-Invasive Physiological Measurements, Vol. 2* (P. Rolfe, ed.), Academic Press, pp. 131–177
14. Milner, A.D. (1970) *The Respiratory Jacket. Lancet*, **i**, 80
15. Milledge, J.S. and Stott, M. (1977) Inductive plethysmography: a new respiratory transducer (Proceedings). *J. Physiol.*, **267**, 4–5
16. Wright, B.M. and Callan, K. (1979) A new respiratory recording and monitoring system. In *ISAM*, Academic Press, pp. 329–335
17. Lewin, J.E. (1969) *An apnoea alarm mattress. Lancet*, **ii**, 667
18. Beardsmore, C.S. *et al.* (1980) Some problems of oesophageal pressure measurement in the newborn. In *Fetal and Neonatal Physiological Measurements* (P. Rolfe, ed.), Pitman Medical, pp. 278–283
19. Rolfe, P., Martin, M., Williams, D., Walters, R. Yamakoshi, K. and Tanaka, S. (1992) In-vivo sensors: haemocompatibility. In *Advances in In-vivo Sensors* (A.J.P. Turner, ed.), Cranfield Press, pp. 83–96
20. Goddard, P.J., Keith, I., Marcovitch, H., Rolfe, P. and Scopes, J.W. (1972) A catheter-tip oxygen electrode: experience in newborn infants with respiratory distress. *Arch. Dis. Childh.*, **47**, 675
21. Goddard, P.J., Keith, I., Marcovitch, H., Roberton, N.R.C., Rolfe, P. and Scopes, J.W. (1974) The use of a continuously recording intravascular oxygen electrode in the newborn. *Arch. Dis. Childh.*, **49**, 853–860
22. Conway, M., Durbin, G.M., Ingram, D. *et al.* (1976) Continuous monitoring of arterial oxygen tension using a catheter-tip polarographic electrode in infants. *Pediatrics*, **57**, 244–250
23. Zhang, S., Wright, G., Kingston, M.A. and Rolfe, P. (1996) Improved performance of intravascular $pO_2$ sensor incorporating poly(MPC-co-BMA) membrane. *Med. & Biol. Engng & Comput.*, **34**, 313–315
24. Peterson, J.L., Golstein, S.R., Fitzgerald, R.V. and Buckhold, K.K. (1980) Fibre-optic pH probe for physiological use. *Anal. Chem.*, **52**, 864–869
25. Peterson, J.L., Fitzgerald, R.V. and Buckhold, K.K. (1984) Fibre-optic probe for in-vivo measurement of oxygen partial pressure. *Anal. Chem.*, **56**, 62–67
26. Rolfe, P. (1990) In-vivo chemical sensors for intensive-care monitoring. *Med. Biol. Eng. Comput.*, **28**, B34–B47
27. Thunstrom, A.M., Stafford, M.J. and Severinghaus, J.W. (1979) A two temperature, two $Po_2$ method of estimating the determinants of $tcPo_2$. In *Continuous Transcutaneous Blood Gas Monitoring* (A. Huch, R. Huch and J.F. Lucey, eds.) Alan R. Liss Inc. pp. 167–182
28. Lubbers, D.W. (1979) Cutaneous and transcutaneous $Po_2$ and $Pco_2$ and their measuring conditions. In *Continuous Transcutaneous Blood Gas Monitoring* (A. Huch, R. Huch and J. Lucey, eds.) Alan R. Liss Inc., pp. 13–31.
29. Golden, S.M. (1981) Skin craters: a complication of transcutaneous oxygen monitoring. *Pediatrics*, **67**, 514–516
30. Evans, N.J. and Rutter, N. (1986) Reduction of skin damage from transcutaneous oxygen electrodes using a spray-on dressing. *Arch. Dis. Childh.*, **61**, 881–884

31. Yoshiya, I., Shimada, Y. and Tanaka, K. (1980) Spectrophotometric monitoring of arterial oxygen saturation in the fingertip. *Med. Biol. Eng. Comput.*, **18**, 27–32

32. Turner, M.J., Davies, V.A., De Ravel, T.J.L., Rothmber, A.D. and Macleod, I.M. (1991) Dynamic performance required of transcuders for measuring pressure and flow in mechanically ventilated infants. In *Fetal and Neonatal Physiological Measurement* 217–222.

33. Shaffer, T.H., Wolfson, M.R. and Greenspan, J.S. (1991) Pulmonary function testing in the critically ill neonate. In *Fetal and Neonatal Physiological Measurement* 199–205

34. Levene, M.I. and Evans, D.H. (1983) Continuous measurement of subarachnoid pressure in the severely asphyxiated newborn. *Arch. Dis. Childh.*, **58**, 1013–1015

35. Lundberg, N. (1960) Continuous recording and control of ventricular fluid pressure in neurosurgical practice. *Acta. Psychiatr. Neurol. Scand.*, **36** (Suppl. 149), 1–193

36. Levene, M.I. and Evans, D.H. (1986) Direct measurement of intracranial pressure in the newborn. In *Neonatal Physiological Measurements* (P. Rolfe, ed.), Butterworths, pp. 174–179

37. Robinson, R.O., Rolfe, P. and Sutton, P. (1977) Non-invasive method for measuring intra-cranial pressure in normal newborn infants. *Dev. Med. Child. Neurol.*, **19**, 305–308

38. Vidyasagar, D. and Raju, T.N.K. (1977) A simple non-invasive technique of measuring intracranial pressure in the newborn. *Pediatrics*, **59**, 957–961

39. Horbar, J.D., Yeager, S., Philip, A.G.S. and Lucey, J.F. (1980) Effect of application force on non-invasive measurements of intracranial pressure. *Pediatrics*, **66**, 455–457

40. Whitelaw, A.G.L. and Wright, B.M. (1982) A pneumatic applanimeter for intracranial pressure measurements. *J. Physiol.*, **336**, 3–4

41. Kaiser, A.M., Whitelaw, S.G.L. and Besag, F.M.C. (1986) An evaluation of fontanelle pressure measurements. In *Neonatal Physiological Measurements* (P. Rolfe, ed.), Butterworths, pp. 167–173

42. Rochefort, M.J., Rolfe, P. and Wilkinson, A.R. (1986) New fontanometer for continuous estimation of intracranial pressure in the newborn. *Arch. Dis. Childh.*, **62**, 152–155

43. Rolfe, P., Persson, B. and Zetterstrom, R. (1983) An appraisal of techniques for studying cerebral circulation in the newborn. *Acta. Paediatr. Scand.* (Suppl. 331), 5–13

44. Tarassenko, L. and Rolfe, P. (1984) Electrical impedance tomography: a new method to image the head continuously in the newborn. In *Proceedings of the 6th Nordic Meeting on Medical and Biological Engineering* (Ake Oberg, ed.), IFMBE, pp. 84–88

45. Tarassenko, L. and Rolfe, P. (1984) Imaging distributions of electrical resistivity: an alternative approach. *Electron. Lett.*, **20**, 547–575

46. Murphey, D., Tarassenko, L., Barry, J. and Rolfe, P. (1986) Digital processing of the impedance plethysmogram. In *Progress Reports on Electronics in Medicine and Biology* (K. Copland, ed.), Institution of Electronic and Radio Engineers, pp. 217–224

47. Rolfe, P., Wickramasinghe, Y., Thorniley, M.S. *et al.* (1992) Fetal and neonatal cerebral oxygen monitoring with NIRS: theory and practice. *Early Hum. Dev.*, **29**, 269–273

48. Hope, P.L., Costello, A.M. de L., Cady, E.B. *et al.* (1986) Cerebral metabolism in newborn infants studied by phosphorus nuclear magnetic resonance spectroscopy. In *Neonatal Physiological Measurements* (P. Rolfe, ed.), Butterworths, pp. 382–389

49. Rea, P.A., Crowe, J., Wickramasinghe, Y. and Rolfe, P. (1985) Non-invasive optical methods for the study of cerebral metabolism in the human newborn: a technique for the future? *J. Med. Eng. Technol.*, **9**, 160–166

50. Wickramasinghe, Y.A.B.D., Thorniley, M.S. and Rolfe, P. (1989) Non-invasive near infra-red spectroscopy (NIRS) for neonatal and fetal monitoring of cerebral oxygenation. In *Fetal and Neonatal Physiological Measurements III* (G. Gennser *et al.*, eds.), Dept. of O. & G., Malmo, pp. 33–37

51. Thorniley, M.S., Wickramasinghe, Y.A.B.D., Tomlinson, A., Houston, R. and Rolfe, P. (1991) Application of near infra-red spectroscopy for clinical monitoring. *Med. Biol. Eng. Comput.*, **29**, 289

52. Livera, L.N., Wickramasinghe, Y.A.B.D., Spencer, S.A., Rolfe, P. and Thorniley, M.S. (1992) Cyclical fluctuations in cerebral blood volume. *Arch. Dis. Childh.*, **67**, 62–63

53. Crowe, J., Rea, P.A., Wickramasinghe, Y.A.B.D. and Rolfe, P. (1986) Towards non-invasive monitoring of cerebral metabolism. In *Neonatal Physiological Measurements* (P. Rolfe, ed.), Butterworths, pp. 150–156

54. Wickramasinghe, Y.A.B.D., Crowe, J.A. and Rolfe, P. (1985) Optical method adaptable for cerebral monitoring in the newborn. *Med. Biol. Eng. Comput.*, **23**, 468–468

55. Wickramasinghe, Y.A.B.D., Crowe, J.A. and Rolfe, P. (1986) Laser source and detector with signal processor for a near infra-red medical application. In *Progress Reports in Medicine and Biology* (K. Copeland, ed.), Institution of Electronic and Radio Engineers, pp. 209–215

56. Wickramasinghe, Y.A.B.D., Crowe, J.A. and Rolfe, P. (1986) Near infra-red technique for monitoring metabolism and blood oxygen saturation. In *Proceedings of the Eighth Annual Conference of the IEEE Engineering in Medicine and Biology Society*, pp. 1172–1174

57. Jobsis, F.F. (1977) Non-invasive infra-red monitoring of cerebral and myocardial oxygen sufficiency and circulatory parameters. *Science*, **198**, 1264–1267

58. Wyatt, J.S., Cope, M., Delpy, D.T., Wray, S. and Reynolds, E.O.R. (1986) Quantification of cerebral

oxygenation and haemodynamics in sick newborn infants by near infra-red spectroscopy. *Lancet*, **ii**, 1063–1066

59. Brazy, J.E., Lewis, D.V., Mitnick, M.H. and Jobsis, F.F. (1985) Non-invasive monitoring of cerebral oxygenation in preterm infants: preliminary observations. *Pediatrics*, **75**, 217–225

60. Wyatt, J.S., Edwards, A.D., Azzopardi, D. and Reynolds, E.O.R. (1989) Magnetic resonance and near infra-red spectroscopy for investigation of perinatal hypoxicischaemic brain injury. *Arch. Dis. Childh.*, **64**, 953–963

61. Rolfe, P., Wickramasinghe, Y. and Thorniley, M.S. (1991) The potential of near infra-red spectroscopy for detection of fetal cerebral hypoxia. *Eur. J. Obstet. Gynecol.*, **42**, S24–S28

62. Vaughan, D.L., Russell, G.I., Thorniley, M.S. *et al.* (1993) Changes in oxygenation status in renal ischaemia, monitored using near infra-red spectroscopy (NIRS). *Clin. Sci.*, **82**(3), 14

63. Rolfe, P. (1976) Arterial oxygen measurement in the newborn with intravascular transducers. In *IEE Medical Electronics Monographs* (Hill and Watson, eds.) Vol. 4, nos. 18–22, pp. 126–158

64. Parker, D., Delpy, D. and Reynolds, E.O.R. (1979) Single electrochemical sensor for transcutaneous measurement of $Po_2$ and $Pco_2$. In *National Foundation – Birth Defects: Original Article Series* (A. Huch, R. Huch and J.F. Lucey, eds.) Vol. XV (4) pp. 109–116

65. Miller, D.L. and Oliver, T.K. (1966) Body temperature in the immediate neonatal period: the effect of reducing thermal losses. *Am. J. Obstet. Gynecol.*, **94**, 964–969

66. Johanson, R.B., Rolfe, P., Spencer, A., Malla, D.S. and Jones, P. (1992) The effect of post delivery care on neonatal body temperature. *Acta. Paediatr. Scand.*, **81**(11), 859–863

67. Johanson, R.B., Rolfe, P. and Spencer, A. (1993) A survey of technology and temperature control on a neonatal unit in Nepal. *J. Trop. Paediatr.*, **27**, 112–115

68. Togawa, T. (1979) Non-invasive deep body temperature measurement. In *Non-invasive Physiological Measurements*, Vol. 1, Academic Press, pp. 261–277

69. Fox, R.H. and Solman, A.J. (1971) A new technique for monitoring the deep body temperature in man from the intact skin surface. *J. Physiol.*, **212**, 8–10P

70. Togawa, T. (1973) Medical thermometer making use of zero heat flow method. *Rep. Inst. Med. Dent. Eng.*, **7**, 75–83

# 10

# Jaundice

Neena Modi

Jaundice is common in the low birth weight baby in whom, unlike the mature neonate, it may persist for up to 4 weeks. Approximately 60% of babies of less than 2000 g birth weight develop a serum bilirubin in excess of 170 $\mu$mol l$^{-1}$ [1] with peak levels on the fourth and fifth days of life. Current management, with early therapeutic intervention at lower bilirubin levels, makes it difficult to assess the natural history of jaundice in infants weighing less than 1000 g.

## Physiology

Physiological jaundice in the term infant results primarily from a combination of increased bilirubin production and immaturity of the hepatic functions of uptake, conjugation and excretion [2]. In preterm infants increased bilirubin production, due to ineffective erythropoiesis and accelerated turnover of non-erythropoietic haem such as the cytochromes, does not appear to be as important [2]. However bruising does occur more readily; preterm red blood cells have a life span of approximately 40 days [3] in contrast to 70 days in the term infant [4] and 120 days in the adult; a hypocaloric intake is common in the first few days of life and the slow intestinal transit time increases the effect of the enterohepatic circulation. Of hepatic functions, the major deficiency in the preterm infant is immaturity of UDP-glucuronyl transferase activity [2]. Though rhesus alloimmunization may pose a

significant problem, the red blood cells of very immature infants have a reduced AB antigenicity [3] and these infants are unlikely to develop haemolysis in the presence of ABO incompatibility. Racial variability in susceptibility to haemolysis secondary to ABO incompatibility, as seen in full term babies, has not been assessed in preterm infants.

## Toxicity

The yellow staining of the cerebral nuclei, originally termed kernicterus by Schmorl [5], is believed to be the pathological correlate of bilirubin encephalopathy, a phrase coined by Zetterstrom and Ernster [6] to describe the clinical syndrome of bilirubin toxicity. Clinical manifestations of bilirubin neurotoxicity, both acute and long-term, and pathological findings present a relatively clear picture in the mature infant, but a simple extrapolation to the extremely immature baby has not proved possible. In this group the risk posed by hyperbilirubinaemia is a matter of current controversy [7–9].

### Acute manifestations

In the term infant, acute bilirubin toxicity is manifest as initial lethargy and hypotonia, followed by irritability, hypertonia, temperature instability, convulsions and opisthotonos, and it may progress to death [10]. Clinical assessment of ELBW babies is difficult. In sick infants the possible influences upon behavioural changes are numerous and cannot reliably be attributed to changes in bilirubin concentration.

### Late sequelae

The classical syndrome of post-icteric encephalopathy – the tetrad of high frequency hearing loss, impairment of upward gaze, athetoid cerebral palsy and dental dysplasia [11] – is rarely seen in extremely low birth weight survivors, nor does a conclusive picture emerge from attempts to evaluate the risk of brain damage due to hyperbilirubinaemia from follow-up studies. Though the spectrum of bilirubin-related brain damage probably does include subtle manifestations [12], the absence of a distinctive syndrome makes it difficult to attribute a given abnormality of the brain to bilirubin toxicity rather than to some other adverse influence. Duara *et al.* [13], in a follow-up study to detect sensorineural hearing loss in infants discharged from a tertiary care centre, found that birth weight of less than 1500 g, perinatal asphyxia and respiratory illness emerged as significant risk factors, but a serum bilirubin exceeding 225 $\mu$mol l$^{-1}$ did not. Conversely Bergman *et al.* [14], in a study of bilateral hearing loss in surviving infants with a birth weight of <1500 g, found that maximum serum bilirubin emerged as a significant predictor on multivariate testing. They also point out that as 61% of the infants with hearing loss had no additional disability, the influence of hypoxia, ischaemia or haemorrhage was unlikely to have been contributory.

Pape *et al.* [15], in a follow-up study of 43 infants of birth weight <1000 g of whom only one had a serum bilirubin in excess of 255 $\mu$mol l$^{-1}$, found no association between peak serum bilirubin and poor neurological outcome. Other authors, studying a wider range of low birth weight infants, also found no significant association between serum bilirubin and developmental outcome [16–19]. Hyman *et al.* [20] and Koch *et al.* [21] found such an association only with total serum bilirubin levels in excess of 340 $\mu$mol l$^{-1}$. Naeye [22] and Scheidt *et al.* [23] described an association at levels of total serum bilirubin from 120 $\mu$mol l$^{-1}$ and 170 $\mu$mol l$^{-1}$. The latter authors, however, failed to present convincing evidence in those born weighing <1500 g and, in addition, stated

that 'birth weight and gestational age appear to be more powerful determinants of poor test performance than maximum serum bilirubin'.

Clinical studies of the past must be interpreted with caution. No allowance was made or, given the knowledge of the day, could have been made, for obvious confounders such as the adverse effect on neurological outcome of hypoxia, ischaemia and haemorrhage. Though associations between hyperbilirubinaemia of varying degree and poor outcome may exist, association should not be allowed to imply causation. It has been shown, for example, that infants with intraventricular haemorrhage have higher serum bilirubin levels [24]. Developmental studies have further drawbacks in that the long follow-up period inevitably results in high drop out rates and as small changes in outcome are being studied in the face of many variables, only an extremely large study would have the statistical power to detect significance.

A recent prospective, national, survey of preterm infants in the Netherlands showed that at a corrected age of 2 years children with minor and major handicaps had had a significantly greater maximal serum bilirubin concentration than children with normal neurodevelopmental outcome [25]. Further, a consistent increase in prevalence of handicaps was found for each 50 $\mu$mol l$^{-1}$ increase in maximum serum bilirubin concentration. However, a further analysis of the same cohort found no effect unless periventricular haemorrhage had been present during the neonatal period [26]. Data from the United States National Institute of Child Health and Human Development (NICHD) randomized phototherapy trial, in which approximately 500 of the babies born at <2000 g were followed up for 6 years [27], has shown that although phototherapy reduced peak bilirubin levels significantly, this intervention did not reduce the incidence of motor deficits or cerebral palsy. There was also no effect on IQ scores.

## Pathological findings

Following the recognition of a serum bilirubin of 340 $\mu$mol l$^{-1}$ as the level requiring intervention in the full term baby with haemolytic disease, reports appeared suggesting increased susceptibility to bilirubin toxicity in preterm infants [28–30]. The impetus to intervene earlier was provided by accounts of postmortem kernicterus in immature babies without haemolysis, with peak total serum bilirubin levels of less than 340 μmol l$^{-1}$ [31–33]. Ritter *et al.* [34] described an infant who had had a peak serum bilirubin of 45 μmol l$^{-1}$ and Gartner *et al.* [35], two babies who had not been jaundiced. These postmortem diagnoses vary in the extent to which various histological changes such as neuronal degeneration, demyelination and gliosis were demonstrated in addition to macroscopic staining and the extent to which these features reflect clinical morbidity is therefore unclear [36,37]. Macroscopic staining may simply represent bilirubin uptake by previously damaged neural tissue, a point which was recognized in the early accounts of kernicterus [38]. Yellow staining has now been produced experimentally in rats without associated EEG evidence of encephalopathy [39]. Turkel *et al.* [40], comparing 32 matched pairs of infants with and without yellow staining of the basal ganglia, found no significant difference in 'risk factors', clinical course and bilirubin levels between the two groups and concluded that yellow staining could not be equated with clinical toxicity. Additionally, the absence of staining may not preclude clinical disease: Perl *et al.* [41] have demonstrated acute clinical toxicity suggestive of classical bilirubin encephalopathy in newborn rabbits without staining. The conclusion in the ELBW infants must be that the incidence of bilirubin toxicity cannot be assessed from postmortem findings.

## Risk factors

'Risk factors' such as acidosis, asphyxia, hypercarbia and hypothermia were purported to increase the likelihood of bilirubin encephalopathy [31–33,35] in the preterm infant. It is notable that these studies all related to ill babies and took no account of other possible influences leading to an adverse outcome. Attempts to define infants at greater risk on the basis of the presence of 'risk factors' have proved unsuccessful [34,42–44] but decisions regarding intervention points in clinical practice often incorporate the presence or absence of such factors and the level of free or unbound bilirubin. The rationale for this lies in current concepts regarding the mechanism of bilirubin toxicity.

## Free bilirubin

Bilirubin depresses cellular respiration, uncouples oxidative phosphorylation at mitochondrial level [6,45] and inhibits numerous enzyme systems. Two theories exist to explain the initial toxic step, believed to be the passage of bilirubin into neural tissue. The free bilirubin theory is based on the hypothesis that the albumin/bilirubin complex in plasma is nondiffusible and that therefore only free bilirubin is toxic with albumin exerting its protective effect so long as its molar concentration is more than that of bilirubin. The increased vulnerability of very immature infants may in part be due to albumin levels that are lower and a low bilirubin binding capacity [46,47]. Sulphonamides, which are known to increase the toxicity of bilirubin [48], displace bilirubin from albumin and the higher risk of toxicity in haemolytic compared to non-haemolytic jaundice is attributed to competitive binding by haematin. Free fatty acids, also bound by albumin, are increased during hypoxia, hypothermia, hypoglycaemia and sepsis. Serious illness in preterm babies is associated with a reduced bilirubin binding capacity and affinity and an increased risk of postmortem kernicterus [49]. Attempts have therefore been made to correlate free bilirubin levels or assessment of bilirubin binding capacity and bilirubin affinity with clinical outcome with a view to using such measurements in deciding intervention points. This has proved a disappointing exercise, not least because of the number of binding tests in use, of which Cashore [50] has provided a useful review.

Zamet *et al.* [51] found an association between free bilirubin and kernicterus diagnosed clinically and at postmortem examination, and furthermore an increased susceptibility in preterm infants to raised free bilirubin concentration. Odell *et al.* [19], studying infants of less than 1500 g birth weight at the age of five years, found a significant correlation between neurological abnormalities and the saturation of serum proteins. Nakamura *et al.* [52] have shown abnormalities in the auditory brainstem-evoked responses in term neonates to be related to the level of unbound bilirubin. However, Ritter *et al.* [34], also using a postmortem diagnosis of kernicterus in a study of infants born weighing <1500 g, found no difference in free bilirubin between those affected and those not affected. In so far as a practical application is concerned, the concept of a stable concentration of free bilirubin that may be reliably measured would appear simplistic: albumin binding is reversible with bound and free bilirubin molecules continuously undergoing exchange. Certain other observations are also inconsistent with the free bilirubin theory alone; analbuminaemic humans do not develop kernicterus [53] and the concentration of bilirubin in the brains of Gunn rats does not correlate with serum free bilirubin.

### Blood–brain barrier

The second theory proposes that all that is necessary are the appropriate physical conditions at cell membrane level permitting the passage of albumin bound bilirubin – the opening of the blood–brain barrier hypothesis. Barrier 'opening' occurs in several disease states such as meningitis, hyperosmolality and hypoxia and may be produced experimentally [54]. Though there is evidence to support the widely held belief that the blood–brain barrier matures with postnatal age [55], classical kernicterus has developed in older infants and children with glucose-6-phosphate deficiency and Crigler–Najjar syndrome. Albumin bound bilirubin may be shown to enter the brain during experimental opening [56]. However, whether any ensuing brain dysfunction is due to bilirubin itself or whether it is due to the underlying pathological precipitant, with bilirubin merely serving as a coloured marker of opening, is undecided. Wennberg and Hance [39], have shown that bilirubin staining in a rat model, without EEG changes of encephalopathy, occurred when the blood–brain barrier was open but that blood–brain barrier opening in association with an increased free bilirubin concentration maximized the risk of encephalopathy. Ives *et al.* [57], using $^{31}$P nuclear magnetic spectroscopy, showed bilirubin, in conjunction with hyperosmolar blood–brain barrier opening, to have a disruptive effect *in vivo* on cerebral energy metabolism.

A question that has not been examined to date is that of variations in cell susceptibility to

a given bilirubin load under varying clinical conditions.

## Objective assessment of neurological function

Little exists in the way of objective assessment of neurological function in the neonate. Abnormalities in the acoustic properties of the cry of hyperbilirubinaemic infants have been found [58] and recently there has been interest in the role of brain-evoked responses. Abnormalities in auditory-evoked responses attributable to hyperbilirubinaemia have been documented in otherwise well infants [52,59,60]. Of interest is that each of these authors stress both the variability of susceptibility and the transient nature of the abnormality. The latter observation suggests an initial reversible phase of bilirubin toxicity. Ahlfors *et al.* [61], studying rhesus primate newborns, while stressing variable susceptibility, also described a progressive pattern to auditory brainstem response changes and presented limited data obtained from nuclear magnetic resonance spectroscopy, supporting a global toxic effect of hyperbilirubinaemia.

Given the wide variations in susceptibility, the occurrence of an initial reversible phase of toxicity and the numerous additional insults infants may be exposed to, it would appear that evidence of acute cerebral dysfunction holds the best promise for the objective assessment of bilirubin toxicity against which criteria for treatment may be evaluated.

## Management

Unfortunately, despite these reservations regarding assessment of toxicity and chiefly because of the unsubstantiated spectre of minimal brain damage [11], clinical practice has evolved into intervention at lower and lower levels of total serum bilirubin, culminating in the advocacy of prophylactic phototherapy for high-risk groups [62,63] and has also seen the proliferation of charts and nomograms which use a selection of criteria to decide intervention points. The rationality of current clinical practice must therefore be questioned.

The extent of current confusion regarding management is revealed by Robertson *et al.* [64] who showed that no agreement exists between five methods used to decide when to perform exchange transfusion. Commonly used charts are those introduced by Gartner [63] and Maisels [65] and formulae considered incorporate total bilirubin, bilirubin binding capacity, total albumin and birth weight. Of these methods, only one, the Gartner chart, has been subjected to any evaluation [66]. A fall in the postmortem prevalence of kernicterus over two periods, 1966–1967 and 1971–1976, was described. The authors attributed this to the introduction, at the start of the second period, of a more aggressive policy of management. Prophylactic phototherapy was used for infants of <1500 g birth weight and exchange transfusion performed in infants weighing less than 1250 g at a total serum bilirubin of 220 µmol l$^{-1}$, if the clinical course was uncomplicated and 170 µmol l$^{-1}$, if one of several risk factors was present. Unfortunately, such a study provides far from conclusive answers. Kernicterus in this series was defined loosely as yellow discoloration of cerebral nuclei with or without histological changes and therefore subject to the criticisms discussed above. Neonatal intensive care has become considerably more sophisticated over the periods in question and a historical study cannot allow for changes in outcome secondary to improvements in care rather than lower serum bilirubin levels.

### Implications for current practice and research

In conclusion, there is little objective basis to current management criteria. In the ELBW infant, the incidence of bilirubin encephalopathy cannot be assessed from postmortem findings. Follow-up studies have not provided, and are unlikely to provide, an objective correlation between jaundice and developmental outcome because of the difficulty of mounting a study with sufficient statistical power and because so much of current treatment has now become firmly established. Both free bilirubin and factors opening the blood–brain barrier influence the development of encephalopathy. The question of variations in brain cell susceptibility, both regional and under differing clinical conditions, has not to date been addressed. The best promise for the future lies with the development of methods of assessing acute cerebral dysfunction.

Rather than aggressive treatment of low levels of bilirubin, attention would be better paid to more intensive monitoring and stabilization of perfusion, temperature, blood gas, hydration and acid–base variables. Given, however, that such management has entered medical lore, controlled trials of early versus late intervention are now ethically unacceptable.

Best guess advice to the clinician caring for infants of <1000 g is to start phototherapy at a total serum bilirubin level of 100–150 µmol l$^{-1}$, ensuring it is maximally effective phototherapy (see below). Prophylactic phototherapy is of no benefit [67]. Further it should be noted that bilirubin is a potent natural antioxidant. Recently, the hypothesis that low levels of bilirubin have a physiologically important protective effect against oxidant damage, has been raised [68]. Guidelines for exchange transfusion are even more difficult, but in the presence of effective phototherapy and the absence of active haemolysis, it is unlikely to be of benefit at a total serum bilirubin of less than 250 µmol l$^{-1}$.

## Obstructive jaundice

The level of conjugated bilirubin does not normally exceed 40 µmol l$^{-1}$ in the ELBW infant but, when seen, occurs most often in infants who have received total parenteral nutrition for over three weeks. The precise reason is unclear but several theories have been advanced. Hughes *et al.* [69] suggested that cholestasis is secondary to the suppression of trophic gut hormones due to the absence of enteral nutrition. Absent enteral nutrition is also associated with mucosal atrophy [70] which, in the extremely immature infant, may further increase intestinal permeability to hepatotoxins [71]. The neonate has been described as being in a state of 'physiological cholestasis' [72] with a reduced rate of bile synthesis and excretion and this may lower the threshold for further cholestasis. Liver biopsies show both hepatocellular injury and bile duct proliferation as seen in biliary atresia [73]. Long-term sequelae such as fibrosis or cirrhosis appear rare and when described have occurred following periods of total parenteral nutrition exceeding 6 months or in association with abdominal sepsis [74,75]. The early introduction of enteral feeds even in small volume may prevent this complication and a possibility for the future is the administration of trophic gastrointestinal hormones when prolonged total parenteral nutrition is necessary. Cholelithiasis has also been described as a possible complication of parenteral nutrition [76]. Other causes of a conjugated hyperbilirubinaemia are well described and investigation should follow the lines suggested for mature neonates [77]. Phototherapy should not be used in the presence of obstructive jaundice as the accumulation and degradation of pigmented photoproducts will result in the bronze baby syndrome [78].

# Treatment of unconjugated jaundice

## Phototherapy

The use of light to clear unconjugated bilirubin was first described by Cremer *et al.* in 1958 [79,80]. It is now the method of choice for the initial treatment of jaundice in the neonate, though there remain several areas of uncertainty as to its mode of action and optimal application.

When light is used therapeutically, the prescription should specify wavelength, irradiance and duration of exposure and documentation of these parameters should form part of standard nursery procedure. The visible spectrum extends from 380 to 770 nm with the blue-green spectrum – the area of interest as regards phototherapy – from 425 to 550 nm. Irradiance is a measure of radiant flux impinging on a unit area, or power density. It should not be confused with illuminance which is the radiant flux visible waveband as perceived by a standard human eye. Irradiance is measured by a spectroradiometer and expressed in mW cm$^{-1}$; illuminance, the objective measure of the sensation of brightness, is measured by a light meter and expressed in footcandles or lux. Though only an approximation, as the actual irradiance impinging on the baby will vary with time due to changing ambient illumination and changes in the position of the baby, the product of duration of exposure and irradiance will give a measure of the total radiant energy to which an infant has been exposed.

## Mode of action

Native bilirubin, 4Z, 15Z bilirubin IXa [81] is composed of four pyrrole rings. Phototherapy was initially assumed to act via the photo-oxidation of bilirubin to water-soluble breakdown products such as mono and dipyrroles. It appears that though photo-oxidation does occur during phototherapy [82] it is not the most important mode of action. The most rapid photochemical reaction is the formation of unstable, reversible configurational isomers of bilirubin that are polar and therefore able to be excreted directly in bile where they appear as a native unconjugated bilirubin. A non-reversible isomer termed lumirubin is also formed, though at a slower rate [83].

When using phototherapy it is important to avoid exposing an infant to wavelengths of light of no therapeutic benefit in clearing bilirubin, but which might have significant effects of their own. An obvious example is the filtering out of ultraviolet and infrared light. The optimal wavelengths for phototherapy in the human newborn baby are currently a matter for debate. Although the absorption spectrum for bilirubin *in vitro* centres around 460 nm, at which wavelength bilirubin absorbs maximally, the action spectrum defining the wavelengths most effective in producing the desired therapeutic effect is dependent *in vivo* on many factors such as competitive absorption by other compounds, skin penetration and the rate of clearance of the various photoproducts. The action spectrum for bilirubin clearance *in vivo* is still not known. Additionally, species differences exist and data pertaining to the Gunn rat model cannot be directly extrapolated to the human neonate. Blue wavelengths (425–475 nm) are undoubtedly effective in clearing bilirubin; what is not known is whether other, possibly safer, wavelengths are also effective. When phototherapy is commenced the formation of configurational isomers of bilirubin, the major photoproduct in the human neonate [84,85], proceeds rapidly reaching photoequilibrium and a stable concentration, but excretion proceeds slowly with a serum half-life of 15 hours [84]. The formation of lumirubin, the non-reversible structural isomer of bilirubin, is slower but excretion is more rapid (serum half-life <2 hours [84]) and takes place both in bile and urine. It has therefore been proposed [86,87] that the ideal light source for phototherapy should promote lumirubin formation and green light has been suggested as effective in this respect [86–88].

## Optimal use

There are several ways in which to increase the effectiveness of phototherapy: the emission spectra of lamps used must include therapeutic wavelengths in effective dose – a suitable irradiance is a minimum of 1 mW cm$^{2-1}$ in the 425–475 nm waveband – and as a saturation effect is believed to exist, 3 mW cm$^{2-1}$ (60 μW cm$^{2-1}$ nm$^{-1}$) should not be exceeded [89,90]. The rate-limiting factor would appear to be the excretion of photoproducts into bile and possibly urine. Irradiance may be increased by ensuring that the baby is not covered in unnecessary clothing, by nursing near a window and by decreasing the distance between the light source and the baby. Recently the delivery of phototherapy through a fibreoptic blanket placed beneath the baby has been shown to be both efficacious and acceptable to parents [91]. Failure to achieve an adequate irradiance, especially when nursing ELBW infants in radiant heat cradles, has been shown to be responsible for therapeutic failures [92]. Changes in line voltage may decrease light emission and the output from both fluorescent tubes and halogen lamps decays with time and should be checked regularly.

Phototherapy is more effective the higher the bilirubin concentration [93]. In babies with an initial serum bilirubin concentration of greater than 250 μmol l$^{-1}$, an approximate decline of 30–40% should be achieved after 24 hours of appropriate phototherapy. Prophylactic phototherapy has not been shown to be of benefit [67]. Intermittent phototherapy has been advocated as both efficient and involving less exposure to light [93,94] but as the spectral band most efficient in producing DNA breaks is that from 420 to 500 nm, precisely the band that bilirubin best absorbs [95], increasing the number of light cycles during which breaks occur and dark cycles during which repair occurs might in theory increase the risk of wrongly repairing a break [96]. However, neither permanent cellular damage nor carcinogenesis has been attributable to phototherapy.

## Hazards

Though numerous theoretical and experimental hazards exist [97,98] no serious toxicity attributable to phototherapy has been seen in all the years of its use. Babies have, however, been exposed to a large variety of light intensities and wavelengths, all loosely termed phototherapy, without further specification. It is not surprising that babies exposed to conventional phototherapy have manifest no serious side-effects – it is possible to receive more radiant energy from exposure to sunlight than from many a conventional unit. Any rational consideration of the question of toxicity must take into account the precise characteristics of the light used. With the increasing use of high intensity, narrow spectra the problem of toxicity may have to be reconsidered.

It is important to point out here that the constant high intensity ambient lighting that many tiny neonates are exposed to for prolonged periods poses a significant health hazard in its own right regardless of additional phototherapy. Effects on biological rhythms, infant behaviour and the development of retinopathy of prematurity have all been described [99,100]. In practice, precautions to be observed during phototherapy include careful temperature monitoring especially when using halogen lamps, shielding of eyes and compensation for the increased fluid lost, principally as insensible water but occasionally in the ELBW infant, as increased stool water as well, of the order of 30–60 ml kg$^{-1}$ day$^{-1}$.

## Exchange transfusion

Exchange transfusion remains the definitive treatment for unconjugated hyperbilirubinaemia. It is, however, a hazardous procedure, perhaps all the more so as certain sequelae may not be immediately evident. A standard two-volume exchange transfusion (two volume = twice circulating blood volume, i.e. 85 ml kg$^{-1}$ doubled = 170 ml kg$^{-1}$) will exchange over 90% of the infant's blood and should reduce the serum bilirubin by approximately 50%. The exchange may be performed as a push–pull procedure via the umbilical vein or artery or as a continuous withdrawal via a central vessel with concurrent continuous infusion via a vein. The latter is the preferred technique as it is likely to result in less haemodynamic fluctuation. If the umbilical vein is used, the catheter tip must be positioned in the inferior vena cava and should not be used if wedged in a hepatic branch vessel. During push–pull exchange each cycle of input and output should take a minimum of 5 min, withdrawing and infusing slowly. Each aliquot should not exceed 5 ml kg$^{-1}$ [101]. Too rapid a rate of exchange results in a progressive fall in blood pressure. The ELBW baby (and ideally all babies) undergoing an exchange transfusion should have continuous monitoring of heart rate, blood pressure, central venous pressure, blood gases and temperature. Blood glucose, packed cell volume (PCV) and serum bilirubin, calcium, sodium and potassium should be checked before, during and after exchange. The blood used should be less than 48 hours old, cytomegalovirus negative, microbiologically screened and partially packed with a PCV of 50–60%. For rhesus incompatibility use low titre O negative blood cross-matched against maternal serum or rhesus negative blood of the same ABO group as the baby cross-matched against baby's serum. Though a theoretical risk of graft versus host disease exists and has infrequently been described [102], in practice it does not appear necessary to irradiate donor blood.

Following exchange transfusion the infant's platelet count is likely to be low, but platelets should not be transfused unless there is evidence of disseminated intravascular coagulation or active bleeding, manifest as oozing, from venepuncture sites. The 24–48 hours following exchange transfusion requires careful monitoring, especially in rhesus alloimmunized or hydropic infants. These babies are initially hypoalbuminaemic to varying degrees and after exchange, with the consequent improvement in intravascular oncotic pressure, interstitial fluid is progressively drawn into the circulation. The intravascular volume may expand sufficiently to result in acute left ventricular failure and catastrophic pulmonary haemorrhage. A careful watch should therefore be kept on the central venous pressure after exchange and any rise above 10 cmH$_2$O (7.4 mmHg) should be treated by venesection and intravenous frusemide. Pulmonary haemorrhage, in particular, is invariably due to left ventricular failure and should be treated by venesection and not with further transfusion of blood.

## Other methods

Adjunctive methods of managing hyperbilirubinaemia include earlier feeding to promote the passage of meconium and earlier provision of fluid and calories [103] to prevent dehydration and acidosis. Methods which have not gained widespread acceptance have been reviewed by Maisels [104] and include phenobarbitone to induce glucuronyl transferase activity, infusions of albumin to augment the bilirubin binding capacity, riboflavin (a singlet oxygen generator) used concomitantly with phototherapy to increase the photo-oxidative route of bilirubin clearance, vitamin E used in haemolytic jaundice to reduce red cell breakdown by increasing membrane stability and absorbent materials such as cholestyramine and agar to trap unconjugated bilirubin in the upper intestine, thus reducing the effect of the enterohepatic circulation.

Other avenues continue to be investigated. The first clinical trials of the administration of metalloprotoporphyrins, which lower bilirubin levels by inhibiting the haem–oxygenase system and thereby slowing the conversion of haem to bilirubin, to human neonates have now been reported [105] and appear promising.

---

**Practical points**

1. The risks of bilirubin toxicity have probably been overestimated.
2. The majority of very low birth weight babies who are neurologically impaired were not severely jaundiced.
3. There is little objective evidence to support current management of non-haemolytic hyperbilirubinaemia in neonates.
4. Unless better evidence emerges regarding the relationship between bilirubin levels and adverse outcome, rational recommendations for reducing serum bilirubin cannot be made.
5. Phototherapy is very effective, but only when used properly.
6. The best promise for future understanding of the role of bilirubin in neurological impairment lies with the development of methods to detect acute cerebral dysfunction.

# References

1. Brown, K.A., Kim, M.H., Wu, P. *et al.* (1985) Efficacy of phototherapy in prevention and management of neonatal hyperbilirubinaemia. *Pediatrics*, **75**(Suppl), 393–400

2. Gartner, L.M., Lee, L.S., Vaisman, S.L. *et al.* (1977) Development of bilirubin transport and metabolism in the newborn rhesus monkey: Part I. The functional basis of physiological jaundice in the newborn. Part II. Effect of prenatal and neonatal administration of phenobarbital. *J. Pediatr.*, **90**, 513–531

3. Mollison, P.L. (1983) *Blood Transfusion in Clinical Medicine*, 7th edn., Blackwell Scientific Publications, Oxford, p. 105.

4. Pearson, H.A. (1967) Lifespan of the fetal red blood cell. *J. Pediatr.*, **70**, 166–171

5. Schmorl, G. (1903) Zur kentniss des icterus neonatorum. *Verh. Deutsche. Pathol.*, **6**, 109

6. Zetterstrom, R. and Ernster, L. (1956) Bilirubin, an uncoupler of oxidative phosphorylation in isolated mitochondria. *Nature*, **178**, 1335

7. Levine, R.L. (1979) Bilirubin: worked out years ago? *Pediatrics*, **64**, 380–385

8. Lucey, J.F. (1982) Bilirubin and brain damage – a real mess. *Pediatrics*, **69**, 381–382

9. McDonagh, A.F. (1985) 'Like a shrivelled blood orange' – bilirubin, jaundice and phototherapy. *Pediatrics*, **75**, 443–455

10. Van Praagh, R. (1961) Diagnosis of kernicterus in the neonatal period. *Pediatrics*, **28**, 870–876

11. Perlstein, M.A. (1960) The late clinical syndrome of posticteric encephalopathy. *Pediatr. Clin. N. Am.*, **7**, 665–687

12. Hansen, T., Sagvolden, T. and Bratlid, D. (1986) Transient hyperbilirubinaemia causes long term changes in the open field behaviour of young rats. (Abstract) *Pediatr. Res.*, **20**, 462A

13. Duara, S., Suter, C.M., Bessard, K. *et al.* (1986) Neonatal screening with auditory brainstem responses: results of follow up audiometry and risk factor evaluation. *J. Pediatr.*, **108**, 276–281

14. Bergman, I., Hirsch, I.P., Fria, T.S. *et al.* (1985) Cause of hearing loss in the high risk premature infant. *J. Pediatr.*, **106**, 95–101

15. Pape, K.E., Buncic, R.J., Ashby, S. *et al.* (1978) The status at two years of low birth weight infants born in 1974 with birth weights less than 1000 g. *J. Pediatr.*, **92**, 253–260

16. Shiller, J.G. and Silverman, W.A. (1961) 'Uncomplicated' hyperbilirubinaemia of prematurity: the lack of association with neurological deficit at three years of age. *Am. J. Dis. Child.*, **101**, 587–592

17. Crichton, J.U., Dunn, H.J., McBurney, A.K. *et al.* (1972) Long term effects of neonatal jaundice on brain function in children of low birth weight. *Pediatrics*, **49**, 656–670

18. Wishingrad, L., Cornblath, M., Takakuwa, T. *et al.* (1965) Studies of non-haemolytic hyperbilirubinaemia in premature infants. I. Prospective randomised selection for exchange transfusion with observations on the levels of serum bilirubin with and without exchange transfusion and neurologic evalution one year after birth. *Pediatrics*, **36**, 162–172

19. Odell, G.B., Storey, G.N. and Rosenberg, L.A. (1970) Studies in kernicterus III. The saturation of serum proteins with bilirubin during neonatal life and its relationship to brain damage at five years. *J. Pediatr.*, **76**, 12–21

20. Hyman, C.B., Keaster, J., Hanson, V. *et al.* (1969) CNS abnormalities after neonatal hyperbilirubinaemia: a prospective study of 405 patients. *Am. J. Dis. Child.*, **117**, 395–405

21. Koch, C.A., Jones, D.V., Dine, M.S. *et al.* (1950) Hyperbilirubinaemia in preterm infants: a follow up study. *J. Pediatr.*, **55**, 23–29

22. Naeye, R.L. (1978) Amniotic fluid infections, neonatal hyperbilirubinaemia and psychomotor impairment. *Pediatrics*, **62**, 497–503

23. Scheidt, P.C., Mellits, E.D., Hardy, J.B. *et al.* (1977) Toxicity of bilirubin in neonates. Infant development during the first year in relation to maximum neonatal serum bilirubin concentration. *J. Pediatr.*, **91**, 292–297

24. Lucey, J.F., Pasnick, M. and Horbar, J.F. (1982) Hyperbilirubinaemia and intracranial haemorrhage in low birth weight infants. *Pediatr. Res.*, **16**, 336A

25. van de Bor, M., van Zeben-van der AA T.M., Verloove-Vanhorick, S.P., Brand, R. and Ruys J.H. (1989) Hyperbilirubinaemia in preterm infants and neurodevelopmental outcome at 2 years of age: results of a national collaborative study. *Pediatrics*, **83**, 915–920

26. van der Bor, M., Veen, S., Ens-Dokkum, M., Schreuder, A.M., Brand, R. and Verloove-Vanhorick, S.P. (1990) Hyperbilirubinaemia in preterm infants and neurodevelopmental outcome at 5 years of age. *Pediatr. Res.*, **27**, 259A

27. Scheidt, P.C., Bryla, D.A. and Nelson, H.B. (1988) NICHD phototherapy clinical trial: Six year follow up results. *Pediatr. Res.*, **23**, 455A

28. Aidin, R., Corner, B. and Tovey, G. (1950) Kernicterus and prematurity. *Lancet*, **i**, 1153–1154

29. Zuelzer, W.W. and Mudgett, R.T. (1950) Kernicterus: aetiologic study based on an analysis of 55 cases. *Pediatrics*, **6**, 452–474

30. Harris, R.C., Lucey, J.F. and MacLean, J.R. (1958) Kernicterus in premature infants associated with low concentrations of bilirubin in plasma. *Pediatrics*, **21**, 875–883

31. Stern, L. and Denton, R.L. (1965) Kernicterus in small premature infants. *Pediatrics*, **35**, 483–485

32. Ackerman, B.D., Dyer, G.Y. and Leydorf, M.M. (1970) Hyperbilirubinaemia and kernicterus in small premature infants. *Pediatrics*, **45**, 918–925

33. Keenan, W.J., Perlstein, P.H., Light, I.J. *et al.* (1972) Kernicterus in small sick premature infants receiving phototherapy. *Pediatrics*, **49**, 652–655

34. Ritter, D.A., Kenny, J.D., Norton, H.J. *et al.* (1982) A

prospective study of free bilirubin and other risk factors in the development of kernicterus in premature infants. *Pediatrics*, **69**, 260–266

35. Gartner, L.M., Snyder, R.N., Chabon, R.S. *et al.* (1970) Kernicterus: high incidence in premature infants with low serum bilirubin concentrations. *Pediatrics*, **45**, 906–917

36. Ahdab-Barmada, M. (1983) Neonatal kernicterus: neuropathologic diagnosis. In *Hyperbilirubinaemia in the Newborn (Report on the 85th Ross Conference on Paediatric Research)* (R.L. Levine and M.J. Maisels, eds), Ross Laboratories, Columbus, Ohio, pp. 2–10

37. Turkel, S.B. (1963) Clinical and pathological correlations with kernicterus and yellow pulmonary membranes. In *Hyperbilirubinaemia in the Newborn (Report of the 85th Ross Conference on Paediatric Research)* (R.L. Levine and M.J. Maisels, eds), Ross Laboratories, Columbus, Ohio, pp. 11–18

38. Gerrard, J. (1952) Kernicterus. *Brain*, **75**, 526–570

39. Wennberg, R.P. and Hance, A.J. (1986) Experimental bilirubin encephalopathy: importance of total bilirubin, protein binding and blood–brain barrier. *Pediatr. Res.*, **20**, 789–792

40. Turkel, S.B., Miller, C.A., Guttenberg, M.E. *et al.* (1982) A clinical pathological reappraisal of kernicterus. *Pediatrics*, **69**, 267–272

41. Perl, H., Nijjar, A., Ebara, H. *et al.* (1982) Bilirubin toxicity without CNS staining. *Pediatr. Res.*, **16**, 303A

42. Turkel, S.B., Guttenberg, M.E., Moynes, D.R. *et al.* (1980) Lack of identifiable risk factors for kernicterus. *Pediatrics*, **66**, 502–506

43. Kim, M.H., Yoon, J.J., Sher, J. *et al.* (1980) Lack of predictive indices in kernicterus: a comparison of clinical and pathologic factors in infants with or without kernicterus. *Pediatrics*, **66**, 852–858

44. Cashore, W.J. and Oh, W. (1982) Unbound bilirubin and kernicterus in low birth weight infants. *Pediatrics*, **69**, 481–485

45. Wennberg, R.P., Pal, N. and Bessman, S.P. (1986) Effects of blood–brain barrier disruption and bilirubin on cerebral metabolism. *Pediatr. Res.*, **20**, 469A

46. Kapitulnik, J., Horner-Mibashan, R., Blondheim, S.H. *et al.* (1975) Increase in bilirubin binding affinity of serum with age of infant. *J. Pediatr.*, **86**, 442–445

47. Ebbesen, F. and Nyboe, J. (1983) Postnatal changes in the ability of plasma albumin to bind bilirubin. *Acta Paediatr. Scand.*, **72**, 665–670

48. Silverman, W.A., Anderson, D.H., Blanc, W.A. *et al.* (1956) A difference in mortality rate and incidence of kernicterus in premature infants allotted to two prophylactic antibacterial regimens. *Pediatrics*, **18**, 616–624

49. Cashore, W.J. (1980) Free bilirubin concentrations and bilirubin binding affinity in term and preterm infants. *J. Pediatr.*, **96**, 521–527

50. Cashore, W.J. (1983) Bilirubin binding tests. In *Hyperbilirubinaemia in the Newborn (Report of the 85th Ross Conference on Paediatric Research)* (R.L.

Levine and M.J. Maisels, eds), Ross Laboratories, Columbus, Ohio, pp. 101–115

51. Zamet, P., Nakamura, H., Perez-Robles S. *et al.* (1975) The use of critical levels of birth weight and 'free bilirubin' as an approach for the prevention of kernicterus. *Biol. Neonate*, **26**, 274–282

52. Nakamura, H., Takada, S., Shimabuku, R. *et al.* (1985) Auditory nerve and brainstem responses in newborn infants with hyperbilirubinaemia. *Pediatrics*, **75**, 703–708

53. Carmode, E.J., Lyster, D.M. and Israels, S. (1975) Analbuminaemia in a neonate. *J. Pediatr.*, **86**, 862–867

54. Rapoport, S.I. (1983) Reversible osmotic opening of the blood–brain barrier for experimental and therapeutic purposes. In *Hyperbilirubinaemia in the Newborn (Report of the 85th Ross Conference on Paediatric Research)* (R.L. Levine and M.J. Maisels, eds), Ross Laboratories, Columbus, Ohio, pp. 116–124

55. Lee, C., Stonestreet, B.S., Outerbridge, E. *et al.* (1986) Postnatal maturation of the blood–brain barrier for unbound bilirubin in piglets. *Pediatr. Res.*, **20**, 353A

56. Levine, R.L., Fredricks, W.R. and Rapoport, S.I. (1982) Entry of bilirubin into the brain due to opening of the blood–brain barrier. *Pediatrics*, **69**, 255–259

57. Ives, N.K., Bolas, N.M. and Gardiner, R.M. (1989) The effects of bilirubin on brain energy metabolism during hyperosmolar opening of the blood–brain barrier: an *in vivo* study using $^{31}$P nuclear magnetic resonance spectroscopy. *Pediatr. Res.*, **26**, 356–361

58. Golub, H.L. and Corwin, M.J. (1982) Infant cry: a clue to diagnosis. *Pediatrics*, **69**, 97–201

59. Stein, L., Ozdamar, O., Kraus, N. *et al.* (1983) Follow up of infants screened by auditory brainstem response in the neonatal intensive care unit. *J. Pediatr.*, **103**, 447–453

60. Perlman, M., Fainmesser, P., Sohmer, H. *et al.* (1983) Auditory nerve brainstem evoked responses in hyperbilirubinaemic infants. *Pediatrics*, **72**, 658–664

61. Ahlfors, C.E., Bennett, S.H., Shoemaker, C.T. *et al.* (1986) Changes in auditory brainstem response associated with intravenous infusion of unconjugated bilirubin into infant rhesus monkeys. *Pediatr. Res.*, **20**, 511–515

62. Lucey, J. (1972) Neonatal jaundice and phototherapy. *Pediatr. Clin. N. Am.*, **19**, 827–839

63. Gartner, L. (1983) Jaundice and liver disease. In *Behrmann's Neonatal-Perinatal Medicine: Diseases of the Fetus and Infant* (A.A. Fanaroff and R.J. Martin, eds), C.V. Mosby, St. Louis, pp. 753–784

64. Robertson, A.F., Karp, W.B., Davis, H.C. *et al.* (1983) Predicting the need for exchange transfusion in newborn infants. *Clin. Pediatr.*, **22**, 533–536

65. Maisels, M.J. (1972) Bilirubin. *Pediatr. Clin. N. Am.*, **19**, 447–501

66. Pearlman, M.A., Gartner, L.M., Lee, K. *et al.* (1978) Absence of kernicterus in low birth weight infants from 1971 through 1976: comparison with findings in 1966 and 1967. *Pediatrics*, **62**, 460–464

67. Curtis-Cohen, M., Stahl, G.E., Costarino, A.T. *et al.*

(1985) Randomized trial of prophylactic phototherapy in the infant of very low birth weight. *J. Pediatr.*, **107**, 121–124

68. Benaron, D.A. and Bowen, F.W. (1991) Variation of initial serum bilirubin rise in newborn infants with type of illness. *Lancet*, **338**, 78–81

69. Hughes, C.A., Talbot, I.C., Ducker, D.A. *et al.* (1983) Total parenteral nutrition in infancy: effect on the liver and suggested pathogenesis. *Gut*, **24**, 241–248

70. Hughes, C.A. and Dowling, R.H. (1980) Speed of onset of adaptive mucosal hypoplasia and hypofunction in the intestine of parenterally fed rats. *Clin. Sci.*, **59**, 317–327

71. Tanner, M.S., Stocks, R.J. and McNeish, A.S. (1984) Adaptation to extrauterine life – a commentary. In *Neonatal Gastroenterology, Contemporary Issues* (M.S. Tanner and R.J. Stocks, eds), Intercept Publications, Newcastle upon Tyne, pp. 209–210

72. Balistreri, W.F., Heubi, J.E. and Suchy, F.J. (1983) Immaturity of the enterohepatic circulation in early life: factors predisposing to 'physiologic' maldigestion and cholestasis. *J. Pediatr. Gastroenterol. Nutr.*, **2**, 346–354

73. Dahms, B.B. and Halpin, T.C. (1981) Serial liver biopsies in parenteral nutrition-associated cholestasis of early infancy. *Gastroenterology*, **81**, 136–144

74. Peden, V.H., Witzleben, C.L. and Skelton, M.A. (1971) Total parenteral nutrition. *J. Pediatr.*, **78**, 180–181

75. Cohen, C.C. and Olsen, M.M. (1981) Pediatric total parenteral nutrition. *Arch. Pathol. Lab. Med.*, **105**, 152–156

76. Whitington, P.F. and Black, D.D. (1980) Cholelithiasis in premature infants treated with parenteral nutrition and furosemide. *J. Pediatr.*, **97**, 647–649

77. Johnston, D.I. (1984) Neonatal cholestasic jaundice. In *Neonatal Gastroenterology, Contemporary Issues* (M.S. Tanner and R.J. Stocks, eds), Intercept Publications, Newcastle upon Tyne, pp. 139–153

78. Onishi, S., Itoh, S., Isobe, S. *et al.* (1982) Mechanism of development of bronze baby syndrome in neonates treated with phototherapy. *Pediatrics*, **69**, 273–276

79. Cremer, R.J., Perryman, P.W. and Richards, D.H. (1958) Influence of light on the hyperbilirubinaemia of infants. *Lancet*, **i**, 1094–1097

80. Dobbs, R.H. and Cremer, R.J. (1975) Phototherapy. *Arch. Dis. Childh.*, **50**, 833–836

81. Ennever, J.F. (1986) Phototherapy in a new light. *Pediatr. Clin. N. Am.*, **33**, 603–620

82. Lightner, D.A., Linnane, W.P. and Ahlfors, C.E. (1984) Bilirubin photooxidation products in the urine of jaundiced neonates receiving phototherapy. *Pediatr. Res.*, **18**, 696–700

83. McDonagh, A.F., Palma, L.A. and Lightner, D.A. (1982) Phototherapy for neonatal jaundice: stereospecific and regioselective photoisomerization of bilirubin bound to human serum albumin and NMR characterisation of intramolecular cyclized photoproducts. *J. Am. Chem. Soc.*, **104**, 6867–6869

84. Ennever, J.F., Knox, K., Denne, S.C. *et al.* (1985) Phototherapy for neonatal jaundice: in vivo clearance of bilirubin photoproducts. *Pediatr. Res.*, **19**, 205–208

85. Costarino, A.T., Ennever, J.F., Baumgart, S. *et al.* (1985) Bilirubin photoisomerization in premature neonates under low and high dose phototherapy. *Pediatrics*, **75**, 519–522

86. Pratesi, R., Agati, G., Fusi, F. *et al.* (1985) Laser investigation of bilirubin – photobilirubin photoconversion. *Pediatr. Res.*, **19**, 166–171

87. Ennever, J.F., Knox, I. and Speck, W.T. (1986) Differences in bilirubin isomer composition in infants treated with green and white light phototherapy. *J. Pediatr.*, **109**, 119–122

88. Vecchi, C., Donzelli, G.P., Sbrana, G. *et al.* (1986) Phototherapy for neonatal jaundice: clinical equivalence of fluorescent green and 'special' blue lamps. *J. Pediatr.*, **108**, 452–456

89. Tan, K.L. (1982) The pattern of bilirubin response to phototherapy for neonatal hyperbilirubinaemia. *Pediatr. Res.*, **16**, 670–674

90. Modi, N. and Keay, A.J. (1983) Phototherapy for neonatal hyperbilirubinaemia: the importance of dose. *Arch. Dis. Childh.*, **58**, 406–409

91. Schuman, A.J. and Karush, G. (1992) Fiberoptic versus conventional home phototherapy for neonatal hyperbilirubinaemia. *Clin. Pediatr. Phila.*, **31**, 345–352

92. Bonta, B.W. and Warshaw, J.B. (1976) Importance of radiant flux in the treatment of hyperbilirubinaemia: failure of overhead phototherapy units in intensive care units. *Pediatrics*, **57**, 502–506

93. Jahrig, K., Jahrig, D. and Meisel, P. (1982) Dependence of the efficiency of phototherapy on plasma bilirubin concentration. *Acta Paediatr. Scand.*, **71**, 293–299

94. Lau, S.P. and Fung, K.P. (1984) Serum bilirubin kinetics in intermittent phototherapy of physiological jaundice. *Arch. Dis. Childh.*, **59**, 892–894

95. Sideris, E.G., Papageorgiou, G.C., Charalampous, S.C. *et al.* (1981) A spectrum response study on single strand DNA breaks, sister chromatid exchanges and lethality induced by phototherapy lights. *Pediatr. Res.*, **15**, 1019–1023

96. Speck, W.T., Santella, R.M. and Rosenkranz, H.S. (1977) Intermittent phototherapy: effect on intracellular DNA. *Pediatr. Res.*, **11**, 542A

97. Cohen, A.N. and Ostrow, J.D. (1980) New concepts in phototherapy: photoisomerization of bilirubin IXa and potential toxic effects of light. *Pediatrics*, **65**, 740–750

98. Sisson, T.R.C. and Vogl, T.P. (1982) Phototherapy of hyperbilirubinaemia. In *The Science of Photomedicine* (J.D. Regan and J.A. Parrish, eds), Plenum Press, New York and London, pp. 477–509

99. Sisson, T.R.C. (1981) Molecular basis of hyperbilirubinaemia and phototherapy. *J. Invest. Dermatol.*, **77**, 158–161

100. Glass, P., Avery, G.B., Kolinjavadi, N. *et al.* (1985) Effect of bright light in the hospital nursery on the incidence of retinopathy of prematurity. *N. Engl. J. Med.*, **313**, 401–404

101. Aranda, J.V. and Sweet, A.Y. (1977) Alterations in blood pressure during exchange transfusion. *Arch. Dis. Childh.*, **52**, 545–548
102. Cochran, W.D. (1978) Increasing safety of exchange transfusions. *Pediatr. Res.*, **12**, 462
103. Wu, P.Y., Hodgman, J.E., Kirkpatrick, B.V. *et al.* (1985) Metabolic aspects of phototherapy. *Pediatrics*, **75**(Suppl), 427–433
104. Maisels, M.J. (1992) Neonatal jaundice. In *Effective Care of the Newborn Infant* (J.C. Sinclair and M.B. Bracken, eds), Oxford University Press, Oxford, pp. 507–561
105. Kappas, A., Drummond, G.S., Manola, T., Petmezaki, S. and Valaes, T. (1988) Sn-protoporphyrin use in the management of hyperbilirubinaemia in term newborns with direct Coombs-positive incompatibility. *Pediatrics*, **81**, 485–497

# 11

# Enteral feeding

Anthony Williams and Sally Mitton

Twenty years have elapsed since Heird *et al.* demonstrated the importance of feeding small babies by calculating their 'caloric reserve' from data about fetal body composition [1]. Assuming this to be the body non-protein energy (mainly fat) plus one-third of body protein, it was calculated that a 1000 g infant might be expected to survive only 4 days without food. In contrast, a full term baby might survive 1 month and an adult 3 months under similar conditions. Few now would disagree that nutrition influences the survival of small babies; indeed, current interest increasingly focuses not just on the relationship between early nutrition and survival but on the quality of developmental outcome and long-term health [2]. Unfortunately, the urgency to meet nutritional requirements is matched by numerous physiological, metabolic and technical constraints which mean that few babies weighing under 1000 g at birth are wholly enterally fed. Early parenteral nutrition (Chapter 12) is essential for most such babies but here we shall show the importance of commencing enteral nutrition at the earliest opportunity.

## Physiology of enteral feeding in the very immature baby

### The anatomy of the gastrointestinal tract

The fetal gastrointestinal tract is anatomically complete at 24 weeks' gestation [3]. Feeding animals at birth triggers both hyperplasia and hypertrophy of the gut mucosa, and there is some evidence that homologous milk is most effective in this regard [4]. Nothing appears to be known about the influence of extreme premature birth on this phenomenon or the time course of adaptation in human infants.

### Gastrointestinal motility

Early amniographic studies showed that fetal intestinal transit is present from around 28 weeks' gestation [5]. Subsequent manometric studies in preterm infants have since confirmed that coordinated peristaltic activity in the small bowel (characterized by the 'migrating motor complex') is unlikely to be present at birth before 34 weeks' gestation, when coordinated sucking and swallowing reflexes develop [6]. Enteral feeding appears to accelerate the appearance of coordinated peristaltic activity, regardless of postconceptional age [7], and also has advantageous effects on the gut endocrine system, promoting biliary flow.

### The gut vasculature and blood flow

The transition to extrauterine life is accompanied by a reversal of the high pulmonary and the relatively low systemic vascular resistance of the fetus. Concomitant with this is the rise in $Po_2$ of blood supplying the gut from the intrauterine value of 19–22 mmHg. Fetal circulatory pathology has important influences on splanchnic blood flow after birth.

## *Effects of abnormal fetal aortic blood flow patterns*

The fetus with intrauterine growth retardation and absent end diastolic flow is at greater risk of necrotizing enterocolitis [8]. The absence or reversal of end diastolic flow in the fetal aorta or umbilical artery (ascertained by Doppler ultrasound measurement) increases this risk independently of growth retardation, gestational age or perinatal asphyxia [9]. Circulatory redistribution in the hypoxic fetus increases blood velocity and decreases pulsatility indices in the cerebral circulation but reduces velocity and increases impedance in the aorta [10], paralleling animal observations that flow to vital organs (brain and heart) is spared at the expense of flow to the splanchnic, renal and pulmonary beds. The intriguing question remains as to whether the predisposition to necrotizing enterocolitis in infants who have absent aortic end-diastolic flow *in utero* is due to the perfusion abnormalities before or after birth, or both. A recent study comparing small-for-gestational-age (SGA) infants with both gestational-age and weight-matched controls confirmed that abnormalities persist postnatally and advised caution when enterally feeding severely growth retarded babies with evidence of fetal hypoxia [11]. Superior mesenteric and coeliac artery flow velocities were significantly reduced in the SGA group compared to the gestation matched group on the first day of life. In a subgroup of SGA infants, with absent end-diastolic aortic flow antenatally, the reductions were significantly greater than in controls or in SGA babies with conserved fetal end-diastolic aortic flow. Even on day seven of life the SGA group still had reduced superior mesenteric flows compared to the gestation matched group though similar numbers in both groups were being fed enterally. It was proposed that the vascular response to feeding seen in normally grown infants might be impaired in SGA infants.

## *Effects of feeding on gut blood flow*

Blood flow velocity, and by implication flow, in coeliac and superior mesenteric arteries rose after the first enteral feed [12] in preterm infants of appropriate weight for gestation (AGA), median weight (range) 1248 (910–2480 g) and gestational age 29 (27–36) weeks. Increases were not correlated with postconceptional, gestational and postnatal ages or birth weight, suggesting that the same situation probably pertains in extremely low birth weight (ELBW) infants (<1000 g).

## *Effects of drugs on gut blood flow*

Indomethacin (0.2 mg kg$^{-1}$) impairs midgut blood flow in the premature infant already compromised by a patent ductus arteriosus; an effect which is ameliorated when indomethacin is given slowly over 30 minutes rather than as a bolus [13]. In two infants who had repeated measurements of superior mesenteric blood velocity, the vasoconstricting effects of indomethacin decreased progressively with the second and third doses. This was also noted in an infant who did not have a patent duct, suggesting that indomethacin affects the splanchnic circulation directly and independently of ductal haemodynamic influences, a proposition supported by animal studies.

## Mucosal macromolecular permeability

Increased amounts of β-lactoglobulin can be detected in serum of babies less than 33 weeks' gestation, suggesting that mucosal permeability is greater [14]. Furthermore, recent animal studies suggest that bacterial translocation across the gut is enhanced by parenteral as opposed to enteral nutrition, possibly as a result of glutamine deficiency during parenteral nutrition [15]. The sequelae of systemic exposure to cow's milk antigens are uncertain. Basophils of very low birth weight infants (VLBW) fed preterm formula showed latent anaphylactic sensitization when challenged [16] but this does not necessarily imply later allergic disease. It is probable that VLBW with family history of atopy who are fed formula, but not breast milk, are more likely to develop allergic disease, particularly eczema [17].

## Aims of enteral feeding

The principal aim of enteral feeding is supply of nutrients to achieve growth. However, the terms *feeding* and *nutrition* are not synonymous when applied to newborn infants, particularly the very immature. In these babies, feeding has additional roles particularly in perinatal adaptation and host defence. Many can be achieved by feeding sub-nutritional quantities of milk.

## Growth of infants weighing <1000 g at birth

The obvious and ultimate aim of enteral feeding is the provision of sufficient nutrients to facilitate adequate growth. Prompt resumption of rates of intra-uterine growth in weight and length, as reflected by birth weight and length centiles, remain the most widely acknowledged measure of growth adequacy [18], though tissue deposited in the quest to meet this objective may differ from that deposited by the fetus [19].

### *Weight gain*

Until recently, growth charts suitable for the assessment of extremely low birth weight infants, particularly those of 24–28 weeks' gestation have not been available. Furthermore, available charts have seemed to overestimate the size at birth even of those infants more than 28 weeks' gestation. This probably reflected the increasing tendency to intervention at delivery by using Caesarean section for growth-retarded infants. Suitable growth charts for immature infants need, therefore, to be based on spontaneous deliveries of certain gestation among a geographically defined population. Charts based on deliveries in a particular centre [20] may reflect inclusion of tertiary care referrals and local obstetric practice more than optimal patterns of intrauterine growth. Two data sets based on United Kingdom births have been published, one from Sheffield [21] and one from five centres, principally in East Anglia [22]. Neither is truly population-based, though the Sheffield dataset comes closer, and only the second refers to spontaneous births alone, perhaps explaining the marked difference between estimates of the 3rd percentile after 28 weeks (Table 11.1). The weight data used to extend the Gairdner–Pearson charts commonly used in British nurseries (available from Castlemead Publications) to 24 weeks of gestation were those of Lucas *et al.* [22].

Using birth weight data, the specific growth rate of a fetus growing along the 50th centile of Keen and Pearse between 24 and 36 weeks has been calculated [23] as $16.2 \, \text{g kg}^{-1} \, \text{day}^{-1}$. However, when using this figure to interpret the relative rate of *extrauterine* growth, it is important to bear two things in mind. First, the specific growth rate of an infant growing along the 10th centile will apparently be bigger since the denominator is smaller. The converse will be true for one growing along the 90th centile. Second, changes in body composition at birth, particularly the contraction in extracellular fluid volume (Chapter 12) mean that the denominator (body weight) is both quantitatively and qualitatively different to the fetal model.

### *Anthropometric assessment*

Linear growth assessment has been a neglected aspect of growth monitoring in the immature baby, presumably because crown–heel measurement requires a certain amount of handling. Knemometry has recently been shown to be a useful alternative. An electronic knemometer with resolution of 0.01 mm and precision of 1.8 mm (standard deviation of a sequence of five measurements) has been applied to

**Table 11.1 Birth weight (g) by centile of babies of 24–31 weeks' gestation born in the UK. Lucas *et al.* data exclude interventive deliveries. 3rd and 97th centiles of Keen and Pearse calculation from mean (SD).**

| Gestation (weeks) | Keen and Pearse [21] | | | Lucas et al. [22] | | |
|---|---|---|---|---|---|---|
| | *3rd* | *50th* | *97th* | *3rd* | *50th* | *97th* |
| 24 | 431 | 685 | 939 | — | — | — |
| 25 | 500 | 738 | 976 | 550 | 760 | 970 |
| 26 | 572 | 904 | 1236 | 630 | 890 | 1150 |
| 27 | 671 | 1037 | 1403 | 720 | 1020 | 1320 |
| 28 | 788 | 1206 | 1624 | 815 | 1160 | 1505 |
| 29 | 804 | 1332 | 1860 | 920 | 1300 | 1680 |
| 30 | 913 | 1467 | 2021 | 1030 | 1450 | 1870 |
| 31 | 1004 | 1580 | 2156 | 1145 | 1605 | 2065 |

measure knee–heel distance in infants <1000 g [24]. These data confirm that linear growth proceeds even during postnatal weight loss in some babies. It has also been shown that linear growth rates are significantly reduced in infants with chronic lung disease, particularly those treated with steroids [25]. The electronic knemometer is expensive but we have found that little precision is sacrificed when the simple analogue slide rule based on a published device for measuring foot length [26] is used. The standard deviation (SD) for a sequence of repeated measurements was 2.5 mm [27] and the device can also be used to measure foot length with similar precision.

Further information about accretion of muscle and fat could be provided by measurement of mid-arm circumference (SD of repeated measurements 0.21 cm), particularly if skinfolds are measured as well, but published data are few [28]. Thickness of the triceps skinfold 15 s after applying the caliper ($TrSkf_{15}$) shows some correlation with body water content whereas the reading at 60 s ($TrSkf_{60}$) reflects fat [29]. The coefficient of variation for measurement of skinfold thickness with Harpenden calipers is about 5% and data are available from 24 weeks onwards [30].

### Long-term growth of VLBW infants

Methodological problems in the study of long-term growth include incomplete follow-up of cohorts leading to the selection of survivors with the greatest early or long-term problems, exclusion of cases who fail to thrive and cross-sectional rather than longitudinal analysis of data [31]. This may induce bias as yesterday's survivors are likely to have been larger and healthier than current ones. Geographically defined cohorts are rare [32] but more likely to be free of case-selection bias.

ELBW babies appear less likely to show complete catch-up growth than those <1500 g (VLBW). For example, a study of the survivors of intensive care in one British neonatal unit [33] showed that 18% of VLBW babies were below the third percentile for weight and 8% were below the third percentile for length at the age of two years. The comparable statistics for ELBW babies were 37% and 20% respectively. At the age of one year, however, 67 per cent of ELBW babies had been below the third percentile for weight and 33% below that for

length. A small study of 500–750 g survivors [31] suggested that catch-up might occur after the age of 5 years though fewer children were included at the older ages, which could have led to bias. A Hungarian study reporting follow-up of ELBW infants to the age of 12 years observed that 28% were still under the third percentile for weight and 12% under that for height [34]. The balance of evidence available from long-term studies of ELBW survivors therefore suggests that average size remains small relative to that of term infants.

The cause of later short stature in extremely premature infants is not well understood at present. Some information suggests that low-birth-weight babies fed human milk in the early weeks are significantly shorter at the age of eighteen months than those who were fed low-birth-weight formula [35]. The presence of metabolic bone disease in the neonatal period increased the risk, suggesting that early mineral deficiency is the important precursor. It has been suggested that early mineral deficiency might program slower bone growth at a critical stage of development, in the interests of later calcium and phosphorus economy.

### Feeding and neurodevelopmental outcome

Currently available evidence on the relationship between early diet and neurodevelopmental outcome of low birth weight infants favours the use of human milk. Contrary to popular belief, there was no significant difference in developmental quotient at nine months between very low-birth-weight infants fed banked human milk or preterm formula as *sole* diets [36]. Furthermore, provision of maternal milk resulted in a statistically significant advantage in Bayley scale assessment at 18 months of age after adjustment for confounding demographic and perinatal factors [37]. At the age of 7 years, low-birth-weight infants fed their own mothers' milk showed an advantage of 8.3 points in IQ which was again independent of other demographic and perinatal factors [38]. It has been argued that this reflects an important difference between the composition of human milk and artificial formula, possibly in the concentration of long chain polyunsaturated (*n*-3) fatty acids, but there are insufficient data at present to exclude behavioural correlates of breast feeding as the important influence. Nevertheless, supplementation of artificial formulae with the 22-carbon *n*-3 fatty acid docosahexaenoic acid improved visual cortical function among formula-fed infants weighing 1000–1500 g at birth, approximating it to that of infants fed human milk [39].

### Enteral feeding as a stimulus to postnatal gut adaptation

Even when morbidity or physiological immaturity constrain the volume of food provided, enteral feeding is generally to be encouraged as a strategy complementary to parenteral feeding. *Minimal enteral feeding* – the provision of amounts of milk as small as $0.5$ ml kg$^{-1}$ h$^{-1}$ – has been shown to change the endocrine environment of the gut [40], to hasten the tolerance of enteral feeds, to reduce the incidence of the cholestasis associated with parenteral nutrition, and to lower peak levels of unconjugated bilirubin [41,42]. There is some evidence that using human milk rather than low-birth-weight formula leads to more rapid tolerance of enteral feeds [43], but the mechanism underlying this is unclear. It could reflect more rapid gastric emptying on account of the lower osmolality of human milk [44], though the ability of milk constituents such as growth factors to induce histological and functional changes could be relevant (page 113). Half-strength formula has been used when it is unavailable [42].

### Enteral feeding and host defences

The composition of human milk would suggest that it has an important role in neonatal host defence but clinical studies are few. Although the anti-infective properties of human milk have been clearly demonstrated in low-birth-weight infants [45–47], only data about necrotizing enterocolitis specifically apply to very immature babies. One study found necrotizing enterocolitis six to ten times more commonly among low-birth-weight babies fed formula than among those fed human milk but the effect seemed less marked in very preterm babies (25–27 weeks) than in more mature growth-retarded ones [48]. A case–control study, however, revealed significant protection in babies of 29 weeks' gestation or less [49].

### Other advantages of early commencement of enteral feeding

Some nutrients can be provided more reliably by the enteral route as the formulation of parenteral nutrition regimens still presents some technical problems. These particularly include calcium, phosphorus, vitamin A and trace elements. Postponement of enteral feeding with the intention of reducing morbidity is generally unjustified (though specific groups of growth retarded infants may benefit; page 114). A study comparing transpyloric feeding with parenteral nutrition in infants weighing 750–1500 g found that any reduction in the risk of necrotizing enterocolitis was outweighed by a higher risk of septicaemia and reversible liver dysfunction in the parenterally fed group [50].

## Practical aspects of feeding

### Human milk or formula?

For all the reasons set out above and elsewhere [51] we recommend that the mother's own milk should be used to feed enterally babies under 1000 g at birth. It is better tolerated than formula, morbidity (particularly related to NEC) is reduced, and there is evidence of later neurodevelopmental advantage though there may be a small penalty in final height. Encouraging lactation has the added advantage of more closely involving parents in the care of their baby.

We use the mother's own milk in the sequence in which it has been expressed colostrum, transitional milk, mature milk without processing it or testing it microbiologically. The only supplement we add to the milk is phosphorus. If the mother's own milk is not available we use banked human milk (donor milk) until 150 ml kg$^{-1}$ d$^{-1}$ is tolerated. We then switch to preterm formula. At present there is no evidence that one brand of preterm formula has any advantage over another; all those marketed in the United Kingdom conform to the European Society of Gastroenterology and Nutrition Guidelines [52,53].

### Providing human milk

Provision of milk presents greater problems for the mother of the extremely low birth weight infant, particularly when geographical separation in a tertiary care centre is prolonged. Mothers of small babies delivered electively are often ill themselves after delivery and unable to express milk in the early days. Human milk banks have a role in providing a microbiologically safe product in these circumstances but the number of banks has fallen in recent years [54], principally as the result of concern about the possible transfer of human immunodeficiency virus (HIV). It is known, however, that HIV is inactivated by heat treatment (56° or 63° C for 30 minutes) [55,56]. If this is combined with exclusion of high-risk donors and serological testing for HIV antibody [57], which does not appear to deter donors [54], safety can be assured.

Encouragement of maternal lactation is essential even when banked human milk is available. Apart from provision of consistent advice and frequent expression, important aspects of support include the avoidance of bottle feeds and facilitation of skin-to-skin (kangaroo) care. A study in which babies of 560–1500 g were randomised to conventional incubator nursing or intermittent kangaroo care once they were stable showed that such care was not associated with any significant adverse effects and increased both the incidence of breastfeeding at discharge and its duration [58]. Although all would agree that mothers should be encouraged to put the babies to the breast when they are able to suck, there is some debate about whether offering milk by bottle, when the mother is absent, impairs breastfeeding. No comparative studies of feeding methods are available but many feel that gastric tube feeding or cup-feeding [59] reduces the chance of nipple confusion. Furthermore, the effect on breastfeeding of offering pacifiers to encourage non-nutritive sucking is unclear. This is sometimes practised because of reports of increased weight gain [60], possibly as a result of increased lingual lipase secretion, but fat balance studies have not confirmed this [61].

## Route of administration

Feeding tubes should preferably be passed orally where they may be fixed with tape or by a moulded dental appliance. Nasal tubes, although more easily fixed in larger babies, increase the impedance of the upper airway

and, consequently, the work of breathing [62,63]. Intragastric feeding is simple and more physiological than jejunal feeding which we reserve for babies at risk from aspiration, such as spontaneously breathing babies verging on respiratory failure or babies receiving pharyngeal distending pressure. Studies comparing nasogastric and nasojejunal feeding generally have failed to detect significant benefit in weight gain from the more complex jejunal approach [64,65] and it is important to remember that the gastric phase of digestion is an important contributor to lipolysis in the preterm infant, mediated by lingual lipase.

Care must be taken to avoid gastric distension when feeding small infants as this is associated with decreased lung volume [66] and arterial oxygen tension [67]. Gastro-oesophageal reflux may also complicate enteral feeding and result in apnoea. An oesophageal pH monitoring study detected reflux in 85% of 35 preterm infants (median birth weight 1040 g; range 720–1470 g) [68]. In most cases this was not clinically apparent and was treatable with conventional anti-reflux therapy (feed thickening with Carobel™, Cow & Gate, 0.3–0.6 g 100 ml⁻¹). This should be considered in any infant with apnoeic attacks, particularly because methylxanthine therapy, such as caffeine, tends to exacerbate reflux. Apnoea noted under these circumstances is not usually the result of aspiration but has been attributed to vagal stimulation secondary to oesophagitis and abnormal oesophageal motility. Intermittent positive pressure ventilation via endotracheal tube does not increase the incidence of gastro-oesophageal reflux [69], indicating that enteral feeding during positive pressure ventilation is safe. We withhold enteral feeds for at least 6 hours after endotracheal extubation.

## Volume and frequency of feeding

We commence enteral feeding as soon as possible after birth, once cardiorespiratory status has stabilized, even in those infants who are being mechanically ventilated. Human milk, either pasteurized banked human milk or the mother's own unheated milk is preferred. In the case of the infant weighing <1000 g we begin with 0.5 ml kg⁻¹ h⁻¹ administered by intragastric hourly gavage, aspirating the tube after 6 hours. If the aspirate is greater than

3 ml at this stage we recommend waiting before instilling more milk. Bile-stained (green) aspirates or obvious abdominal distension are indications to stop. If feeds are not tolerated, a small glycerine suppository may be helpful if the infant has not passed meconium. In our experience it is rare for the baby paralysed with neuromuscular relaxants to tolerate enteral feeds reliably, but there may be some advantage in instilling small quantities to promote gastrointestinal adaptation since amounts of feed as small as 0.65 ml kg$^{-1}$ each *day* have resulted in maturation of the gut endocrine response to feeding [40]. When small volumes of feed are consistently tolerated we increase the volume very gradually, continuing with hourly gavage feeds, and do not consider it necessary to continue with parenteral nutrition once a daily volume of 120 ml kg$^{-1}$ has been attained. Vitamin supplements are commenced at this stage. We increase the volume of feed to a maximum of 200 ml kg$^{-1}$ day$^{-1}$ as tolerated.

Continuous nasogastric feeds are popular in some units but sedimentation of fat and adsorption to the material of syringe and tubing presents a problem. This is well recognized but it is worth noting that the smaller the infant, the greater the dead space of the administration system as a proportion of total intake and, consequently, the greater the potential energy loss. The neuroendocrine correlates of continuous and bolus intragastric feeding are quite different [70] but the clinical consequences of this observation are unknown.

### Vitamin and iron supplements

We give 400 µg/kg of vitamin K (Konakion MM Roche) intravenously at birth to all babies under 36 weeks of gestation.

Once 120 ml kg$^{-1}$ day$^{-1}$ enteral feeds are tolerated we commence a proprietary multivitamin supplement (0.6 ml Abidec™). Intake of vitamin A is much better assured by the oral route as the amount in some parenteral vitamin solutions is very low and most is adsorbed to infusion tubing or photodegraded. This could be particularly important in infants <1000 g as vitamin A deficiency has been linked causally to chronic lung disease in one study [71] (but not in another [72]). We give extra vitamin D (as 600 units calciferol) to

babies <1500 g at birth, making their total daily intake 1000 units day$^{-1}$ (allowing for 400 units in 0.6 ml Abidec™).

We do not give vitamin E supplements as no benefit has been proven, nor do we give folic acid supplements though ESPGAN recommended up to 65 µg kg$^{-1}$ day$^{-1}$ [52]. Currently there are early concerns that vitamin C intake may be excessive in some very low birth weight babies, reducing plasma ferroxidase activity and theoretically predisposing to free radical injury. Plasma vitamin C levels of unsupplemented babies fed pasteurized human milk are nevertheless low [73] and transient tyrosinaemia of the newborn has been observed in such circumstances.

We do not commence iron supplements earlier than 4 weeks of age and often postpone them until later as we maintain the haemoglobin concentration of oxygen dependent babies at more than 12 g dl$^{-1}$ (packed cell volume >40%) by repeated transfusion, thus increasing iron stores *pari passu* with growth. As it seems likely that erythropoietin will be used increasingly in such babies, earlier iron supplementation may become necessary in the future. It is important to bear in mind, however, both the effect of the free ferrous ion (Fe$^{2+}$) on growth of *E coli* and its propensity to promote free radical damage in the gut together with the free hydroxyl ion OH$^{-}$ (Weiss reaction). There is also a possibility that iron supplements alter the absorption and metabolism of other trace minerals, particularly copper [74] and zinc [75]. We provide 2 mg kg$^{-1}$ day$^{-1}$ of elemental iron (as iron edetate, Sytron™) to a maximum of 15 mg day$^{-1}$ [52].

### Supplementation of human milk

The only supplement we add *routinely* to human milk is phosphorus. There is good evidence from a randomized controlled study of babies weighing <1250 g that a supplement of 50 mg daily prevents radiologically apparent metabolic bone disease [76]. We add a smaller amount initially, 13 mg day$^{-1}$ phosphorus (as 0.5 ml buffered phosphate solution, McCarthy's) which should approximate the calcium/phosphorus ratio of breast milk to 1.4:1. A plasma phosphate concentration of <1.5 mmol l$^{-1}$ suggests phosphorus deficiency and the efficacy of phosphorus supplementation can be monitored, if desired, by measurement of the calcium and phosphorus content of the urine. Many babies fed unsupplemented human milk show no phosphorus excretion and hypercalciuria, indicating that tubular reabsorption is maximal and calcium deposition in bone is limited by phosphorus deficiency. The urine calcium excretion should not exceed 6 mg kg$^{-1}$ day$^{-1}$ and the ratio of calcium phosphorus (expressed in milligrams) in the urine should be <1. It has been claimed that supplements of up to 50 mg P dl$^{-1}$ (as disodium phosphate) and up to 70 mg Ca dl$^{-1}$ (as calcium gluconate) are stable in human milk overnight [77]. Phosphate should be mixed with the milk before calcium is added (see also the section on phosphorus in Chapter 13).

In our opinion the case for *routinely* supplementing the milk of a small baby's own mother with protein has not been established. Banked human milk (collected from donors who have delivered at term) should be used only for short periods to facilitate the early tolerance of enteral feeds whilst maternal milk is unavailable but would require protein supplementation (0.7 g dl$^{-1}$) [78] if used for longer. Energy supplementation, however, is equally important if dripped rather than expressed milk is collected. Where the mother's own milk is concerned it is vital to bear in mind both the range of protein concentration encountered and the possibility that its energy content may also be low. The average protein content of milk supplied by mothers of very low birth weight infants in the first 4 weeks after delivery was 1.5–1.7 g dl$^{-1}$ [79] compared with other values in the literature of 1.7 ± 3.3 [80] and 2.2 ± 5.6 [81] (mean ± SD). Thus, feeding maternal milk at 180–200 ml kg$^{-1}$ day$^{-1}$ can provide, on average, 3.1–4.4 g kg$^{-1}$ day$^{-1}$ of protein (expressed as total nitrogen × 6.38). Addition of a standard 0.7 g protein to 100 ml$^{-1}$ samples of milk at the upper limit of this range could considerably increase this to intakes as high as 5.8 g kg$^{-1}$ day$^{-1}$ which could be too high, particularly if energy intake is low.

We find that it is helpful to consider whether individual babies who are not thriving adequately require supplements of protein or energy, or both. The plasma urea concentration can be a helpful indicator and correlates with quantitative nitrogen excretion [82]. In babies fed human milk, but who are not growing, plasma urea concentrations of <1 mmol l$^{-1}$ tend to be associated with protein deficiency; concentrations consistently exceeding 2 mmol l$^{-1}$ are more suggestive of energy deficiency. In the former case we have successfully supplemented maternal milk with Maxipro™ (Scientific Hospital Supplies, Liverpool, UK). In the latter case we recommend instructing the mother on separate collection of hind milk, which is higher in energy content. If this is not possible we use Duocal™ (same supplier), a supplement containing maltodextrins and fat as long and medium chain triglycerides. Trends in weight gain and plasma urea can be used to monitor treatment.

Some have argued that proprietary *human milk fortifiers* should be added to all maternal milk used to feed VLBW babies. Studies have certainly shown faster rates of weight gain and linear growth without disturbance of metabolic homeostasis in some VLBW infants fed supplemented maternal milk [83] but no large-scale clinical trials from which one can assess adequately benefit and risk in unselected VLBW have yet been undertaken.

### Diet after hospital discharge

Until recently little has been published on the feeding of preterm infants after hospital discharge, despite the fact that many are at this stage showing catch-up growth. A retrospective study of 50 VLBW showed that infants weaned before a postconceptional age of term + 4 months showed no growth advantage nor any difference in total energy intake [84]. We sometimes introduce supplementary foods early if babies, particularly those with chronic respiratory distress, are failing to grow on breast milk or formula alone. However, we would not entertain this before 14 weeks from birth or term + 6 weeks of age, whichever is the later.

Two recent studies have argued that special post-discharge formulae have advantages over standard infant formulae for VLBW infants. The mean weight, length and head circumferences of VLBW babies randomly allocated to a special formula were greater than those of infants fed standard formula but the study was quite small, no information was given about weaning diets, and the major growth differences were apparent only in the first few weeks after discharge [85]. The growth trajectories of the two groups of infants were parallel thereafter. Subsequent studies have shown the bone mineral density of infants fed the special formula to be significantly greater at 3 and 9 months of age [86].

# Problems associated with feeding

## Early feeding of growth retarded babies

Babies who have had absent or reversed end-diastolic flow detected in the fetal aorta or umbilical artery are at increased risk of necrotizing enterocolitis (NEC) (p. 114) and enteral feeds should be introduced cautiously. A study including historical controls suggested that oral administration of vancomycin (15 mg kg$^{-1}$, eight hourly for six doses) reduced the incidence of NEC in babies considered at-risk, though the criteria used to identify such babies were unclear [87]. It is debatable whether delaying introduction of enteral feeds post-natally reduces the incidence of NEC or merely postpones presentation. In one of the largest studies of factors correlated with NEC undertaken [48] there was an interaction between age at introduction of feeds and the type of milk administered: the incidence of NEC was reduced when formula feeds but not human milk feeds were delayed. Evidence that formula-fed babies are at significantly greater risk of NEC was discussed above, making provision of breast milk essential for those at high risk of NEC. Historically controlled studies [88] and some [89,90], but not all [91,92], case–control studies have also identified a relationship between NEC and the rate at which enteral feeds are increased.

In practice, we delay the introduction of enteral feeds by 5 days in babies in whom there was absent fetal umbilical artery end-diastolic flow, ten when flow was reversed. We use human milk only, give vancomycin for 48 hours before enteral feeding and increase the feeds as tolerated but no more quickly than 30 ml kg$^{-1}$ day$^{-1}$. Controlled studies are urgently needed in this area.

## Failure to thrive in bronchopulmonary dysplasia (BPD)

Bronchopulmonary dysplasia is a common problem in the very immature infant, as many as 85% of those under 750 g at birth may be affected. Resting energy expenditure is significantly greater [93] but it is uncertain whether this reflects altered body proportions or increased work of breathing. Failure to thrive in BPD is most likely to result from energy deficiency and calorie supplements are often used. Caution is nevertheless advised as increased carbohydrate load will increase respiratory quotient to >1, thereby increasing $V_{CO_2}$ and minute volume. Thus, there are theoretical grounds for preferring fat supplements, if absorbed. Careful attention to the calcium and phosphorus nutrition of babies with BPD is also desirable for loop diuretics promote calciuresis and reduced bone mineralization will increase the compliance of the thoracic cage.

The most severe growth failure in BPD is seen among babies treated with corticosteroids. Energy supplements have not been shown to be helpful under these circumstances and, as treated infants are already catabolizing lean tissue, protein supplements might well be deleterious, increasing demands on the immature metabolic and excretory pathways involved in nitrogen elimination [94].

---

**Practical points**

1. Early enteral feeding is beneficial to the development of the gut and should be viewed as complementary to parenteral feeding.
2. Delaying the initiation of *formula* feeds is appropriate for a small number of babies at increased risk of necrotizing enterocolitis by virtue of abnormal blood flow in the umbilical artery/fetal aorta. Delay may be unnecessary if human milk is used.
3. Human milk is more rapidly tolerated than formula and is associated with a reduced risk of necrotizing enterocolitis.
4. Gastric tubes should be sited orally rather than nasally. This is particularly important where respiratory function is impaired.
5. It is unnecessary to prescribe commercial 'fortifiers' for the majority of babies fed their own mother's milk.
6. Energy and protein supplementation is unhelpful for babies who fail to thrive during dexamethasone therapy. It may increase $V_{CO_2}$ and thus be deleterious to respiratory function.

# References

1.  Heird, W.C., Driscoll, J.M., Schullinger, J.N., Grebin, B. and Winters, R.W. (1972) Intravenous alimentation in pediatric patients. *J. Pediatr.*, **80**, 351–372

2.  Lucas, A. (1991) Programming by early nutrition in man. In *The Childhood Environment and Adult Disease. CIBA Foundation Symposium 156*. Wiley, Chichester, pp. 38–55

3.  Lebenthal, E. and Leung, Y.K. (1989) Feeding the premature and compromised infant: gastrointestinal considerations. *Pediatr. Clin. N. Am.*, **25**, 215–238

4.  Heird, W.C., Schwartz, S.M. and Hansen, I.H. (1984) Colostrum induced enteric mucosal growth in beagle puppies. *Pediatr. Res.*, **18**, 512–515

5.  McLain, C.R. (1963) Amniography studies of the gastrointestinal motility of the human fetus. *Am J. Obstet. Gynecol.*, **68**, 1079–1087

6.  Bissett, W.M., Watt, J.B., Rivers, R.P.A. and Milla, P.J. (1988) Ontogeny of fasting small intestinal motor activity in the human infant. *Gut*, **29**, 483–488

7.  Bissett, W.M., Watt, J., Rivers, R.P.A. and Milla, P.J. (1989) Postprandial motor response of the small intestine to enternal feeds in preterm infants. *Arch. Dis. Childh.*, **64**, 1356–1361

8.  Hackett, G.A., Campbell, S., Gamsu, H., Cohen-Overbeck, T. and Pearce, J.M.F. (1987) Doppler studies in the growth retarded fetus and prediction of neonatal necrotising enterocolitis, haemorrhage and neonatal morbidity. *Br. Med. J.*, **294**, 13–16

9.  Malcolm, G., Ellwood, D., Devonald, K., Beilby, R. and Henderson-Smart, D. (1991) Absent or reversed end diastolic flow velocity in the umbilical artery and necrotising enterocolitis. *Arch. Dis. Childh.*, **66**, 805–807

10. Billardo, C.M., Nicolaides, K.H. and Campbell, S. (1990) Doppler measurements of fetal and uteroplacental circulations: relationships with umbilical venous gases measured at cordocentesis. *Am J. Obstet. Gynecol.*, **162**, 115–120

11. Kempley, S.T., Gamsu, H.R., Vyas, S. and Nicolaides, K. (1991) Effects of intrauterine growth retardation on postnatal visceral and cerebral blood flow velocity. *Arch. Dis. Childh.*, **66**, 1115–1118

12. Gladman, G., Sims, D.G. and Chiswick, M.L. (1991) Gastrointestinal blood flow velocity after the first feed. *Arch. Dis. Childh.*, **66**, 17–20

13. Coombs, R.C., Morgan, M.E.I., Durbin, G.M., Booth, I.W. and McNeish, A.S. (1990) Gut blood flow velocities in the newborn: effects of patent ductus arteriosus and parenteral indomethacin. *Arch. Dis. Childh.*, **65**, 65–71

14. Roberton, D.M., Paganelli, R., Dinwiddie, R. and Levinsky, R.J. (1982) Mild antigen absorption in the preterm and term neonate. *Arch. Dis. Childh.*, **57**, 369–372

15. Alverdy, J.C., Aoys, E. and Moss, G.S. (1988) Total parenteral nutrition promotes bacterial translocation across the gut. *Surgery*, **104**, 185–190

16. Lucas, A., McLaughlan, P. and Coombs, R.R.A. (1984) Latent anaphylactic sensitisation of infants of low birth weight to cows' milk protein. *Br. Med. J.*, **289**, 1254–1256

17. Lucas, A., Brooke, O.G., Morely, R., Cole, T.J. and Bamford, M.F. (1990) Early diet of preterm infants and development of allergic or atopic disease: randomised prospective study. *Br. Med. J.*, **300**, 837–840

18. American Academy of Pediatrics, Committee on Nutrition (1985) Nutritional needs of low-birth-weight infants. *Pediatrics*, **75**, 976–986

19. Reichman, B., Chessex, P., Putet, G. *et al.* (1981) Diet, fat accretion and growth in premature infants. *N. Engl. J. Med.*, **305**, 1495–1500

20. Brooke, O.G. and McIntosh, N. (1984) Birthweights of infants born before 30 weeks' gestation. *Arch. Dis. Childh.*, **59**, 1189–1190

21. Keen, D.V. and Pearse, R.G. (1985) Birthweight between 14 and 42 weeks' gestation. *Arch. Dis. Childh.*, **60**, 440–446

22. Lucas, A., Cole, T.J. and Gandy, G.M. (1986) Birthweight centiles reappraised. *Early Hum. Dev.*, **13**, 313–322

23. Shaw, J.C.L. (1988) Growth and nutrition of the very preterm infant. *Br. Med. Bull.*, **44**, 984–1009

24. Michailsen, K.F., Skov, L., Badsberg, J.H. and Jorgensen, M. (1991) Short term measurement of linear growth in preterm infants: validation of a hand-held knemometer. *Pediatr. Res.*, **30**, 464–468

25. Gibson, A.T., Pearse, R.G. and Wales, J.K.H. (1993) Chronic lung disease, dexamethasone and linear growth in neonates. In *Proceedings of the Nutrition Society*, **52**, 225A.

26. James, D.K., Dryburgh, E.H. and Chiswick, M.L. (1979) Foot length – a new and potentially useful measurement in the neonate. *Arch. Dis. Childh.*, **54**, 226–230

27. Prins, I. (1995) Anthropometry in the newborn: a clinical review. *Pediatric Rev. Commun.*, **8**, 157–170

28. Georgieff, M.K., Mills, M.M., Zempel, C.M. and Pi-Nian, C. (1989) Catch-up growth, muscle and fat accretion and body proportionality of infants one year after newborn intensive care. *J. Pediatr.*, **114**, 288–292

29. Thornton, C.J., Shallon, D.L., Hunter, M.A. and Brans, Y.W. (1982) Dynamic skinfold measurements: a non-invasive estimate of neonatal extracellular water content. *Pediatr. Res.*, **16**, 989–994

30. Vaucher, Y.E., Harrison, G.G., Udall, J.N. and Morrow, G. (1984) Skinfold thickness in North American infants 24–41 weeks' gestation. *Hum. Biol.*, **56**, 713–731

31. Hirata, T., Epcar, J.T. and Walsh, B.A. (1983) Survival and outcome of infants 501 to 750 grams: a 6-year experience. *J. Pediatr.*, **102**, 741–748

32. Saigal, S., Rosenbaum, P., Stotskopf, B. and Milner, R. (1982) Follow-up of infants 501–1500 gram birthweight delivered to residents of a geographically defined region with intensive perinatal care facilities. *J. Pediatr.*, **100**, 606–613

33. Brothwood, M., Wolke, D., Gamsu, H. and Cooper, D. (1988) Mortality, morbidity, growth and development of babies weighing 501–1000 grams and 1001–1500 grams at birth. *Acta. Paediatr. Scand.*, **77**, 10–18

34. Vekerdy-Lakatos, Z., Lakatos, L. and Ittzes-Nagy (1989) Infants weighing 1000 g or less at birth. Outcome at 8–11 years of age. *Acta. Paediatr. Scand.*, **360** (Suppl.), 62–71

35. Lucas, A., Brooke, O.G., Baker, B.A., Bishop, N. and Morley, R. (1989) High alkaline phosphatase activity and growth in preterm neonates. *Arch. Dis. Childh.*, **64**, 902–909

36. Lucas, A., Morley, R., Cole, T.J. *et al.* (1989) Early diet in preterm babies and developmental status in infancy. *Arch. Dis. Childh.*, **64**, 1570–1578

37. Morley, R., Cole, T.J., Powell, R. and Lucas, A. (1988) Mother's choice to provide breast milk and developmental outcome. *Arch. Dis. Childh.*, **63**, 1382–1385

38. Lucas, A., Morley, R., Cole, T.J., Lister, G. and Leeson-Payne, C. (1992) Breast milk and subsequent intelligence quotient in children born preterm. *Lancet*, **339**, 261–264

39. Uauy, R., Birch, D., Birch, E., Tyson, J. and Hoffman, D.R. (1990) Effect of omega-3 fatty acids on retinal function of very low-birth weight neonates. *Pediatr. Res.*, **28**, 485–492

40. Lucas, A., Bloom, S.R. and Aynsley-Green, A. (1986) Gut hormones and minimal enteral feeding. *Acta Paediatr. Scand.*, **75**, 719–723

41. Slagle, T.A. and Gross, S.J. (1988) Effect of early low-volume enteral substrate on subsequent feeding tolerance in very low birth weight infants. *J. Pediatr.*, **113**, 526–531

42. Dunn, L., Hulman, S., Weiner, J. and Kliegmann, P. (1988) Beneficial effects of early hypocaloric enteral feeding on neonatal gastrointestinal function: preliminary report of a randomised trial. *J. Pediatr.*, **112**, 622–629

43. Lucas, A. (1987) AIDS and human milk bank closures. *Lancet*, **i**, 1092–1093

44. Cavell, B. (1979) Gastric emptying in preterm infants. *Acta. Paediatr. Scand.*, **68**, 725–730

45. Naryanan, I., Prakash, K., Bala, S., Verma, R.K. and Gufral, V.V. (1980) Partial supplementation with expressed breast milk for the prevention of infection in low-birth weight infants. *Lancet*, **ii**, 561–563

46. Naryanan, I., Prakash, K., Prabhakar, A.K. and Gujral, V.V. (1982) A planned prospective evaluation of the anti-infective property of varying quantities of expressed human milk. *Acta. Paediatr. Scand.*, **71**, 441–445

47. Naryanan, I., Prakash, K., Murthy, N.S. and Gujral, V.V. (1984) Randomised controlled trial of effect of raw and Holder pasteurised human milk and of formula supplements on incidence of neonatal infection. *Lancet*, **ii**, 1111–1112

48. Lucas, A. and Cole, T.J. (1990) Breast milk and neonatal necrotising enterocolitis. *Lancet*, **336**, 1519–1523

49. Beeby, P.J. and Jeffery, H. (1992) Risk factors for necrotising enterocolitis: the influence of gestational age. *Arch. Dis. Childh.*, **67**, 432–435

50. Glass, E.J., Hume, R., Lang, M.A. and Forfar, J.O. (1984) Parenteral nutrition compared with transpyloric feeding. *Arch. Dis. Childh.*, **59**, 131–135

51. Williams, A.F. (1993) Human milk and the preterm baby. *Br. Med. J.*, **306**, 1628–1629

52. European Society for Paediatric Gastroenterology and Nutrition, Committee on Nutrition of the Preterm Infant (1987) Nutrition and feeding of preterm infants. *Acta. Paediatr. Scand.*, **336** (Suppl.), 1–14

53. Wharton, B.A. (1987) *Nutrition and Feeding of Preterm Infants*. Blackwell, Oxford

54. Balmer, S.E. and Wharton, B.A. (1992) Human milk banking at Sorrento Maternity Hospital, Birmingham. *Arch. Dis. Childh*, **67**, 556–559

55. Eglin, R.P. and Wilkinson, A.R. (1987) HIV infection and pasteurisation of breast milk. *Lancet*, **i**, 1092–1093

56. Orloff, S.L., Wallingford, J.C. and McDougal, J.S. (1993) Inactivation of human immunodeficiency virus Type I in human milk. Effects of intrinsic factors in human milk and of pasteurisation. *J. Hum. Lact.*, **9**, 13–17

57. Department of Health and Social Security (1988) *HIV Infection, Breastfeeding and Human Milk Banking.* HMSO, London

58. Whitelaw, A., Heisterkamp, G., Sleath, K., Acolet, D. and Richards, M. (1988) Skin to skin contact for very low birthweight infants and their mothers. *Arch. Dis. Childh.*, **63**, 1377–1381

59. Giroux, J.D., Sizun, J. and Alix, D. (1991) L'alimentation à la tasse chez le nouveau né. *Arch. Franc. Pediatr.*, **48**, 737–740

60. Bernbaum, J.C., Pereira, G.R., Watkins, J.B. and Peckham, G.J. (1983) Non-intrusive sucking during gavage feeding enhances growth and maturation in premature infants. *Pediatrics*, **71**, 41–45

61. de Curtis, M., McIntosh, N., Ventura, V. and Brooke, O. (1986) Effect of non-nutritive sucking on nutrient retention in preterm infants. *J. Pediatr.*, **109**, 888–890

62. Stocks, J. (1980) Effects of nasogastric tubes on nasal resistance during infancy. *Arch. Dis. Childh.*, **55**, 17–21

63. van Someren, V., Linnett, S.J., Stothers, J.K. and Sullivan, P.G. (1984) An investigation into the benefits of resisting nasoenteric feeding tubes. *Pediatrics*, **74**, 379–383

64. Laing, I.A., Lang, A., Callaghan, O. and Hume, R. (1986) Nasogastric compared with nasoduodenal feeding in low birthweight infants. *Arch. Dis. Childh.*, **61**, 138–141

65. Beddis, I. and McKenzie, S. (1979) Transpyloric feeding in the very low birth weight infant (1500 g). *Arch. Dis. Childh.*, **54**, 213–217

66. Pitcher-Wilmott, R., Shutack, J.G. and Fow, W.W. (1979) Decreased lung volume after nasogastric feeding of neonates recovering from respiratory distress. *J. Pediatr.*, **95**, 119–121

67. Herrell, N., Martin, R.J. and Farnaroff, A. (1980)

Arterial oxygen tension during nasogastric feeding in the preterm infant. *J. Pediatr.*, **96**, 914–916

68. Newell, S.J., Booth, I.W., Morgan, M.E.I. *et al.* (1989) Gastro-oesophageal reflux in preterm infants. *Arch. Dis. Childh.*, **64**, 780–786

69. Newell, S.J., Morgan, M.E.I., Durbin, G.M. *et al.* (1989) Does mechanical ventilation precipitate gastro-oesophageal reflux during enternal feeding? *Arch. Dis. Childh.*, **64**, 1352–1355

70. Aynsley-Green, A., Adrian, T.E. and Bloom, S.R. (1982) Feeding and the development of enteroinsular hormone release in the preterm infant: effects of continuous gastric infusion of human milk compared with boluses. *Acta. Paediatr. Scand.*, **71**, 379–383

71. Shenai, J.P., Kennedy, K.A., Chytil, F. and Stahlman, M.T. (1987) Clinical trial of vitamin A supplementation in infants susceptible to bronchopulmonary dysplasia. *J. Pediatr.*, **111**, 269–277

72. Pearson, E., Bose, C., Snidow, T. *et al.* (1992) Trial of vitamin A supplementation in very low birth weight infants at risk for bronchopulmonary dysplasia. *J. Pediatr.*, **121**, 420–427

73. Heinonen, K., Mononen, I., Mononen, T., Parviainen, M., Penttila, I. and Launiala, K. (1986) Plasma vitamin C levels are low in premature infants fed human milk. *Am. J. Clin. Nutr.*, **43**, 923–924

74. Barclay, S.M., Aggett, P.J., Lloyd, D.J. and Duffty, P. (1991) Reduced erythrocyte superoxide dismutase activity in low birth weight infants given iron supplements. *Pediatr. Res.*, **29**, 297–301

75. Solomons, N.W. (1986) Competitive interaction of iron and zinc in the diet. Consequences for human nutrition. *J. Nutr.*, **116**, 927–935

76. Holland, P.C., Wilkinson, A.R., Diez, J. and Lindsell, D.R.M. (1990) Prenatal deficiency of phosphate, phosphate supplementation and rickets in very low birthweight infants. *Lancet*, **335**, 697–701

77. Salle, B., Senterre, J., Putet, G. and Rigo, J. (1986) Effects of calcium and phosphorus supplementation on calcium retention and fat absorption in preterm infants fed pooled human milk. *J. Pediatr. Gastroenterol.*, **5**, 638–642

78. Williams, A.F. (1987) How should we use banked human milk? In *New Aspects of Nutrition in Pregnancy, Infancy and Prematurity* (M. Xanthou, ed.), Elsevier, pp. 117–127

79. Lucas, A. and Hudson, G.J. (1984) Preterm milk as a source of protein for low birthweight infants. *Arch. Dis. Childh.*, **59**, 831–836

80. Lemons, J.A., Moye, L.L., Hall, D. and Simmons, M. (1982) Differences in the composition of preterm and term human milk during early lactation. *Pediatr. Res.*, **16**, 113–117

81. Gross, S.J., David, R.J., Baumann, L. and Tomarelli, R.M. (1980) Nutritional composition of milk produced by mothers delivering preterm. *J. Pediatr.*, **96**, 641–644

82. Polberger, S.K.T., Axelsson, I.E. and Räihä, N.C.R. (1990) Urinary and serum urea as indicators of protein metabolism in very low birthweight infants fed varying human milk protein intakes. *Acta. Paediatr. Scand.*, **79**, 737–742

83. Kashyap, S., Schulze, K.F., Forsyth, M., Dell, B., Ramakrishna, R. and Heird, W.C. (1990) Growth, nutrient retention and metabolic response of low birthweight infants fed supplemented and unsupplemented preterm human milk. *Am. J. Clin. Nutr.*, **52**, 254–262

84. d'Souza, S.W., Vale, J., Sims, D.G. and Chiswick, M.L. (1985) Feeding, growth and biochemical studies in very low birthweight infants. *Arch. Dis. Childh.*, **60**, 215–218

85. Lucas, A., Bishop, N.J., King, F.J. and Cole, T.J. (1992) Randomised trial of nutrition for preterm infants after discharge. *Arch. Dis. Childh.*, **67**, 324–327

86. Bishop, N.J., King, F.J. and Lucas, A. (1993) Increased bone mineral content of preterm infants fed with a nutrient enriched formula after discharge from hospital. *Arch. Dis. Childh.*, **68**, 573–578

87. Ng, P.C., Dear, P.R.F. and Thomas, D.F.M. (1988) Oral vancomycin in prevention of necrotising enterocolitis. *Arch. Dis. Childh.*, **63**, 1390–1393

88. Goldman, H.I. (1980) Feeding and necrotising enterocolitis. *Am. J. Dis. Child.*, **134**, 553–555

89. McKeown, R.E., Marsh, D., Amarnath, U. *et al.* (1992) Role of delayed feeding and feeding increments in necrotising enterocolitis. *J. Pediatr.*, **121**, 764–770

90. Anderson, D.M. and Kliegman, R.M. (1991) The relationship of neonatal alimentation practices to the occurrence of endemic necrotising enterocolitis. *Am. J. Perinatol.*, **8**, 62–67

91. Frantz, I.D. III, L'Heureux, P., Engel, R.P. and Hunt, C.E. (1975) Necrotising enterocolitis. *J. Pediatr.*, **86**, 259–263

92. Ryder, R.W., Shelton, J.D. and Guinan, M.E. (1980) Necrotising enterocolitis: a prospective multicentre investigation. *Am. J. Epidermiol.*, **112**, 113–123

93. Kurzner, S.I., Garg, M., Bautista, D.B. *et al.* (1988) Growth failure in bronchopulmonary dysplasia: elevated metabolic rates and pulmonary mechanics. *J. Pediatr.*, **112**, 73–80

94. Williams, A.F. and Jones, M.G. (1992) Dexamethasone increases plasma amino acid concentrations in bronchopulmonary dysplasia. *Arch. Dis. Childh.*, **67**, 5–9

# 12

# Intravenous nutrition

Victor Yu

Extrauterine survival for extremely low birth weight (ELBW, <1000 g) babies depends on the maintenance of nutrition after birth with intravenous nutrition and a successful transition to enteral nutrition. A survey of neonatal units in the USA published in 1985 showed that 80% of units used intravenous nutrition exclusively in the first week for ELBW babies [1]. Data from a more recent survey published in 1991 showed that over 80% of survivors with a birth weight of 500–1500 g received intravenous nutrition for a mean of 19 days (range 12–26 days) [2]. It is the purpose of this chapter to review the principles and practice of intravenous nutrition in these high-risk babies.

## Fluid and nutrient requirements

### Fluid

The mean postnatal weight loss in babies born at 26–29 weeks' gestation was reported to be 12–15% of birth weight, while those born at 25 weeks or less had a mean loss of about 20% [3]. A randomized controlled trial (RCT) was conducted in babies with a birth weight of 750–1500 g utilizing two intravenous regimes: one which allowed 1–2% loss of birth weight per day to a maximum loss of 8–10%, versus one which allowed 3–5% loss per day to a maximum of 13–15% [4]. Neonatal mortality and morbidity was similar in the two groups, indicating that the gradual loss of 15% of birth weight in the first week after birth is safe. Some studies have suggested that this weight loss resulted from fluid loss [5,6] while others have suggested that it resulted from tissue loss caused by catabolism [7,8]. One study demonstrated that the observed postnatal weight changes in babies receiving intravenous nutrition reflect changes in their interstitial volume [9].

ELBW babies in the first 1–2 weeks after birth have excessive transepidermal water loss [10], secondary to an underdeveloped stratum corneum prior to cornification [11]. Their insensible water loss (IWL) can range from 50 ml kg$^{-1}$ day$^{-1}$ to over 150 ml kg$^{-1}$ day$^{-1}$ depending on environmental factors. The use of radiant warmers and/or phototherapy [12], an increase in ambient temperature [13], nursing under conditions of forced convection [14] and intravenous nutrition [15] increase IWL by 40–60%. The use of plastic heat shields [16,17], plastic blankets [17,18] and a high ambient humidity [19] decrease IWL by 30–60%. If preterm babies are nursed in maximally humidified incubators, their intravenous requirement is not too different from that of term babies: 60–80 ml kg$^{-1}$ day$^{-1}$ increasing to 100–120 ml kg$^{-1}$ day$^{-1}$ over the first week [4]. If the ambient humidity is only 50%, it is advisable to start at 100 ml kg$^{-1}$ day$^{-1}$ increasing to 150 ml kg$^{-1}$ day$^{-1}$ [20]. However, when measures to reduce IWL are not taken, intravenous requirements for some ELBW babies may exceed 200 ml kg$^{-1}$ day$^{-1}$. Serial assessment of hydration status is mandatory, using clinical and laboratory parameters (see Chapter 8, Table 8.1).

## Energy

ELBW babies have low energy reserves because they have diminished glycogen stores in the liver and reduced fat deposits. However, they also have a low basal metabolic rate of 130 kJ kg$^{-1}$ day$^{-1}$ (about 30 kcal kg$^{-1}$ day$^{-1}$) when nursed in a thermoneutral environment with minimal activity. Allowing for the energy cost of intermittent cold stress and physical activity, an intravenous input of 200 kJ kg$^{-1}$ day$^{-1}$ (about 50 kcal kg$^{-1}$ day$^{-1}$) is sufficient to match ongoing expenditure but does not provide additional energy required for growth.

The energy cost of growth is about 20 kJ (5 kcal) per gram of tissue increment [21]. This includes the specific dynamic action of intravenous nutrition which is about 13% of basal metabolic rate or 10% of the energy infused [22]. To achieve the equivalent of third trimester intrauterine weight gain (14 g kg$^{-1}$ day$^{-1}$), an additional energy intake of 300 kJ kg$^{-1}$ day$^{-1}$ (about 70 kcal kg$^{-1}$ day$^{-1}$) is theoretically required. Intravenously fed babies, compared to those who are enterally fed, begin to grow at a lower energy intake because faecal losses are negligible, thermoneutrality is more carefully controlled and physical activity is reduced with minimal handling. Thus, even though the optimal energy intake for a rapidly growing preterm baby is 500 kJ kg$^{-1}$ day$^{-1}$ (about 120 kcal kg$^{-1}$ day$^{-1}$), a growth rate and nitrogen accretion similar to *in utero* values can be sustained by intravenous nutrition when an intake of 340 kJ kg$^{-1}$ day$^{-1}$ (80 kcal kg$^{-1}$ day$^{-1}$) has been reached, provided that an appropriate amount of nitrogen is infused [23,24].

## Glucose

Almost all ELBW babies require intravenous glucose during the first few days after birth to prevent hypoglycaemia. The risk, however, is of hyperglycaemia and glucosuria [25,26] in particular those with hyaline membrane disease [27]. Hyperglycaemia during glucose infusion results from persistent endogenous hepatic glucose production due to an insensitivity of hepatocytes to insulin [28,29]. To minimize the risk of hyperglycaemia in ELBW babies, glucose infusion should begin at a rate of 6–8 g kg$^{-1}$ day$^{-1}$ (4–6 mg kg$^{-1}$ min$^{-1}$). Since glucose tolerance improves with increasing postnatal age, the glucose infusion rate can in most babies be increased progressively to 18–20 g kg$^{-1}$ day$^{-1}$ (12–14 mg kg$^{-1}$ min$^{-1}$) by the second or third week after birth [30].

It is advisable to maintain a serum glucose of below 8 mmol l$^{-1}$. The level at which brain metabolism is compromised and the risk of intracranial haemorrhage is increased, is unknown. Nevertheless, hyperglycaemia has been defined as a serum glucose above 8 mmol l$^{-1}$ [26] when glucosuria commonly appears [25]. Although osmotic diuresis has been shown to be uncommon with glucosuria [25,28], the glucose infusion rate should be reduced in the presence of hyperglycaemia. Insulin therapy is recommended in those who remain hyperglycaemic even at a lowered glucose infusion rate of 8 g kg$^{-1}$ day$^{-1}$ (6 mg kg$^{-1}$ day$^{-1}$) [31], starting at a continuous insulin infusion rate of 0.05 units kg hour [32]. A randomized clinical trial in ELBW babies with glucose intolerance has shown that insulin administration can improve glucose intake and weight gain [33].

## Nitrogen

The goal of early intravenous nutrition is to infuse sufficient energy and nitrogen to prevent catabolism and achieve positive nitrogen balance. However, at energy intakes of below 200 kJ kg$^{-1}$ day$^{-1}$ (50 kcal kg$^{-1}$ day$^{-1}$), equivalent to a glucose infusion rate of 12 g kg$^{-1}$ day$^{-1}$ (9 mg kg$^{-1}$ min$^{-1}$), increasing amounts of the infused amino acids are oxidized to meet endogenous energy needs and less remain for tissue synthesis. A negative nitrogen balance of about 10 mmol kg$^{-1}$ day$^{-1}$ has been documented before amino acids were commenced, equivalent to a daily loss of 3% of the body's protein in the first 3 days after birth [34]. However, those who received an amino acid intake of about 1.8 g kg$^{-1}$ day$^{-1}$ and an energy intake of 190 kJ kg$^{-1}$ day$^{-1}$ (45 kcal kg$^{-1}$ day$^{-1}$) within the first day of birth had a nitrogen retention rate of 9 mmol kg$^{-1}$ day$^{-1}$. This early introduction of intravenous amino acids to achieve positive nitrogen balance has been shown to be well tolerated and not to result in an elevation in plasma amino acid levels even in sick preterm babies [35].

The intravenous nitrogen intake required to achieve nitrogen retention equal to the fetal accretion rate at 24–36 weeks' gestation ($24$ mmol kg$^{-1}$ day$^{-1}$) depends on a number of factors such as energy intake, the type of amino acids, vitamin and mineral cofactors, and the patient's clinical status. Crystalline amino acids have a higher bioavailability compared to protein hydrolysates and have replaced the latter as the nitrogen source in intravenous nutrition [36]. Amino acids in the form of L-stereoisomers, preferred to the metabolically inactive D-stereoisomers which are prone to excessive urinary loss, have a nitrogen retention rate of over 70% of the amount infused [24,37]. Thus, an intravenous nitrogen intake of $32$ mmol kg$^{-1}$ day$^{-1}$, equivalent to $3.3$ g kg$^{-1}$ day$^{-1}$ of amino acids or $2.8$ g kg$^{-1}$ day$^{-1}$ of protein, will result in duplication of intra-uterine nitrogen accretion rates.

## Amino acids

The optimal composition of an amino acid solution for ELBW babies is unknown. Oral requirements of normal babies cannot be extrapolated to intravenous intake, because the role of the gastrointestinal tract and liver in selective absorption, anabolism or catabolism of the ingested amino acid before systemic distribution has not been adequately studied. Furthermore, a formula appropriate for a term baby is not necessarily suitable for a preterm baby, especially one who is ELBW. The reference standard against which to assess the plasma aminogram in babies on intravenous nutrition remains arbitrary. Control subjects from which these standards were derived vary from unfed term babies, breastfed term babies, breastfed preterm babies to formula-fed preterm babies. Since plasmafree amino acids represent only 1% of the baby's total amino acid pool, an aminogram is probably an inappropriate measure of amino acid deficiency or excess. Intravenous requirements and tolerance of essential and non-essential amino acids are not well defined in the ELBW baby and concerns remain that imbalances may result in abnormal aminograms, altered growth or deleterious effect on the developing central nervous system.

Amino acid solutions based on the composition of breast milk [38], compared with those based on the composition of egg protein [39], result in a more favourable aminogram and a lower risk of high plasma phenylalanine levels

[40]. Amino acid solutions designed for paediatric patients are more suitable for preterm babies [41,42]. Cysteine [43] and taurine [44] have been added to new amino acid solutions under development, as they are considered to be essential in preterm babies. New amino acid solutions have also been developed using the engineering technique of optimization, in which the composition is derived from calculations based on a large body of plasma amino acid data from patients given a variety of intravenous amino acid solutions. Preterm babies show good tolerance for these 'designer' amino acid solutions [37,45]. The metabolic capacity of preterm babies for intravenously delivered amino acids is better than commonly thought [37,45] and in general, their plasma aminograms are comparable to those found in term babies fed human milk [46,47].

## Fat

Intravenous fat is the main non-protein energy source in intravenous nutrition. Glucose and fat have similar nitrogen sparing effects in intravenously-fed babies under steady-state conditions [48,49]. Both soyabean and safflower emulsions are well tolerated though the optimal ratio of linoleic and linolenic acid is believed to lie between that present in the two oil emulsions [50]. Essential fatty acid deficiency is prevented by as little as $0.5$ mg kg$^{-1}$ day$^{-1}$ of a soyabean emulsion [51] and $0.3$ mg kg$^{-1}$ day$^{-1}$ of a safflower emulsion [52]. New intravenous fat preparations which contain medium-chain triglycerides have been shown to result in a lower serum cholesterol compared to emulsions with long-chain triglycerides of soyabean or safflower origin [53].

Preterm babies have poor intravenous fat tolerance compared to term babies [54], especially those who are ELBW [55], due more to deficient cellular uptake and utilization of free fatty acids than low lipoprotein lipase activity [56]. Carnitine is essential for optimal fatty acid oxidation as it facilitates their transport across the mitochondrial membrane. Preterm babies are born with low carnitine depots and have limited capacity for carnitine biosynthesis. They develop low blood and tissue carnitine levels while on intravenous nutrition with carnitine-free solutions. Short-term studies on the effects of carnitine gave inconsistent results. However, carnitine supplementation has been shown to improve fat utilization in babies on prolonged intravenous nutrition [57] and is therefore recommended for those who have been on total intravenous nutrition for longer than 4 weeks [58].

In ELBW babies, it is usual to commence intravenous fat on a dose not exceeding $1 \, g \, kg^{-1} \, day^{-1}$. This should be increased stepwise over several days to a dose not exceeding $3 \, g \, kg^{-1} \, day^{-1}$. The basis for this practice is that metabolic adaptation is slow when changing from a high-glucose to a high-fat intravenous nutrition regimen [59]. The cautious introduction of intravenous fat, even as early as on the first day after birth, has been shown to be well tolerated with no increase in adverse effects [60]. The use of a 20% fat emulsion which has a lower phospholipid/ triglyceride ratio than a 10% emulsion (0.06 versus 0.12) is associated with a lower plasma triglyceride level and less accumulation of cholesterol and phospholipids in low-density lipoproteins [61]. Two RCTs comparing a continuous fat infusion regimen with an intermittent infusion regimen, have shown that a continuous infusion results in less fluctuation in serum lipid levels and a lower incidence of clinical and metabolic complications [55,62]. Plasma turbidity, assessed by visual inspection or nephelometry, does not reliably detect excess serum lipid concentration [63]. Triglyceride measurements are required and if the levels exceed $1.7 \, mmol \, l^{-1}$, it is necessary to reduce or interrupt the fat infusion until normal triglyceride levels are regained [64,65].

Caution has been expressed on the early use of intravenous fat because of its association with increased and prolonged respiratory difficulty [66] and incidence of chronic lung disease [67]. However, studies have shown that oxygenation and pulmonary function were not impaired unless the fat infusion rate exceeded $6–7 \, g \, kg^{-1} \, day^{-1}$ [68–70]. Since excess free fatty acids compete with bilirubin for binding to albumin, it has been recommended that the free fatty acid to albumin ratio be kept below six [71] and that babies should receive no more than $1 \, g \, kg^{-1} \, day^{-1}$ of intravenous fat if their serum bilirubin level is greater than $170 \, \mu \, litre^{-1}$ when their serum albumin is $30 \, g \, l^{-1}$ [72]. However, fat emulsion is also capable of binding unconjugated bilirubin [73] and no effect on total or unbound serum bilirubin was detected with fat infusions of up to $4 \, g \, kg^{-1} \, day^{-1}$ [74]. It has been recommended that fat infusions be reduced to $2 \, g \, kg^{-1} \, day^{-1}$ in preterm babies with sepsis who have a reduced fat oxidation rate [75]. Although an association between intravenous fat administration and coagulase-negative staphylococcal bacteraemia in babies has been reported [76], studies have not shown an impairment of immune function in babies on intravenous nutrition [77–79].

## Minerals and trace elements

The high IWL in ELBW babies is responsible for most cases of hypernatraemia in the first week after birth. Early hyponatraemia in preterm babies has been shown to be due to inappropriate arginine vasopressin release associated with periventricular haemorrhage, pneumothorax or hyaline membrane disease [80]. The same study suggested that a sodium intake of $1 \, mmol \, kg^{-1} \, day^{-1}$ is adequate in the first week before diuresis sets in. Late hyponatraemia in preterm babies is due to limited tubular sodium reabsorption [81], for which a sodium intake of $>5–10 \, mmol \, kg^{-1} \, day^{-1}$ is sometimes required. An intravenous potassium intake of $1–2 \, mmol \, kg^{-1} \, day^{-1}$ is generally recommended even though potassium should be withheld in ELBW babies during the first three days after birth when they are at risk of developing nonoliguric hyperkalaemia due to immature distal tubular function [82,83]. An intravenous chloride intake of at least $2–3 \, mmol \, kg^{-1} \, day^{-1}$ is required to achieve fetal accretion rate, but it should not exceed $6 \, mmol \, kg^{-1} \, day^{-1}$ above which there is an

**Table 12.1  Recommendations for intravenous minerals and trace elements in preterm babies (mol kg$^{-1}$ 24h$^{-1}$) [86]**

| | |
|---|---|
| Sodium | 3–5 mmol |
| Chloride | 3–5 mmol |
| Potassium | 1–2 mmol |
| Calcium[a] | 1.5–2.2 mmol |
| Phosphorus[a] | 1.5–2.2 mmol |
| Magnesium | 0.3–0.4 mmol |
| Zinc | 6–8 μmol |
| Copper | 0.3–0.6 μmol |
| Selenium | 13–25 nmol |
| Manganese | 18–180 nmol |
| Iodide | 8 nmol |
| Chromium | 4–8 nmol |
| Molybdenum | 2–10 nmol |

[a]Based on a 120–150 ml kg$^{-1}$ 24h$^{-1}$ fluid intake of a solution which contains 1.3–1.5 mmol dl$^{-1}$ of calcium and phosphorus (molar ratio 1:1)

increased risk of hyperchloraemic metabolic acidosis [84].

To maintain short-term homeostasis, an intravenous calcium intake of 1 mmol kg$^{-1}$ day$^{-1}$ after birth can prevent early neonatal hypocalcaemia in preterm babies without depressing their parathyroid activity [85]. However, the infusion rate calculated to match the intrauterine accretion rate of calcium is more than twice that amount. Table 12.1 summarizes recommendations on intravenous minerals and trace elements based on guidelines for preterm babies published by the American Society for Clinical Nutrition [86] and recent reviews on intravenous nutrition in the newborn baby [87]. If supplemental intravenous nutrition is administered as an adjunct to enteral feeding or if total intravenous nutrition is administered for a period of not more than 2 weeks, no trace elements need to be added except for zinc [86]. Modifications to the recommended doses of trace elements are required in the following circumstances: zinc supplements should be increased with excessive gastrointestinal losses. Copper and manganese supplements should be withheld in the presence of cholestasis, and selenium supplements should be withheld when renal function is impaired. Iron, molybdenum and fluoride supplements need to be considered with long-term total intravenous nutrition which exceeds 6 months in duration.

## Vitamins

The provision of vitamins in intravenous nutrition is determined by what is commercially available. MVI-Paediatric in the dose of 2 ml g$^{-1}$ day$^{-1}$ body weight, up to a maximum of 5 m g$^{-1}$, has been recommended to best suit the ELBW baby's requirements. Nevertheless, one study has shown that its use is associated with a low level of vitamin A and high levels of most of the B vitamins [86]. During intravenous administration, about 80% of vitamin A and 30% of vitamins D and E are lost because of adherence to plastic tubing and photodegradation, especially during phototherapy [88,89]. However, this can be minimized by adding the vitamin preparation into the fat emulsion instead of the amino acid–glucose mixture. One study has demonstrated that the vitamin A loss is reduced from 80% to 10% by this procedure [90].

## Practical considerations

### Preparation

A variety of computer programs have been written to improve the efficiency and safety of intravenous nutrition by facilitating doctor's prescriptions, providing automatic physiological safety and precipitation checks, and increasing the ease of nutritional data retrieval [91–97]. Preparation of intravenous solutions should be carried out by the pharmacist under a laminar flow hood with terminal filtration using a 0.22 μm filter, before delivery to the neonatal unit.

### Delivery

For peripheral vein delivery, short Teflon catheters remain functional significantly longer than steel needles with no increase in complications [98,99]. Percutaneous central venous catheterization has been successfully applied to ELBW babies [100,101]. Although this technique is preferred to the surgical cutdown approach [102], the Broviac catheter developed for long-term intravenous nutrition has also been used in ELBW babies [103,104]. Heparin (1 unit ml$^{-1}$) added to the infusate, reduces significantly the incidence of phlebitis and thrombosis of both peripheral [105] and central venous catheters [106]. Parenteral nutrition has also been administered routinely through umbilical arterial catheters in babies who require arterial access for blood gas monitoring in the first 2 weeks of age [107,108]. Compared to central venous catheters, the umbilical arterial route of administration has been found to be equal in efficacy and safety [107].

### Monitoring

Daily body weight and weekly body length and head circumference measurements are usually carried out during intravenous nutrition though some neonatal units also measure triceps skinfold thickness and mid-upper-arm circumference as part of their growth assessment. Strict fluid balance, 6–12 hourly urine and blood glucose, and daily plasma sodium, potassium, calcium, creatinine and acid–base determinations, are recommended before optimal glucose, amino acid and fat intake is achieved or during periods of metabolic instability. This routine can be reduced to once or twice weekly when the baby is metabolically stable. Weekly measurements of plasma magnesium, phosphorus, total and direct bilirubin, alkaline phosphatase, albumin, and liver enzymes, are also recommended during intravenous nutrition. Most neonatal units do not routinely monitor plasma triglycerides, amino acids, trace elements or ammonia.

## Benefits of intravenous nutrition

RCTs have shown that total or supplemental intravenous nutrition, compared to enteral feeding supplemented only with a glucose–electrolyte mixture, results in a significantly earlier and faster weight gain [108–111]. The weight gain during intravenous nutrition has been shown to be a result of tissue accretion rather than water retention [112,113]. Routine use of intravenous nutrition has enabled postnatal weight gain consistently above intrauterine growth rate after 2 weeks of age for babies born at 29 weeks' gestation, after 3 weeks of age for those born at 26–28 weeks and after 4 weeks of age for those born at 24–25 weeks [3]. An improvement in early growth is associated with a lower incidence of growth failure in late infancy [114]. However, the importance of achieving adequate postnatal nutrition in ELBW babies, given intravenously if necessary, in regards to their long-term somatic growth and brain development, requires further studies.

Intravenous nutrition, which permits the cautious and gradual introduction of enteral feeding, can minimize the risk of aspiration pneumonia [108], cardiorespiratory disturbances [115] and necrotizing enterocolitis [116–118]. Those who are on prolonged assisted ventilation have been found to tolerate the introduction of enteral feeding better and have a shorter convalescent period following a period of intravenous nutrition [119].

## Hazards of intravenous nutrition

### Infections and technical complications

The incidence of catheter-related bacterial [120] and fungal [121] sepsis in babies on intravenous nutrition ranges from 8% to 45%, with staff training playing a key role in its prevention [122]. Serious complications of central venous catheterization which have been described include superior or inferior vena cava obstruction, cardiac arrhythmia or tamponade, intracardiac thrombi, pleural effusion or chylothorax, pulmonary embolism, Budd–Chiari syndrome, and hydrocephalus secondary to jugular vein thrombosis. Though these problems could be avoided with peripheral vein delivery, frequent insertions of peripheral venous catheters could lead to excessive handling of the baby and extravasation could lead to serious tissue necrosis and subcutaneous calcium deposition.

### Metabolic complications

Aluminium accumulation in babies on intravenous nutrition has been documented and although its clinical consequences are unclear, attention should be given to minimize if possible aluminium contamination of the infusates [123]. The risks associated with the use of intravenous fat should be avoidable if the precautions described in the early part of this chapter are followed.

Cholestatic jaundice is uncommon with short-term total intravenous nutrition of less than 2 weeks, but up to 80% of those who required total intravenous nutrition for more than 2 months have been reported to develop cholestasis [124]. Some of the proposed mechanisms include immaturity of the hepatobiliary system [125], prolonged fasting [126], impaired bile secretion and bile salt formation [127], coexisting sepsis [128], underlying medical conditions associated with hypoxia or gastrointestinal conditions requiring surgery [129], taurine deficiency [130], excessive amino acid and glucose intake [131,132] and deficiency of antioxidants such as vitamin E [133]. Another hypothesis that intravenous fat is associated with cholestasis, cannot be confirmed [134]. The administration of oral gentamicin [135] and intravenous metronidazole [136] in babies on prolonged intravenous nutrition have been found to be protective against cholestasis, suggesting possible involvement of intestinal flora in the pathogenesis of this condition. With few exceptions, cholestasis resolves when enteral feeding is commenced but it is known to progress to biliary cirrhosis [137] and liver failure [138]. Rapid recovery following phenobarbitone therapy [139] and biliary irrigation [140] has been reported.

Intravenous nutrition is contraindicated in babies with fulminating sepsis prior to adequate stabilization with antibiotic and supportive treatment. It should also be withheld in babies with severe circulatory instability or acute renal failure.

## Transition to enteral feeding

Enteral feeding is necessary for adaptation to extrauterine nutrition through its trophic effects on the gastrointestinal tract and its physiological effects on gastrointestinal exocrine and endocrine secretion and motility [141]. Comparing intravenously fed young animals with those who were enterally fed, growth failure of the stomach, small intestine and pancreas and a decrease in disaccharidase activity in the proximal small intestine mucosa have been demonstrated [142]. Human studies have shown that enteral feeding is associated with a higher nitrogen turnover reflecting rapid gut growth [143] as well as normal gastric acid secretion [144]. Glucagon stimulates bile flow and in the absence of enteral feeding, babies secrete extremely dilute bile which possibly explains the cholestasis associated with prolonged total intravenous nutrition [145]. Intravenously fed babies also have significantly fewer immunoglobulin-containing intestinal plasma cells than those who are enterally fed [146].

Instead of prolonged total intravenous nutrition, the early use of subnutritional quantities of milk to supplement intravenous nutrition is therefore recommended [118,147]. Two RCTs have been conducted to compare early (2–7 days) and late (9–18 days) introduction of enteral feeding. They showed that those who received early low-volume enteral feeds had better feed tolerance, reached full enteral feeding faster, had less indirect hyperbilirubinaemia, cholestatic jaundice and osteopenia of prematurity, and had a shorter hospital stay [148,149]. Therefore, enteral feeds should be commenced whenever possible within one week after birth. As tolerance improves, the milk volume can be increased gradually over the ensuing days or weeks, during which period the intravenous route is relied upon to supply the balance of nutrients necessary for optimal growth and development.

---

**Practical points**

1. The risk of hyperglycaemia can be reduced by commencing at a low glucose infusion rate of 6–8 g kg$^{-1}$ day$^{-1}$ and increasing progressively over a 2-week period to 18–20 g kg$^{-1}$ day$^{-1}$.

2. The early introduction of 1–2 g kg$^{-1}$ day$^{-1}$ of intravenous amino acids in the first 3 days after birth is well tolerated and beneficial in achieving positive nitrogen balance.

3. Conflicting opinions exist regarding the safety of intravenous fat commenced in the first few days after birth. This controversy awaits resolution evidence from randomized clinical trials.

4. Intravenous vitamins should be added into the fat emulsion to reduce loss from adherence to plastic tubing and photodegradation.

5. Percutaneous central venous catheterization is now routinely used to deliver intravenous feeding. Staff training plays a key role in prevention of catheter-related sepsis.

6. 'Sub-nutritional' quantities of enteral feeding should begin within 1 week of birth. Supplemental intravenous feeding has significant benefits over total intravenous feeding, including earlier transition to enteral feeds and less cholestatic jaundice.

## References

1. Churella, H.R., Bachhuber, W.L. and MacLean, W.C. Jr. (1985) Survey: methods of feeding low birth weight infants. *Pediatrics*, **76**, 243–249

2. Hack, M., Horbar, J.D., Malloy, M.H. *et al.* (1991) Very low birthweight outcomes of the National Institutes of Child Health and Human Development Neonatal Network. *Pediatrics*, **87**, 587–597

3. Gill, A., Yu, V.Y.H., Bajuk, B. and Astbury, J. (1986) Postnatal growth in infants born before 30 weeks' gestation. *Arch. Dis. Childh.*, **61**, 549–553

4. Lorenz, J.M., Kleinman, L.I., Kotagal, U.R. and Reller, M.D. (1982) Water balance in very low birth weight infants: relationship to water and sodium intake and effect on outcome. *J. Pediatr.*, **101**, 423–432

5. Shaffer, S.G., Bradt, S.K. and Hall, R.T. (1986) Postnatal changes in total body water and extracellu-

lar volume in the preterm infant with respiratory distress syndrome. *J. Pediatr.*, **109**, 509–514

6. Bauer, K. and Versmold, H. (1989) Postnatal weight loss in preterm neonates <1500 g in isotonic dehydration of the extracellular volume. *Acta Paediatr. Scand.*, **360**, 37–42

7. Van der Wagen, A., Okken, A., Zweens, J. and Zijlstra, W.G. (1985) Composition of postnatal weight loss and subsequent weight gain in small for dates newborn infants. *Acta Paediatr. Scand.*, **74**, 57–61

8. Georgieff, M.K., Amarnath, U.M. and Mills, M.M. (1989) Determinants of arm muscle and fat accretion during the first postnatal month in preterm newborn infants. *J. Pediatr. Gastroenterol. Nutr.*, **9**, 219–224

9. Bauer, K., Bovermann, G., Roithmaier, A., Gotz, M., Proiss, A. and Versmold, H.T. (1991) Body composition, nutrition, and fluid balance during the first two weeks of life in preterm neonates weighing less than 1500 grams. *J. Pediatr.*, **118**, 615–620

10. Rutter, N. and Hull, D. (1979) Water loss from the skin of term and preterm babies. *Arch. Dis. Childh.*, **54**, 858–868

11. Hammerlund, K., Sedin, G. and Stromberg, B. (1983) Transepidermal water loss in newborn infants. Relation to gestational age and postnatal age in appropriate and small for gestational age infants. *Acta Paediatr. Scand.*, **72**, 721–728

12. Wu, P.Y.K. and Hodgman, J.E. (1974) Insensible water loss in preterm infants: changes with postnatal development and non-ionizing radiant energy. *Pediatrics*, **54**, 704–718

13. Bell, E.F., Gray, J.C., Weinstein, M.R. and Oh, W. (1980) The effects of thermal environment on heat balance and insensible water loss in low birth weight infants. *J. Pediatr.*, **96**, 452–459

14. Okken, A., Blijham, C., Franz, W. and Bohn, E. (1982) Effects of forced convection of heated air on insensible water loss and heat loss in preterm infants in incubators. *J. Pediatr.*, **101**, 108–112

15. Marks, K.H., Farrell, T.P., Friedman, Z. and Maisels, M.J. (1979) Intravenous alimentation and insensible water loss in low birth weight infants. *Pediatrics*, **63**, 543–546

16. Fanaroff, A.A., Wald, M., Gruber, H.S. and Klaus, M.H. (1972) Insensible water loss in low birth weight infants. *Pediatrics*, **50**, 236–245

17. Baumgart, S., Engle, W.D., Fox, W.W. and Polin, R.A. (1981) Effect of heat shielding on convective and evaporative heat loss and on radiant heat transfer in the premature infants. *J. Pediatr.*, **99**, 948–956

18. Baumgart, S. (1984) Reduction of oxygen consumption, insensible water loss and radiant heat demand with use of a plastic blanket for low birth weight infants under radiant warmers. *Pediatrics*, **74**, 1022–1028

19. Harpin, V.A. and Rutter, N. (1985) Humidification of incubators. *Arch. Dis. Childh.*, **60**, 219–224

20. Nash, M.A. (1981) The management of fluid and electrolyte disorders in the baby. *Clin. Perinatol.*, **8**, 251–262

21. Reichman, B.L., Chessex, P., Putet, G. *et al.* (1982) Partition of energy metabolism and energy cost of growth in the very low birth weight infants. *Pediatrics*, **69**, 446–451

22. Rubecz, I. and Mestyan, J. (1973) Energy metabolism and intravenous nutrition of premature infants. *Biol. Neonate*, **23**, 45–58

23. Zlotkin, S.H., Bryan, M.H. and Anderson, G.H. (1981) Intravenous nitrogen and energy intakes required to duplicate *in utero* nitrogen accretion in prematurely born human infants. *J. Pediatr.*, **99**, 115–120

24. Chessex, P., Zebiche, H., Pineault, M., Lopage, D. and Dallaire, L. (1985) Effect of aminoacid composition of parenteral solutions on nitrogen retention and metabolic response in very low birth weight infants. *J. Pediatr.*, **106**, 111–117

25. Stonestreet, B.S., Rubin, L., Pollak, A., Cowett, R.M. and Oh, W. (1980) Renal functions of low birth weight infants with hyperglycemia and glucosuria produced by glucose infusion. *Pediatrics*, **66**, 561–567

26. Louik, C., Mitchell, A.A., Epstein, M.F. and Shapiro, S. (1985) Risk factors for neonatal hyperglycemia associated with 10% dextrose infusion. *Am. J. Dis. Child.*, **139**, 783–786

27. Lilien, L.D., Rosenfield, R.L., Baccaro, M.M. and Phildes, R.S. (1979) Hyperglycemia in stressed small premature babies. *J. Pediatr.*, **94**, 454–459

28. Pollak, A., Cowett, R.M., Schwartz, R. and Oh, W. (1978) Glucose disposal in low birth weight infants during steady state hyperglycemia: effects of exogenous insulin administration. *Pediatrics*, **61**, 546–549

29. Cowett, R.M., Anderson, G.E., Maguire, C.A. and Oh, W. (1988) Ontogeny of glucose homeostasis in low birth weight infants. *J. Pediatr.*, **112**, 462–465

30. Yu, V.Y.H., James, B.E., Hendry, P.G. and MacMahon, R.A. (1979) Glucose tolerance in very low birthweight infants. *Aust. Paediatr. J.*, **15**, 147–151

31. Ostertag, S.G., Jovanovic, L., Lewis, B. and Auld, P.A.M. (1986) Insulin pump therapy in the very low birth weight infant. *Pediatrics*, **78**, 625–630

32. Binder, N.D., Raschko, R.K., Benda, G.I. and Reynolds, J.W. (1989) Insulin infusion with parenteral nutrition in extremely low birthweight infants with hyperglycemia. *J. Pediatr.*, **114**, 273–280

33. Collins, J.W. Jr., Hoppe, M., Brown, K., Edidin, D.V., Padbury, J. and Ogata, E.S. (1991) A controlled trial of insulin infusion and parenteral nutrition in extremely low birth weight infants with glucose intolerance. *J. Pediatr.*, **118**, 921–927

34. Saini, J., MacMahon, P., Morgan, J.B. and Kovar, I.Z. (1989) Early parenteral feeding of amino acids. *Arch. Dis. Childh.*, **64**, 1362–1366

35. Rivera, A. Jr., Bell, E.F., Stegink, L.D. and Ziegler, E.E. (1989) Plasma amino acid profiles during the first three days of life in infants with respiratory distress syndrome: effect of parenteral amino acid supplementation. *J. Pediatr.*, **115**, 465–468

36. Duffy, B., Gunn, T., Collinge, J. and Pencharz, P.

(1980) The effect of varying protein quality and energy intake on the nitrogen metabolism of parenterally fed low birthweight (<1600 g) infants. *Pediatr. Res.*, **15**, 1040–1044

37. Heird, W.C., Hay, W., Helms, R.A., Storm, M.C., Kashyap, S. and Dell, R.B. (1988) Pediatric parenteral amino acid mixture in low birth weight infants. *Pediatrics*, **81**, 41–50

38. Coran, A.G. and Drongowski, R.A. (1987) Studies on the toxicity and efficacy of a new amino acid solution in pediatric parenteral nutrition. *J. Parent. Ent. Nutr.*, **11**, 368–377

39. Anderson, G.E., Bucher, D., Friis-Hansen, B., Nexo, E. and Olesen, H. (1983) Plasma amino acid concentrations in newborn infants during parenteral nutrition. *J. Parent. Ent. Nutr.*, **7**, 369–373

40. Puntis, J.W., Ball, P.A., Preece, M.A., Green, A., Brown, G.A. and Booth, I.W. (1989) Egg and breast milk based nitrogen sources compared. *Arch. Dis. Childh.*, **64**, 1472–1477

41. Rosenthal, M., Sinha, S., Laywood, E. and Levene, M. (1987) A double blind comparison of a new paediatric amino acid solution in neonatal total parenteral nutrition. *Early Hum. Dev.*, **15**, 37–146

42. Helms, R.A., Christensen, M.L., Mauer, E.C. and Storm, M.C. (1987) Comparison of a pediatric versus standard amino acid formulation in preterm babies requiring parenteral nutrition. *J. Pediatr.*, **110**, 466–470

43. Malloy, M.H., Rassin, D.K. and Richardson, C.J. (1984) Total parenteral nutrition in sick preterm infants: effects of cysteine supplementation with nitrogen intakes of 240 and 400 mg/kg/day. *J. Pediatr. Gastroenterol. Nutr.*, **3**, 239–244

44. Thornton, L. and Griffin, E. (1991) Evaluation of a taurine containing amino acid solution in parenteral nutrition. *Arch. Dis. Childh.*, **66**, 21–25

45. Imura, K., Okada, A., Fukui, Y. *et al.* (1988) Clinical Studies on a newly devised amino acid solution for babies. *J. Parent. Ent. Nutr.*, **12**, 496–504

46. Clark, D., Henderson, M., Smith, M. and Dear, P.R.F. (1989) Plasma amino acid concentrations in parenterally fed preterm infants. *Arch. Dis. Child.*, **64**, 939–942

47. Hanning, R.M. and Zlotkin, S.H. (1989) Amino acid and protein needs of the baby: effect of excess and deficiency. *Semin. Perinatol.*, **13**, 131–141

48. Rubecz, I., Mestyan, J., Varga, P. and Klujber, L. (1981) Energy metabolism, substrate utilization and nitrogen balance in parenterally fed postoperative babies and infants. *J. Pediatr.*, **98**, 42–46

49. Pineault, M., Chessex, P., Bisaillon, S. and Brisson, G. (1988) Total parenteral nutrition in the newborn: impact of the quality of infused energy on nitrogen metabolism. *Am. J. Clin. Nutr.*, **47**, 298–304

50. McClead, R.E. Jr., Meng, H.C., Gregory, S.A., Budde, C. and Sloan, H.R. (1985) Comparison of the clinical and biochemical effect of increased linolenic acid in a safflower oil intravenous fat emulsion. *J. Pediatr. Gastroenterol. Nutr.*, **4**, 234–239

51. Tashiro, T., Ogato, H., Yokoyama, H., Mashima, Y. and Itoh, K. (1976) The effect of fat emulsion (Intralipid) on essential fatty acid deficiency in infants receiving intravenous alimentation. *J. Pediatr. Surg.*, **11**, 505–515

52. Cooke, R.J., Zee, P. and Yeh, Y. (1985) Safflower oil emulsion administration during parenteral nutrition in the preterm infant. Effect on essential fatty acid status. *J. Pediatr. Gastroenterol. Nutr.*, **4**, 799–803

53. Lima, L.A.M., Murphy, J.F., Stansbie, D., Rowlandson, P. and Gray, O.P. (1988) Neonatal parenteral nutrition with a fat emulsion containing medium chain triglycerides. *Acta Paediatr. Scand.*, **77**, 332–339

54. Shennan, A.T., Bryan, M.H. and Angel, A. (1977) The effects of gestational age on Intralipid tolerance in newborn infants. *J. Pediatr.*, **91**, 134–137

55. Brans, Y.W., Andrew, D.S., Carillo, D.W., Dutton, E.B., Menchaca, E.M. and Puleo-Scheppke, B.A. (1990) Tolerance of fat emulsions in very low birthweight babies: effect of birthweight on plasma lipid concentrations. *Am. J. Perinatol.*, **7**, 114–117

56. Rovamo, L.M., Nikkila, E.A. and Raivio, K.O. (1988) Lipoprotein lipase, hepatic lipase, and carnitine in premature infants. *Arch. Dis. Childh.*, **63**, 140–147

57. Helms, R.A., Whitington, P.F., Mauer, E.C., Catarau, E.M., Christensen, M.L. and Borum, P.R. (1986) Enhanced lipid utilization in infants receiving oral L-carnitine during long-term parenteral nutrition. *J. Pediatr.*, **109**, 984–988

58. Christensen, M.L., Helms, R.A., Mauer, E.C. and Storm, M.C. (1989) Plasma carnitine concentration and lipid metabolism in infants receiving parenteral nutrition. *J. Pediatr.*, **115**, 794–798

59. Chessex, P., Gagne, G., Pineault, M., Vaucher, J., Bisaillon, S. and Brisson, G. (1989) Metabolic and clinical consequences of changing from high-glucose to high-fat regimens in parenterally fed newborn infants. *J. Pediatr.*, **115**, 992–997

60. Gilbertson, N., Kovar, I.Z., Cox, D.J., Crowe, L. and Palmer, N.T. (1991) Introduction of intravenous lipid administration on the first day of life in the low birth weight baby. *J. Pediatr.*, **119**, 615–623

61. Haumont, D., Deckelbaum, R.J., Richelle, M. *et al.* (1989) Plasma lipid and plasma lipoprotein concentrations in low birth weight infants given parenteral nutrition with twenty or ten percent lipid emulsion. *J. Pediatr.*, **115**, 787–793

62. Kao, L.C., Cheng, M.H. and Warburton, D. (1984) Triglycerides, free fatty acids, free fatty acids/albumin molar ratio, and cholesterol levels in serum of babies receiving long-term lipid infusions: controlled trial of continuous and intermittent regimes. *J. Pediatr.*, **104**, 429–435

63. Sehreiner, R.L., Glick, M.R., Nordschow, C.D. and Gresham, E.L. (1979) An evaluation of methods to monitor infants receiving intravenous lipids. *J. Pediatr.*, **94**, 197–200

64. Paust, H., Schroder, H., Park, W., Jakobs, C. and Frauendienst, G. (1983) Fat elimination in parenterally fed low birthweight infants during the first two weeks of life. *J. Parent. Ent. Nutr.*, **7**, 557–559

65. Cooke, R.J., Yeh, Y., Gibson, D., Debo, D. and Bell, G.L. (1987) Soybean oil emulsion administration during parenteral nutrition in the preterm infant: effect on essential fatty acid, lipid and glucose metabolism. *J. Pediatr.*, **111**, 767–773

66. Hammerman, C. and Aramburo, M.J. (1988) Decreased lipid intake reduces morbidity in sick premature babies. *J. Pediatr.*, **113**, 1983–1988

67. Cooke, R.W.I. (1991) Factors associated with chronic lung disease in preterm infants. *Arch. Dis. Childh.*, **66**, 76–779

68. Adamkin, D.H., Gelke, K.N. and Wilderson, S.S. (1985) Influence of intravenous fat therapy on tracheal effluent phospholipids and oxygenation in severe respiratory distress syndrome. *J. Pediatr.*, **106**, 122–124

69. Brans, Y.W., Dutton, E.B., Andrew, D.S., Menchaca, E.M. and West, D.L. (1986) Fat emulsion tolerance in very low birth weight babies: effect on diffusion of oxygen in the lungs and on blood pH. *Pediatrics*, **78**, 79–84

70. Lloyd, T.R. and Boucek, M.M. (1986) Effect of Intralipid on the neonatal pulmonary bed: an echocardiac study. *J. Pediatr.*, **108**, 130–133

71. Andrew, G., Chan, G. and Schiff, D. (1976) Lipid metabolism in the baby. II The effects of Intralipid on bilirubin binding in vitro and in vivo. *J. Pediatr.*, **88**, 279–284

72. Heird, W.C. (1981) Use of intravenous fat emulsions in pediatric patients. *Pediatrics*, **68**, 738–743

73. Thaler, M.M. and Wennberg, R.P. (1977) Influence of intravenous nutrients on bilirubin transport. II Emulsified lipid solutions. *Pediatr. Res.*, **11**, 167–171

74. Brans, Y.W., Ritter, D.A., Kenny, J.D., Andrew, D.S., Dutton, E.B. and Carillo, D.W. (1987) Influence of intravenous fat emulsion on serum bilirubin in very low birthweight infants. *Arch. Dis. Child.*, **62**, 156–160

75. Park, W., Paust, H., Brosicke, H., Knoblack, G. and Helge, H. (1986) Impaired fat utilization in parenterally fed low birth weight infants suffering from sepsis. *J. Parent. Ent. Nutr.*, **10**, 627–630

76. Freeman, J., Goldman, D.A., Smith, N.E., Sidebottom, D.G., Epstein, M.F. and Platt, R. (1990) Association of intravenous lipid emulsion and coagulase-negative staphylococcal bacteremia in neonatal intensive care units. *N. Engl. J. Med.*, **323**, 301–308

77. English, D., Roloff, J.S., Lukens, J.N., Parker, P., Greene, H.L. and Ghishan, F.K. (1981) Intravenous lipid emulsions and human neutrophil function. *J. Pediatr.*, **99**, 913–916

78. Helms, R.A., Herrod, H.G., Burckart, G.J. and Christensen, M.L. (1983) E-rosette formation, total T-cells, and lymphocyte transformation in infants receiving intravenous safflower oil emulsion. *J. Parent. Ent. Nutr.*, **7**, 541–545

79. Osmani, S.S., Harper, R.G. and Usmani, S.F. (1988) Effect of a lipid emulsion (Intralipid) on polymorphonuclear leukocyte functions in the baby. *J. Pediatr.*, **113**, 132–136

80. Rees, L., Shaw, J.C.L., Brook, C.G.D. and Forsling, M.L. (1984) Hyponatraemia in the first week of life in preterm infants. II Sodium and water balance. *Arch. Dis. Childh.*, **59**, 423–429

81. Al-Dahhan, J., Haycock, G.B., Chantler, C. and Stimmler, L. (1983) Sodium homeostasis in mature and immature babies. I Renal aspects. *Arch. Dis. Child.*, **58**, 335–342

82. Gruskay, J., Costarino, A.T., Polin, R.A. and Baumgart, S. (1988) Nonoliguric hyperkalemia in the premature infant weighing less than 1000 grams. *J. Pediatr.*, **113**, 381–386

83. Brion, L.P., Schwartz, G.J., Campbell, D. and Fleischman, A.R. (1989) Early hyperkalaemia in very low birthweight infants in the absence of oliguria. *Arch. Dis. Childh.*, **64**, 270–282

84. Groh-Wargo, S., Ciaccia, A. and Moore, J. (1988) Neonatal metabolic acidosis: effect of chloride from normal saline flushes. *J. Parent. Ent. Nutr.*, **12**, 159–161

85. Salle, B.L., David, L., Chopard, J.P., Grafmeyer, D.C. and Renaud, H. (1977) Prevention of early neonatal hypocalcemia in low birth weight infants with continuous calcium infusion: effect on serum calcium, phosphorus, magnesium, and circulating immunoactive parathyroid hormone and calcitonin. *Pediatr. Res.*, **11**, 1180–1185

86. Greene, H.L., Hambridge, K.M., Schanler, R. and Tsang, R.C. (1988) Guidelines for the use of vitamins, trace elements, calcium, magnesium and phosphorus in infants and children receiving total parenteral nutrition: report of the Subcommittee on Paediatric Parenteral Nutrition Requirements from the Committee on Clinical Practice Issues of the American Society for Clinical Nutrition. *Am. J. Clin. Nutr.*, **48**, 1324–1342

87. Yu, V.Y.H. and MacMahon, R.A. (1993) *Intravenous Feeding in the Neonate*. Edward Arnold, London

88. Gilles, J., Jones, G. and Pencharz, P. (1983) Delivery of vitamins A, D and E in parenteral nutrition solutions. *J. Parent. Ent. Nutr.*, **7**, 11–14

89. Smith, J.L., Canham, J.E. and Wells, P.A. (1988) Effect of phototherapy light, sodium bisulfite, and pH on vitamin stability in total parenteral nutrition and mixtures. *J. Parent. Ent. Nutr.*, **12**, 394–402

90. Baeckert, P.A., Greene, H.L., Fritz, I., Oelberg, D.G. and Adcock, E.W. (1988) Vitamin concentrations in very low birth weight infants given vitamins intravenously in a lipid emulsion: measurement of vitamins A, D and E and riboflavin. *J. Pediatr.*, **113**, 1057–1063

91. May, F. and Robbins, G. (1978) A computer program for parenteral nutrition solution preparation. *J. Parent. Ent. Nutr.*, **2**, 646–651

92. Giacoia, G.P. and Chopra, R. (1981) The use of a computer in parenteral alimentation of low birth weight infants. *J. Parent. Ent. Nutr.*, **5**, 329–331

93. Gale, R., Gale, J., Branski, D., Armon, Y., Zelingher, J. and Roll, D. (1983) An interactive microcomputer program for calculation of combined parenteral and enteral nutrition for babies. *J. Pediatr. Gastroenterol. Nutr.*, **2**, 653–658

94. Wilson, F.E., Yu, V.Y.H., Hawgood, S., Adamson, T.M. and Wilkinson, M.H. (1983) Computerised nutritional data management in neonatal intensive care. *Arch. Dis. Childh.*, **58**, 732–736

95. MacMahon, P. (1984) Prescribing and formulating neonatal intravenous feeding solutions by microcomputer. *Arch. Dis. Childh.*, **59**, 548–552

96. Harper, R.G., Carrera, E., Weiss, S. and Luongo, M. (1985) A complete computerized program for nutritional management in the neonatal intensive care nursery. *Am. J. Perinatol.*, **2**, 161–162

97. Yamamoto, L.G., Gainsley, G.J. and Witek, J.E. (1986) Pediatric parenteral nutrition management using a comprehensive user-friendly computer program designed for personal computers. *J. Parent. Ent. Nutr.*, **10**, 535–539

98. Batton, D.G., Maisels, J. and Appelbaum, P. (1982) Use of peripheral intravenous cannulas in premature infants: a controlled study. *Pediatrics*, **70**, 487–490

99. Phelps, S.J. and Helms, R.A. (1987) Risk factors affecting infiltration of peripheral venous lines in infants. *J. Pediatr.*, **111**, 384–389

100. Chathas, M.K., Paton, J.B. and Fisher, D.E. (1990) Percutaneous central venous catheterization. *Am. J. Dis. Child.*, **144**, 1246–1250

101. Nakamura, K.T., Sato, Y. and Erenberg, A. (1990) Evaluation of a percutaneously placed 27-gauge central venous catheter in babies weighing <1200 grams. *J. Parent. Ent. Nutr.*, **14**, 295–299

102. Shulman, R.J., Pokorny, W.J., Martin, C.G., Pettitt, R., Baldaia, L. and Roney, D. (1986) Comparison of percutaneous and surgical placement of central venous catheters in babies. *J. Pediatr. Surg.*, **21**, 348–350

103. Ogata, E.S., Schulman, S., Raffensperger, J., Luck, S. and Rusnak, M. (1984) Caval catheterisation in the intensive care nursery: a useful means for providing parenteral nutrition to the extremely low birthweight infant. *J. Pediatr. Surg.*, **19**, 258–262

104. Warner, B.W., Gorgone, P., Schilling, S., Farell, M. and Ghory, M.J. (1987) Multiple purpose central venous access in infants less than 1000 grams. *J. Pediatr. Surg.*, **22**, 820–822

105. Alpan, G., Eyal, F., Springer, C., Glick, B., Goder, K. and Armon, J. (1984) Heparinization of alimentation solutions administered through peripheral veins in premature infants: a controlled study. *Pediatrics* **74**, 374–378

106. Brismar, B., Hardstedt, C., Jacobson, S., Kager, L. and Malmborg, A. (1982) Reduction of catheter-associated thrombosis in parenteral nutrition by intravenous heparin therapy. *Arch. Surg.*, **117**, 1196–1199

107. Kanarek, K.S., Kuznicki, M.B. and Blair, R.C. (1991) Infusion of total parenteral nutrition via the umbilical artery. *J. Parent. Ent. Nutr.*, **15**, 71–74

108. Yu, V.Y.H., James, B., Hendry, P. and MacMahon, R.A. (1979) Total parenteral nutrition in very low birthweight infants: a controlled trial. *Arch. Dis. Childh.*, **54**, 653–661

109. Bryan, M.H., Wei, P., Hamilton, J.R., Chance, G.W. and Swyer, P.R. (1973) Supplemental intravenous alimentation in low birth weight infants. *J. Pediatr.*, **82**, 940–944

110. Pildes, R.S., Ramamurthy, R.S., Cordero, G.V. and Wong, P.W.K. (1973) Intravenous supplementation of L-amino acids and dextrose in low-birth-weight infants. *J. Pediatr.*, **82**, 945–950

111. Brans, Y.W., Sumners, J.E., Dweck, H.S. and Cassady, G. (1974) Feeding the low birth weight infant: orally or parenterally? Preliminary results of a comparative study. *Pediatrics*, **54**, 15–22

112. Polley, T.Z., Benner, J.W., Rhodin, A., Weintraub, W.H. and Coran, A.G. (1979) Changes in total body water in infants receiving total intravenous nutrition. *J. Surg. Res.*, **26**, 555–559

113. Coran, A.G., Drongowski, R.A. and Wesley, J.R. (1984) Changes in total body water and extracellular fluid volume in infants receiving total parenteral nutrition. *J. Pediatr. Surg.*, **19**, 771–776

114. Georgieff, M.K., Mills, M.M., Lindeke, L., Iverson, S., Johnson, D.E. and Thompson, T.R. (1989) Changes in nutritional management and outcome of very low birth weight infants. *Am. J. Dis. Childh.*, **143**, 82–85

115. Yu, V.Y.H. (1976) Cardiorespiratory response to feeding in newborn infants. *Arch. Dis. Childh.*, **51**, 305–309

116. Eyal, F., Sagi, E., Arad, I. and Avital, A. (1982) Necrotising enterocolitis in the very low birthweight infant: expressed breast milk feeding compared with parenteral feeding. *Arch. Dis. Childh.*, **57**, 274–276

117. Glass, E.J., Hume, R., Lang, M.A. and Forfar, J.O. (1984) Parenteral nutrition compared with transpyloric feeding. *Arch. Dis. Childh.*, **59**, 131–135

118. Unger, A., Goetzman, B.W., Chan, C., Lyons, A.B. and Miller, M.F. (1986) Nutritional practices and outcome of extremely premature infants. *Am. J. Dis. Child.*, **140**, 1027–1033

119. Moyer-Mileur, L. and Chan, G.M. (1986) Nutritional support of very low birth weight infants requiring prolonged assisted ventilation. *Am. J. Dis. Child.*, **140**, 929–932

120. Beganovic, N., Verloove-Vanhorick, S.P., Brand, R. and Ruys, J.H. (1988) Total parenteral nutrition and sepsis. *Arch. Dis. Childh.*, **63**, 66–89

121. Weese-Mayer, D.E., Fondriest, D.W., Brouilette, R.T. and Shulman, S.T. (1987) Risk factors associated with candidemia in the neonatal intensive care unit: a case control study. *Pediatr. Infect. Dis. J.*, **6**, 190–196

122. Puntis, J.W., Holden, C.E., Smallman, S., Finkel, Y., George, R.H. and Booth, I.W. (1991) Staff training: a key factor in reducing intravascular catheter sepsis. *Arch. Dis. Childh.*, **66**, 335–337

123. Koo, W.W.K., Kaplan, L.A., Bendon, R. *et al.* (1986) Response to aluminium in parenteral nutrition during infancy. *J. Pediatr.*, **109**, 877–883

124. Beale, E.F., Nelson, R.M., Bucciarelli, R.L., Donnelly, W.H. and Eitzman, D.V. (1979) Intrahepatic cholestasis associated with parenteral nutrition in premature infants. *Pediatrics*, **64**, 342–347

125. Merritt, R.J. (1986) Cholestasis associated with total parenteral nutrition. *J. Pediatr. Gastroenterol. Nutr.*, **5**, 9–22

126. Rager, R. and Finegold, M.J. (1975) Cholestasis in immature newborn infants: is parenteral alimentation responsible? *J. Pediatr.*, **86**, 264–269

127. Sondheimer, J.M., Bryan, H., Andrews, W. and Forster, G.G. (1978) Cholestatic tendencies in premature infants on and off parenteral nutrition. *Pediatrics*, **62**, 984–989

128. Kubota, A., Okada, A., Nezu, R., Kamata, S., Imura, K. and Takagi, Y. (1988) Hyperbilirubinemia in babies associated with total parenteral nutrition. *J. Parent. Ent. Nutr.*, **12**, 602–606

129. Bell, R.L., Ferry, G.D., Smith, E.O. *et al.* (1986) Total parenteral nutrition related cholestasis in infants. *J. Parent. Ent. Nutr.*, **10**, 356–359

130. Cooper, A., Betts, J.M., Pereira, G.R. and Zeigler, M.M. (1984) Taurine deficiency in the severe hepatic dysfunction complicating total parenteral nutrition. *J. Pediatr. Surg.*, **19**, 462–466

131. Vileisis, R.A., Inwood, R.J. and Hunt, C.E. (1980) Prospective controlled study of parenteral nutrition associated cholestatic jaundice: effects of protein intake. *J. Pediatr.*, **96**, 893–897

132. Sankaran, K., Berscheid, B., Verma, V., Zakhary, G. and Tan, L. (1985) An evaluation of total parenteral nutrition using Vamin and Aminosyn as protein base in critically ill preterm infants. *J. Parent. Ent. Nutr.*, **9**, 439–442

133. Berger, H.M., Den Ouden, A.L. and Calame, J.J. (1985) Pathogenesis of liver damage during parenteral nutrition: is lipofuscin a clue? *Arch. Dis. Childh.*, **60**, 774–776

134. Black, D.D., Suttle, E.A., Whitington, P.F., Whitington, G.L. and Korones, S.D. (1981) The effect of a short-term total parenteral nutrition on hepatic function in the human baby: a prospective randomised clinical study demonstrating alteration of hepatic canalicular function. *J. Pediatr.*, **99**, 445–449

135. Spurr, S.G., Grylack, L.J. and Mehta, N.R. (1989) Hyperalimentation associated neonatal cholestasis: effect of oral gentamicin. *J. Parent. Ent. Nutr.*, **13**, 633–636

136. Kubota, A., Okada, A., Imura, K. *et al.* (1990) The effect of metronidazole on TPN-associated liver dysfunction in babies. *J. Pediatr. Surg.*, **25**, 618–621

137. Pereira, G.R., Sherman, M.S., DiGiacomo, J., Zieler, M., Roth, K. and Jacobowski, D. (1981) Hyperalimentation induced cholestasis. *Am. J. Dis. Child.*, **135**, 842–845

138. Postuma, R. and Trevenen, C.L. (1979) Liver disease in infants receiving total parenteral nutrition. *Pediatrics*, **63**, 110–115

139. South, M. and King, A. (1987) Parenteral nutrition associated cholestasis: recovery following phenobarbitone. *J. Parent. Ent. Nutr.*, **11**, 208–209

140. Cooper, A., Ross, A.J. III, O'Neil, J.A., Bishop, H.C., Templeton, J.M. and Ziegler, M.M. (1985) Resolution of intractable cholestasis associated with total parenteral nutrition following biliary irrigation. *J. Pediatr. Surg.*, **20**, 772–774

141. Lucas, A., Bloom, S.R. and Aynsley-Green, A. (1983) Metabolic and endocrine effects of depriving preterm infants of enteral nutrition. *Acta Paediatr. Scand.*, **72**, 245–249

142. Goldstein, R.M., Hebiguchi, T., Luk, G.D. *et al.* (1985) The effects of total parenteral nutrition on gastrointestinal growth and development. *J. Pediatr. Surg.*, **20**, 785–791

143. Duffy, B. and Pencharz, P. (1986) The effect of feeding route (IV or oral) on the protein metabolism of the baby. *Am. J. Clin. Nutr.*, **43**, 108–111

144. Hyman, P.E., Feldman, E.J., Ament, M.E., Bryne, W.J. and Euler, A.R. (1983) Effect of enteral feeding on the maintenance of gastric acid secretory function. *Gastroenterology*, **84**, 341–345

145. Al-Rabeeah, A., Thurston, O.G. and Walker, K. (1986) Effect of total parenteral nutrition on biliary lipids in babies. *Can. J. Surg.*, **29**, 289–291

146. Knox, W.F. (1986) Restricted feeding and human intestinal plasma cell development. *Arch. Dis. Childh.*, **61**, 744–749

147. LaGamma, E.F., Ostertag, S.G. and Birenbaum, H. (1985) Failure of delayed oral feedings to prevent necrotizing enterocolitis. *Am. J. Dis. Child.*, **139**, 385–389

148. Dunn, L., Hulman, S., Weiner, J. and Kliegman, R. (1988) Beneficial effects of early hypocaloric enteral feeding on neonatal gastrointestinal function: preliminary report of a randomized trial. *J. Pediatr.*, **112**, 622–629

149. Slagle, T.A. and Gross, S.J. (1988) Effect of early low-volume enteral substrate on subsequent feeding tolerance in very low birth weight infants. *J. Pediatr.*, **13**, 526–531

# 13

# Calcium and phosphorus metabolism, rickets and bone mineral content

## Neil McIntosh

Mineralization of the fetus occurs continuously and logarithmically and calcification of the skeleton is radiologically demonstrable from the eighth week of pregnancy [1]. Because of the logarithmic accumulation, infants born significantly early, e.g. at 28 weeks' or less gestation, will have a considerable deficit in mineral compared to the full term baby. These very preterm infants now survive frequently and it is evident that provision of calcium and phosphorus is not only extremely inadequate postnatally but that the immaturity of the gastrointestinal tract further reduces the effective supply by relatively poor absorption mechanisms.

## Maternal mineral supply in the last trimester

The skeleton of a newborn term infant contains about 25 g calcium and 16 g phosphate and about 80% of this is transferred to the fetus during the last 3 months of pregnancy [2]. This represents a flux of 6.5 mmol day$^{-1}$ of calcium and 4.6 mmol day$^{-1}$ of phosphorus and is a considerable proportion of the maternal dietary intake. The fetal plasma calcium exceeds the maternal (as does the fetal phosphate) and it is thought that there is active transfer of calcium to the fetus across the placenta; 80% of the calcium transferred finds its way back to the mother [3].

However the neonatologist decides to feed the ELBW infant and whatever the food chosen, the calcium and phosphorus intake will be considerably less than the accumulation of these elements across the placenta during the last 3 months of pregnancy (Table 13.1). Most infants born at 28 weeks' gestation or less will require a period – sometimes extended – of intravenous feeding. These regimens will supply usually between 50 and 70% of the bone mineral (calcium and phosphorus) required [4–7]. The solubility product of calcium and phosphate in intravenous feeding solutions restricts a further increase of the concentrations. Breast milk is extremely deficient in mineral content and, although the milk from the mothers of preterm infants may have higher concentrations of some minerals, Atkinson et al. [8] could show no significant difference in bone mineral, and the variable content of the constituents as a whole makes this food very inadequate [9]. The preterm infant formulae acknowledge that the very immature infant requires a large amount of bone mineral and their concentrations have been increased very significantly. If the absorption of these formulae was complete, the small baby would receive an adequate supply for bone mineralization, but our own data on babies of less than 1000 g birth weight show that although phosphorus absorption is good by the second week of life even in the most immature infants (70–80% of ingested), the calcium absorption is very poor for a long time. Thus these babies at 30 days of age are only retaining between 30 and 50% of their enteral calcium intake (depending on the food given)

**Table 13.1    Calcium and phosphate intake and retention data in the perinatal period**

|  | Calcium (mg) | Phosphate (mg) | Calcium (mmol) | Phosphate (mmol) |
|---|---|---|---|---|
| Transplacental intake kg$^{-1}$ 24h$^{-1}$ in the last three months of pregnancy [26] | 140 | 70 | 3.5 | 2.3 |
| Intake from typical intravenous feeding regime at 150 ml kg$^{-1}$ 24h$^{-1}$ [4] | 45 | 23 | 1.1 | 0.8 |
| Intake per day by breast-fed infant fed at 200 ml kg$^{-1}$ 24h$^{-1}$ | 45–70 | 23–28 | 1.1–1.8 | 0.8–0.9 |
| Retention per day by breast-fed infant fed at 200 ml kg$^{-1}$ 24h$^{-1}$ (day 30 data) [10] | 13.5–21 | 20–24 | 0.34–0.53 | 0.7–0.8 |
| Intake per day by preterm formula-fed infant at 200 ml kg$^{-1}$ 24h$^{-1}$ (preterm SMA) | 150 | 80 | 3.8 | 2.6 |
| Retention per day by preterm formula-fed infant fed at 200 ml kg$^{-1}$ 24h$^{-1}$ (day 30 data) [10] | 75 | 56 | 1.9 | 1.8 |

[10]. A full term formula with its low mineral content would be inappropriate now for the feeding of the ELBW infant.

## Neonatal hypocalcaemia

Prematurity predisposes to early neonatal hypocalcaemia [11]. In our own unit, despite anticipating the fall in calcium and routinely using calcium gluconate in the first 3 days of life, 37% of 171 infants of less than 1000 g birth weight have over the last 5 years dropped their serum calcium levels to less than 1.65 mmol l$^{-1}$, though these infants have rarely been symptomatic. We have not seen any cases of late neonatal hypocalcaemia or neonatal tetany, probably because our routine feeding is largely with expressed breast milk and the serum biochemistry is closely monitored.

### Early neonatal hypercalcaemia and hypophosphataemia

The inadequate supply of mineral to the extremely immature infant was postulated by Lyon *et al.* [12] to be the cause of hypercalcaemia seen in the second week of life. This hypercalcaemia, seen in ten infants of less than 1000 g birth weight, was always associated with extreme hypophosphataemia. It was suggested that even the immature infant, when faced with the need for phosphate for essential metabolic processes, will extract this mineral from bone. The extraction of phosphate will be accompanied by extraction of calcium

which leads to both hypercalcaemia and hypercalciuria. The addition of extra phosphate to the diet (given as sodium dihydrogen phosphate to breast milk) reversed the

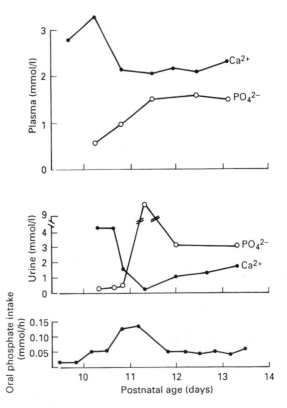

**Figure 13.1** Hypercalcaemia, hypercalciuria and hypophosphataemia all normalized in an infant of 6.0 g given extra oral phosphate on the tenth and eleventh days of life

hypophosphataemia, hypercalcaemia and hypercalciuria (Figure 13.1). It is suggested that all infants weighing less than 1000 g (and probably those less than 1250 g) should receive phosphate supplements from the third day of life when early neonatal hypocalcaemia has resolved. Our own practice is to give 1 ml of buffered sodium phosphate (BP) daily even from the first day of life mixed with the breast milk that they receive in small quantities enterally, no matter how small and sick (our only contraindication is a congenital intestinal abnormality). This provides the baby with an intake of 0.83 mmol of phosphate in addition to that in the milk and the supplemental parenteral nutrition. The extra oral phosphate is given while the infant is on breast milk (but not formula) and is less than 1500 g in actual weight. We believe that radiological morphology is at least objective and the wrist should be X-rayed at 2-week intervals beginning from the age of 3 weeks.

## Rickets in ELBW infants

### Incidence

At St. George's Hospital, London, between 1981–1985, the incidence of radiological rickets in infants of less than 1000 g birth weight is more than 50% if they survive for more than 28 days (Table 13.2).

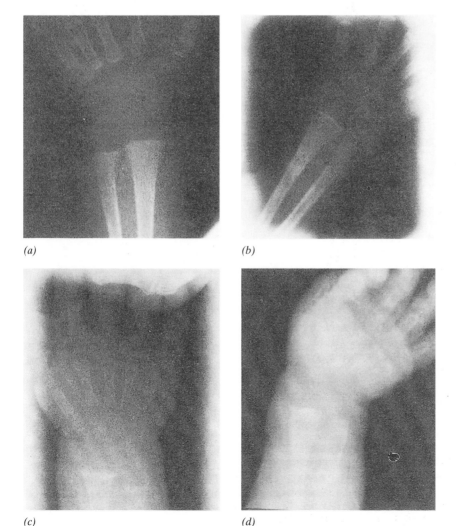

**Figure 13.2** Radiological rickets: *(a)* grade 0; *(b)* grade 1; *(c)* grade 2; *(d)* grade 3; (see Table 13.3 for description)

*(a)*

*(b)*

*(c)*

*(d)*

**Table 13.2   Incidence of rickets of prematurity (Koo grades 2 and 3) [27] in babies of <1000 g birth weight managed at St. George's Hospital Neonatal Unit who survived for more than 28 days**

|  | 1981 | 1982 | 1983 | 1984 | 1985 |
|---|---|---|---|---|---|
| No. of cases | 7 | 8 | 11 | 13 | 12 |
| Percentage incidence | 47 | 44 | 50 | 42 | 56 |

**Table 13.3   Radiological grading of rickets of prematurity described by Koo *et al.* [27]**

| Grade | Description |
|---|---|
| 1 | Loss of dense white line at the metaphysis, increased submetaphyseal lucency and thinning of the cortex |
| 2 | Irregularity and fraying, cupping and splaying, i.e. the changes of rickets |
| 3 | Changes of rickets with evidence of fractures |

## Diagnosis

The incidence depends on the method of diagnosis. All infants of this birth weight have a raised serum alkaline phosphatase and 75% have obvious radiological osteopenia [13]. The few studies available using photon absorptiometry invariably showed mineral deficiency [14,15]. However, although this technique allows considerable sophistication at quantifying the mineral deficit, it is not measuring or identifying classical changes. This, and the fact that most units do not have the method available, make it more likely that the diagnosis will be made on biochemical or radiological criteria. The alkaline phosphatase level in the serum has been suggested as a screening test for the diagnosis [16]. The levels are always high, being directly related to the gestation of the infant [17] and the type of food [10]. A comparison of maximum serum alkaline phosphatase concentrations with the radiological grading of rickets (shown in Figure 13.2 and described in Table 13.3) shows considerable overlap of levels in infants without radiological changes and in those with classical radiological signs (Figure 13.3).

## Aetiology

Although Von Sydow in 1946 suggested that rickets was due to calcium deficiency [18], most early workers assumed that it was a problem associated with the supply of, or metabolism of vitamin D. Between 1981 and 1983 at St. George's Hospital, despite an intake of 2000 units of vitamin D daily from the seventh day of life, 54% of infants with a birth weight of less than 1000 g developed radiological rickets and at the time of diagnosis they had high circulating levels of 25-hydroxycholecalciferol [19]. In 1981 we treated half the cases with alphacalcidol in case there was a problem of 1α-hydroxylation by the kidney but these cases healed at the same rate as those untreated.

Shortly afterwards, others demonstrated high levels of 1,25-dihydroxycholecalciferol [20,21] and although it is possible that there may be end organ insensitivity to the active hormone, it seems more likely that the major factor in the aetiology is a deficiency of mineral substrate [22]. The provision of adequate calcium and phosphorus in the diet is therefore an important goal in these infants. It should also be noted that the use of loop diuretics such as frusemide may lead to calcium loss in the urine which may exaggerate substrate deficiency.

It would appear that the osteopenia that is obvious radiologically in 75% of the babies in our unit with a birth weight of less than 1000 g and that is implied to be universally present by the few studies on preterm babies using photon absorp-

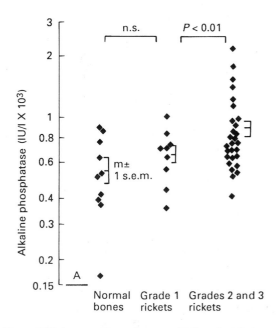

**Figure 13.3** A comparison of serum alkaline phosphatase levels with the radiological grading of rickets described in Table 13.3. A = laboratory upper limit of normal for children

tiometry [14,15], is not only a consequence of poor mineral supply in the weeks after birth but is likely to be particularly related to the demineralization process that goes on in the first 2 weeks as the infants try to maintain their serum phosphate concentration at an adequate level for essential metabolic processes (*see* p. 138).

## Complications

If rickets of prematurity heals itself with time, should we worry about it? The development of spontaneous fractures cannot be pleasant for the baby and this complication was seen in 17% of our cases between 1981 and 1983. We have never knowingly seen the development of rachitic respiratory distress [23] but the undermineralization of the rib cage must reduce the efficiency of respiration.

## Treatment

The prevention of rickets must be the goal but we have had remarkably little success. From 1981 to 1983 inclusive, 2000 units daily of vitamin D from the seventh day of life did not prevent rickets. In 1984, reduction of vitamin D to 1000 units daily from the first day and the addition of phosphate supplements (0.83 mmol 24h$^{-1}$) reduced the incidence but not significantly. In 1985, the addition of calcium 1.62 mmol 24h$^{-1}$ to this regime was associated with an increase, though again this was not significant [24]. The routine feeding of these ELBW infants has always been with expressed breast milk, and it is likely that the mineral intake is insufficient even with the added minerals. Seino *et al.* [25] suggested that the incidence could be reduced by the use of alphacalcidol but only 3 infants in their series had a birth weight of <1000 g. Our own experience in a small number of cases suggests that once the radiological changes are apparent, the use of alphacalcidol does not increase the natural rate of healing [19]. Since the study of this small series we have not used additional vitamin D therapy to heal the condition.

## The measurement of bone mineral content (BMC) and collagen

The measurement of BMC has helped clarify the dietary and mineral requirements of the very immature infant.

## Methodology

### Bone mineral

Single beam photon absorptiometry has been most commonly used. Though non-invasive in the classical sense, and subjecting the infant to only small radiation doses when compared to those given by neutron activation analysis and computerized tomography, it still suffers from the necessity for the small and potentially unstable newborn infant to travel to moderately sophisticated equipment [28–30]. The better sensitivity of dual photon absorptiometry has been offset in the neonate by the long scan times required using a gadolinium 153 source. The replacement of gadolinium with an X-ray source to give dual energy X-ray absorptiometry (DEXA, bone densitometry [31,32]) and relatively short scanning times looks promising for the future though the equipment for total body DEXA is still complex and expensive. There is no data yet available on extremely low birth weight infants. The use of dual *exposure* X-ray densitometry [33,34] using an ordinary mobile X-ray machine allows repeated measurements on even the sickest infants in their incubators. Although the sensitivity of measurement is slightly less than with DEXA, this technique is potentially widely available to neonatologists [33].

### Results of BMC measurements

Single photon absorptiometry has been most widely used in the last ten years but is still only available in academic centres. It has shown that small-for-gestational-age babies have poorly mineralized bones compared to those appropriate for gestational age of the same gestation [35,36]. The ELBW infant on reaching term has a bone mineral content on average about 60% that of the full term infant [37–39] but this reduction, which is more in infants fed human milk [39], can be offset by mineral supplementation [40]. Even without supplementation the BMC quickly catches up so that there is no difference from the equivalent full term infant at 1 to 2 years of age [37,39]. The mechanism for the rapid BMC catch up after 40 weeks' gestation [38,41] in the ex-preterm baby is not understood – the full term infant does not have this rapid accumulation of bone mineral at this time.

## Collagen

The bone matrix contains 40% of body collagen, and 13% of collagen is hydroxyproline. Osteoblastic activity and endogenous collagen metabolism are reflected by urinary hydroxyproline excretion. Greer *et al.* showed a significant positive correlation between the linear growth rate in infants (and to a lesser extent weight gain) and urinary hydroxyproline excretion: the excretion was higher in infants on either fortified human milk or formula compared to human milk alone [42]. Surprisingly, the urinary hydroxyproline excretion did not correlate with BMC. This may have been because the evaluation was comparatively short term and any change in BMC would have been difficult to demonstrate.

More recently urinary excretions of pyrodinoline and deoxypyrodinoline, the cross-linking amino acids of collagen, have been suggested as measures of collagen turnover but we are aware of no data in ELBW infants [43].

---

**Practical points**

1.  Calcium gluconate BP supplementation is warranted at 1 ml kg$^{-1}$ day$^{-1}$ over the first 3 days of life to attenuate early neonatal hypocalcaemia.
2.  Beware of hypercalcaemia in the first two weeks of life due to inadequate phosphate intake (supplement if necessary).
3.  Monitoring for osteopenia is more easily done by weekly alkaline phosphatase estimations. This should particularly be done in babies on unsupplemented human milk. X-rays of the wrist done from 3 weeks of age at 2 week intervals provide more objective evaluation. (Look for the traditional bone changes of rickets.)
4.  Phosphate supplements (buffered sodium phosphate BP 1 ml kg$^{-1}$ day$^{-1}$) equivalent to 0.83 mmol of phosphate ml$^{-1}$ should be offered to all infants where the alkaline phosphatase rises above 1000 units l$^{-1}$.
5.  Consideration should be given to calcium and phosphate mineral supplementation in all infants solely on human milk until term equivalent gestation.

---

## References

1.  Hamilton, W.J. (ed.) (1976) *Textbook of Human Anatomy*, 2nd edn, Macmillan, London
2.  McCance, R.A. and Widdowson, E.M. (1961) Mineral metabolism of the foetus and newborn. *Br. Med. Bull.*, **176**, 132–136
3.  Ramberg, C.F., Delivoria-Papadopoulos, M., Crandell, E.D. and Kronfeld, D.S. (1973) Kinetic analysis of calcium transport across the placenta. *J. Appl. Physiol.*, **35**, 682–688
4.  Shaw, J.C.L. (1973) Parenteral nutrition in the management of sick low birthweight infants. *Pediatr. Clin. N. Am.*, **20**, 333–358
5.  Cockburn, F. (1976) Complete intravenous feeding of the newborn. *Clin. Endocrinol. Metab.*, **5**, 191–219
6.  Wretland, A. (1972) Complete intravenous nutrition. Theoretical and experimental background. *Nutr. Metab.*, **14** (Suppl. 1), 57
7.  Fomon, S.J. (1974) *Infant Nutrition*, 2nd edn, W.B. Saunders, Philadelphia
8.  Atkinson, S.A., Anderson, G.H. and Bryan, M.H. (1980) Human milk: comparison of the nitrogen composition in the milk from mothers of premature and full term infants. *Am. J. Clin. Nutr.*, **33**, 811–815
9.  Hibberd, C.M., Brooke, O.G., Carter, N.D., Haug, M. and Harzas, G. (1982) Variation in the composition of breast milk during the first five weeks of lactation: implications for feeding of preterm infants. *Arch. Dis. Childh.*, **57**, 658–662
10. Lyon, A.J. and McIntosh, N. (1984) Calcium and phosphorus balance in extremely low birthweight infants in the first six weeks of life. *Arch. Dis. Childh.*, **59**, 1145–1150
11. Tsang, R.C. and Oh, W. (1970) Neonatal hypocalcemia in low birthweight infants. *Pediatrics*, **45**, 773–781
12. Lyon, A.J., McIntosh, N., Wheeler, K. and Brooke, O.G. (1984) Hypercalcaemia in extremely low birthweight infants. *Arch. Dis. Childh.*, **59**, 1141–1144
13. McIntosh, N., Williams, J.E., Lyon, A.J. and Wheeler, K.A. (1984) Diagnosis of rickets of prematurity. *Lancet*, **ii**, 869
14. Steichen, J.J., Gratton, T.L. and Tsang, R.C. (1980) Osteopenia of prematurity: the cause and possible treatment. *J. Pediatr.*, **96**, 528–534
15. James, J.R., Congdon, P.J., Truscott, J., Horsman, A. and Arthur, R. (1986) Osteopenia of prematurity. *Arch. Dis. Childh.*, **61**, 871–876
16. Kovar, I., Mayne, P. and Barltrop, D. (1982) Plasma alkaline phosphatase activity: a screening test for rickets in preterm neonates. *Lancet*, **i**, 308–310
17. Glass, E.J., Hume, R., Hendry, G.M.A., Strange, R.C. and Forfar, J.O. (1982) Plasma alkaline phosphatase activity of prematurity. *Arch. Dis. Childh.*, **57**, 373–376
18. Von Sydow, G. (1946) A study of the development of rickets in premature infants. *Acta Paediatr. Scand.*, **33** (Suppl. 2), 5–122
19. McIntosh, N., Livesey, A. and Brooke, O.G. (1982)

Plasma 25-hydroxyvitamin D and rickets in infants of extremely low birthweight. *Arch. Dis. Childh.*, **57**, 848–850

20. Rowe, J.C., Wood, D.H., Rowe, D.W. and Raisz, L.G.(1979) Nutritional hypophosphataemic rickets in a premature infant fed breast milk. *N. Engl. J. Med.*, **300**, 293–297

21. Steichen, J.J., Tsang, R.C., Greer, F.R., Ho, M. and Hug, G. (1981) Elevated serum 1,25-hydroxyvitamin D concentration in rickets of very low birthweight infants. *J. Pediatr.*, **99**, 293–298

22. Day, G.M., Chance, G.W., Radde, I.C. *et al.* (1975) Growth and mineral metabolism in very low birthweight infants. II. Effects of calcium supplementation on growth and divalent ions. *Pediatr. Res.*, **9**, 568

23. Glasgow, J.F.T. and Thomas, P.S. (1977) Rachitic respiratory distress in small preterm infants. *Arch. Dis. Childh.*, **52**, 268–273

24. De Curtis, M., Nicholson, S., Fenton, T., Gibson, P. and McIntosh, N. (1986) Failure of mineral supplementation to reduce the incidence of rickets of prematurity in infants weighing less than 1000 g at birth. *Pediatr. Res.*, **20**, 98

25. Seino, Y., Ishii, T., Shimotsuji, T., Ishida, M. and Yabuuchi, H. (1981) Plasma active vitamin D concentration in low birthweight infants with rickets and its response to vitamin D treatment. *Arch. Dis. Childh.*, **56**, 628–632

26. Shaw, J.C.L. (1976) Evidence for defective skeletal mineralization in low birthweight infants: the absorption of calcium and fat. *Pediatrics*, **57**, 16–25

27. Koo, W.W.I., Gupta, J.M., Nayanar, V.V., Wilkinson, M. and Posen, S. (1982) Skeletal changes in preterm infants. *Arch. Dis. Childh.*, **57**, 447–552

28. Cameron, J.R., Mazess, R.B. and Sorenson, J.A. (1968) Precision and accuracy of bone mineral determination by direct photon absorptiometry. *Invest. Radiol.*, **3**, 141–150

29. Minton, S.D., Steichen, J.J. and Tsang, R.C. (1979) Bone mineral content in term and preterm appropriate-for-gestational-age infants. *J. Paediatr.*, **95**, 1037–1042

30. Greer, F.R., Lane, J., Weiner, S. and Mazess, R.B. (1983) An accurate and reproducible absorptiometric technique for determining bone mineral content in newborn infants. *Paediatr. Res.*, **17**, 259–262

31. Braillon, P.M., Salle, B.L., Brunet, J., Glorieux, F.H., Delmas, P.D. and Meunier, P.J. (1992) Dual energy X-ray absorptiometry measurement of bone mineral content in newborns: validation of the technique. *Pediatr. Res.*, **32**, 77–80

32. Venkataraman, P.S. and Ahluwalia, B.W. (1992) Total bone mineral content and body composition by X-ray densitometry in newborns. *Pediatrics*, **90**, 767–770

33. Lyon, A.J., Hawkes, D.J., Doran, M., McIntosh, N. and Chan, F. (1989) Bone mineralisation in preterm infants measured by dual energy radiographic densitometry. *Arch. Dis. Childh.*, **64**, 919–923

34. William, J.R., Davidson, F., Menon, G. and McIntosh N. (1994) A portable dual energy X-ray absorptiometry technique for the measurement of bone mineral in preterm infants. *Paediatr. Res.*, **36**, 351–357

35. Minton, S.D., Steichen, J.J. and Tsang, R.C. (1983) Decreased bone mineral content in small-for-gestational-age infants compared with appropriate-for-gestation-age infants: normal serum 25-hydroxyvitamin D and decreasing parathyroid hormone. *Pediatrics*, **71**, 383–388

36. Pohlandt, F. and Mathers, N. (1989) Bone mineral content of appropriate and light for gestational age preterm and term newborn infants. *Acta Paediatr. Scand.*, **78**, 835–839

37. Horsman, A., Ryan, S.W., Congdon, P.J., Truscott, J.G. and James, J.R. (1989) Osteopenia in extremely low birthweight infants. *Arch. Dis. Childh.*, **64**, 485–488

38. Pittard, W.B., Geddes, K.M., Sutherland, S.E., Miller, M.C. and Hollis, B.W. (1990) Longitudinal changes in the bone mineral content of term and premature infants. *Am. J. Dis. Child.*, **144**, 36–40

39. Schanler, R.J., Burns, P.A., Abrams, S.A. and Garza, C. (1992) Bone mineralization outcomes in human milk-fed preterm infants. *Pediatr. Res.*, **31**, 583–586

40. Moyer-Mileur, L., Chan, G.M. and Gill, G. (1992) Evaluation of liquid or powdered fortification of human milk on growth and bone mineralization status of preterm infants. *J. Pediatr. Gastroenterol. Nutr.*, **15**, 370–374

41. Congdon, P.J., Horsman, A., Ryan, S.W., Truscott, J.G. and Durward, H. (1990) Spontaneous resolution of bone mineral depletion in preterm infants. *Arch. Dis. Childh.*, **65**, 1038–1042

42. Greer, F.R., Chen, X. and McCormick, A. (1991) Urinary hydroxyproline: relationship to growth, bone mineral content and serum alkaline phosphatase level in premature infants. *J. Pediatr. Gastroenterol. Nutr.*, **13**, 176–181

43. Branca, F., Robins, S.P., Ferro-Luzzi, A. and Golden, M.H.N. (1992) Bone turnover in malnourished children. *Lancet*, **340**, 1493–1496

# 14

# Haematology and transfusion

## I. HAEMATOLOGY

### Elizabeth Letsky and Irene Roberts

There are marked differences between fetal and adult red cells, and in the first few weeks of life many changes occur in the composition of the circulating blood. Only by 6 months of age has a stable population of red cells been established with characteristics which persist into adult life.

All newborn infants experience a fall in haemoglobin concentration in the first few weeks but this fall is greater and earlier in preterm infants; frequently this means that a transfusion must be considered. The indications for blood transfusion in small babies are not well defined. Some infants tolerate very low levels of haemoglobin with none of the accepted signs of tissue anoxia while others are clinically ill.

Tissue oxygenation depends on cardiopulmonary function, concentration and composition of haemoglobin and the position of the haemoglobin–oxygen dissociation curve. Tissue oxygenation in the small preterm infant is adequate but is relatively poorly adapted for postnatal existence [1]. True anaemia at any time in life is present when the demand of tissues for oxygen, in order to maintain normal metabolism, exceeds the ability to delivery oxygen to the tissues.

To establish whether or not true anaemia is present and whether transfusion is indicated, some knowledge of the normal physiology and potential of the adaptive processes in the very small preterm infant is required.

## The pathophysiology of anaemia of prematurity

### Erythropoietin

Maternal erythropoietin does not cross the placenta. Fetal erythropoiesis is controlled by erythropoietin produced by the fetus; high concentrations have been observed in the amniotic fluid and fetal blood in pregnancies complicated by severe erythroblastosis fetalis [2]. Elevated levels of erythropoietin have also been found in cord blood of babies who have had stressful birth or have suffered hypoxia *in utero*, including infants of hypertensive mothers and those with intrauterine growth retardation [3,4]. However, the fetal production of erythropoietin in response to hypoxia or anaemia is poor compared with that of older infants or adults; this probably prevents accelerated erythropoiesis and hyperviscosity of the blood in the healthy fetus [5].

The preterm infant retains this poor response to hypoxic stimuli even though such infants do produce some erythropoietin in response to a fall in haemoglobin concentration. The limited production of erythropoietin, together with the greatly shortened red-cell life-span, appear to be the principal cause of the refractory anaemia of the preterm infant.

Prematurity is a major factor in erythropoietin response, the least mature babies having the lowest levels of erythropoietin [6] in spite of low haemoglobin concentration, high affinity of oxygen for haemoglobin and clinical hypoxia.

ELBW infants appear to have an inadequate haemopoietic response to anaemia-related tissue hypoxia. This may be due to a shift in the site of erythropoietin production [5]. In many mammalian species, including man, erythropoietin is produced in the liver in fetal life and there is a gradual shift to renal production of erythropoietin in the perinatal period. This fetal production of erythropoietin is much less sensitive to tissue hypoxia than that produced in the kidney, but this has not been confirmed in the human fetus. Human adult renal and hepatic erythropoietins have been shown to be structurally identical [7].

Recombinant erythropoietin (EPO) has been shown to stimulate erythroid proliferation *in vitro* [8]. The conclusion that the anaemia of prematurity results from inadequate erythropoietin production and that there are circulating erythroid progenitors [9] has led to the use of recombinant human EPO as a therapeutic and prophylactic agent in the management of the anaemia of prematurity. However, this strategy has not had the strikingly successful outcome observed in those patients treated with EPO for the anaemia of chronic renal failure.

## Clinical trials of erythropoietin for anaemia of prematurity

The mixed results obtained in a variety of reported pilot studies and more recently from randomized controlled trials have been well reviewed [10]. The clinical use of EPO in the preterm infant has been an important but confusing issue [11–25b] and perhaps deserves a little more detailed comment (Table 14.1).

One of the earliest published pilot studies came from Halpcrin and colleagues, 1991 [11]. Treatment was not started until 21 to 33 days of life and the dose given of 75–300 units EPO $kg^{-1}$ $week^{-1}$ was relatively small. All patients showed an increase in reticulocytes but an increase in haematocrit was variable and not universal and in some infants a secondary decrease was observed. The effect of EPO was limited by a number of factors, the most important of which was iron deficiency, the serum iron and ferritin showing a rapid

**Table 14.1   Summary of clinical trials of erythropoietin in anaemia of prematurity**

| Trial | No. of infants | | Mean gesta-tional age (weeks) | Age at start (days) | Duration of Rx (weeks) | Dose (units EPO $kg^{-1}$ $week^{-1}$) | No. of Transfusions | | Oral Fe dose mg $kg^{-1}$ $day^{-1}$ |
|---|---|---|---|---|---|---|---|---|---|
| | EPO | Placebo | | | | | EPO | Placebo | |
| Halperin 1991 [11] | 14 | — | 31 | 21–33 | 4 | 75–300 | 3 | — | 2–5 |
| Beck *et al.* 1991 [12] | 16 | — | 29 | 24–48 | 4 | 10–200 | 4 | — | 3 |
| Shannon *et al.* 1991 [13] | 10 | 10 | 27 | 10–35 | 6 | 200 | 6 | 8 | 3 |
| Obladen 1991 [14] | 43 | 50 | 30 | 4 | 4 | 70 | 30 | 34 | 2 |
| Shannon *et al.* 1992 [15] | 4 | 4 | 28 | 8–28 | 6 | 500–1000 | 1 | 3 | 3–6 |
| Ohls & Christensen 1991 [16] | 10 | 9 | 28 | 45 ± 15 | 3 | 700 | 0 | 5 | 2 |
| Carnielli *et al.* 1992 [17] | 11 | 11 | 30 | 2 | <8 | 1200 | NA | NA | 3 |
| Soubasi *et al.* 1993 [18] (C) | 16 | 12 | 28 | <7 | 6 | 300 | No difference | | 3 |
| Soubasi *et al.* 1993 [18] (U) | 9 | 7 | 30 | <7 | 6 | 300 | 3 | 6 | 3 |
| Bechensteen *et al.* 1993 [19] | 14 | 15 | 30 | 21 | 4 | 300 | 0 | 4 | 6–9 |
| Messer *et al.* 1993 [20] | 31 | 20 | 30 | 10 | 6 | 300–900 | 6 | 9 | 3–8 |
| Emmerson *et al.* 1993 [21] | 15 | 8 | 30 | 8 | 5 | 100–300 | 7 | 7 | 6 |
| Maier *et al.* 1994 [22] | 121 | 120 | 29 | 3 | 6 | 750 | 60 | 81 | 2 |
| Meyer *et al.* 1994 [23] | 40 | 40 | 30 | 14–56 (mean 27) | 6 | 600 | 7 | 21 | 2–6 |
| Ohls *et al.* 1995 [25] | 10 | 10 | 27 | 1 | 2 | 1400 | 2 | 14 | 2–6 |
| Shannon *et al.* 1995 [25b] | 77 | 80 | 27 | 23–24 | 6 | 700 | 1.1 | 1.6 | 3–6 |

EPO = erythropoietin
C = Complications
U = No complications

decrease after commencement of therapy. The consensus opinion of this study was that therapy was started too late and too little EPO was given.

The first randomized trial reported by Shannon *et al.* [13] showed no improvement in haematocrit or need for transfusion due to the low dose of EPO and iron deficiency. In this group's second study [15] more EPO was given (500–1000 units $kg^{-1}$ $week^{-1}$) with adequate iron supplements. The increased haematocrit and reticulocyte counts in the treated group led to a large multicentre trial of erythropoietin (500 units $kg^{-1}$ $week^{-1}$) in the USA of 157 infants (mean gestational age 27 weeks, mean birth weight 924 g) [25b]. This confirmed the safety of EPO in such babies and showed a significant, but very small reduction both in the mean number of transfusions per infant (1.1 vs 1.6; $P = 0.046$) and the mean volume of red cells transfused (16.5 ml vs 23.9 ml; $P = 0.023$). This does suggest some benefit for EPO but it is of note that the transfusion requirement in this study appears very low and this may reflect the fact that EPO was not started until a mean of 23–24 days after birth.

The other large randomized trial completed to date [22] comes from the European multicentre Erythropoietin Study Group and involved 12 centres in six European countries. In contrast to the US study, only 25% of the 241 patients evaluated weighed less than 1000 g and 50% weighed more than 1250 g. The success rate, assessed by lack of need for transfusion and haematocrit never falling below 32%, was 4.1% in controls and 27.5% in EPO group ($P = 0.008$). The results were broadly similar in the smaller randomized controlled trial by Meyer *et al.* [23] in babies <1500 g (mean 1059 g) in which they also found significantly fewer transfused babies in the EPO treated group (six babies vs. 17 babies in the treatment vs. placebo groups). The success of EPO in this study may have been related to the small amount of blood taken for routine tests during the 6 weeks of the study – only 7.6 ± 1.7 ml in the treated cases and 8.1 ± 2.3 ml in the control subjects. Taken together these studies show a small but significant benefit for EPO in reducing transfusion requirements in relatively well preterm infants including those with birth weights below 1000 g [24]. However, the majority of these studies have not included sick preterm infants or those with birthweights <1000 g.

Two recent studies, both small but randomized and controlled, have tried to address this. Ohls *et al.* carried out a placebo-controlled trial of high dose (1400 units $kg^{-1}$ $week^{-1}$) in 20 VLBW with a mean birthweight of around 1200 g [25]. These were 'sick' infants receiving mechanical ventilation and EPO was given by daily intravenous infusion starting within 3 days of birth and continuing for 2 weeks. EPO significantly and quite dramatically reduced the number of transfusions (two vs 14 per infant; EPO vs placebo). This study also confirmed the safety and efficacy of the intravenous route of administration as used by Carnielli et al [17]. The most recent study in ELBW infants, also by Ohls *et al.* [26], was confined to infants with birthweights of <750 g: the mean birthweight was 662 g with a mean gestational age at birth of 24.7 ± 3 weeks. The babies were treated either with placebo (n = 11) or with 200 units $kg^{-1}$ of EPO daily (n = 13) by iv infusion for 2 weeks beginning within 72 hours of birth. The EPO-treated babies received significantly fewer transfusions than the babies receiving placebo (4.7 vs 7.5; $P<0.05$) adding further weight to their earlier study which suggested a modest effect of EPO even in sick VLBW infants provided it is given early and in a sufficiently high dose. Indeed, the study by Soubasi *et al.* also indicated that doses of EPO which were of some benefit in well preterm newborns had no effect in reducing the transfusion requirements of sick babies of a similar gestational age and birthweight [18].

However, in appraising all of these studies, we have to bear in mind that there has been a fall in transfusion rate in recent years independent of the use of r-Hu EPO. Treatment with surfactant, modern ventilation, small blood losses for monitoring and conservative transfusion practices have all limited the need for r-Hu EPO. In addition, one must address the side-effects and the cost of this therapy, the latter being very difficult to assess accurately. The cost of EPO has to be weighed against that of repeated transfusion. A comparison of the EPO treated and control patients in the Zurich centre of the European trial assessed the cost of the EPO treated as 1262 US dollars as opposed to 1203 US dollars in the control infants. A small, recently reported controlled trial [25] of the use of higher doses of r-Hu EPO in the first 2 weeks of life also concluded that this resulted in fewer transfusions and was cost effective. In the UK the NHS cost of a 1000 u vial of r-Hu EPO is £9.00. The current cost of an 'octopus' multisatellite unit of blood is £160.00.

### Side-effects of erythropoietin

(i) Neutropenia and sepsis: although *in vitro* data suggest that erythropoietin suppresses granulopoiesis there was no evidence of significant neutropenia in the controlled trials. However, in the European multicentre trial there was an increased (non-significant) incidence of infection. They suggested that this may be due to depletion of iron stores or the number of subcutaneous injections.

(ii) Sudden Infant Death Syndrome: Several cases have been reported in infants treated with r-Hu EPO [21] but the controlled trials show no increase in SIDS.

(iii) Poor weight gain: This has been reported in some studies but not in others and probably reflects the increased protein and calorie needs arising from the stimulation of erythropoiesis. Indeed, where infant's diet has been modified to achieve optimal protein and iron balance EPO convincingly reduced transfusion requirements [19].

In summary, the main problems with the studies of erythropoietin for anaemia of prematurity are the low doses in early trials, the lack of uniformity of dosage schedules, variable and inadequate iron supplementation, the small numbers of infants in each study and the small numbers of infants under 1000 g. While many questions remain to be answered [27–31], some recommendations from all these studies are possible. To achieve maximum efficiency enough erythropoietin has to be given and it should probably be started early: during the first 7 to ten days of life. For 'well' preterm infants not requiring mechanical ventilation at the end of the first week of life doses of EPO of 750–900 units kg$^{-1}$ week$^{-1}$ for 6 weeks can significantly reduce transfusion requirements. For 'sick' VLBW infants, particularly for those with birthweights below 750 g, administration of higher doses of EPO by daily intravenous infusion is the only regimen shown to be effective. In order to allow the maximal

response increased iron supplements must be administered and may be given orally or intravenously [32]. However, at best, this therapy will only be an adjunct to supportive therapy in the VLBW infant and will not replace, although it may reduce, the need for red cell transfusion [33].

## Availability of oxygen and special problems of demand and supply

Tissue oxygen availability depends on arterial oxygen saturation, the concentration of haemoglobin and the position of the haemoglobin–oxygen dissociation curve. These are all different in VLBW infants. Arterial oxygen saturation is frequently low because of diseases of the lung and apnoeic attacks. The concentration and type of haemoglobin is different from a term baby.

### Developmental changes in haemoglobins

There are embryonic, fetal and adult haemoglobins. The three embryonic haemoglobins – Hb Gower 1 and 2 and Hb Portland – disappear by 12 weeks' gestation; they are probably restricted to the immature red cells produced in the yolk sac (Table 14.2).

Fetal haemoglobin, HbF ($\alpha_2\gamma_2$) can be detected in the blood from embryos of 6–12 weeks' gestation.

From the time when hepatic erythropoiesis is established HbF ($\alpha_2\gamma_2$) forms the major respiratory pigment throughout intrauterine life, but from as early as 8–10 weeks' gestation it is possible to detect about 5–10% of haemoglobin HbA ($\alpha_2\beta_2$). Between 32 and 36 weeks'

Table 14.2 **Globin chain composition of human haemoglobins**

| Haemo-globin | Globin composition | Site of production | State of development |
|---|---|---|---|
| Gower 1 | $\zeta_2\epsilon_2$ | | Embryo |
| Gower 2 | $\alpha_2\epsilon_2$ | Yolk sac | Embryo |
| Portland | $\zeta_2\gamma_2$ | | Embryo |
| Fetal | $\alpha_2\gamma_2$ | | Embryo |
| Fetal | $\alpha_2\gamma_2$ | Liver | Fetus |
| Adult | $\alpha_2\beta_2$ | Bone marrow | Fetus |
| HbA$_2$ | $\alpha_2\delta_2$ | | Fetus |
| Fetal | $\alpha_2\gamma_2$ | Bone marrow | Adult |
| Adult | $\alpha_2\beta_2$ | | Adult |
| HbA$_2$ | $\alpha_2\delta_2$ | | Adult |

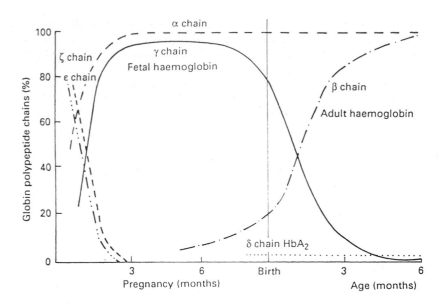

**Figure 14.1** Developmental changes in human haemoglobins

gestation the production of HbA increases and there is a sharp decline in HbF production (Figure 14.1). HbF makes up less than 10% of haemoglobin at 3 months of age and has fallen to the adult level of less than 1% by 6 months to 1 year.

The decline of fetal haemoglobin in the neonatal period appears to be strictly regulated. The switch from HbF to HbA synthesis occurs around 32 weeks' gestation [34]; it is not related to birth, but it is based on post-conceptional age. Babies at 32–34 weeks have a mean of 90% HbF; at term it is around 70–80%.

The efficiency of oxygen delivery to the tissues is directly related to the interactions of haemoglobin with 2,3-diphosphoglycerate (2,3-DPG). High concentrations of 2,3-DPG push the oxygen dissociation curve to the right and facilitate oxygen delivery to the tissues. The reduction in the oxygen affinity of HbF by interaction with 2,3-DPG is only a fraction of that produced by the same concentration of 2,3-DPG with HbA. The effect of this reduced reaction of HbF with 2,3-DPG ensures that the oxygen affinity of fetal blood does not drop below that of its mother. This helps binding of oxygen from the maternal circulation in the placenta villi. More than half of the oxygen bound in the placenta by the fetal blood can be released to fetal tissue because the tissue oxygen levels in the fetus are much lower than those in the maternal tissues.

In the first few weeks of extrauterine life, there is a progressive increase in the delivery of oxygen to the tissues. There is a gradual replacement of HbF by HbA, an increase in 2,3-DPG which shifts the oxygen dissociation curve to the right, and, of course, increased availability of oxygen. The net result of these changes is that, although the haemoglobin level in the term infant falls from 17 to 11 g dl$^{-1}$ in the first 12 weeks of life, the oxygen delivery to the tissues at 3 months is greater than that in the newborn infant.

However, the infant under 1000 g is unlikely to have reached 32 weeks' postconception and therefore the switch to predominant β globin chain production has not even begun and it may be some weeks later before significant amounts of HbA are produced [35,36]. This compromises the delivery of oxygen to the tissues by preventing the shift of the oxygen dissociation curve to the right.

### Haemoglobin concentration

Cord haemoglobin values for preterm infants (17.5 ± 1.6 g dl$^{-1}$) do not vary significantly from those observed at term.

Dependent upon the amount of placental transfusion and transient haemoconcentration due to poor oral fluid intake, a brief rise in haemoglobin is often seen during the first 24 hours of life. The haemoglobin returns to the original concentration of birth by the end of the first week, and there is then a progressive fall over 4–12 weeks. The rapidity of fall and the nadir of haemoglobin concentration vary inversely with gestational age; the fall results from a reduction in red cell mass and not from haemodilutional effect of a greater plasma volume. The red-cell life-span is even shorter in the preterm infant than at term and there is a marked reticulocytopenia.

The supply of oxygen to the tissues of the healthy neonate is only just adequate. In the very preterm infant this marginal oxygen supply often fails. Superimposed on the multiple causes of anaemia in the baby under 1000 g are the sampling blood losses essential for the monitoring and intensive management of such small birth weight babies. Iatrogenic blood letting is probably the major cause of anaemia in such infants [37].

### Haematinics

The ELBW infant is more prone to develop nutritional deficiencies than the term infant because of rapid growth and diminished resources. Factors that can accelerate the anaemia of prematurity are iron, folate and vitamin $B_{12}$ and vitamin E deficiency [38].

#### *Iron*

Although iron transport to the fetus is unidirectional with ratio of maternal:fetal serum ferritin concentrations of 1:2 to 1:4 and there are adequate fetal iron stores even in cases of maternal iron deficiency, there is some evidence that there is a reduced red-cell mass in the offspring of iron-deficient mothers; iron stores, although high by adult standards, are reduced in these infants compared to those born to iron-replete mothers [39]. The fetus normally recruits 75 mg iron kg body weight$^{-1}$; iron status will be related to birth weight and maturity [40].

The role of iron in the pathogenesis of the anaemia of prematurity has excited interest for almost 50 years. As a result of innumerable investigations a clearer picture has emerged from the initial confusion. Iron deficiency is not likely to play a part in the early anaemia of prematurity unless there has been perinatal blood loss or repeated blood sampling [41]. It follows that the administration of medicinal iron will not prevent the initial fall in haemo-

globin. However, unless the premature infant is given iron supplements some time in the first 2–4 months of life, anaemia (the so-called late anaemia of prematurity) inevitably develops from iron deficiency. The time of the anaemia will depend on the initial haemoglobin level and the rate of growth. In general, infants with normal haemoglobin levels at birth will have depleted their iron stores and therefore limited the rate of haemoglobin synthesis by the time they have doubled their birth weight [40]. Approximately 75% of the infant's total body iron is contained in the haemoglobin of the circulating and developing red cells; those who are anaemic at birth have reduced iron reserves [42].

There is now a consensus that all premature infants, and particularly those weighing less than 1500 g at birth, require supplemental iron to prevent the development of late anaemia due to iron deficiency [42].

Iron supplements in VLBW infants should be started on the 15th day of life in the following dosage regime [40]:

3 mg kg 24h$^{-1}$ for infants of 1000–1500 g birth weight
4 mg kg 24h$^{-1}$ for those <1000 g birth weight

Many preterm babies are now receiving EPO and they may need more iron (up to 9 mg kg$^{-1}$ day$^{-1}$; see Table 14.1). For those not yet on enteral feeds, intravenous iron (1 mg kg daily) has been used successfully [32]. Ideally iron supplements should be continued for at least 12–15 months after birth [38] although this is probably not necessary in bottle-fed babies if infant formula with a high iron content (15 mg l$^{-1}$) is used [43]. If the infant is receiving adequate vitamin E in relation to polyunsaturated fat in the diet then the early introduction of supplemental iron causes no adverse effects.

It is important to give these supplements. Iron deficiency may have long-term effects on the fetus, neonate and developmental parameters in the first few years of life which are not anything to do with the Hb concentration and oxygen carrying capacity of red cells. Animal experimentation has shown that early iron deficiency [44] irreversibly affects brain iron control and distribution which results in neuro-transmitter and behavioural alterations. Iron deficiency has been shown in the human infant to be associated with psychomotor delays in many studies. Careful follow-up studies have shown that even after haematological corrections the cognitive disadvantages persist at 5 to 6 years of age. It is therefore very important to prevent iron deficiency during early development in the preterm infant with appropriate supplementation [44].

### Vitamin E

Alpha-tocopherol (vitamin E) is a fat soluble dietary factor first shown to be required for successful reproduction in rats and now known to be an essential nutrient for man. Adults do not readily become deficient in vitamin E because there is α-tocopherol in foodstuffs. Vitamin E deficiency has been described in the neonate, especially those who are preterm [45]. This is because all newborn infants have relative tocopherol deficiency; the smaller the infant at birth the greater the lack of vitamin E.

A mother at term has a vitamin E level around 0.9 mg 100 ml$^{-1}$ whereas her baby's value is only 0.2 mg 100 ml$^{-1}$. Term infants with a birth weight of 3500 g have vitamin E body stores of 20 mg while infants with a birth weight of 1000 g have only 3 mg. There is a relationship between the maternal level of vitamin E and that of her infant but a newborn infant never has a value in excess of 0.6 mg 100 ml$^{-1}$, which is the lowest limit of normal for older children and adults.

Vitamin E is a potent antiperoxidant at the cellular level; its deficiency results in an increased rate of cell membrane lipid peroxidation which can lead to a shortening of the red-cell life-span and a haemolytic anaemia.

The dietary requirement for vitamin E increases when the intake of polyunsaturated fatty acids (PUFA) increases. Although the breastfed infant quickly attains normal adult levels, there is considerable variability in the vitamin E status in artificially fed infants. This results in part from the PUFA content of the artificial formulae. Most infant formulae contain quantities of linoleic acid, an 18-carbon fatty acid with two unsaturated double bonds, that are in excess of the quantities found in breast milk.

The first reports of the association of vitamin E deficiency with haemolytic anaemia in the premature neonate came from the USA in the late 1960s. These infants were aged 6–10 weeks and had been fed proprietary formulae with a high PUFA content [46,47]. The administration of vitamin E to affected infants resulted in a prompt increase in the haemoglobin level and a fall in the reticulocyte count.

It is clear that the severity of the haemolysis in the premature infant was related to the level of vitamin E and the PUFA content of the diet (E/PUFA ratio). The lack of reports from the UK is probably a reflection of the lower PUFA content of our proprietary formulae at that time and hence a higher E/PUFA ratio.

It became evident through the passage of time that it was not just the high PUFA and low vitamin E content of the diet which were predisposing factors to haemolysis in the premature infant. Iron acts as a catalyst in the non-enzymatic auto-oxidation of unsaturated fatty acids and can result in the peroxidation of red cell membrane lipids. It has been shown that iron-fortified formulae can trigger a haemolytic anaemia in the infant who receives large quantities of PUFA with inadequate amounts of vitamin E [48].

The incidence of vitamin E deficiency haemolytic anaemia varied from nursery to nursery and was always rare in the UK. It should be appreciated that vitamin E deficiency may contribute to the magnitude of the physiological anaemia in all non-supplement premature infants. The commercial formulae have, for the most part, corrected the potential problem by reducing the content of linoleic acid and increasing the concentration of vitamin E. Breast milk has a very low content of linoleic acid.

The problem of the triad of factors (iron, PUFA and vitamin E levels) contributing to anaemia in the premature infants is now well recognized and haemolysis can thus be prevented by:

(1) A delay in introduction of iron.
(2) Vitamin E can be administered to overcome the malabsorption of the natural vitamin.
(3) Formulae with a low PUFA content, or human milk, can be fed to small premature infants.

The removal or correction of just one of the contributing triad will prevent any significant haemolysis or anaemia in the premature neonate [49], but no haematological difference between infants supplemented with 0.25 units oral vitamin E daily and a control group has been shown.

### Folic acid

Serum and red cell folate levels are higher in the newborn than in the normal adult regardless of birth weight or gestation, but fall quickly to levels which are often below the normal adult levels within several weeks of birth. This fall occurs more rapidly in the preterm infant, subnormal levels being reached within the first few weeks of life, whereas low levels do not develop in the term infant until after six months of age. Controlled studies, however, have failed to demonstrate any alteration in the early anaemia of prematurity by giving routine folate supplementation. The normal premature infant absorbs folic acid easily and although there is no general recommendation for the prophylactic use of folic acid in the newborn, a dietary provision of 20–50 $\mu$g 24h$^{-1}$ would ensure sufficiency [50].

There is an increased risk of megaloblastic anaemia occurring in the neonate of a folate-deficient mother, especially if delivery is preterm. The pathogenesis of the development of such an anaemia is shown in Figure 14.2.

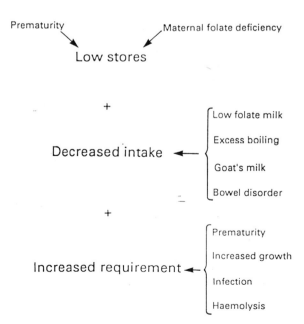

**Figure 14.2** The factors which contribute to the development of megaloblastic anaemia due to folate deficiency in infancy

The young infant's requirement for folate has been estimated at 20–50 $\mu$g 24h$^{-1}$ (4–10 times the adult requirement) on a weight basis. Serum and red cell folates are consistently higher in cord than in maternal blood, but the premature infant is in severe negative folate balance because of high growth rate and reduced intake. The usual fall in serum and red cell folate in the preterm neonate, and even in the absence of other complicating factors, may result in megaloblastic anaemia. This can be prevented by giving supplements of 50 $\mu$g 24h$^{-1}$ [51].

In those infants whose dietary intake would be predictably poor, such as the very immature or those with chronic diarrhoea or recurrent infections, it would appear wise to give parenteral folic acid.

### Vitamin B$_{12}$

Serum B$_{12}$ levels in all neonates are generally higher than in maternal serum. This is the result of active transfer of vitamin B$_{12}$ across the placenta to the fetus at the expense of maintaining maternal vitamin B$_{12}$ serum levels. This makes little impact on the mother's own reserves because adult stores are of the order of 300 $\mu$g or more and vitamin B$_{12}$ stores in the newborn infant are about 50 $\mu$g [52].

Because of these low storage reserves and because of poor dietary intake of vitamin B$_{12}$ during the period of rapid growth, most premature infants will have lower than normal adult levels by the fourth or fifth month of life. However, a deficiency of vitamin B$_{12}$ is not related to the early anaemia of prematurity and the haemoglobin, red cell counts and haematocrit are similar in premature infants who are deficient or replete for vitamin B$_{12}$. The recommended oral intake of vitamin B$_{12}$ in low birth weight infants is the same as in term infants. Sufficient vitamin B$_{12}$ is present both in breast milk and in all types of infant formula. Additional supplements of vitamin B$_{12}$ are therefore unnecessary even in premature infants.

### Protein

Protein synthesis and turnover are increased in preterm infants because of their very high metabolic rates. Adequate protein is necessary for healthy haemopoiesis and therefore dietary requirements for protein must be increased in these immature infants.

It has been shown [53] that human milk proteins promote general growth and erythropoiesis in VLBW infants. The beneficial effect, particularly on erythropoiesis promoting higher haemoglobin concentration in the early weeks of life, appears to be dependent on the human origin of this protein, and an uptake of 4 g kg$^{-1}$ daily which is double the usual intake.

# Haemostasis and thrombosis in the baby under 1000 g

Normal haemostasis is determined by the interaction between the vessel wall, platelets, procoagulation factors, naturally occurring anticoagulants and fibrinolysis.

The haemostatic mechanisms of the ELBW infant cannot be considered in isolation. The haemostatic system is immature in the healthy term neonate with little reserve capacity to deal with the stresses of delivery or the immediate postnatal period. Constant changes occur in the components of these systems over the first few weeks of life and the haemostatic mechanisms are not mature by adult standards until 6 to 9 months of age. These changes are dependent not only on the postnatal age but also on the gestational age [54,55].

Although the healthy term infant can maintain haemostatic competence, physiological and pathological stimuli may tip the balance in the direction of either thrombosis or haemorrhage, particularly in the preterm infant. Acquired haemostatic disorders are by far the greatest problem on the special care baby unit but genetic disorders can present in the first weeks of life. The differentiation between physiological values of haemostatic components and inherited deficiency can be very difficult. In addition, the small size of the infant and the unique haematological parameters present a technical challenge both in obtaining suitable specimens and developing microtechnology in the laboratory [56]. The alterations in the haemostatic system in the sick preterm infant can only be interpreted with a knowledge of normal physiology in the development and prenatal periods. A brief overview of healthy and disordered haemostasis in the newborn infant follows. For further information of this complex subject the reader is referred to some reviews [57,58,59].

## Developmental haemostasis

### Platelets

Platelets are present in the circulation in the fetus from 7 weeks' gestation onwards. There appears to be little difference between platelet counts in term and preterm infants, as long as they are healthy. Sick preterm infants often develop moderate, and sometimes severe, thrombocytopenia depending on the cause (Table 14.3). The normal neonatal platelet count lies in the adult range. Although platelet function tests *in vitro* are impaired due, it is thought, to a basic developmental defect in

**Table 14.3** Causes of neonatal thrombocytopenia

| | |
|---|---|
| Inherited | Megakaryocytic hypoplasia |
| | TAR (thrombocytopenia Absent Radii) Syndrome |
| | Fanconi's pancytopenia (occasionally in newborn period) |
| | Myeloproliferative disease (Down's syndrome) |
| | Osteopetrosis |
| | Wiskott–Aldrich syndrome and variants |
| | Bernard–Soulier syndrome |
| | May–Hegglin anomaly |
| Immune disorders | Maternal idiopathic thrombocytopenia (ITP) |
| | Maternal systemic lupus erythematosus (SLE) |
| | Drug-induced |
| | Alloimmune |
| Consumption disorders | Disseminated intravascular coagulation (DIC) |
| | Large vessel thrombosis |
| | Necrotizing enterocolitis |
| | Thrombotic thrombocytopenic purpose (TTP) |
| | Giant haemangioma |
| | Hyperviscosity syndrome |
| Infection | Bacterial: sepsis, congenital syphilis |
| | Viral: CMV, herpes simplex, rubella |
| | Other: toxoplasmosis |
| Drugs | Maternal: tolbutamide, thiazide diuretics |
| | Infant: Intralipid, tolazoline |
| Other | Intrauterine growth retardation |
| | Maternal hypertension/pre-eclampsia |
| | Congenital leukaemia |
| | Post-exchange transfusion |
| | Metabolic disorders |
| | Neonatal cold injury |

membrane, the bleeding time in normal term and preterm infants is the same or slightly shorter than in adults or older children if appropriately modified equipment is used.

## Clotting factors

Visible evidence of clotting of fetal blood has been observed as early as 12 weeks' gestation [60]. Concentrations of clotting factors have been studied in cord blood of term and preterm infants at birth, but there are profound changes in the baby at and during birth and the levels obtained will be affected by these changes. Factor VIII:C levels are 30–50% higher in vaginally delivered infants as opposed to those delivered by Caesarean section. Fibrinogen, factor V and factor VIII levels are within the normal range in term and preterm infants. Cord plasma shows a prolonged thrombin and repti-lase time, suggesting an altered function of fibrinogen, but there is still controversy regarding the existence of a structurally distinct fetal fibrinogen.

Studies on the factor VIII:C – von Wille-brand factor (VWF) complex show that the newborn factor VIII complex is elevated in both term and preterm infants. In addition VWF levels remain elevated until 3 months of age, suggesting that this elevation is not just a reaction to the process of delivery [54].

Concentrations of factors II, VII, IX and X, the vitamin K-dependent procoagulants, are reduced in both term and preterm infants. Compared to adult levels the percentage increases from approximately 30% at 24 weeks' gestation to 50% at term. There is also a defect of the γ carboxylation of the glutamic acid residues caused by the deficiency of vitamin K [60].

Factors XI, XII – prekallikrein (PK) and high molecular weight kininogen (HMWK) –

are the so-called contact factors. These are reduced by adult standards with concentrations of 20–30% in the preterm infant and 20–50% at term. These levels are not associated with significant haemorrhage in adults, but may be a major cause of a prolonged in vitro partial thromboplastin time (PTT) in the normal neonate (Table 14.4) [60,61,62].

## Anticoagulants

The five major naturally occurring anticoagulants are α2-macroglobulins, antithrombin III, protein C, protein S and the newly identified cofactor for activated protein C (Factor V Leiden).

α2-macroglobulin depends upon reticuloendothelial clearance to exert its physiological role rather than inactivation. It complexes with serine proteases including the procoagulants thrombin, Xa, IXa and kallikrein. Although there are normal levels by adult standards in the neonate, the effect may be reduced because of the immaturity of the reticuloendothelial system.

Antithrombin III levels are reduced in newborn infants. They rise from levels of below 30% of adult values in preterm infants to 60% at term. However, these low levels, which can be associated with a thrombotic tendency in adults, are balanced by the lower levels of vitamin K dependent procoagulants which antithrombin III inhibits. The newborn infant is thought therefore not to be a thrombotic risk because of the low levels of antithrombin III. On the other hand the vitamin K dependent anticoagulants – protein C and its cofactor protein S – are reduced by adult standards in the newborn infant. The role of these factors is to inactivate factors V and VIII: two of the major rate-limiting steps in blood clotting. These factors are at normal or increased adult concentrations in both term and preterm infants. The physiological imbalance between factors V and VIII and protein C may be a cause for the thrombotic tendency in the newborn infant.

A genetic tendency to thrombosis has recently been shown in families showing a mutation in the Factor V gene (Factor V Leiden) which results in impaired inactivation of Factor Va by activated protein C [63]: so-called activated protein C resistance (APCR). Many studies have now shown that APCR is the most frequent genetic abnormality associated with thrombosis in young adults.

**Table 14.4** Neonatal haemostasis: screening tests [62]

|  | Preterm infant (≈27–30 weeks) | Term infant | Adult |
|---|---|---|---|
| Bleeding time (min) | within normal range | within normal range | 2–10 |
| PTT (s) | 70–110 | 40–60 | 35–45 |
| PT (s) | 17–29 | 12–20 | 12–14 |
| TT (s) | 20–28 | 18–24 | 15–19 |
| Fibrinogen (g/l) | 2–4 | 2–4 | 2–4 |

Data are lacking concerning the normal activity of APC cofactor in the neonate. One study has shown that activity of this factor may be increased in normal neonates [64]. This will limit the ability of the standard functional APC cofactor assay to diagnose thrombophilia in the neonate.

### Fibrinolytic system

The newborn infant, whether mature or preterm, demonstrates an overall increased fibrinolytic activity which lasts for several hours, probably due to increased activator activity. This is in spite of levels of plasminogen ranging from 25% for preterm to 50% in term infants. Sick infants, with the additional stress of disseminated intravascular coagulation or RDS frequently deplete their fibrinolytic potential. In healthy infants plasminogen reaches normal adult levels by approximately 2 weeks of age. Because newborn plasminogen has been demonstrated to be defective in its function it has been suggested that infusions of plasminogen may help in reducing the severity of RDS. Normal infants do not show increased levels of fibrinogen degradation products if the blood is collected properly. Elevated levels of fibrinogen degradation products are seen frequently in sick infants.

In summary, previable fetuses, less than 24 weeks' gestation, do show a bleeding tendency which is associated with poor development of the entire mechanism of haemostasis including vessels, platelets and coagulation factors, but thriving, clinically stable preterm infants at 26–29 weeks appear to show no bleeding tendency even if subjected to major surgery. Screening tests for coagulation yield values for clotting factors and platelets within the currently minimal haemostatic levels for older children and adults [62,65].

Thrombotic complications, in contrast, are frequently seen in association with low levels of coagulation inhibitors in both the healthy and ill preterm infant. The widely reported increased bleeding and clotting tendencies, together with significantly abnormal coagulation tests, are seen primarily in sick preterm infants.

Thus, healthy preterm infants do not bleed excessively, but have extremely limited reserves to compensate for a decrease in procoagulants. Sick infants have an increased tendency to bleed due to the many pathological conditions sometimes triggering disseminated intravascular coagulation which complicates their first few weeks of life.

### Haemostasis, hepatic maturity and haemorrhagic disease of the newborn

The liver is the site of synthesis of plasminogen, antithrombin III, the contact factors (XII, XI, high molecular weight kininogen and prekallikrein) and the vitamin K dependent factors (II, VII, IX, X and protein C). The preterm infant shows moderate deficiencies of all of these factors which appear to be gestationally dependent; they increase in concentration as the infant matures. All preterm infants require parenteral vitamin K at birth to prevent the fall in prothrombin activity during the second and third day of life and to protect them against development of classic haemorrhagic disease of the newborn [66].

During recent years knowledge of the pathogenesis of haemorrhagic disease of the newborn (HDN) and its association with vitamin K deficiency has increased considerably but it is still not fully understood [67,68]. It is useful to classify the disorder into three clinical syndromes: early, classic and late [69].

There are wide variations in preparation, routes and dosage schedules for vitamin K prophylaxis both between countries and within countries. VLBW infants are most likely to receive intravenous vitamin K which has not been implicated in the cancer controversy. However, it is very important that the doses should be repeated at appropriate intervals because it is becoming clear that the probable slow release effect of a single intramuscular administration is not apparent with either oral or intravenous administration.

### Disseminated intravascular coagulation (DIC)

This is always a secondary phenomenon. Laboratory evidence and clinical expression of DIC are not infrequent findings in the sick newborn infant because triggers of the process such as hypoxia, acidosis, hypothermia, poor tissue perfusion and hypotension quickly develop in the course of neonatal disease whatever its origin, particularly in the preterm infant. The severity of clinical expression is compounded by immaturity, limiting the ability to produce coagulation factors to replace those consumed and the fact that the poorly developed reticuloendothelial system is unable to clear efficiently the products of coagulation such as fibrinogen degradation products.

DIC in the neonate is frequently associated with maternal hypertension and shock, placental abruption, placentae praevia and also with a dead twin fetus [70]. Postnatal associations include both bacterial and viral infection, respiratory distress syndrome, erythroblastosis fetalis, necrotizing enterocolitis and hyperviscosity.

The most practical and useful tests for diagnosis and day-to-day management of DIC in the newborn are the platelet count, prothrombin and thrombin times (PT and TT) with fibrinogen concentration and fibrinogen degradation products (Table 14.4). The management must depend on successful elimination of the trigger and will vary accordingly, but it is sometimes necessary to replace coagulation factors with fresh frozen plasma and occasionally exchange transfusion is indicated. Platelets are not usually severely depressed except in association with sepsis, and platelet transfusions are rarely required in this situation. Indeed, their use may have been harmful in the past in providing free thromboplastin and a continuing trigger for DIC [71].

### Haematological manifestations in offspring of mothers with pre-eclampsia and intrauterine growth retardation (IUGR)

The haemostatic status of the fetus and newborn may be affected by the placental damage which occurs in association with severe pre-eclampsia and IUGR. Significant numbers of infants whose mothers have the HELLP (haemolysis, elevated liver enzymes and low platelet count) syndrome and pre-eclampsia have been shown to have thrombocytopenia [72,73]. In addition to thrombocytopenia many infants show significant neutropenia at birth. Recent studies have shown that these changes are due to reduced production of platelets and neutrophils respectively, due to reduced numbers of their progenitor cells [74].

The reported coagulation factor changes in infants of hypertensive mothers are variable, although decreased platelets seem to be a constant finding [70]. These infants should be monitored closely for evidence of infection,

DIC and thrombotic complications for which they appear to be at increased risk and managed appropriately.

### Thrombocytopenia

There are many causes of neonatal thrombocytopenia (Table 14.3). The most usual mechanisms for decreased platelets in the newborn are either increased destruction and consumption as seen in DIC, particularly associated with infection and immunological disorders [75] or reduced platelet production as seen in IUGR and infants of hypertensive mothers [74].

Immune thrombocytopenias in the neonate are relatively acute and transitory and depend on transplacental passage of maternal IgG anti-platelet antibodies and will therefore be dealt with a little more fully here.

The management of immune thrombocytopenia in the newborn is different for each type and therefore the pathogenesis must be clearly established so that the correct and optimum therapy can be instituted [76–78].

With auto-immune thrombocytopenia (AITP) the maternal platelet count can vary from normal to profound thrombocytopenia depending on activity of disease, response to therapy and whether or not the spleen has been removed.

Severity of thrombocytopenia in the fetus is difficult to assess, but a direct correlation has been shown between maternal platelet associated IgG and affected infants [79]. As far as the fetus and newborn infant is concerned this disease is relatively benign compared with alloimmune thrombocytopenia.

Alloimmune thrombocytopenia may be associated with delivery of a very small infant. It is a much less common disorder and is due in the vast majority of cases to maternal antibodies directed against the human platelet antigen HPA[1] (also known as PI[A1]), the mother being HPA[1] negative and her fetus carrying paternally derived HPA[1] antigens. In this condition the mother's platelet count is normal but she has free identifiable specific antiplatelet antibodies in her serum. These IgG antibodies cross the placenta and fix to the glycoprotein receptor areas of the fetal platelets and seriously interfere with platelet function. It is probably for this reason that serious spontaneous intracranial haemorrhage may occur *in utero* before delivery and as early as 18–20 weeks' gestation. However, there is also evidence that anti-HPA[1A] antibodies can in some cases inhibit platelet progenitor cells and this may contribute to the severity of the thrombocytopenia [80].

Alloimmune thrombocytopenia can occur in the first pregnancy and will recur in subsequent pregnancies. The first affected pregnancy cannot be predicted unless epidemiological studies are being carried out [81] but it is important to identify the couple at risk if an otherwise healthy infant is born with thrombocytopenia so that future pregnancies can be managed optimally. Before delivery an affected fetus can be identified by finding the specific antibodies in the mother's serum and thrombocytopenia in a fetal cord blood sample. In this situation intravenous IgG immunoglobulin administration to the mother may have a beneficial effect, it is thought to block the passage across the placenta of specific IgG antibodies [82]. Favourable reports from USA have not been reproduced in European centres.

Some fetuses have been treated by HPA[1] negative platelet transfusions before delivery [83]. These should not be given unless it can be established that the fetus has not sustained any serious bleeding *in utero* before treatment. Sometimes, such fetal treatment provokes preterm labour. At Queen Charlotte's we have successfully treated several infants with serial weekly intrauterine platelet transfusions from 24 weeks up to 34 weeks' gestation but the outcome has to be weighed against the considerable cumulative hazard to the fetus of each intrauterine transfusion. We have not found either maternally or fetally administered i.v. IgG to raise the fetal platelet count [84].

Delivery should be by the most atraumatic route possible. There is a relatively high mortality rate in this condition compared with idiopathic thrombocytopenia purpura [76] and those who survive may have serious long-term morbidity if appropriate measures have not been taken. The treatment of neonatal alloimmune thrombocytopenia is with donor HPA[1A] negative platelet concentrates. Maternal platelets, because of their rapid availability, although widely recommended in the past are not now thought to be optimum therapy [78]. Facilities for collecting and washing the platelets will be limited to a few specialist units. Residual maternal HPA[1A] antibody will not be beneficial

and there is the additional hazard of graft-versus-host disease if the platelets are not irradiated. In an emergency, a random platelet donor transfusion will have a transient beneficial effect until HPA[1A] negative platelets are available.

Paradoxically, immune thrombocytopenia may become worse in the first few days after birth in both alloimmune and autoimmune types, although the source of antibody has been cut off. This may be due to HPA[1A] antibody-mediated inhibition of platelet progenitor cells [80] but is probably due to the development of the reticuloendothelial circulation, particularly in the spleen. The splenic circulation is not established at delivery, but after a few days it will more effectively remove coated platelets from the circulation. Mild thrombocytopenia may continue for several weeks although normal platelet counts are usually achieved by the end of the first month of life. Active treatment is rarely required after the first week or so of life. The greatest hazard is passed once delivery has been successfully negotiated.

## Thrombosis

The preterm infant is particularly susceptible to acquired thrombotic lesions, both in the presence and absence of indwelling catheters [85]. It is difficult to know whether the apparent increasing incidence is due to the use of more searching and accurate diagnostic methods or due to changing modes of therapy and support in the special care baby unit [86].

### Risk factors for neonatal thrombosis

Three major factors contribute to the formation of thrombin according to Virchow's postulates:

(1) Abnormalities of vessel wall.
(2) Disturbances of blood flow.
(3) Changes in blood coagulability.

Only those factors of particular significance in the ELBW infant will be referred to.

### Abnormalities of the vessel wall

A wide variety of maternal disorders, including hypertension, may result in thrombin formation in fetal placental veins. Chorion thrombi are of importance because they may embolize to fetal vessels.

If the ductus does not undergo its normal involutional change, thrombin may form within the vessel and provide a source of emboli to both systemic and pulmonary circulations.

Intravascular catheters both provide a foreign surface and may injure the vessel wall in which they are placed, exposing collagen and releasing thromboplastin. They are frequently associated with thromboembolism.

Endothelial damage provoked by localized or generalized hypoxaemia may well initiate thrombosis as will the endothelial damage occurring in the course of septicaemia. These are well-known triggers of DIC, but may also cause localized thrombosis.

### Changes in blood coagulation and fibrinolysis

Normal physiological changes in neonatal haemostasis, as described above, do not seem to predispose the healthy infant to thrombotic complications. Low levels of antithrombin III are balanced by low levels of procoagulant factors against which antithrombin III is directed. However, there is a discrepancy between the low levels of protein C in the neonate compared with the normal to high levels of factors V and VIII. Hereditary protein C deficiency in its heterozygous form is associated with a thrombotic tendency later in life. Severe or homozygous protein C deficiency is associated with massive thromboembolism and recurrent purpura fulminans in the neonate. Although successful management with protein C concentrate followed by warfarin therapy has been reported, this genetic condition is usually rapidly fatal [87]. Of particular interest here is the fact that neonatal protein C levels as measured by immunological methods may be undetectable in the sick preterm infant with thrombosis. The protein C levels will subsequently rise to normal levels as the infant recovers and matures [86]. These infants therefore have acquired not genetic deficiency of protein C.

A similar situation may occur in heterozygotes for ATIII deficiency making it difficult to distinguish between inherited and acquired disease. Only follow-up and family studies [86] will clarify the picture.

It is not estimated whether or to what degree any of the special features of normal neonatal haemostasis contribute to the thrombotic tendency in the sick newborn infant. In contrast, convincing demonstrations of the role of vascular damage and disturbances of blood flow in the development of thrombosis have been made by several groups.

### Thrombosis associated with the use of indwelling catheters

There is a potential risk of initiating thrombosis by the use of indwelling catheters in the neonate irrespective of the vessel catheterized. The vast majority of thromboses in the neonatal period are catheter related.

#### Umbilical artery catheters

Umbilical artery catheterization is common in the sick newborn and has been associated with severe thromboembolic phenomena [88] requiring aggressive intervention in 1% of cases. The incidence of subclinical thrombosis is much higher and can be detected by ultrasound and/or at autopsy in 20–95% of infants with umbilical artery catheters.

Sequelae of clinically evident thrombosis include renal hypertension, necrotizing enterocolitis, peripheral gangrene, and even paraplegia [85]. Follow-up studies in small groups of children up to the age of 4 years have not revealed any sequelae of clinically silent catheter-induced thromboses.

Prevention of catheter-related thrombosis is an important but controversial issue. It is current practice to use heparin at a rate of 1–10 units or more per hour in many preterm neonatal units. Although catheter patency has been shown to improve when heparin is given in doses of 100–200 units $kg^{-1}$ $day^{-1}$, the effect on incidence of catheter-related thrombosis is still not established. There is also the hazard of bleeding when heparin is given in doses of 5–10 units $kg^{-1}$ $h^{-1}$ in the ELBW infant. Current evidence suggests that low-dose heparin should not be used routinely to prevent thrombosis in preterm infants with catheters.

#### Umbilical vein catheters

It is generally believed that umbilical vein catheters carry a greater risk of thrombosis than arterial catheters, but this has never been demonstrated in a prospective trial.

Misplacement of the catheter and rapid infusion of hyperosmolar solutions increase the incidence of thrombosis. The incorrect placement of the catheter in the portal or hepatic vein may lead to hepatic necrosis. Portal vein thrombosis resulting in portal hypertension has also been described.

Splenic vein thrombosis has been described as a late complication of umbilical catheterization. The patients present with splenomegaly and gastric and oesophageal varices.

Immediate clinical signs of thrombosis associated with umbilical vein catheterization are slight or absent in contrast to those associated with umbilical artery catheterization.

In order to reduce the risk of hepatic necrosis and portal vein thrombosis the tip of the catheter should be placed correctly in the inferior vena cava and its position checked by ultrasound before hyperosmolar fluids are infused.

### Principles of treatment of neonatal thrombosis [59,70,85]

There is no generally accepted protocol for management of neonatal thrombosis. The actions will be influenced by the site and the size of the thrombus and the time elapsing between the occlusion of vessels and restoration of blood flow either by vessel recanalization or by establishment of efficient collaterals. Symptomatic thromboses associated with catheterization can be minimized by: avoiding repeated attempts at placing catheters; and removing catheters at the first sign of compromised circulation, reduced pulses or colour change [58,86].

#### Management of established thrombosis
Any catheter with which thrombosis is suspected on clinical grounds should be removed as soon as possible. It is always safer to proceed to catheter removal without awaiting confirmation of thrombosis unless this can be performed without delay. Other measures which may help include warming of the affected or contralateral limb.

The majority of cases will respond to removal of the catheter but if there is no improvement within two hours of removal,

therapeutic heparin should be commenced. If there continues to be severe compromise of the circulation or deterioration, antithrombotic therapy should be commenced immediately without waiting for improvement.

#### Heparin
Heparin in adult practice is used whether in primary prevention of thrombosis or in the secondary prevention of thrombus extension. Objective evidence of the beneficial role of heparin in treatment of neonatal thrombosis is largely anecdotal. The haemostatic system of the newborn infant is unique and it is not certain whether the rules for efficient heparinization in adults can be applied. Laboratory monitoring is difficult because the *in vitro* coagulation times are already prolonged and rapidly become infinite with very small doses of heparin. The generally accepted guidelines are based on individual experience and have not been substantiated by controlled trials. The actual loading dose recommended is 50–100 units $kg^{-1}$. Maintenance levels of 0.3–0.5 units $ml^{-1}$ are achieved by doses of 16–35 units $kg^{-1}$ $h^{-1}$ and this should be administered by continuous infusion. Duration of therapy depends on clinical state and may vary from a few days to several weeks.

It is important that every special care baby unit has its own locally prepared protocol with which all the staff involved are familiar. Successful management depends on continuing close communication, cooperation and understanding between the cot side and the laboratory. A well-tried dosage schedule for the neonate under 28 weeks' gestation suggests a bolus dose of heparin 25 units $kg^{-1}$ and a maintenance of 15 units $kg^{-1}$ $h^{-1}$.

Ideally the control of dosage should be carried out using a heparin assay aiming for 0.3–0.5 units $ml^{-1}$. Alternatively the PTT can be used keeping the prolongation 1.5 – 2 × normal.

Neonates are usually relatively heparin resistant due to rapid heparin clearance and low levels of ATIII and may require higher maintenance doses to achieve the required heparin assay/PTT results.

Failure to achieve anticoagulation may require ATIII supplementation though this has not been a problem in our experience or that of others [58]. Bleeding complications are rare even if the *in vitro* therapeutic limits are exceeded. The heparin should be given for a minimum of 48 hours. If there has been sustained improvement it can be discontinued but should be given until the clot has cleared and circulation re-established.

Mild to moderate occlusion can probably be managed with heparin alone, but with extensive thrombosis with critical impairment of blood flow, many centres would attempt to lyse the clot with fibrinolytic agents.

### Fibrinolytic agents

Available drugs include urokinase, streptokinase and tissue plasminogen activator (tPA). Confirmation of large vessel thrombosis by angiography or ultrasound is a prerequisite for the use of fibrinolytic therapy.

tPA is theoretically more clot specific in its action and therefore less likely to be associated with systemic fibrinolysis with consequent coagulation factor depletion and bleeding. However, it has only been used in small numbers of neonates and its safety profile remains to be established. Of concern is the well recognized incidence of fatal cerebral bleeds in adults given tPA, suggesting that it should be used with great caution in neonates. A recent innovation has been to try local tPA leaving the catheter *in situ*, but there are insufficient data to recommend this mode of therapy.

Both streptokinase and urokinase also stimulate fibrinolysis by activating plasminogen. Urokinase may be preferable to streptokinase in neonates since it has a linear dose–response curve. Urokinase and streptokinase lyse all clots (they work best in small newly-formed clots) and should not be used within 10 days of surgery or a significant bleed or if the baby has a pre-existing bleeding problem. When thrombolytic agents are being given, arterial puncture and invasive procedures, including intramuscular injections, should be avoided.

Considerably higher dosage may be tolerated and needed in the neonate compared with that in adults. A loading dose of 4000 units kg$^{-1}$ given intravenously over 10 min should be followed by a continuous infusion of 4000–6000 units k$^{-1}$ h$^{-1}$ but should be increased if necessary within hours until improved perfusion of the affected part is achieved. The duration of useful therapy in newborns is as uncertain as the dosage, but may be continued for more than the usual 72 hours. If the thrombin time is not prolonged by the generation of fibrinolytic degradation products then heparin may be added also to prevent extension of the thrombus. The degree of thrombolysis will be determined by the age of the thrombus, its location and plasminogen levels.

Laboratory testing should be performed before administering urokinase to establish baselines. Thereafter regular monitoring is required. Suitable rapid tests are measurement of fibrinolytic degradation products and fibrinogen levels. Very low fibrinogen levels would indicate urgent readjustment of the dose.

### Surgery

In adult arterial thrombosis if the clot is not removed by endarterectomy the thrombosis tends to recur. This is not so in the smaller thrombi seen in neonates. In addition, the very small size of vessels in this age group makes surgical intervention difficult. Surgery is usually reserved for resection of non-viable tissue.

# References

1. Holland, B.M. and Wardrop, C.A.J. (1991) Oxygen transport in blood, haematinics and blood cell component therapy in the neonate. In *Neonatal Clinical Pharmacology and Therapeutics* (G. Rylance, J. Arander and D. Harvey, eds), Butterworths, Oxford, pp. 211–223

2. Thomas, R.M., Channing, C.E., Cotes, P.M. *et al.* (1983) Erythropoietin and cord blood haemoglobin in the regulation of human fetal erythropoiesis. *Br. J. Obstet. Gynaecol.*, **90**, 795–800

3. Ruth, V., Widness, J.A., Clemons, G. and Raivio, K.O. (1990) Postnatal changes in serum immunoactive erythropoietin in relation to hypoxia before and after birth. *J. Pediatr.*, **116**, 950–954

4. Rollins, M.D., Maxwell, A.P., Afrasiabi, M., Halliday, H.L. and Lappin, T.R.J. (1993) Cord blood erythropoietin, pH, $Pa_{O_2}$ and haematocrit following Caesarean section before labour. *Biol. Neonate*, **63**, 147–152

5. Dallman, P.R. (1984) Erythropoietin and the anemia of prematurity. *J. Pediatr.*, **105**, 756–757

6. Brown, M.S., Garcia, J.F., Phibbs, R.H. and Dallman, P.R. (1984) Decreased response of plasma immunoreactive erythropoietin to 'available oxygen' in anemia of prematurity. *J. Pediatr.*, **105**, 793–798

7. Jacobs, K., Shoemaker, C., Rudersdorf, R. *et al.* (1985) Isolation and characterization of genomic and cDNA clones of human erythropoietin. *Nature*, **313**, 806–810

8. Sieff, C.A., Emerson, S.G., Mufson, A., Gesner, T.G. and Nathan, D.G. (1986) Dependence of highly enriched human bone marrow progenitors on hemopoietic growth factors and their response to recombinant erythropoietin. *J. Clin. Invest.*, **77**, 74–81

9. Shannon, K.M., Naylor, G.S., Torkildson, J.C. *et al.* (1987) Circulating erythroid progenitors in the anemia of prematurity. *N. Engl. J. Med.*, **317**, 728–733

10. Strauss, R.G. (1995) Erythropoietin in the pathogenesis and treatment of neonatal anemia. *Transfusion*, **35**, 68–73

11. Halperin, D.S. (1991) Use of recombinant erythropoietin in treatment of the anemia of prematurity. *Am. J. Pediatr. Hematol. Oncol.*, **13**, 351–363

12. Beck, D., Masserey, E., Meyer, M. and Calame, A. (1991) Weekly intravenous administration of recombinant human erythropoietin in infants with the anaemia of prematurity. *Eur. J. Pediatr.*, **150**, 767–772

13. Shannon, K.M., Mentzer, W.C., Abels, R.I. *et al.* (1991) Recombinant human erythropoietin in the anemia of prematurity: results of a placebo-controlled pilot study. *J. Pediatr.*, **118**, 949–955

14. Obladen, M., Maier, R., Segerer, H. *et al.* (1991) Efficacy and safety of recombinant human erythropoietin to prevent the anaemias of prematurity. European Randomized Multicenter Trial. *Contrib. Nephrol.*, **88**, 314–326

15. Shannon, K.M., Mentzer, W.C., Abels, R.I. *et al.* (1992) Enhancement of erythropoiesis by recombinant human erythropoietin in low birth weight infants: a pilot study. *J. Pediatr.*, **120**, 586–592

16. Ohls, R.K. and Christensen, R.D. (1991) Recombinant erythropoietin compared with erythrocyte transfusion in the treatment of anemia of prematurity. *J. Pediatr.*, **119**, 781–788

17. Carnielli, V., Montini, G., Da Riol, R. *et al.* (1992) Effect of high doses of human recombinant erythropoietin on the need for blood transfusions in preterm infants. *J. Pediatr.*, **121**, 98–102

18. Soubasi, V., Kremenopoulos, G., Diamandi, E. *et al.* (1993) In which neonates does early recombinant human erythropoietin treatment prevent anemia of prematurity? Results of a randomized, controlled study. *Pediatr. Res.*, **34**, 675–679

19. Bechensteen, A.G., Haga, P., Halvorsen, S. *et al.* (1993) Erythropoietin, protein, and iron supplementation and the prevention of anaemia of prematurity. *Arch. Dis. Childh.*, **69**, 19–23

20. Messer, J., Haddad, J., Donato, L. *et al.* (1993) Early treatment of premature infants with recombinant human erythropoietin. *Pediatrics*, **92**, 519–523

21. Emmerson, A.J., Coles, H.J., Stern, C.M. and Pearson, T.C. (1993) Double blind trial of recombinant human erythropoietin in preterm infants. *Arch. Dis. Childh.*, **68**, 291–296

22. Maier, R.F., Obladen, M., Scigalla, P. *et al.* (1994) The effect of epoetin beta (recombinant human erythropoietin) on the need for transfusion in very-low-birth-weight infants. European Multicentre Erythropoietin Study Group. *N. Engl. J. Med.*, **330**, 1173–1178

23. Meyer, M.P., Meyer, J.H., Commerford, A. *et al.* (1994) Recombinant human erythropoietin in the treatment of the anemia of prematurity: results of a double-blind, placebo-controlled study. *Pediatrics*, **93**, 918–923

24. Phibbs, R.H. and Keith, J.F. III. (1994) Recombinant Human Erythropoietin (r-HuEPO) stimulates Erythropoiesis and reduces Transfusions in Preterm Infants. *Neonatology*, 248A

25. Ohls, R.K., Osborne, K.A., Christensen, R.D. (1995) Efficacy and cost analysis of treating very low birth weight infants with erythropoietin during their first two weeks of life: A randomized, placebo-controlled trial. *J. Pediatr.*, **126**, 421–426

25b. Shannon, K.M., Keith, J.F., Mentzer, W.C. *et al.* (1995) Recombinant human erythropoietin in the treatment of the anemia of prematurity: results of a double-blind placebo-controlled study. *Pediatr.*, **95**, 1–8

26. Stockmann, J.A. II (1988) Erythropoietin: off again, on again. *J. Pediatr.*, **112**, 906–908

27. Shannon, K.M. (1990) Anemia of prematurity: progress and prospects. *Am. J. Pediatr. Hematol. Oncol.*, **12**, 14–20

28. Fernandes, C.J., Hagan, R., Frieberg, A. *et al.* (1994) Erythropoietin in very preterm infants. *J. Paediatr. Child. Health*, **30**, 356–359

29. Lachance, C., Chessex, P., Fouron, J.C. *et al.* (1994) Myocardial, erythropoietic, and metabolic adaptations to anemia of prematurity. *J. Pediatr.*, **125**, 278–282

30. Christensen, R.D., Hunter, D.D., Ohls, R.K. (1994) Pilot study comparing recombinant erythropoietin alone with erythropoietin plus recombinant granulocyte-macrophage colony-stimulating factor for treatment of the anemia of prematurity. *J. Perinatol.*, **14**, 110–113

31. Ohls, R.K., Li, Y., Trautman, M.S., Christensen, R.D. (1994) Erythropoietin production by macrophages from preterm infants: implication regarding the cause of the anemia of prematurity. *Pediatr. Res.*, **35**, 169–170

32. Dallman, P.R. (1993) Anemia of prematurity: the prospects for avoiding blood transfusions by treatment with recombinant human erythropoietin. *Adv. Pediatr.*, **40**, 385–403

33. Stamatoyannopoulos, G. and Nienhuis, A.W. (1993) Haemoglobin switching. In *The Molecular Basis of Blood Diseases* (G. Stamatoyannopoulos, A.W. Nienhuis, P. Majerus and H. Varmus, eds), W.B. Saunders, Philadelphia, pp. 107–154

34. Phillips, H., Holland, B.M., Jones, J.G. *et al.* (1988) Definitive estimate of rate of haemoglobin switching: measurement of per cent Hb.F in neonatal reticulocytes. *Pediatr. Res.*, **23**, 595–597

35. Bard, H. and Prosmanne, J. (1982) Postnatal fetal and adult hemoglobin synthesis in preterm infants whose birthweight was less than 1000 grams. *J. Clin. Invest.*, **70**, 50–52

36. Blanchette, V.S. and Zipursky, A. (1984) Assessment of anaemia in newborn infants. *Clin. Perinatol.*, **11**, 489

37. Oski, F.A. (1979) Nutritional anaemias. *Semin. Perinatol.*, **3**, 381–395

38. Fenton, V., Cavill, I. and Fisher, J. (1977) Iron stores in pregnancy. *Br. J. Haematol.*, **37**, 145–149

39. Siimes, M.A. (1981) Pathogenesis of iron deficiency in infancy. In *Iron Nutrition Revisited: Infancy, Childhood, Adolescence (Report on the 82nd Conference on Pediatric Research)* (F.A. Oski and H.A. Pearson, eds), Ross Laboratories, Columbus, Ohio, pp. 96–108

40. Lundstrom, U., Siimes, M.A. and Dallman, P.R. (1977) At what age does iron supplementation become necessary in low birthweight infants? *J. Pediatr.*, **91**, 878–883

41. Dallman, P.R., Yip, R. and Oski, F.A. (1991) Iron deficiency and related nutritional anemias. In *Hematology of Infancy and Childhood, 4th edn.* (D.G. Nathan and F.A. Oski, eds), W.B. Saunders, Philadelphia, pp. 413–450

42. Hall, R.T., Wheeler, R.E., Benson, J., Harris, G. and Rippetoe, L. (1993) Benefit from formula containing high iron content (15 mg/L) versus low (3 mg/L) during initial hospitalization to infants less than 1800 g birth weight. *Pediatrics*, **92**, 409–414

43. Walter, T. (1994) Effect of iron-deficiency anaemia on cognitive skills in infancy and childhood. *Baillières Clinical Haematology*, **7**, 815–827

44. Sutton, A.M., Harvie, A., Cockburn, F. *et al.* (1985) Copper deficiency in the pre-term infant of very low birth weight. *Arch. Dis. Childh.*, **60**, 644

45. Ehrenkranz, R.A. (1980) Vitamin E and the neonate. *Am. J. Dis. Child.*, **134**, 1157–1166

46. Hassan, H., Hashim, S.A., Van Itallie, T.B. and Sebrell, W.H. (1966) Syndrome in premature infants associated with low plasma vitamin E levels and high polyunsaturated fatty acid diet. *Am. J. Clin. Nutr.*, **19**, 147–157

47. Oski, F.A. and Barness, L.A. (1967) Vitamin E deficiency: a previously unrecognised cause of hemolytic anemia in the premature infant. *J. Pediatr.*, **70**, 211–220

48. Melhorn, D.K., Gross, S. and Childers, G. (1971) Vitamin E-dependent anaemia in the premature infant. I. Effects of large doses of medicinal iron. *J. Pediatr.*, **79**, 569–580

49. Zipursky, A., Brown, R.T., Watts, J. *et al.* (1987) Oral vitamin E supplementation for the prevention of anemia of the premature infant: a controlled trial. *Pediatrics*, **79**, 61–68

50. Committee on Nutrition, American Academy of Pediatrics (1985) Nutritional needs of low birthweight infants. *Pediatrics*, **75**, 976

51. Haworth, C. and Evans, D.I.K. (1981) Nutritional aspects of blood disorders in the newborn. *J. Hum. Nutr.*, **35**, 323–334

52. Roberts, P.D., James, H., Petrie, A., Morgan, J.O. and Hoffbrand, A.V. (1973) Vitamin $B_{12}$ status in pregnancy among immigrants to Britain. *Br. Med. J.*, **iii**, 67–72

53. Ronnholm, K.A.R. and Siimes, M.A. (1985) Haemoglobin concentration depends on protein intake in small preterm infants fed human milk. *Arch. Dis. Child.*, **60**, 99–104

54. Andrew, M., Paes, B., Milner, R. *et al.* (1987) Development of the human coagulation system in the full-term and preterm infant. *Blood*, **70**, 165–172

55. Andrew, M., Paes, B., Milner, R. *et al.* (1988) Development of the human coagulation system in the healthy premature infant. *Blood*, **72**, 1651–1657

56. Andrew, M. and Johnston, M. (1991) An approach to the infant with impaired haemostasis. In *Blood Coagulation and Haemostasis – A Practical Guide. 4th edn.* (J.M. Thomson, ed.), Churchill Livingstone, Edinburgh, pp. 209–259

57. Gibson, B.E.S. (1991) Normal and disordered coagulation. In: *Fetal and Neonatal Haematology* (I.M. Hann, B.E.S. Gibson and E.A. Letsky, eds), Baillière Tindall, London, pp. 123–188

58. Hathaway, W.E. (1992) Haemostatic and thrombotic problems in the fetus and neonate. In *Haemostasis and Thrombosis in Obstetrics and Gynaecology* (I.A. Greer, A.G.G. Turpie and C.D. Forbes, eds), Chapman & Hall, London, pp. 525–557

59. Hathaway, W.E. (1987) Haemostatic disorders in the newborn. In *Haemostasis and Thrombosis, 2nd edn*, (A.L. Bloom and D.P. Thomas, eds), Churchill Livingstone, Edinburgh, pp.

60. Corrigan, J.J. Jnr. (1989) Neonatal coagulation disorders. In *Perinatal Hematology* (B.P. Alter, ed.), Churchill Livingstone, Edinburgh, pp. 165–193

61. Rivers, R.P.A. (1991) Neonatal coagulation disorders. In *Perinatal Haematological Problems.* (T.L. Turner, ed.), John Wiley and Sons, Chichester, pp. 137–175

62. Stevens, R.F. (1987) Congenital and acquired coagulation defects. In *Practical Paediatric Haematology* (R.F. Hinchliffe and J.S. Lilleyman, eds), John Wiley and Sons, Chichester, pp. 281–315

63. Svensson, P.S. and Dahlbäck, B. (1994) Resistance to activated protein C as a basis for venous thrombosis. *N. Engl. J. Med.*, **330**, 517–522

64. Manco-Johnson, M., Nuss, R., Jacobson, L. and Hathaway, W. (1994) Activated protein C cofactor activity is increased in neonates. *Blood*, **84** (Suppl 1), 85a

65. Barnard, D.R., Simmons, M.A. and Hathaway, W.E. (1979) Coagulation studies in extremely premature infants. *Pediatr. Res.*, **13**, 1330–1335

66. Lane, P.A. and Hathaway, W.E. (1985) Vitamin K in infancy. *J. Pediatr.*, **106**, 351–359

67. Shearer, M.J. (1995) Vitamin K, *Lancet.* **345**, 229–234

68. Thorp, J.A., Gaston, L., Caspers, D.R. and Pal, M.L. (1995) Current concepts and controversies in the use of Vitamin-K. *Drugs*, **49**, 376–387

69. Hathaway, W.E. (1987) New insights on vitamin K. *Hematol. Oncol. Clin. N. Am.*, **1**, 367–379

70. Hathaway, W.E. and Bonnar, J. (1987) *Hemostatic Disorders of the Pregnant Woman and Newborn Infant*, John Wiley and Sons, Chichester

71. Sharp, A.A. (1977) Diagnosis and management of disseminated intravascular coagulation. *Br. Med. Bull.*, **33**, 265–272

72. Weinstein, L. (1982) Syndrome of hemolysis elevated liver enzyme and low platelet count. A severe consequence of hypertension in pregnancy. *Am. J. Obstet. Gynecol.*, **142**, 159–167

73. Thiagarajah, S., Bourgeois, F.J., Harbert, G.M. and Caudle, M.R. (1984) Thrombocytopenia in eclampsia: associated abnormalities and management principles. *Am. J. Obstet. Gynecol.*, **150**, 1–7

74. Murray, N.A. and Roberts, I.A.G. (1995) Platelet production in pre-term neonates. *Pediatr. Res.* (In Press)

75. Andrew, M. and Kelton, J. (1984) Neonatal thrombocytopenia. *Clin. Perinatol.*, **11**, 359–391

76. Burrows, R.F. and Kelton, J.G. (1993) Fetal thrombocytopenia and its relation to maternal thrombocytopenia. *N. Engl. J. Med.*, **320**, 1463–1466

77. Bussel, J., Kaplan, C., McFarland, J. and the Working Party on Neonatal Immune Thrombocytopenia of the Neonatal Hemostasis Subcommittee of the Scientific and Standardization Committee of the ISTH. (1991) Recommendations for the evaluation and treatment of neonatal autoimmune and alloimmune thrombocytopenia. *Thromb. Haemos.*, **65**, 631–634

78. Pillai, M. (1993) Platelets and pregnancy. *Br. J. Obstet. Gynaecol.*, **100**, 201–204

79. Samuels, P., Bussel, J.B., Braitman, L.E. *et al.* (1990) Estimation of the risk of thrombocytopenia in the offspring of pregnant women with presumed immune thrombocytopenic purpura. *N. Engl. J. Med.*, **323**, 229–235

80. Warwick, R.k Vaughan, J., Murray, N., Lubenko, A. and Roberts, I. (1994) In vitro culture of colony forming unit-megakaryocyte (CFU-MK) in fetal alloimmune thrombocytopenia. *Br. J. Haematol.*, **88**, 874–877

81. Blanchette, V.S., Chen, L., Salomon de Friedberg, Z. *et al.* (1990) Alloimmunization to the PI^A1 platelet antigen. Results of a prospective study. *Br. J. Haematol.*, **74**, 209–215

82. Bussel, J.B., Berkowitz, R.L., McFarland, J.G., Lynch, L. and Chitkara, U. (1988) Antenatal treatment of neonatal alloimmune thrombocytopenia. *N. Engl. J. Med.*, **319**, 1374–1378

83. Daffos, F., Forestier, F., Muller, J.Y. *et al.* (1984) Prenatal treatment of allo-immune thrombocytopenia. *Lancet*, **ii**, 632

84. Weiner, E., Zosmer, N., Bajoria, R. *et al.* (1994) Direct fetal administration of immunoglobulins: another disappointing therapy in alloimmune thrombocytopenia. *Fetal Diagn. Ther.*, **9**, 159–164

85. Schmidt, B. and Zipursky, A. (1984) Thrombotic disease in newborn infants. *Clin. Perinatol.*, **11**, 461–488

86. Manco-Johnson, M.J. (1990) Diagnosis and management of thrombosis in the neonatal period. *Semin. Perinatol.*, **14**, 393–402

87. Seligsohn, U., Berger, A., Abend, M. *et al.* (1984) Homozygous protein C deficiency manifested by massive venous thrombosis in the newborn. *N. Engl. J. Med.*, **310**, 559–562

88. Vailas, G.N., Brouillette, R.T., Scott, J.P. *et al.* (1986) Neonatal aortic thrombosis: recent experience. *J. Pediatr.*, **109**, 101–108

# II. BLOOD TRANSFUSION

## Charles Wardrop and Barbara Holland

The vital need to maximize potential oxygen delivery is recognized universally in critical care medicine. The blood, along with the cardiovascular system and lungs, represents one of the three key components in oxygen delivery. However, understanding and manipulation of the blood in this context has lagged behind appraisal and management of the heart and lungs in sick patients, especially in those requiring critical care [1–3]. Anaemia limits maximal oxygen delivery [4].

## The blood's functions in oxygen transport

### Oxygen carriage

Oxygen carrying capacity, *per unit volume of blood*, is represented by the haemoglobin concentration or haematocrit (HCT). Each of these represents a ratio of cells/plasma. Because of plasma volume fluctuation, HCT does not predict red cell volume (RCV) or blood volume (BV) (see Figure 14.3). The

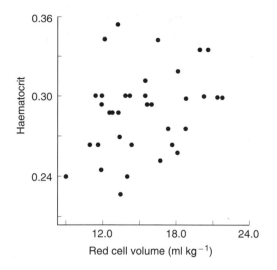

**Figure 14.3** Correlation between haematocrit and red cell volume in infants before red cell transfusion for the refractory anaemia of prematurity [3]

red cells is 0.55. The total circulating RCV gives the $O_2$ *carrying capacity in the circulation.*

## Systemic and pulmonary perfusion

Systemic and pulmonary perfusion is governed by the BV. Figures 14.4 and 14.5 show the relationships respectively between the RCV and HCT and BV and also that sub-normal RCV is almost invariably associated with hypovolaemia. In full term babies, a reduction from normal in BV of as little as 7% results in compensatory increases in cardiac output. This may critically compromise the sick infant. This has not been studied in the sick ELBW infant, but tiny babies are unlikely to withstand oligovolaemia better than mature babies.

## Maintenance of vascular endothelial nutrition and functional integrity

When this is impaired, components of plasma (water, salt, and albumin) extravasate to the interstitial fluid. Plasma volume in the circulation therefore fluctuates and falls, with consequent haemoconcentration so that the HCT may appear normal, or only slightly low. This masks the hypovolaemia and red-cell lack. This is demonstrable only by measurement of the

HCT associated with maximal oxygen delivery potential, which depends on interactions between the rheological (flow) properties of the red cells and blood viscosity, is higher in the neonate than in later life. The optimal HCT for maximal oxygen delivery by autologous (fetal)

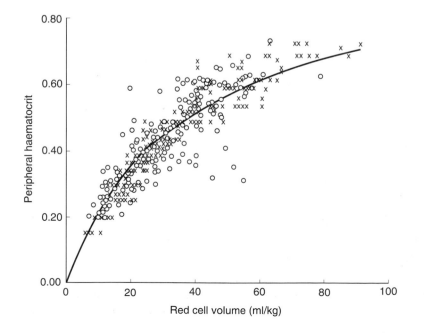

**Figure 14.4** Relationship between red cell volume and peripheral blood HCT in adults and neonates [16]

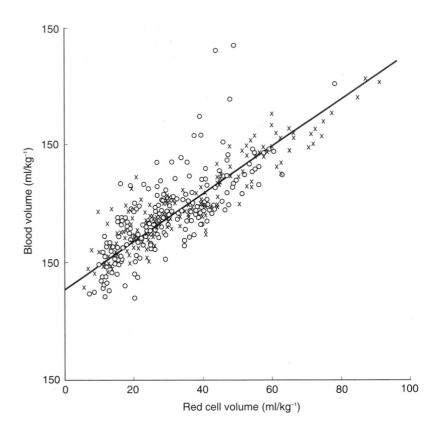

**Figure 14.5** Relationship between red cell volume and blood volume in adults and neonates (○) [16]

blood volume parameters, RCV and plasma volume [5–7].

## Management of tiny babies

The blood of the ELBW infant in current management is, typically, compromised in each of the above three functions. Detailed laboratory evaluation of the blood [5–7] is desirable, regarding its ability to fulfil its physiological functions in the individual patient. The ELBW infant, like other critical care patients of all ages, suffers from impaired respiratory and often cardiac function. These disabilities impair oxygen delivery as well as organ and tissue perfusion. These impairments represent a large part of the fundamental pathogenesis of complications of preterm delivery. Thus, optimization of the blood, in terms not only of HCT but also total circulating volume, is clearly of paramount importance in promoting oxygen delivery and minimizing complications stemming from microcirculatory failure. In

addition, complications after preterm delivery may be prevented or ameliorated by enhancement, at birth, of BV and HCT [8,9]. This can be achieved by allowing placentofetal transfusion in larger, vaginally-delivered infants of <33 weeks' gestation at birth [10]; this may also be true of the ELBW infant.

### The importance of euvolaemia at birth

Adaptive processes and functions dependent on adequacy of the blood in terms of volume and flow include:

(1)   Immediate postnatal lung adaptation through vascular [11] and airways expansion.
(2)   Maintenance of physiological intracranial blood flow, volume and perfusion so as to minimize the risk of hypoxic-ischaemic brain injury.

Evidence is accumulating of reduced morbidity, complications and costs in newborn preterm infants in whom the blood can be manipulated therapeutically so as to approach the physiologically-predicted requirements. For example, by placentofetal transfusion [10–13] at birth and by adequate donor blood transfusion to minimize recurring need. Fears of polycythaemia [14] or of damage to the intracranial circulation [15] dictate caution. More research and development work is needed in placental (autologous) and donor blood transfusion in sick ELBW infants.

The RCV requirement for oxygen delivery may be predicted [16]. We estimate this to be approximately 50 ml kg$^{-1}$ at birth in the ELBW infant, with a BV of approximately 100 ml kg$^{-1}$.

In present management, RCV and BV in many ELBW infants at birth are clearly suboptimal for oxygen delivery and tissue perfusion, in agreement with earlier reports [5–9].

These findings, just after birth, probably reflect the almost invariable practice of immediate cord clamping at preterm delivery. This is done misguidedly, though in good faith, so as to facilitate efforts in achieving cardiopulmonary resuscitation and reduce the risk of hypothermia. Immediate cord clamping deprives the baby of oxygen carrying capacity and BV. This produces a more marked deficiency of blood in the ELBW infant because, although the volume of blood in the fetoplacental circulation at 30 weeks' gestation has been estimated at 105–115 ml kg$^{-1}$ fetal weight, only half of this volume of blood is in the fetus at this stage of *in utero* development, compared with two-thirds at term [17]. However, because of immediate postnatal opening up of the lung vasculature, there is an obvious acute need for expansion of the newborn's blood volume to 'fill' both the substantially expanded pulmonary [11] and systemic circulation. Perinatal blood losses worsen this hypovolaemia.

## Management during intensive care

Detailed studies addressing the means of achieving optimization of the circulation have not yet been reported. Until such research and development has been carried out, we depend on the application of physiological principles, as well as observations and clinical practices reported in less preterm infants [18–22].

We suggest that ensuring optimal O$_2$ carrying capacity by the blood in infants with respiratory insufficiency is crucial to the defences against respiratory failure, indeed against multi-organ failure. We recommend that, during intensive management, the HCT is kept at the upper normal limit for a term infant [23], using partially packed red cells in autologous (donor) plasma (Table 14.5). It is most important to recognize that the optimum HCT of 0.55 (regarding both O$_2$ carrying capacity and viscosity) is higher at birth in neonates, especially if very preterm, than in adults: 0.45 is usually regarded as optimum for adults.

It is important to recall that the ELBW infant's blood is very rich in haemopoietic progenitor cells [24], which are necessary for the infant's haemopoietic and immunological constitution in the course of normal development. Denial or losses of this blood limits the body's endowment of haemopoietic progenitors, and may impair the development of immune competence. During postnatal management of the ELBW baby and of more mature preterm infants, an aggregate tally of investigative and spontaneous blood losses and replacement transfusion, shows that it is common for two or three 'exchange transfusions' to be performed, depending on the level of intensive care [22,25]. This means that large numbers of haemopoietic progenitor cells in the circulation of the ELBW baby are removed and are not replaced by transfused stored blood, which is devoid of haemopoietic progenitor cells. The full consequences of these stem cell losses have yet to be studied, but common sense suggests that we must learn how to optimize placentofetal transfusion at birth and then minimize subsequent blood losses in the ELBW infant.

We believe that, in assessing the adequacy of the blood, the variable individual need for O$_2$, must be taken into account. For example, ELBW infants with bronchopulmonary disease (BPD) have higher O$_2$ requirements so need augmented O$_2$ carrying capacity and BV, to supply the enhanced O$_2$ needs of their respiratory and cardiac muscles.

### Practical opportunities for optimization of the ELBW infant's blood

Practical points in attaining rational blood management of importance in ELBW babies include the following.

### *Placentofetal transfusion at birth*

Immediate cord clamping is likely to be especially detrimental in such infants of shortest gestation. Consideration of the proportions of blood in the placenta, umbilical vessels and fetus respectively at low gestation, suggest that a longer period may be required for transfer of blood to the baby [26,27], at least a 30-second delay, with the baby held as low as possible during resuscitation. Meanwhile, uterine contraction should be encouraged, possibly using an intravenous oxytoxic agent given to the mother before the cord is clamped.

Studies are urgently needed to determine appropriate management of placental transfusion for ELBW babies. This represents a very major opportunity for optimization of $O_2$ carrying capacity, BV and haemopoietic progenitor cells from birth.

### *Donor blood transfusion*

Adequate 'dosage' of donor blood, when necessary, is important so as to avoid undertransfusion and minimize the need for repeated transfusions. This recurring need for transfusion and multiple donor exposures depends on continued ventilator dependence. That leads to continued sampling losses and failure to ensure that the maximum safely tolerable volume of donor blood is transfused on each occasion a transfusion is judged necessary. The infective and other consequences of multiple blood donor exposure are not trivial. These have been well described [20–22,28,29].

### Transfusion triggers

It should be noted that the published indicators of the need for transfusion are not based on controlled studies. Also, they are not necessarily adequate as transfusion triggers in ELBW babies. However, such indicators represent reasonable starting points in devising rational protocols for transfusions.

There is an urgent need for studies to define appropriate transfusion triggers not only for ELBW babies but also all preterm infants. It is equally important that appropriate transfusion targets are defined by physiological parameters. The target in transfusion represents the desired HCT and BV and the end of that stage of the transfusion.

**Table 14.5**  Blood components used for transfusion in NICU/SCBU

| | |
|---|---|
| Whole blood partially packed red blood cells | red cells in autologous plasma HCT 0.35–0.60 |
| Packed red blood cells | red cells in plasma/xoids HCT 0.55–0.90 |
| Recommended | Partially packed red blood cells, HCT 0.55–0.60 in autologous plasma |

Suggested guidelines for considering donor blood transfusion include:

(1)  Replace blood losses totalling 10% of an assumed blood volume, i.e. typically a loss of 5–10 ml kg$^{-1}$. Use multiple packs, single donor, with red cells in autologous plasma, HCT 0.35–0.60. This reduces donor exposures [30,31]. Avoid the use of fully-packed red cells, which fail to make good any lack of plasma and may lead to regional hyperviscosity.

(2)  Maintain a central (arterial or venous) blood HCT of greater than 0.40–0.45 in infants who are ventilated. We suggest HCT 0.55, using partially-packed red cells, with a donor HCT of approximately 0.50 (see Table 14.5).

(3)  In babies breathing room air, with clinical signs of anaemia, maintain an arbitrary HCT of greater than 0.35 but less than 0.50. If apparently asymptomatic and tolerating feeds, transfusion may not be needed [32]. However, the need for adequacy of the blood is increased in association with clinical complications causing increased $O_2$ *need*. We recommend aiming for a post-transfusion target HCT at the upper limit of normal. Use partially-packed cells as above.

## Summary

The ELBW baby's autologous placental blood is best in terms of providing adequate $O_2$ carrying capacity and BV as well as haemopoietic progenitor cells. The $O_2$ association characteristics of autologous blood are an advantage to those babies with respiratory difficulties, facilitating $O_2$ loading in the lungs. The rheologic advantages of the fetal red cells over transfused cells are also important.

Therefore, to ensure optimal placentofetal transfusion, delay (with the baby held below the placenta) cord clamping for at least 30 seconds, in vaginally delivered infants. In Caesarean section cases, a longer delay may be needed during resuscitation. Uterine contraction should be encouraged before the cord is clamped [27].

ELBW babies are likely to be hypovolaemic at birth and during a period of intensive care. Monitor core–peripheral temperature, peripheral perfusion and blood pressure. When necessary, replace with blood and plasma, maintaining HCT at approximately 0.50 (do not exceed 0.60). Blood losses for sampling in the ELBW baby are relatively massive. Consider every sample: is it really necessary? *Replace* when a maximum of 10% has been lost. HCT may not fall despite the large losses, and therefore cannot be used as a guide to transfusion volume. Hypervolaemic polycythaemia is desirable in physiological theory and from investigative observations, in infants with lung disease.

On each transfusion give the maximum tolerated donor blood volume. Each transfusion has a (small) infective risk, so volumes such as 20–30 ml kg$^{-1}$ may be given using single-donor multiple packs.

## References

1. Wardrop, C.A.J., Holland, B.M. and Jones, J.G. (1996) Red cell physiology. In *Pediatrics and Perinatology, the Scientific Basis*, 2nd edn. (P.D. Gluckman and M.A. Heymann, eds), Edward Arnold, London, pp. 868–876
2. Hinds, C. and Watson, D. (1995) Manipulating haemodynamics and oxygen transport in critically ill patients. *New Engl. J. Med.*, **333**, 1-74–1075
3. Wardrop, C.A.J., Holland, B.M., Jacobs, S. *et al.* (1992) Optimization of the blood for oxygen transport and tissue perfusion in critical care. *Postgrad. Med. Journal.*, **68**, (Suppl. 2), S2–S6
4. Woodson, R.D. (1984) Hemoglobin concentration and exercise capacity. *Am. Rev. Respir. Dis.*, **129**, Suppl, S72–S75
5. Hudson, I., Cavill, I.A.J., Holland, B.M. *et al.* (1990) Biotin labelling of red cells in the measurement of red cell volume in preterm infants. *Pediatr. Res.*, **28**, 199–202
6. Wynn, R.F., Dixon, S.A., Al-Ismail, S.A. *et al.* (1995) Flow cytometric determination of pretransfusion red cell volume. *Br. J. Haematol.*, **59**, 620–622
7. Phillips, H.M., Holland, B.M., Abdel-Moy, A. *et al.* (1986) Determination of red cell mass in assessment and management of anaemic babies needing blood transfusion. *Lancet*, **i**, 882–884
8. Hudson, I.R.B., Holland, B.M., Jones, J.G. *et al.* (1990) First-day red cell volume predicts outcome in preterm infants. *Pediatr. Res.*, **27**, 273–81
9. Faxelius, G., Raye, J., Gutberlet, R. *et al.* (1977) Red cell volume measurements an acute blood loss in high risk newborn infants. *J. Pediatr.*, **90**, 273–281
10. Kinmond, S., Aitchison, T.C., Holland, B.M. *et al.* (1993) Umbilical cord clamping and preterm infants: A randomised trial. *Br. Med. J.*, **306**, 172–175
11. Jaykka, S. (1958) Pulmonary capillary erection. *Acta Paediatrica.*, **47**, 484–500
12. Dunn, P.M. (1989) Perinatal factors influencing adaptation to extrauterine life. In *Advances in Gynecology and Obstetrics, 5, Pregnancy and Labor. Proc. 12th World Congr. Obstet. and Gynec., Rio de Janeiro, Oct. 1988* (P. Belfort, J.A. Pinotti and T.K.A.B. Eskes, eds), Parthenon, Carnforth, Lancs, p. 15
13. Nelle, M., Zilow, E.P., Kraus, M. *et al.* (1993) The effects of Leboyer delivery on blood viscosity and other hemorheologic parameters in term neonates. *Am. J. Obstet. Gynecol.*, **169**, 189–193

---

**Practical points**

1. Remember that the blood is part of the oxygen transport system.
2. The baby's own blood is best, therefore allow placental transfusion.
3. Minimize blood losses particularly to the laboratory. Consider each investigation. Can the information be obtained by other means, such as transcutaneous monitoring?
4. Maintain red cell volume and blood volume when blood loss approaches 10%. On each occasion a transfusion is given, ensure the maximum safe volume is given to minimize the total number of transfusions. Use partially-packed donor cells in autologous plasma to obviate regional hyperviscosity.
5. Consider subcutaneous rEPO, 750 units kg$^{-1}$ per week, which will reduce the need for transfusion in babies who do not have large blood losses. Adequate nutrition is vital for active erythropoiesis.
6. The future aim is to reduce or obviate blood transfusion by maximizing placental transfusion, minimizing blood losses and judicious use of rEPO.

14.  Mentzer, W.M. (1978) Polycythaemia and the hyperviscosity syndrome in newborn infants. *Clin. Haematol.*, **7**, 63–74

15.  Goldberg, R.N., Chung, D., Goldman, S.L. *et al.* (1980) The association of rapid volume expansion and intraventricular hemorrhage in the preterm infant. *J. Pediatr.*, **96**, 1060–1063

16.  Jones, J.G., Holland, B.M., Hudson, I.R.B. *et al.* (1990) Total circulating red cells versus haematocrit as the primary descriptor of oxygen transport by the blood. *Br. J. Haematol.*, **76**, 288–294

17.  Brace, R. (1993) Regulation of blood volume in utero. In *Fetus and Neonate, Physiology and Clinical Applications. 1: The Circulation* (M.A. Hanson, J.A.D. Spencer and C.H. Rodeck, eds), Cambridge University Press, Cambridge, pp. 75–99

18.  Roberton, N.R.C. (1987) Top up transfusions in neontes. *Arch. Dis. Childh.*, **62**, 984–986

19.  Widness, J.A., Seward, V.J., Kromer, I.J. *et al.* (1996) Changing patterns of red blood cell transfusion in very low birth weight infants. *J. Pediatr.*, **129**, 680–687

20.  Blanchette, V.S., Hume, H.A. *et al.* (1991) Guidelines for auditing pediatric blood transfusion practices. *Am. J. Dis. Child.*, **145**, 787–796

21.  BCSH Blood Transfusion Task Force (1994) Guidelines for administration of blood products: transfusion of infants and neonates. *Transfus. Med.*, **4**, 63–69

22.  Strauss, R.G. (1991) Transfusion therapy in neonates. *Am. J. Dis. Child.*, **145**, 904–911

23.  Nathan, D.G. and Oski, F.A. (1987) *Hematology of Infancy and Childhood.* W.B. Saunders, Philadelphia

24.  Shannon, K.M., Naylor, G., Torkildsen, J.C. *et al.* (1987) Circulating erythroid progenitors in the anemia of prematurity. *N. Engl. J. Med.*, **317**, 728–733

25.  Obladen, M., Sachsenweger, M., Stahnke, M. *et al.* (1988) Blood sampling in very-low-birthweight infants on different intensive care levels. *Eur. J. Pediatr.*, **147**, 399–404

26.  Linderkamp, O.L. (1982) Placental transfusion: determinants and effects. *Clin. Perinatol.*, **9**, 55–592

27.  Rabe, H., Wacker, A. and Schulze, E.A. (1997) A study on late cord clamping in preterm babies born <32 gestational weeks. *J. Obstet. Gynecol.*, **17** (Suppl. 2), 541.

28.  Strauss, R.G. (1992) Autologous transfusions for neonates using placental blood. *Am. J. Dis. Child.*, **146**, 21–22

29.  Moraff, G. and Luban, N.L.C. (1992) Prevention of transfusion-associated graft-versus-host disease. *Transfusion*, **32**, 102–103

30.  Wood, A., Wilson, N., Skacel, P. *et al.* (1995) Reducing donor exposure in preterm infants requiring multiple blood transfusion. *Arch. Dis. Childh.*, **72**, F29–F33

31.  Lee, D.A., Slagle, T.A., Jackson, T.M. *et al.* (1995) Reducing blood donor exposures in low birth weight infants by the use of older, unwashed packed red blood cells. *J. Pediatr.*, **126**, 280–286

32.  Lanchance, C., Chessex, P., Fouron, J. *et al.* (1994) Myocardial, erythropoietic and metabolic adaptations to anemia of prematurity. *J. Pediatr.*, **125**, 278–282

# 15

# Infection

**Michael Hall and Robert Ironton**

The majority of ELBW babies are at increased risk of infection and the illness is often severe for a number of reasons:

(1) Preterm delivery may have resulted from maternal infection, such as chorioamnionitis, which exposes the fetus to infection before or at delivery.
(2) Preterm babies, particularly those below 28 weeks' gestation, are immunologically immature.
(3) They will inevitably be nursed in an environment which harbours potential microbial pathogens.
(4) They are likely to receive forms of treatment, and undergo invasive procedures, which increase their chances of acquiring sepsis, particularly caused by opportunistic micro-organisms.
(5) They are likely to suffer conditions such as the respiratory distress syndrome, and chronic lung disease which may mask the signs of sepsis.

## Incidence

Sepsis rates in ELBW infants have been regarded both as a primary outcome measure for studies of therapy, such as the administration of intravenous immunoglobulin, and as a secondary outcome measure in interventions such as the administration of vitamin E, surfactant and steroids. The incidence of 'culture positive sepsis' in these studies has ranged from 0% [1] to 50% [2]. However, the number of babies in some of these studies has been small, the definition of sepsis has not always been clear and the study periods have varied from less than 28 days to several months. More specific information from the USA has been provided in a report from the National Institute of Child Health and Human Development (NICHD) Neonatal Network, which detailed various outcomes for very low birth weight babies admitted to the seven participating neonatal units during the year from November 1987 to October 1988 [3]. The outcome data shown in Table 15.1 were collected until death or discharge. Remarkably similar frequencies of septicaemia and meningitis were reported for 1990 from the Vermont–Oxford Trials Network (VOTN) [4], although it would appear that survival rates were higher in these

**Table 15.1 Incidence (%) of sepsis, necrotizing enterocolitis and survival by birth weight (NICHD 1987–1988) [3]**

|  | Birth weight (g) | | |
| --- | --- | --- | --- |
|  | 501–750 (n=349) | 751–1000 (n=382) | 1001–1500 (n=1034) |
| Pneumonia | 9 | 10 | 6 |
| Septicaemia | 22 | 25 | 13 |
| Meningitis | 2 | 3 | 1 |
| Urinary tract infection | 4 | 6 | 3 |
| Necrotizing enterocolitis | 3 | 9 | 7 |
| Survived | 34 | 66 | 90 |

**Table 15.2   Frequency (%) of sepsis, necrotizing enterocolitis, steroid treatment and survival by birth weight (Vermont–Oxford trials network database project 1990) [4]**

|  | Birth weight (g) | | | |
|---|---|---|---|---|
|  | 501–750 (n=526) | 751–1000 (n=726) | 1001–1250 (n=820) | 1251–1500 (n=889) |
| Sepsis[a] | 26 | 22 | 15 | 8 |
| Meningitis | 1 | 2 | 1 | 1 |
| Necrotizing enterocolitis | 9 | 7 | 6 | 5 |
| Steroids for chronic lung disease | 30 | 26 | 12 | 10 |
| Survived[b] | 47 | 80 | 92 | 95 |

[a]Recovery of a pathogen from at least one blood culture or recovery of a potential pathogen from two separate blood cultures obtained within 24 hours.
[b]Status at time of discharge.

centres, possibly reflecting an increased use of surfactant (Table 15.2). The difference in survival may also be relevant to the higher frequency of necrotizing enterocolitis (NEC) in the 501–750 g group in the VOTN report.

Thus, when the effect of survival is taken into account, babies weighing less than 1000 g are much more likely to suffer septicaemia than larger infants; the incidence of meningitis and urinary infections is low in all groups of very low birth weight babies.

Are these infections important? In such small babies, who often suffer from several serious coexisting conditions, it is often difficult to know whether a baby has died *with* a condition or *from* that condition. The 1994 OPCS mortality statistics (Tables 15.3 & 15.4) show that, in England and Wales, only 21 ELBW babies were recorded as dying as a result of infection during the neonatal period [5]; however, the risk of ELBW babies dying

**Table 15.3   Neonatal deaths, England and Wales, 1994 [5]**

|  | All births | <1000 grams birthweight |
|---|---|---|
| Livebirths | 664,256 | 2855 |
| Deaths (all causes) | 2724 | 1050 |
| Antepartum infections | 14 | 3 |
| Infections | 95 | 18 |

**Table 15.4   Postneonatal deaths, England and Wales, 1994 [5]**

|  | All births | <1000 grams birthweight |
|---|---|---|
| Livebirths | 664,256 | 2855 |
| Deaths (all causes) | 1331 | 155 |
| Antepartum infections | 14 | 3 |
| Infections | 199 | 28 |

from infection in the neonatal period was much higher than that of all babies with an odds ratio for death from infection of 45.5 (95% confidence interval 28.3–72.1). This suggests that they are much more vulnerable to the effects of sepsis. In this postneonatal period only two deaths were attributed primarily to infection (Table 15.4). It does seem that ELBW babies in the UK have a considerable ability to resist the effects of severe sepsis, presumably as a result of both their own immunological defences and the care which they receive.

## The ELBW infant: the compromised host

In a contaminated environment the human organism's ability to prevent and combat serious infection is dependent upon:

(1)   surface barriers,
(2)   the innate or non-specific immune response,
(3)   specific immune responses.

Recognized deficiencies in the defences of ELBW infants underlie their susceptibility to infection and may suggest therapeutic manoeuvres to enhance their survival.

### Surface barriers

Infants are rapidly colonized with a variety of organisms following birth. Organisms acquired vaginally during birth put the infant at risk from early-onset sepsis. The ELBW infant requiring intensive care is exposed to an extended range of pathogens and is tended by a number of carers each of whom may contribute to the infant's flora [6–8]. The neonate's skin is functionally and anatomically immature [9] but even in the ELBW infant it acts as an effective barrier to invasion by micro-organisms. Occasionally certain strains of bacteria appear that are more invasive or virulent and may circulate within neonatal units. An example was the appearance in the 1960s of *Staphylococcus aureus* phage type 80/81 which caused a high rate of invasive disease in neonatal nurseries. It was suggested that this particular organism could traverse intact skin [10]. The ELBW infant's skin is extremely fragile and easily traumatized creating portals for bacterial invasion. The skin's protection is breached by the need for the numerous invasive procedures that accompany modern intensive care. The prolonged use of umbilical catheters and central venous lines is a major factor in the spectrum of sepsis seen in the ELBW infant [11–14].

Various aspects of the ELBW infant's gastrointestinal tract are likely to predispose to invasive sepsis. Enteric feeding is often delayed in these infants and as a result the normal evolution of an enteric flora is disturbed [15]. Antibiotic treatment and the presence of antibiotic-resistant organisms in the unit further modifies the acquired enteric flora [16,17]. This provides a reservoir of potential pathogens, with effects on the pattern of acquired sepsis [18]. The ELBW infant has difficulty in maintaining a low gastric pH [19] and this is further compromised by continuous or frequent bolus feeds buffering gastric acid and the use of H2-receptor antagonists resulting in reduced bactericidal activity within the stomach allowing more ingested organisms to reach the small bowel or to cause respiratory infection following reflux [20,21]. Milk that has been banked or stored is likely to have increased bacterial counts. If nasojejunal feeding is utilized the stomach acidity will be by-passed altogether. The reduced intestinal peristalsis of the preterm infant [22], coupled with low bile acid levels, promotes multiplication of these organisms. The preterm infant is deficient in IgA, reducing the gut's defences, and the important contribution provided by breast milk may not be available to the ELBW infant [23].

The lining of the respiratory tract is compromised by prolonged endotracheal intubation and suction resulting in abnormal ciliary movement [24]. The respiratory tract becomes extensively colonized with organisms which may lead to bacteraemic episodes [25].

The front-line barrier defences against invasion by micro-organisms are less effective in the ELBW infant. Micro-organisms are more likely to gain access to subepithelial tissues where the inflammatory, phagocytic and immune mechanisms must come into play to prevent further progression of infection.

## The innate immune system

### *Phagocytes*

Phagocytic cells are present from an early stage of embryogenesis. By 8 weeks' gestation neutrophils and monocytes can be found in the fetal liver and by 16 weeks in the spleen [26]. Absolute numbers of circulating neutrophils are increased in the neonate (both term and preterm) but the reserve or storage pool available in times of challenge is reduced and easily depleted and such depletion is associated with a higher mortality during sepsis [27–32]. In addition, neonatal neutrophils show a number of functional deficiencies, for example in chemotaxis, phagocytosis and bactericidal killing, particularly when put under stress such as hypoxia or sepsis [33–36]. Tissue macrophages are similarly immature in their responses [37].

### *Complement*

The complement system plays a crucial role in the defence against microbial organisms. It is involved in opsonization and lysis of bacterial membranes. Some components of the complement system are detectable as early as 8 weeks of fetal life [38] and all the significant components are detectable by 20 weeks [38,39]. Levels correlate with gestational age, most components reaching 50% of adult levels at term although C8 and C9 levels are only 10–20% adult levels [40,41]. Infants aged below 32 weeks' gestation have significantly reduced complement levels [42].

In summary, deficiencies in the numbers of available neutrophils, their reduced ability to migrate out of the circulation, reduced opsonization due to low complement and immunoglobulin (see below) levels and inefficient bactericidal activity at times of stress limit the ELBW infants' innate immune defences.

## Specific immune responses

Lymphocytes are the cellular basis of specific immunity. They have their origins in pluripotent stem cells first detectable in the blood islands of the yolk sac that migrate to the liver in early embryonic life [43].

### T lymphocytes

T lymphocyte precursors migrate from bone marrow and liver to colonize the thymus around 8 weeks' gestation and subsequent development occurs within the thymus itself [44]. By 17 weeks' gestation the architecture and cell distribution within the thymus is virtually identical to that of the adult [45]. Mature cells expressing the TCR-CD3 surface complex are present by this stage, migrating to secondary lymph organs around the body and when appropriately activated will define the subsequent immune response via lymphokine production. Functionally, evidence of T cell activity can be detected at an early stage of fetal development. Mixed lymphocyte responses can be demonstrated in the thymus by 12 weeks' and in blood by 14 weeks' gestation [46–49]. By mid-gestation, T cell function is developed sufficiently to suppress potential graft-versus-host reactions arising from *in utero* blood transfusions of adult blood containing mature lymphocytes. Delayed type hypersensitivity reactions, such as the development of positive Mantoux reactions following BCG vaccination have been demonstrated in the preterm infant.

While T cell function can be demonstrated there are clear indications that neonatal T cell function is altered compared to that of adults. Neonatal T cells proliferate in response to mitogens as effectively as adult cells, but their ability to produce certain lymphokines is reduced [50–53]. With respect to stimulation of B cell immunoglobulin synthesis both helper and suppressor functions can be demonstrated within the neonatal T cell population [52] but in comparison to later life the balance between enhancing and suppressor cell activity appears to be biased towards suppression in the neonatal period [54].

### Cell mediated cytotoxicity

Neonatal T cell-mediated cytotoxic activity is diminished. Cytotoxicity of fetal blood is absent before approximately 20 weeks' gestation, with minimal activity noted before the last trimester [55]. In term neonates, the cytotoxic potential of T cells is reduced to around 50% of that of adult cells [56–58].

Natural killer (NK) cells are differentiated lymphocytes with certain T cell characteristics that are able to lyse target cells expressing foreign antigen and do not require prior antigen processing by cells of the innate system [69,70]. Neonates have a similar number of NK cells at birth to adults [71]. Earlier in gestation NK cells are rarer but can be detected at 8 to 13 weeks of gestation [67,72,73]. These early NK cells, however, are immature and surface characteristics of mature NK cells have not been detected before about 27 weeks' gestation [64]. There appears to be a progressive increase in cytolytic function throughout late fetal and early postnatal life [65]. Deficiencies in cytolytic activity may, at least in part, be due to failure to respond to, and/or reduced, cytokine signals [66,67].

## B lymphocyte development and immunoglobulin synthesis

The earliest detectable cell of the B lymphocyte lineage, the pre-B cell, is found in fetal liver by 7–8 weeks' gestation [68]. True B cells, characterized by the expression of membrane-bound immunoglobulins on their surface, are first seen around 10 weeks' gestation and rapidly increase in numbers so that by 15–18 weeks' gestation the absolute number of B lymphocytes in blood, liver, spleen and bone marrow is equivalent to those found in adults [69]. B cell development gradually switches from the liver to bone marrow in parallel with other aspects of haematopoiesis and by 30 weeks pre-B cells are undetectable in the liver [68].

The earliest B cells found express only IgM on their surface. This confers on them a functional immaturity which is thought necessary for the development of tolerance to self-antigens [70,71]. From 11 to 12 weeks onwards cells appear expressing multiple immunoglobulin types on their surface, mainly IgM and IgD, but IgG and IgA are also found. These apparently mature B cells migrate through the circulation to the lymph nodes and the spleen. Early B cell maturation appears to occur largely independent of either antigen or T lymphocytes. The ability to recognize antigen and secrete antibody however is dependent on T lymphocytes and the development of thymic maturation [68,72,73]. The differentiation into an antibody producing plasma cell requires specific antigen recognised by the B cells' surface immunoglobulin in the presence of competent T cells.

*In vitro* studies have demonstrated that fetal lymphocytes are capable of both IgM and IgG production from around 20 weeks' gestation [74] and some IgM is often detected in vivo by this time [75]. Antibody produced in response to congenital infection has been demonstrated from around 20 weeks' gestation [76,77]. Fetal immunoglobulin synthesis is predominantly IgM with little if any IgG and no IgA. The lack of fetal IgG and IgA production is in part due to immaturity of T cell function [54] but even in the presence of adult T cells, fetal B cell immunoglobulin synthesis, particularly IgG and IgA, production is deficient compared to adult responses [78–80].

The reduced capacity for antibody production in the fetal and neonatal period does not seem to be one of failure of antigen recognition. Although the neonatal repertoire of antibody diversity is reduced compared to the adult [81], it has been suggested that as early as midgestation sufficient diversity exists within the human B-cell population to recognize virtually any antigen determinant likely to be met. The deficiency in antibody producing capability in fetal and neonatal life is due to functional immaturity of both B and T lymphocytes and differing balances of regulatory (helper/suppressor) T cells that exist in the fetus compared to the adult [83]. This is illustrated by the fact that lymphocytes isolated from umbilical cord blood can suppress the normally observed proliferation of adult lymphocytes in response to antigenic stimulation [43].

Due to the functional immaturities of the lymphocyte population and its highly protected environment with minimal exposure to foreign antigen, the fetus produces little immunoglobulin of its own [83]. Even in a normal term infant humoral immunity would be profoundly deficient if it were not for placental transfer of maternal IgG to the fetus. Due to this transfer, term neonates have IgG levels (around 1000 mg dl$^{-1}$) equivalent to or higher than maternal levels [38,84]. Placental IgG transfer occurs throughout gestation but initially in relatively small amounts. At birth, IgG levels are proportional to gestational age [85,86]. Before 28 weeks, IgG levels are less than half those found at full term [85,87,88] and infants under 1000 g have substantially lower IgG levels (mean about 250 mg dl$^{-1}$) at birth than babies of 1000–1500 g [89]. There is a progressive fall in IgG levels over the first 3 months, with the under 1000 g babies reaching levels as low as 50 mg dl$^{-1}$ [89–91]. There is no selectivity in placental transfer of IgG subclasses, the levels in cord blood showing the same proportions as those in the mother [92,93].

The ELBW infant's hypogammaglobulaemic state increases the risk of invasive sepsis. Such infants are also at risk from missing out on a further source of passive immunity as supplied by immunoglobulin, particularly IgA, in breast milk. Enteral feeding is often delayed in these infants and breast milk production may fail.

Postnatally neonates show a reduced capacity to synthesize antibody against certain bacterial antigens. In particular antibody responses to the capsular antigens of Group B streptococcus or the capsular polysaccharides of pneumococcus, meningococcus, and *Haemophilus influenzae* are poor and remain so up until about 2 years of age [94,95]. The responses to protein antigens are more mature, although antibody titres may rise slowly in comparison to responses in later life [96,97]. The response to these protein antigens, in particular the response to diphtheria/tetanus/pertussis immunization, has been studied in very preterm infants and at 24 weeks' gestation there is a response ability to these antigens in a way comparable to that of term babies [97–99].

The ELBW infant's immune system is deficient in a number of areas and this, coupled with the lack of prior antigen exposure and the failure of passive protection from the mother, underlies the vulnerability of this category of infant to sepsis.

## Factors influencing immune function in the ELBW infant

### Nutrition

*In utero* nutritional deprivation leading to growth retardation creates a risk for infection independent of any coexisting prematurity. SGA infants have reduced numbers of circulating lymphocytes (both B and T cells) in the neonatal period [100]. T cell function seems particularly susceptible to *in utero* nutritional deprivation [108]. Interestingly, such infants may show disturbances in their immune reactivity for some considerable time [100,102].

McIntosh *et al.* showed that in infants below 1000 g, *in utero* growth retardation was associated with significantly reduced peripheral blood neutrophil counts [103]. Counts were low for the first 2 weeks of postnatal life. In some cases neutrophil counts fall below $1 \times 10^9 l^{-1}$ with presumed consequences for infection risk.

In the older child, protein-energy malnutrition is well recognized as a major risk factor for infection and immune dysfunction is well documented in such children. Postnatally the ELBW infant is clearly at risk nutritionally both in terms of overall intake of protein and calories but also in the intake of specific factors essential for immune function, for example vitamins A and E and trace metals [104]. Unfortunately, the specific requirements of neonates are not well worked out and there are risks involved with supplementation of diets, as was discovered with vitamin E in the 1980s [105]. While it is possible to say that an adequate and balanced nutritional input is required to optimize the immune response, clearly more work is required to define areas where important deficits may occur and perhaps where supplementation might enhance immune function [102,104,106,107]. Enteral feeds, when they can be established, carry less infection risk than parenteral feeds (see below). Breast milk appears to have advantages over formula feeds when considering the risks of necrotizing enterocolitis and it seems likely that it has advantages when considering the risks of nosocomial infection [108,109,110].

## Organisms

The ELBW infant does not seem to be substantially different from heavier infants in the type of organism likely to cause *early-onset sepsis* in the neonatal period. Group B Streptococcus and *E. coli* are the most common organisms detected, followed by a variety of enteric organisms [111]. The real differences are in *late-onset*, nosocomial infection rates which relate to the prolonged periods of intensive care which these infants require.

Most cases of late-onset sepsis (80–90%) are bacterial in origin, with coagulase negative staphylococci (CNS) contributing at least 30% and *Staphylococcus aureus* around 20%; streptococcal species and a variety of Gram-negative organisms make up the rest of the bacterial infections.

In addition to bacteria, however, fungi and viruses, notably *Respiratory Syncitial Virus* (RSV) are more likely to cause life-threatening illnesses than in more mature infants.

### Coagulase-negative staphylococci

Prolonged venous cannulation and endotracheal intubation are the main factors underlying susceptibility to this group of organisms. *Staphylococcus epidermidis* has the ability to adhere to the plastics used for catheters via surface lectins [112]. This organism produces a surface slime material which has anti-inflammatory activity, inhibits immune recognition, hinders phagocytosis and protects against antibiotics [113]. Multiple antibiotic resistance further complicates effective therapy.

### Fungal infections

There have been many case reports of fungal infections over the past 20 years or so, the most frequently isolated organism being *Candida albicans*, but also less common types such as *Malassezia furfur* have been reported [114]. In two large studies fungal organisms accounted for 12% and 16% of infective episodes [115,116]. A recent survey conducted in Leeds found the prevalence of colonization with *Candida spp.* to be 65% in neonates of 28 weeks' gestation or less compared with 26% in neonates of higher gestational age; in this study *Candida albicans* accounted for 95% of the yeast isolates [8]. This increased colonization rate is reflected in true sepsis rates among ELBW babies and in two series, one from the US [117] and the other from the UK [118], 11 of the 15 cases of systemic candidiasis occurred in babies weighing 1000 g or less.

Apart from the duration of antibiotic therapy [119], there are no clearly defined risk factors for fungal sepsis but the use of steroids for the management of hypotension has been reported to be associated with an increased frequency of fungal sepsis [12]. It is also possible that interventions such as the placement of central venous catheters add to the risk of fungal invasion. A particularly difficult therapeutic problem has recently been described in which an ELBW baby developed a renal candidal bezoar causing urinary obstruction at the level of the renal pelvis; the infection was treated by the insertion of a nephrostomy tube and local irrigation with amphotericin B [12]. Two similar cases have occurred on our own unit and in both it seemed likely that the renal candidiasis was acquired from the perineum via umbilical arterial catheters; in both of these cases the infection responded to intravenous antifungal therapy [122].

It is not yet clear whether antifungal prophylaxis is effective in reducing the risk of systemic fungal infection in ELBW babies. A randomized placebo-controlled study of nystatin prophylaxis in babies weighing <1250 g at birth did show lower colonization and infection rates in the group receiving prophylactic nystatin but the frequency of systemic fungal infection in the control group (32%) was much higher than in other studies [123]. In contrast, of the five cases of systemic fungal sepsis reported by Johnson *et al.*, four had received nystatin prophylaxis [11]; further, in the recent Leeds study, antifungal prophylaxis with miconazole gel or nystatin solution during antibiotic therapy did not affect the frequency of yeast colonization among the neonates [8]. It is probable that the efficacy of antifungal prophylaxis for ELBW babies, the group of neonates at most risk of systemic fungal infection, could only be assessed by means of a randomized placebo-controlled multicentre trial.

# The influence of therapeutic interventions

Although there are no forms of therapy which are used only for ELBW babies, there are some which are more frequently applied to this group of neonates than those who are more mature; these include parenteral nutrition, 'antioxidant' therapy, the administration of surfactant into the lungs and the use of steroids for the treatment of chronic lung disease. For many of these agents there has been concern that their use may be associated with an increased risk of sepsis or NEC. Some of the recent information concerning the risk of

sepsis associated with these forms of treatment in ELBW babies is reviewed in this chapter.

## Parenteral nutrition

In addition to the risks imposed by central venous catheters, parenteral nutrition may have specific influences on the immune system. Intravenous lipid emulsions increase exposure to micro-organisms and interfere with the immune system. This has to be contrasted to the enhancing effect of adequate nutrition in these small babies. Freeman *et al.* [124] demonstrated a marked association between the use of lipid emulsions and the onset of coagulase negative staphylococci bacteraemia; the increased risk of infection was independent of central venous catheter use. Crystalline amino acid and dextrose solutions are (perhaps surprisingly) relatively poor growth media for bacteria but may support fungal growth [125]. In contrast, lipid emulsion is an excellent medium for growth of both bacteria and fungal species [126]. Lipids may act as growth media for unusual pathogens. The fungus Malassezia furfur grows well in lipid emulsions and there have been several reports documenting disseminated infection in the premature infant [127,128,129,130]. Lipid emulsions contain particles that are trapped by filters fine enough to prevent bacterial passage. To date, lipid infusions have, therefore, usually been unfiltered, increasing the risk of microbial contamination reaching the infant. Filters suitable for lipid emulsions are becoming available and may go some way to reducing these risks.

There are a number of studies demonstrating altered immune function in the presence of lipid emulsions. Much of this work has been done *in vitro* and with relatively high concentrations of lipid so interpretation has to be cautious. Macrophages, particularly within the reticuloendothelial system, will take up lipid and in high concentration this might be expected to interfere with phagocytic activity. Administration of intravenous lipid over long periods has been shown to increase tumour necrosis factor (TNF) production by macrophages [131]. Lipid emulsions depress lymphocyte proliferative responses and neutrophil function at concentrations often found in the plasma during administration [132–134]. There is no clearly documented clinically significant depression of the immune

**Table 15.5    Incidence of sepsis and necrotizing enterocolitis: effect of vitamin E[a]**

|  | *501–750 g* | | *751–1000 g* | |
| --- | --- | --- | --- | --- |
|  | *Treatment[b]* | *Placebo[b]* | *Treatment[b]* | *Placebo[b]* |
| Early acquired sepsis | 7/28 (25) | 6/28 (21) | 7/44 (16) | 5/45 (11) |
| All sepsis | 10/28 (36) | 6/28 (21) | 13/44 (29) | 8/45 (18) |
| Necrotizing enterocolitis | 1/28 (4) | 3/28 (11) | 2/44 (4) | 3/45 (7) |
| Survived | 8/28 (29) | 7/28 (25) | 32/44 (73) | 37/45 (82) |

[a] Fish *et al.* [140]
[b]Figures in parentheses are percentages

system when using standard low rates of infusion and in the ELBW infant the nutritional gain is likely to outweigh the risks. Efforts to commence adequate enteral nutrition as soon as possible would appear to be a sensible approach so that i.v. lipid use is minimized. An area of future interest will be the differential effects of alternative types of lipids on immune function [134,135].

### Vitamin E

Vitamin E has been investigated as a prophylactic agent in the prevention of various conditions which may affect very preterm babies, including haemolytic anaemia, retinopathy of prematurity, intracranial haemorrhage and chronic lung disease. While earlier studies indicated that vitamin E may provide protection against sepsis [136,137] there has been more recent evidence that vitamin E may increase the risk of sepsis by altering neutrophil function as a result of reduced superoxide anion release [138,139]. In 1985 Johnson *et al.*, who were investigating the use of vitamin E as prophylaxis for retinopathy of prematurity in babies with a birth weight of less than 1500 g, reported a higher incidence of sepsis and NEC in babies who had received vitamin E for 8 or more days. They did not find a direct relationship between serum vitamin E levels and the incidence of sepsis or NEC, although an aim of this study was to maintain serum vitamin E concentrations at the relatively high level of 5 mg dl$^{-1}$ [105]. In this study, for which recruitment had been stratified by birth weight, the highest treatment-related incidence of bacterial or candidal sepsis was found in infants whose birth weight was 1000 g or less, with a 43% sepsis rate for

vitamin E-treated babies compared with 18% for those receiving placebo. There was a significantly higher rate of NEC among vitamin E-treated babies in those weighing 1001–1250 g.

The incidence of sepsis and NEC was also recorded in a subsequent investigation of the use of intramuscular vitamin E as prophylaxis for intra-cranial haemorrhage [140]. In this study, which included only babies whose birth weight was less than 1000 g, no statistically significant association was found between vitamin E treatment and sepsis or NEC (Table 15.5). Although there was a trend towards a higher sepsis rate after the first week of life in babies receiving vitamin E, the mean serum vitamin E levels were lower in the septic babies than in those who did not develop sepsis. The design of this study was markedly different to that of Johnson *et al.*, with mean serum vitamin E levels beyond the first week of life of 2.70 and 2.39 mg dl$^{-1}$ in treated and control groups respectively, compared with median concentrations of 4.9 and 0.7 mg dl$^{-1}$ in the treatment and control groups of the earlier investigation.

On the evidence so far available, the case for a direct relationship between vitamin E prophylaxis and sepsis or NEC in ELBW babies cannot be regarded as proven, particularly in the absence of a relationship between serum vitamin E levels and the occurrence of sepsis. However, the available data do give some cause for concern and it is possible either that the risk of sepsis is not related to serum vitamin levels or that there is a threshold level at which sepsis or NEC become more likely.

### Vitamin A

Another form of anti-oxidant treatment which has excited some interest recently has been that of vitamin A for the prevention of chronic lung disease. In a double-blind randomized placebo-controlled trial, Shenai *et al.* administered vitamin A supplements to babies at risk of developing chronic lung disease [141]. Eligible babies were given a total of 14 intramuscular doses of retinyl palmitate, 2000 units per dose, from 4 to 28 days of life. The mean birth weight of babies in this study was 1006 g for the vitamin A-treated group and 976 g for the controls. A significant reduction in the frequency of bronchopulmonary dysplasia (BPD) was found in the treated group when compared with the saline-treated controls. A secondary outcome measure in this study was the frequency of clinically diagnosed episodes of airway infection, 'confirmed by positive microbiologic cultures of airways secretions'. It was found that airway infection occurred in 11/20 (55%) of control infants compared with only 4/19 (21%) of those who received vitamin A, a difference which was statistically significant at the *P* <0.03 level. While only *Staphylococcus epidermidis* was isolated from the airways secretions of babies receiving vitamin A, multiple organisms were found in the controls, including *S. epidermidis, Staphylococcus aureus, Pseudomonas aeruginosa, Klebsiella pneumoniae, Enterococcus* spp., *Proteus mirabilis* and *Serratia marcescens*. It was suggested in this report that the histopathological changes which occur in the lung and tracheobronchial tree of babies with BPD, and vitamin A deficiency, may explain their predisposition to airway infections. As with some other neonatal studies, this report is difficult to interpret as the incidence of BPD in the control group (85%) is somewhat higher than might have been expected and the incidence in the treated group (45%) was no lower than would have been predicted in unsupplemented babies. There is, therefore, a need for larger randomized controlled studies to determine whether vitamin A supplementation does have a role in the prevention of pulmonary infections in the ELBW baby.

## Steroids

Over the past few years oral and parenteral synthetic steroids, notably dexamethasone, have been used with increasing frequency for the treatment of chronic lung disease of prematurity (CLP). Table 15.2 shows that, in the VOTN study, ELBW babies were more likely to be treated with steroids for CLP than bigger babies. Steroids are also administered to certain categories of expectant mothers for the prevention of the respiratory distress syndrome in preterm babies. One of the potential adverse effects associated with high-dose steroid treatment is sepsis, so most of the published studies concerning steroid treatment in preterm neonates have reported on the incidence of sepsis.

The first full report of a randomized, placebo-controlled trial of dexamethasone for the treatment of chronic lung disease was published in 1983 by Mammel and coworkers [142]. Of the six patients studied, three were ELBW infants and all were reported to have developed septic complications (one case of subacute bacterial endocarditis and two cases of septicaemia) all of which were caused by coagulase-negative staphylococci. However, since all of the patients in this study received both dexamethasone and placebo at different stages of the trial, there was no direct evidence that the sepsis was due to the steroids. Subsequent studies of the use of dexamethasone in the neonatal period have not found convincing evidence of an increased sepsis risk [143,144] although Yeh and co-workers in a recent multicentre controlled trial, found a slight but statistically significant increase in the rates of bacteraemia or clinical sepsis in the steroid-treated group compared with those receiving a placebo and, perhaps of more concern, it was reported that a higher proportion of infants in the dexamethasone group died in the late study period, probably attributable to infection or sepsis [145]. At present, therefore, the majority of studies have not found a link between the use of steroids in the neonatal period and the development of sepsis but the report by Yeh and the finding of an increased risk of fungal infection in babies receiving hydrocortisone [120] are of concern. Given that therapeutic steroids are more likely to be used in ELBW babies this aspect of neonatal care may represent a particular hazard for this group of infants.

## Surfactant

One of the major advances in the management of preterm infants over the past few years has been the introduction of surfactant therapy.

There is now good evidence that preterm infants suffering from the respiratory distress syndrome, including ELBW infants [146–149], are more likely to survive if they receive exogenous surfactant soon after birth. The VOTN reflected management and outcome of very low birth weight babies in 36 neonatal intensive care units (NICUs) in North America, indicating that 64% of neonates weighing 751–1000 g and 57% of those weighing 501–750 g were treated with surfactant in 1990 [4]. There have been concerns that the introduction of foreign substances such as surfactant directly into the respiratory system might predispose the infant to pulmonary infections and there is some evidence from animal experiments that the process of phagocytosis by pulmonary alveolar macrophages [150] might be inhibited by exogenous surfactant. Recent studies on human adult alveolar macrophages have also shown that Exosurf® has an inhibitory effect on endotoxin-induced cytokine secretion [151]. One of the secondary outcome measurements, therefore, in many of the clinical trials of surfactant therapy has been the incidence of sepsis. There have been four published studies to date which have reported on the incidence of sepsis associated with surfactant therapy, in which either all or the majority of the study patients weighed <1000 g at birth. The sepsis rates reported in these studies are shown in Table 15.6. In none of these studies was the sepsis rate significantly different between treatment and control groups but the table does indicate a trend towards a higher sepsis rate associated with the administration of Survanta®. In fact, when the results of all clinical studies with Survanta® were combined the rate of post-treatment sepsis in neonates of all birth weight categories was 20.7% in those treated with Survanta® compared with 16.1% in control neonates, a difference which was statistically significant

**Table 15.6  Frequency of sepsis associated with surfactant treatment**

| Study (Ref) | n | Sepsis rate (%) | |
|---|---|---|---|
| | | Placebo | Treatment |
| Stevenson et al. [146] | 215 | 31 | 34[a] |
| Hoekstra et al. [147] | 428 | 16 | 22[b] |
| Corbet et al. [148] | 410 | 26 | 25[a] |
| Soll et al. [149] | 67 | 23 | 37[b] |
| Average | | 23 | 26 |

[a]Babies received Exosurf®
[b]Babies received Survanta®

(personal communication, Abbott Laboratories). It is not clear whether this does indicate a true increased risk of sepsis or whether the difference can be accounted for, for instance, by the improved survival rate in the treated group. Further, an open surveillance study of Survanta®, after it was made available to 231 neonatal intensive care units in the USA and Canada under a 'treatment investigational new drug' protocol, has shown lower post-treatment sepsis rates than in the controlled trials [152]. Clearly, there is a need for more information concerning the association between sepsis and surfactant therapy and this is an outcome which should continue to be monitored in future clinical trials.

## Necrotizing enterocolitis

In Table 15.7 the frequencies of NEC found in three recent USA studies are presented, in which specific information is available for ELBW babies. These data suggest that, allowing for the effects of survival, ELBW babies are at higher risk of developing NEC than those of higher birth weight, although the level of the

**Table 15.7  Frequency of necrotizing enterocolitis (%) and survival (%) by birth weight**

| Study (Ref) | Birth weight (g) | | | | |
|---|---|---|---|---|---|
| | 501–750 | 751–1000 | 1001–1250 | 1251–1500 | 1001–1500 |
| NICHD [3] | 3 (34) | 9 (66) | — | — | 7 |
| VOTN [4] | 9 (47) | 7 (80) | 6 (92) | 5 (95) | — |
| Fish [140] | 7 (27) | 6 (78) | — | — | — |

Figures in parentheses are percentage surviving

increased risk varies markedly among the studies. The studies of vitamin E discussed above indicate that there may be different risk factors according to the size, or maturity, of the infant. Further support for this concept is provided in a recent paper from Australia. In a study of risk factors for NEC occurring during a 7-year period, it was found that, of the 39 babies of 25–29 weeks' gestation who developed NEC, only 13% were fed with expressed breast milk only, compared with 39% of case-controls; this difference was not found for babies of 30–36 weeks' gestation [153]. It was not clear whether the breast milk referred to included donor milk but it does seem likely that ELBW babies, in particular, are likely to derive some protection against NEC from breast milk. The factors in breast milk which are important in protecting against NEC have not been identified, but in 1988 a study was reported from Vienna in which an oral immunoglobulin preparation, containing 73% IgA and 26% IgG, was orally administered to infants of 800–2000 g birth weight for whom breast milk from their mothers was not available; of the 45 babies (21 treated and 24 controls) in the 800–1300 g category none developed NEC while six of the 70 controls weighing above 800 g developed the condition, compared with none of 64 treated babies. Thus, while this study indicates that oral immunoglobulins may provide some protection against NEC in low birth weight babies, there is no direct evidence that this applies to the ELBW baby [154].

## Prevention and management

The approach to therapy for infection in the ELBW infant consists of efforts to reduce risk, vigorous surveillance with a high index of suspicion and prompt treatment, namely supportive intensive care and early use of appropriate antibiotics. The exact choice of antibiotics will depend upon individual units' policies, the timing of the infection and prior knowledge of the individual's and the unit's flora. A discussion of antibiotic therapy for neonates has been published previously [155]. There is a relative lack of pharmacokinetic data available to guide antibiotic use in the ELBW infant.

General measures to reduce the risk of infection, part of good neonatal care, are essential when caring for the ELBW infant. Attention to reducing spread of organisms from infant to infant via the carers with frequent and adequate handwashing and isolation in incubators are all important but easily overlooked factors. Efforts to reduce skin trauma in the ELBW infant may reduce the portals of entry of organisms. Minimizing invasive procedures similarly reduces infection risk. Introducing and switching over to enteral feeds at an early stage where practically possible is likely to be of benefit, particularly where breast milk is available.

Indwelling lines for vascular access are an inevitable part of caring for the ELBW infant. Centrally placed lines used for parenteral feeding are a major source of secondary sepsis. Scrupulous attention to aseptic technique when placing such lines and when changing infusion fluids is essential. The need to break into lines to change fluids or administer drugs should be minimized. The use of an efficient bacterial filter reduces the likelihood of introducing bacteria [156] but the main portals of entry in relation to cannulas seem to be either migration from the skin along the catheter or, more commonly, contamination of injection ports [157–159]. Different catheter materials may be less conducive to colonization and catheters are now being produced with antibiotics or antiseptics bonded to their surfaces which may turn out to be beneficial [162]. We are not aware of any studies relevant to the ELBW and even in larger patients the benefits of such catheters appear uncertain [163,164]. Insertion of central lines early in the infant's life before significant numbers of skin bacteria have developed might also reduce the incidence of catheter contamination [7]. Low dose heparin in infusion fluids is used to reduce thrombus formation at catheter tips which in turn may reduce bacterial colonization [165], but this can have adverse effects on the stability of the lipid emulsion [165–167]. The increased use of bacterial filters would seem to be a sensible precaution to guard against inadvertent contamination of intravenous fluids. They have the added advantage of functioning as filters for particulate matter as well.

### Immunotherapy

#### *Immunoglobulin prophylaxis*

The knowledge that preterm infants are deficient in immunoglobulin coupled with the availability of non-specific immunoglobulin preparations and their relative ease of use has led to a profusion of studies on the prophylactic use of immunoglobulin in the prevention of neonatal sepsis, particularly late onset, nosocomial infection [168,169]. Interpretation of results has been confounded by varying treatment protocols, different immunoglobulin preparations and the likely variation in the quantity of pathogen specific antibodies in these preparations. The number of clinical studies is rivalled by the number of editorials and reviews written on the subject and we do not propose to review this area in detail. A recent meta-analysis of the field concludes that prophylactic immunoglobulin use is unlikely to be justified given the cost implications and theoretical infection transmission risk [170].

Arguably, if immunoglobulin prophylaxis is to be of benefit, it would be in the ELBW infant where immunoglobulin deficiency is profound. Five studies give the necessary information to determine results specifically for <1000 g infants. Their results are summarized in Table 15.8. Only the studies reported by Fanaroff *et al.* and Baker *et al.* are of sufficient size to have statistical validity: Fanaroff *et al.* found no benefit while Baker *et al.* found evidence for protection. There was no major difference in study design, although Baker *et al.* had an initial increased dosing frequency; the one major difference was in the immunoglobulin preparations used, Sandoglobulin versus Gammagard, respectively. Overall these studies do not provide a convincing argument in favour of immunoglobulin prophylaxis in infants <1000 g. Proponents of the therapy would argue that we still need to find the optimum preparation and dosing schedule but the answers to these questions are going to require very large studies and are likely to remain unresolved for some time. It

seems unlikely that immunoglobulin prophylaxis, at least by itself, is going to be the solution to late-onset sepsis in these infants.

### Immunoglobulin rescue therapy

An alternative to prophylactic administration of non-specific immunoglobulin to at-risk premature infants is the administration of immunoglobulin (either pooled non-specific immunoglobulins or preparations with a high content of specific antibody against the relevant organism) to infants at the point of diagnosing sepsis or possible sepsis as an adjunct to other therapies. Studies have been small but the results are encouraging [170–172]. Specific comment on the ELBW infant is not possible. Particular benefit is likely when the immunoglobulin preparation used has high titres of specific antibody to the infecting organism [173,174] and it is possible that preparations of hyperimmune globulin could be developed against organisms causing neonatal infections [175,176]. Monoclonal antibody production is likely to be a more practical solution and studies in mice have shown that murine monoclonal antibody against the Group B streptococcus is highly protective [177,178]; the technique seems to be effective against other organisms as well [176].

Hyperimmune globulin administration is established in the prevention and amelioration of perinatally acquired infections such as varicella-zoster and hepatitis B. Experience is also being gained with recently introduced preparations with activity against RSV [179, 180]. Available evidence would appear to support the administration of immunoglobulin to the ELBW infant considered septic particularly if the immunoglobulin preparation has high titres of relevant titres of relevant antibodies. However, administration of immunoglobulin may not be without detrimental effects on the recipient's immune system [181–3] and further studies are needed.

### Immunization

An alternative to passive administration of antibody is active immunization. As described above, premature infants show a reasonably adequate, albeit slow, response to immunization with proteinaceous antigens. The ineffective responses to capsular polysaccharide

**Table 15.8    The use of prophylactic intravenous immunoglobulin in the ELBW infant: no. of cases of sepsis/no. of infants in group**

| Study (Ref.) | Immunoglobulin treated | Placebo |
|---|---|---|
| Clapp 1989 [168] | 0/11 | 5/11 |
| Didato 1988 [169] | 3/10 | 1/7 |
| Kinney 1991 [90] | 3/25 | 3/24 |
| Fanaroff 1992 [116] | 126/467 | 131/437 |
| Baker 1992 [115] | 28/84 | 50/97 |

antigens is likely to limit the usefulness of such an approach unless they can be conjugated to a protein carrier, as with *Haemophilus influenzae* vaccine [181]. Clearly the time course of an immunization response lends itself to prophylaxis rather than active treatment of established infection.

### Opsonization

Specific immunoglobulin is an important factor in enhancing opsonization of organisms, but other factors are likely to be limiting in the ELBW infant. Complement components are low in the ELBW infant and are depleted in the face of sepsis. Transfusions of fresh frozen plasma may restore complement activity. There is little information on the potential benefit of plasma infusions either as prophylaxis or in the treatment of acute infection. A practical problem is that plasma complement concentrations are low in stored plasma necessitating relatively large volumes to be infused to make significant differences in levels; circulatory overload may, therefore, be a limiting factor. It would seem to be a reasonable strategy to use plasma as part of the resuscitation of the shocked septic infant.

In adult patients, increasing fibronectin levels have been associated with improved reticuloendothelial function during sepsis [185]. *In vitro* deficiencies of opsonic activity of sera from premature infants can be improved by the addition of fibronectin [186]. Fibronectin can be prepared from human plasma cryoprecipitate. As yet its use is experimental with clinical experience limited to a few small uncontrolled studies in adults. In septic surgical patients, and in adults following massive trauma, increased fibronectin levels improved reticuloendothelial function *in vitro* [187], but so far no consistent clinical benefit has been demonstrated in adult patients.

### Cells

The described deficiencies in the premature infant's white cells, their functional limitations and the ease with which they become depleted has naturally led to attempts to boost immunity with mature granulocyte transfusions. Encouraging results in animal models have led to some limited studies in human neonates [188 192]. The results of these reports taken together suggest that granulocyte transfusions are beneficial and that they may be more effective than pooled immunoglobulin in septic neonates with neutropenia [193]. Lack of further published studies reflects the difficulties in preparing granulocytes for infusion [194] coupled with their significant potential for serious side effects, most notably transmission of viruses and graft-versus-host disease. For the ELBW infant with severe sepsis, who is neutropenic and not responding to other therapies, granulocyte transfusions could be a useful adjunct to therapy if they were available and could be prepared in time. Given the difficulties in using donated white cells this is unlikely to be of use for prophylaxis in the at risk ELBW infant. Enhancing the infant's own white cell function and numbers is likely to be rewarding and practical. In recent years our knowledge of the factors involved in the regulation of blood cell proliferation and in controlling the inflammatory responses of white cells has substantially increased. With many of these factors (e.g. granulocyte colony-stimulating factor and granulocyte-macrophage colony-stimulating factor) now being produced by recombinant technology the way is open to testing their effects in the clinical situation. Early results [195–200] are encouraging, including hints that transplacental therapy might be possible [201] and may herald a breakthrough in the management of the ELBW infant at least as far as susceptibility to infection is concerned.

## Conclusions

The ELBW infant by virtue of its immunological deficiencies and needs for invasive intensive care is extremely vulnerable to sepsis. Currently the mainstays of preventative treatment are scrupulous attention to details of care such as handwashing and aseptic technique, and strategies to shorten periods of invasive procedures such as endotracheal intubation and centrally placed catheters. Treatment requires extreme vigilance to detect septic episodes early and appropriate antimicrobial use. Immunomodulation has exciting potential but is as yet experimental rather than established therapy.

---

**Practical points**

1. The need for prolonged intensive care, with exposure to a range of pathogenic drug-resistant organisms, coupled with prolonged use of intravascular catheters and endotracheal intubation, exposes the ELBW baby to a high risk of acquiring invasive sepsis.
2. The organisms involved include antibiotic-resistant bacteria and fungi.
3. Specific therapies, such as parenteral nutrition, postnatal steroids and the prophylactic use of vitamin E may pose additional risks.
4. Despite these risks, and the immunological immaturity of ELBW babies, documented mortality rates from infections are low.
5. The effectiveness of immune modulation has still to be proven in this group of infants.
6. ELBW babies are also probably at an increased risk of developing NEC when compared with bigger preterm babies, and their risk of developing the condition can be minimized by the use of breast milk in the early stages of enteral feeding.

---

# References

1. Kazzi, N.J., Brans, Y.W. and Poland, R.L. (1990) Dexamethasone effects on the hospital course of infants with bronchopulmonary dysplasia who are dependent on artificial ventilation. *Pediatrics*, **86**, 722–727
2. Harkavy, K.L., Scanlon, J.W., Chowdray, P.K. and Grylack, L.J. (1989) Dexamethasone therapy for chronic lung disease in ventilator- and oxygen-dependent infants: a controlled trial. *J. Pediatr.*, **115**, 979–983
3. Hack, M., Horbar, J.D., Malloy, M.H., Tyson, J.E., Wright, E. and Wright, L. (1991) Very low birth weight outcomes of the National Institute of Child Health and Human Development Neonatal Network. *Pediatrics*, **87**, 587–597
4. The investigators of the Vermont–Oxford trials network database project (1993) The Vermont–Oxford trials network: very low birth weight outcomes for 1990. *Pediatrics*, **91**, 540–545
5. Office for National Statistics: mortality statistics, childhood, infant and perinatal (1994) Series DH3, No. 28. London, The Stationery Office 1995, 157–162
6. Peters, G. and Cashore, W.J. (1990) Infections acquired in the nursery; epidemiology and control. In J.S. Remington and J.O. Klein, eds) *Infectious Diseases of the Fetus and Newborn Infant*, 3rd edn. Saunders, Philadelphia, pp. 1000–1019
7. Keyworth, N., Millar, M.R. and Holland, K.T. (1992) Development of cutaneous microflora in premature neonates. *Arch. Dis. Childh*, **67**, 797–801
8. Sharp, A.M., Odds, F.C. and Evans, E.G.V. (1992) Candida strains from neonates in a special care baby unit. *Arch. Dis. Childh.*, **67**, 48–52
9. Solomon, L.M. and Estetly, N.B. (1983) *Neonatal Dermatology*. Saunders, Philadelphia
10. Quie, P.G. (1990) Antimicrobial defenses in the neonate. *Semin. Perinatol.*, **14**(Suppl.), 2–9
11. Battisti, O., Mitchison, R. and Davis, P.A. (1981) Changing blood culture isolates in a referral neonatal intensive care unit. *Arch. Dis. Childh.*, **56**, 775–778
12. Noel, G.J. and Edelson, P.J. (1984) *Staphylococcus epidermidis* bacteraemia in neonates: further observations and occurrence of focal infections. *Pediatrics*, **74**, 832–837
13. Beganovic, N., Verloove-Van Horick, S.P., Brand, R. and Ruys, J.H. (1988) Total parenteral nutrition and sepsis. *Arch. Dis. Childh.*, **63**, 66–89
14. Decker, M.D. and Edwards, K.M. (1988) Central venous catheter infections. *Pediatr. Clin. N. Am.*, **35**, 579–612
15. Fitzgerald, J.F. (1977) Colonization of the gastrointestinal tract. In *Mead Johnson Symposium on Perinatal and Developmental Medicine*, No. 11. Vail, Colorado
16. Bennet, R., Erikson, M. and Nord, C.E. (1986) Faecal bacterial microflora of newborn infants during intensive care management and treatment with five antibiotic regimes. *Paediatr. Infect. Dis. J.*, **5**, 533–539
17. Guerrant, R.L., Cleary, T.G. and Pickering, L.K. (1990) Microorganisms responsible for neonatal diarrhoea. In *Infectious Diseases of the Fetus and Newborn Infant*, 3rd edn (J.S. Remington and J.O. Klein, eds), Saunders, Philadelphia, 901–980
18. Millar, M.R., Mackay, P., Levene, M. *et al.* (1992) Enterobacteriaceae and neonatal necrotising enterocolitis. *Arch. Dis. Childh.*, **67**, 53–56
19. Harries, J.T. and Fraser, A.J. (1968) The acidity of the gastric contents of premature babies during the first fourteen days of life. *Biol. Neonate*, **12**, 186–193
20. Sondheimer, J.M., Clark, D.A. and Gervaise, E.P. (1985) Continuous gastric pH measurement in young and older healthy preterm infants receiving formula and clear liquid feedings. *J. Pediatr. Gastroenterol. Nutr.*, **4**, 352–355
21. Inglis, T.J.J., Sherratt, M.J., Sproat, L.J., Gibson, J.S. and Hawkey, P.M. (1993) Gastroduodenal dysfunction and bacterial colonisation of the ventilated lung. *Lancet*, **341**, 911–913
22. Bisset, W.M. (1991) Development of intestinal motility. *Arch. Dis. Childh.*, **66**, 3–5
23. Ogra, P.L. and Fishaut, M. (1990) Human breast milk.

In *Infectious Diseases of the Fetus and Newborn Infant*, 3rd edn (J.S. Remington and J.O. Klein, eds), Saunders, Philadelphia, 66–88

24. Friedburg J, and Forle, V. (1987) Acquired bronchial injury in neonates. *Int. J. Pediatr. Otorhinolaryngol.*, **14**, 223–228

25. Storm, W. (1980) Transient bacteraemia following endotracheal suctioning in ventilated newborns. *Pediatrics*, **65**, 487–490

26. Stiehm, E.R. (1975) Fetal defense mechanisms. *Am. J. Dis. Childh.*, **129**, 438–443

27. Erdman, S.H., Christensen, R.D., Bradley, P.O. *et al.* (1982) Supply and release of storage neutrophils. *Biol. Neonate*, **41**, 132–137

28. Christensen, R.D. and Rothstein, G. (1984) Pre- and postnatal development of granulocyte stem cells in the rat. *Pediatr. Res.*, **18**, 599–602

29. Christensen, R.D., Harper, T.E. and Rothestein, G. (1986) Granulocyte-macrophage progenitor cells in term and preterm neonates. *J. Pediatr.*, **109**, 1047–1051

30. Squire, E., Favara, B. and Todd, J. (1979) Diagnosis of neonatal bacterial infection: hematologic and pathologic findings in fatal and nonfatal cases. *Pediatrics*, **64**, 60–64

31. Christensen, R.D. and Rothstein, G. (1980) Exhaustion of mature marrow neutrophils in neonates with sepsis. *J. Pediatr.*, **96**, 316–318

32. Christensen, R.D., Macfarlane, J.L., Taylor, N.L. *et al.* (1982) Blood and marrow neutrophils during experimental group B Streptococcal infection: quantification of the stem cell, proliferative, storage and circulating pools. *Pediatr. Res.*, **16**, 549–553

33. Al-Hadithy, H., Addison, I.E., Goldstone, A.H. *et al.* (1981) Defective neutrophil function in low-birth weight premature infants. *J. Clin. Pathol.*, **34**, 366–370

34. Cairo, M.S. (1989) Neonatal neutrophil host defense. *Am. J. Dis. Child.*, **143**, 40–46

35. Hajjar, F. (1990) Neutrophils in the newborn: normal characteristics and quantitative disorders. *Semin. Perinatol.*, **14**, 374–383

36. Carr, R., Pumford, D. and Davies, J.M. (1992) Neutrophil chemotaxis and adhesion in preterm babies. *Arch. Dis. Childh.*, **67**, 813–817

37. Lu, C.Y. and Unanue, E.R. (1985) Macrophage ontogeny: implications for host defence, T-lymphocyte differentiation and the acquisition of self-tolerance. *Clin. Immunol. Allergy* **5**, 253–269

38. Kohler, P.F. and Farr, R.S. (1966) Elevation of cord over maternal IgG immunoglobulin: evidence for an active placental IgG transport. *Nature* **210**, 1070–1071

39. Colten, H.R. (1985) Complement biosynthesis. *Clin. Immunol. Allergy*, **5**, 287–300

40. Ballow, M., Fung, F., Good, R.A. *et al.* (1974) Developmental aspects of complement components in the newborn. *Clin. Exp. Immunol.*, **18**, 257–266

41. Colten, H.R. (1985) Complement biosynthesis. *Clin. Immunol. Allergy*, **5**, 287–300

42. Kovar, I., Ajina, N.S. and Hurley, R. (1983) Serum complement and gestational age. *J. Obstet. Gynecol.*, **3**, 182–186

43. Wilson, M. (1985) Immunology of the fetus and newborn: lymphocyte phenotype and function. *Clin. Immunol. Allergy*, **5**: 191–234

44. Stutman, O. (1985) Ontogeny of T cells. *Clin. Immunol. Allergy*, **5**, 191–234

45. Rosenthal, P., Rimm, I.J., Umiel, T. *et al.* (1983) Ontogeny of human haemopoietic cells: analysis utilizing monoclonal antibodies. *J. Immunol.*, **31**, 232–237

46. Stites, D.P., Wybran, J., Carr, M.C. and Fudenberg, H.H. (1972) Development of cellular immune competence in man. In: *Ontogeny of Acquired Immunity*, Ciba Foundation Symposium. Elsevier-Excerpta Medica, Amsterdam, pp. 113–129

47. Stites, D.P., Carr, M. and Fudenberg, H.H. (1974) Ontogeny of cellular immunity in the human fetus. Development of responses to phytohemagglutinin and to allogeneic cells. *Cell. Immunol.*, **11**, 257–271

48. Stites, D.P. and Pavia, C.S. (1979) Ontogeny of human T cells. *Pediatrics*, **64** (Suppl.), 795–802

49. Carr, M.C., Stites, D.P. and Fundenberg, H.H. (1973) Dissociation of responses to phytohemagglutin and adult allogenic lymphocytes in human foetal lymphoid tissues. *Nature, New Biol.*, **241**, 279–281

50. Watson, W., Oen, K., Ramdakin, R. *et al.* (1991) Immunoglobulin and cytokine production by neonatal lymphocytes. *Clin. Exp. Immunol.*, **83**, 169–174

51. Miyawaki, T., Seki, H., Taga, K. *et al.* (1985) Dissociated production of interleukin 2 and immune (Y) interferon by phytohaemagglutinin stimulated lymphocytes in healthy infants. *Clin. Exp. Immunol.*, **59**, 505–511

52. Wilson, C.B., Westall, J., Johnston, L. *et al.* (1986) Decreased production of interferon-gamma by human neonatal cells. *J. Clin. Invest.*, **77**, 860–867

53. Wilson, C.B. and Lewis, D.B. (1990) Basis and implications of selectivity diminished cytokine production in neonatal susceptibility to infection. *Rev. Infect. Dis.*, **12** (Suppl. 4), S410–S420

54. Hayward, A.R. and Lawton, A.R. (1977) Induction of plasma cell differentiation of human fetal lymphocytes: evidence for functional immaturity of T and B cells. *J. Immunol.*, **119**, 1213–1217

55. Rayfield, L.S., Brent, L. and Rodeck, C.H. (1980) Development of cell mediated lympholysis in human foetal blood lymphocytes. *Clin. Exp. Immunol.*, **42**, 561–570

56. Granberg, C. and Hirvonen, T. (1980) Cell-mediated lympholysis by fetal and neonatal lymphocytes in sheep and man. *Cell. Immunol.*, **51**, 13–22

57. Toivanen, P., Uksila, J., Leino, A. *et al.* (1981) Development of mitogen responding and natural killer cells in the human fetus. *Immunol. Rev.*, **57**, 89–105

58. Palacios, R. and Anderson, U. (1982) Autologous mixed lymphocyte reaction in human cord blood lymphocytes: decreased generation of helper and cytotoxic T-cell functions and increased proliferative response and induction of suppressor T-cells. *Cell. Immunol.*, **66**, 88–98

59. Stern, P., Gidlund, M., Orn, A. *et al.* (1980) Natural killer cells mediate lysis of embryonal carcinoma cells lacking MHC. *Nature*, **285**, 341–342

60. Bellan, A.H., Quilet, A., Marchiol, C. *et al.* (1986) Natural killer susceptibility of human cells may be regulated by genes in the HLA region on chromosome 6. *Proc. Nat. Acad. Sci.*, **83**, 5688–5692

61. Perussia, B., Starr, S., Abraham, S. *et al.* (1983) Human natural killer cells analysed by B73.1, a monoclonal antibody blocking Fc receptor functions. *J. Immunol.*, **130**, 2133–2141

62. Abo, T., Millar, C.A., Gartland, G.L. *et al.* (1983) Differentiation stages of human natural killer cells in lymphoid tissues from fetal to adult life. *J. Exp. Med.*, **157**, 273–284

63. Uksila, J., Lassilo, O., Hirvonen, T. *et al.* (1983) Development of natural killer cell function in the human fetus. *J. Immunol.*, **130**, 153–156

64. Ueno, Y., Miyawaki, T., Seki, H. *et al.* (1985) Differential effects of recombinant human interferon-Y and interleukin-2 on natural killer cell activity of peripheral blood in early human development. *J. Immunol.*, **135**, 180–184

65. Noble, R.L. and Warren, R.P. (1985) Age-related development of human natural killer cell activity. *N. Engl. J. Med.*, **313**, 641–642

66. Lee, S.M., Suen, Y. and Chang, L. (1996) Decreased interleukin-12 (IL-12) from activated cord versus adult peripheral blood mononuclear cells and up regulation of interferon-gamma, natural killer, and lymphokine-activated killer activity by IL-12 in cord blood mononuclear cells. *Blood*, **88**, 945–954

67. Merrill, J.D., Sigaroudinia, M. and Kohl, S. (1996) Characterisation of natural killer and antibody dependent cellular cytotoxicity of preterm infants against human immunodeficiency virus-infected cells. *Pediatr. Res.*, **40**, 494-5-3

68. Gathings, W.E., Lawton, A.R. and Cooper, M.D. (1977) Immunofluorescent studies of the development of pre-B cells, B-lymphocytes and immunoglobulin isotype diversity in humans. *Eur. J. Immunol.*, **7**, 804–810

69. Lawton, A.R. and Cooper, M.D. (1979) B cell ontogeny: immunoglobulin genes and their expression. *Pediatrics*, **64**(s): 750–757

70. Raff, M.C., Owen, J.T., Cooper, M.D. *et al.* (1975) Differences in susceptibility of mature and immature mouse B lymphocytes to anti-immunoglobulin induced immunoglobulin suppression in vitro: possible implications for B cell tolerance to self. *J. Exp. Med.*, **142**; 1052–1064

71. Metcalf, E.S. and Klinman, N.R. (1977) In vitro tolerance induction of bone marrow cells: a marker for B cell maturation. *J. Immunol.*, **118**, 2111–2116

72. Chen, Y-W., Jacobson, E.B. and Siskind, G.W. (1984) Ontogeny of B lymphocyte function. XV. A role for thymus in the maturation of the capacity of a sub-population of B cells to re-express surface immunoglobulin after treatment with anti-immunoglobulin. *J. Immunol.*, **133**, 1209–1214

73. Coffman, R.L., Seymour, B.W., Lebman, D.A. *et al.* (1988) The role of helper T cell products in mouse B cell differentiation and isotype regulation. *Immunol. Rev.*, **102**, 5–28

74. Lawton, A.R., Self, K.S., Royal, S.A. *et al.* (1972) Ontogeny of B lymphocytes in the human fetus. *Clin. Immunol. Immunopath.*, **1**, 104–121

75. Van Furth, R., Schuit, R.E. and Hijmans, W. (1965) The immunological development of the human fetus. *J. Exp. Med.*, **122**, 1173–1188

76. Silverstein, A.M. and Lukes, R.J. (1962) Fetal response to antigenic stimulus. 1. Plasma cellular and lymphoid reactions in the human fetus to intrauterine infection. *Lab. Invest.*, **11**, 918–932

77. Alford, C.A., Wu, L.Y.F., Blanco, A. *et al.* (1974) Developmental humoral immunity and congenital infections in man. In: *The Immune System and Infectious Diseases* (J. Neter and F. Milgram, eds), S. Karger, Basel, 42–58

78. Tosato, G., Magrath, I.T., Koski, I.R. *et al.* (1980) B cell differentiation and immunoregulatory T cell function in human cord blood lymphocytes. *J. Clin. Invest.*, **66**, 383–388

79. Andersson, U., Bird, A.G., Britton, S. and Palacios, R. (1981) Humoral and cellular immunity in humans studied at the cell level from birth to two years of age. *Imm. Rev.*, **57**, 5–38

80. Hayward, A.R. (1981) Development of lymphocyte responses and interactions in the human fetus and newborn. *Imm. Rev.*, **57**, 39–60

81. Vogler, L.B. and Lawton, A.R. (1985) Ontogeny of B cells and humoral immune functions. *Clin. Immunol. Allergy*, **5**, 235–252

82. Lawton, A.R. (1984) Ontogeny of the immune system. In *Neonatal Infections: Nutritional and Immunologic Interactions* (P.L. Ogra, ed.), Greene & Stratton, Orlando, Florida, pp. 3–20

83. Allansmith, M., McClellan, B.H., Butterworth, M. and Maloney, S.R. (1968) The development of immunoglobulin levels in man. *J. Pediatrics*, **72**, 276–290

84. Kohler, P.F. and Farr, R.S. (1996) Elevation of cord over maternal IgG immunoglobulin: evidence for an active placental IgG transport. *Nature*, **210**: 1070–1071

85. Hobbs, J.R. and Davis, J.A. Serum IgG-globulin levels and gestational age in premature babies. *Lancet*, **1**, 757–759

86. Papadatos, C., Papaevangelou, G., Alexiou, D. and Mendris, J. (1964) Immunoglobulin levels and gestational age. *Biol. Neonate*, **14**, 365–373

87. Evans, H.E., Alpata, S.O. and Glass, L. (1971) Serum immunoglobulin levels in premature and full term infants. *Am. J. Clin. Pathol.*, **56**, 416–418

88. Hyvarinen, M., Zeltzer, P., Oh, W. and Stiehm, E.R. (1973) Influence of gestational age on serum levels of alpha-1 fetoprotein, IgG globulin, and albumin in newborn infants. *J. Paediatr.*, **82**, 430–437

89. Ballow, M., Cates, K.L., Rowe, J.C. *et al.* (1986) Development of the immune system in very low birth

weight (less than 1500 g) premature infants: concentrations of plasma immunoglobulins and patterns of infection. *Pediatr. Res.*, **20**, 899–904

90. Kinney, J., Mundorf, L., Gleason, C. *et al.* (1991) Efficacy and pharmokinetics of immune globulin administration to high-risk neonates. *Am. Dis. Child.*, **145**, 1233–1238

91. Baker, C.J. and Edwards, M.S. (1990) Methods for evaluating the protective activity of intravenous immunoglobulins for neonatal pathogens: entanglement or encouragement? *Pediatrics*, **86**, 995–996

92. Miller, M.E. and Stiehm, E.R. (1983) Immunology and resistance to infection. In *Infectious Diseases of the Fetus and Newborn Infant*, 2nd edn. (J.S. Remington and J.O. Klein, eds), Saunders, Philadelphia, pp. 27–68

93. Oxelius, V.A. and Svenningsen, N.W. (1984) IgG subclass concentrations in preterm neonates. *Acta Paediatr. Scand.*, **73**, 626–630

94. Cowan, M.J., Ammann, A.J., Wara, D.W. *et al.* Pneumococcal polysaccharide immunisation in infants and children. *Pediatrics*, **62**, 721–728

95. Kayhty, H., Somer, H.J., Peltola, H. *et al.* (1981) Antibody response to capsular polysaccharides of groups A and C Neisseria meningitidis and Haemophilus influenzae type b during bacteraemic disease. *J. Infect. Dis.*, **143**, 32–41

96. Smith, R.T., Eitzman, D.V., Catlin, M.E. *et al.* (1964) The development of the immune response. *Pediatrics*, **33**, 1

97. Uhr, J.W., Dancis, J., Franklin, E.C. *et al.* (1962) The antibody response to bacteriophage in newborn premature infants. *J. Clin. Invest.*, **41**, 1509–1513

98. Dancis, J., Osbor, J.J. and Kunz, H.W. (1953) Studies on the immunology of the newborn infant. *Pediatrics*, **12**, 151–156

99. Bernbaum, J.C., Daft, A., Anolik, R. *et al.* (1985) Response of preterm infants to diphtheria-tetanus-pertussis immunization. *J. Pediatr.*, **107**, 184–188

100. Ferguson, A.C., (1978) Prolonged impairment of cellular immunity in children with intrauterine growth retardation. *J. Pediatr.*, **93**, 52–56

101. Wilson, C.B. (1990) Developmental immunology and role of host defences in neonatal susceptibility. In *Infectious Diseases of the Fetus and Newborn Infant*, 3rd edn. (J.S. Remington and J.O. Klein, eds), Saunders, Philadelphia, pp. 17–67

102. Chandra, R.K. (1975) Fetal malnutrition and postnatal immunocompetence. *Am. J. Dis. Child.*, **129**, 450–454

103. McIntosh, N., Kempson, C. and Tyler, R.M. (1988) Blood counts in extremely low birth weight infants. *Arch. Dis. Childh.*, **63**, 74–76

104. Schlesinger, L. and Uauy, R. (1991) Nutrition and neonatal immune function. *Sem. Perinatol.*, **15**, 469–477

105. Johnson, L., Bowen, F.W., Abassi, S. *et al.* (1985) Relationship of prolonged pharmacologic serum levels of vitamin E to incidence of sepsis and necrotising enterocolitis in infants with birth weight 1500 grams or less. *Pediatrics*, **75**, 619–638

106. Carver, J.D., Pimental, B., Cox, W.I. and Berness, L.A. (1991) Dietary nucleotide effects upon immune function in infants. *Pediatrics*, **88**, 359–363

107. Pickering, L.K., Granoff, D.M., Erikson, J.R. *et al.* (1998) Modulation of the immune system by human milk and infant formula containing nucleotides. *Pediatrics*, **101**, 248–249

108. Go, L.L., Albanese, C.T., Watkins, S.C. *et al.* (1994) Breast milk protects the neonate from bacterial translocation. *J. Pediatr. Surg.*, **29**, 1059–1063

109. Ford, H.R., Avanogulu, A., Boechat, P.R. *et al.* (1996) The micro-environment influences the pattern of bacterial translocation in formula-fed neonates. *J. Pediatr. Surg.*, **31**, 486–489

110. el-Mohandes, A.E., Picard, M.B., Simmens, S.J. and Keiser, J.F. (1997) Use of human milk in the intensive care nursery decreases the incidence of nosocomial sepsis. *J. Perinatol.*, **17**, 130–134

111. Weisman, L.E., Stoll, B.J., Kueser, T.J. *et al.* (1992) Intravenous immune globulin therapy for early-onset sepsis in premature neonates. *J. Pediatr.*, **121**, 434–443

112. Peters, G., Locci, R. and Pulverer, G. (1982) Adherence and growth of coagulase-negative staphylococci on surfaces of intravenous catheters. *J. Infect. Dis.*, **146**, 479–482

113. Gray, E.D., Pteres, G., Verstegen, M. *et al.* (1984) Effect of extracellular slime substance from Staphylococcus epidermidis on the human cellular immune response. *Lancet*, **1**, 365–367

114. Faix, R.G., Kovarik, S.M., Shaw, T.R. and Johnson, R.V. (1989) Mucocutaneous and invasive candidiasis among very low birthweight (<1500 g) infants in intensive care nurseries: a prospective study. *Pediatrics*, **83**, 101–107

115. Baker, C.J., Mellish, M.E., Hall, R.T. *et al.* (1992) Intravenous immune globulin for the prevention of nosocomial infection in low-birth-weight neonates. *N. Engl. J. Med.*, **327**, 213–219

116. Fanaroff, A., Wright, E. Koroness, S. and Wright, L. (1992) A controlled trial of prophylactic intravenous immunoglobulin (IVIG) to reduce nosocomial infections in VLBW infants. *Pediatr. Res.*, **31**, 202A

117. Johnson, D.E., Thompson, T.R., Green, T.P. and Ferrieri, P. (1984) Systemic candidiasis in very low-birthweight infants (<1500 grams). *Pediatrics*, **73**, 138–143

118. Smith, H. and Congdon, P. (1985) Neonatal systemic candidiasis. *Arch. Dis. Childh.*, **60**, 365–369

119. Isaacs, D. (1990) Hospital-acquired infections. In *Infection in the Newborn* (J. de Louvois and D. Harvey, eds), Wiley, Chichester, p. 40

120. Botas, C.M., Kurlat, I., Young, S.M. and Sola, A. (1995) Disseminated candidal infections and intravenous hydrocortisone in preterm infants. *Pediatrics*, **95**, 883–7

121. Hitchcock, R.J., Pallett, A., Hall, M.A. and Malone, P.S. (1995) Urinary tract candidiasis in neonates and infants. *Br. J. Urol.*, **76**(2), 252–6

122. Visser, D., Monnens, L., Feitz, W. and Semmekrot, B.

(1998) Fungal bezoars as a cause of renal insufficiency in neonates and infants – recommended treatment strategy. *Clin. Nephrol.,* **49**(3), 198–201

123. Sims, M.E., Yoo, Y., You, H., Salminen, C. and Walther, F.J. (1988) Prophylactic oral nystatin and fungal infections in very-low-birthweight infants. *Am. J. Perinatol.,* **5**, 33–36

124. Freeman, J., Goldmann, D.A., Smith, N.E. *et al.* (1990) Association of intravenous lipid emulsion and coagu-lase-negative Staphylococcal bacteraemia in neonatal intensive care units. *N. Engl. J. Med.,* **323**, 301–308

125. Thompson, B. and Robinson, L.A. (1991) Infection control of parenteral nutrition solutions. *Nutr. Clin. Pract.,* **6**, 49–54

126. Avila-Figueroa, C., Goldmann, D.A. *et al.* (1998) Intravenous lipid emulsions are the major determi-nants of coagulase-negative staphylococcal bacter-emia in very low birth weight newborns. *Pediatr. Infect. Dis. J.,* **17**, 10–17

127. Shek, Y.H., Tucker, M.C., Viciana, A.L. *et al.* (1989) Malassezia furfur – disseminated infection in prema-ture infants. *Am. J. Clin. Pathol.,* **92**, 595–603

128. Surmont, I., Gavilanes, A., Vandepitte, J. *et al.* (1989) Malassezia furfur fungaemia in infants receiving intra-venous lipid emulsions. A rarity or just underesti-mated? *Eur. J. Pediatr.,* **148**, 435–438

129. Weiss, S.J., Schoch, P.E. and Cunha, B.A. (1991) Malassezia furfur fungaemia associated with central venous catheter lipid emulsion infusion. *Heart-Lung,* **20**, 87–90

130. Marcon, M.J. and Powell, D.A. (1992) Human infec-tions due to Malassezia spp. *Clin. Microbiol. Rev.,* **5**, 101–119

131. Gogos, C.A., Zoumbos, N.C., Makri, M. and Kalfar-entzos, F. (1992) Tumor necrosis factor production by human mononuclear cells during total parenteral nutrition containing long-chain triglycerides. *Nutri-tion,* **8**, 26–29

132. Salo, M. (1990) Inhibition of immunoglobulin synthe-sis *in vitro* by intravenous lipid emulsion (Intralipid). *J. Parent. Ent. Nutr.,* **14**, 459–46

133. Sirota, L., Straussberg, R., Notti, I. and Bessler, H. (1997) Effect of lipid emulsion on IL-2 production by mononuclear cells of newborn infants and adults. *Acta Pediatr.,* **86**, 410–403

134. Sedman, P.C., Somers, S.S., Ramsden, C.W. *et al.* (1991) Effects of different lipid emulsions on lympho-cyte function during total parenteral nutrition. *Br. J. Surg.,* **78**, 1396–1399

135. Palmblad, J. (1991) Intravenous lipid emulsions and host defences – A critical review. *Clin. Nutr.,* **10**, 303–308

136. Heinzerling, R.H., Nockels, C.F., Quarles, C.L. *et al.* (1974) Protection of chicks against *E. coli* infection by dietary supplementation with vitamin E. *Soc. Exp. Biol. Med.,* **146**, 279–283

137. Boxer, L., Harris, R. and Baehner, R. (1979) Regula-tion of membrane peroxidation in health and disease. *Pediatrics,* **64** (Suppl), 713–714

138. Prasad, J. (1980) Effect of vitamin E supplementation leukocyte function. *Am. J. Clin. Nutr.,* **33**, 606–608

139. Engle, W.A., Yoder, M.C., Baurley, J.L. *et al.* (1988) Vitamin E decreases superoxide anion production by polymorphonuclear leukocytes. *Pediatr. Res.,* **23**, 245–248

140. Fish, W.H., Cohen, M., Franzek, D., Williams, J.M. and Lemons, J.A. (1990) Effect of intramuscular Vitamin E on mortality and intracranial haemorrhage in neonates of 1000 grams or less. *Pediatrics,* **85**, 578–584

141. Shenai, J.P., Kennedy, K.A., Chytil, F. and Stahlman, M.T. (1987) Clinical trial of vitamin A supplementa-tion in infants susceptible to bronchopulmonary dysplasia. *J. Pediatr.,* **111**, 269–277

142. Mammel, M.C., Johnson, D.E., Green, T.P. and Thompson, T.R. (1983) Controlled trial of dexam-ethasone therapy in infants with bronchopulmonary dysplasia. *Lancet,* **1** (8338) (June 18th), 1356–1358

143. The Collaborative Dexamethasone Trial Group (1991) Dexamethasone therapy in neonatal chronic lung disease: an international placebo-controlled trial. *Pediatrics,* **88**, 421–427

144. Shinwell, E.S., Karplus, M. and Zmora, E. (1996) Failure of early postnatal dexamethasone to prevent chronic lung disease in infants with the respiratory distress syndrome. *Arch. Dis. Child. Fetal Neonatal Ed.,* **74**, F33–37

145. Yeh, T.F., Liu, Y.J., Lsieh, W.S. *et al.* (1997) Early postnatal dexamethasone therapy for the prevention of chronic lung disease in preterm infants with the respiratory distress syndrome. *Pediatrics,* **100**, e3

146. Stevenson, D., Walther, F., Long *et al.* (1992) Ameri-can Exosurf Neonatal Study Group 1. Controlled trial of a single dose of synthetic surfactant at birth in premature infants weighing 500 to 699 grams. *J. Pediatr.,* **120**, S3–12

147. Hoekstra, R.E., Jackson, J.C., Myers, T.F. *et al.* (1991) Improved neonatal survival following multiple doses of bovine surfactant in very premature neonates at risk for Respiratory Distress Syndrome. *Pediatrics,* **88**, 10–18

148. Corbet, A., Bucciarelli, R., Goldman, S., Mammel, M., Wold, D. and Long, W. (1991) US Exosurf Pediatric Study Group 1. Decreased mortality rate among small premature infants treated at birth with a single dose of synthetic surfactant: a multicenter controlled trial. *J. Pediatr.,* **118**, 277–284

149. Soll, R.F., Hoekstra, R.E., Fangman, J.J. *et al.* (1990) Ross Collaborative Surfactant Prevention Study Group. Multicenter trial of single-dose modified bovine surfactant extract (surfactant) for prevention of Respiratory Distress Syndrome. *Pediatrics,* **85**, 1092–1102

150. Taeusch, W., Alleyne, C., Takahashi, A. *et al.* (1989) In *Surfactant for the Treatment of Respiratory Distress Syndrome: Selected Clinical Issues* (D.L. Shapiro and R.H. Notter, eds), A.R. Liss, New York

151. Thomassen, M.J., Meeker, D.P., Antal, J.M., Connors, M.J. and Wiedemann, H.P. (1992) Synthetic surfactant

(Exosurf) inhibits endotoxin-stimulated cytokine secretion by human alveolar macrophages. *Am. J. Respir. Cell. Mol. Biol.*, **7**, 257–260

152. Zola, E.M., Overbach, A.M., Gunkel, H. *et al.* (1993) Treatment investigational new drug experience with Survanta (Beractant). *Pediatrics*, **91**, 546–551

153. Beeby, P.J. and Jeffrey, H. (1992) Risk factors for necrotising enterocolitis: the influence of gestational age. *Arch. Dis. Childh.*, **67**, 432–435

154. Eibl, M.M., Wolff, H.M., Furnkranz, H. and Rosenkranz, A. (1988) Prevention of necrotizing enterocolitis in low-birth-weight infants by IgA-IgG feeding. *N. Engl. J. Med.*, **319**, 1–7

155. Hall, M.A. (1990) Antibiotic policies. In: *Infection in the Newborn* (de Louvois, J., Harvey, D., eds), John Wiley & Sons, Chichester, pp. 127–43

156. Quercia, R.A., Hills, S.Q., Klimer, J.J. *et al.* (1986) Bacteriological contamination of intravenous infusion delivery systems in an intensive care unit. *Am. J. Med.*, **80**, 364–368

157. Salzman, M.B., Isenberg, H.D., Shapiro, J.F. *et al.* (1993) A prospective study of the catheter hub as the portal of entry for micro-organisms causing catheter-related sepsis in neonates. *J. Infect. Dis.*, **167**, 487–490

158. Bozetti, F. (1985) Central venous catheter sepsis. The experience of the Instituto Nazionale Tumori of Milan. *Acta Anaesth. Scand.*, **81** (Suppl), 53–57

159. Linares, J., Sitges Serra A., Garau, J. *et al.* (1985) Pathogenesis of catheter sepsis: a prospective study with quantitative and semi-quantitative cultures of catheter hub and segments. *J. Clin. Microbiol.*, **21**, 357–360

160. Kamal, G.D., Pfaller, M.A., Rempe, L.E. and Jebson, P.J. (1991) Reduced intravascular catheter infection by antibiotic bonding. A prospective, randomised, control trial. *JAMA*, **265**, 2364–2368

161. Thornton, J., Todd, N.J. and Webster, N.R. (1996) Central venous line sepsis in the intensive care unit. A study comparing antibiotic coated catheters with plain catheters. *Anaesthesia*, **51**, 1018–1020

162. Maki, D.G., Stolz, S.M., Wheeler, S. and Marmel, L.A. (1997) Prevention of central venous catheter-related bloodstream infection by the use of an antiseptic-impregnated catheter. A randomized, controlled trial. *Arch. Intern. Med.*, **127**, 257–266

163. Circesi, D.L., Albrecht, R.M., Vokers, P.A. and Scholten, D.J. (1996) Failure of antiseptic bonding to prevent central venous catheter-related infection and sepsis. *Ann. Surg.*, **62**, 641–646

164. Pemberton, L.B., Ross, V., Cuddy, P. *et al.* (1996) No difference in catheter sepsis between standard and antiseptic central venous catheters. A prospective randomised trial. *Arch. Surg.*, **131**, 986–989

165. Bailey, M.J. (1979) Reduction of catheter associated sepsis in parenteral nutrition using low-dose intravenous heparin. *Br. Med. J.*, **1**, 1671–1673

166. Raupp, P., Von Kries, R., Schmidt, E. *et al.* (1988) Incompatability between fat emulsion and calcium plus heparin in parenteral nutrition of premature babies. *Lancet*, **i**, 700

167. Rattenbury, J.M., Timmins, J.G., Cawthorne, E.A. *et al.* (1989) Identification of the cause of separation (creaming) of lipid emulsions in intravenous infusions. *J. Pediatr. Gastroenterol. Nutr.*, **8**, 491–495

168. Clapp, D.W., Kliegman, R.M., Baley, J.E. *et al.* (1989) Use of intravenously administered immune globulin to prevent nosocomial sepsis in low birth weight infants: report of a pilot study. *J. Pediatr.*, **115**, 973–978

167. Hill, H.R. (1991) Is prophylaxis of neonates with intravenous immunoglobulin beneficial? *Am. J. Dis. Child.*, **145**, 1229–1230

168. Hill, H.R. (1991) The role of intravenous immunoglobulin in the treatment and prevention of neonatal bacterial infection. *Semin. Perinatol.*, **15** (Suppl 12), 41–46

169. Didato, M.A., Gioeli, R. and Priolisi, A. (1988) The use of intravenous gamma-globulin for prevention of sepsis in pre-term infants. *Helv. Paediatr. Acta*, **43**, 283–294

170. Jenson, H.B. and Pollock, B.H. (1998) The role of intravenous immunoglobulins for the prevention and treatment of neonatal sepsis. *Semin. Perinatol.*, **22**, 50–63

171. Sideropoulos, D. (1986) Ig therapy in preterm infants with perinatal infections. In *Clinical Use of IVIG* (Morett A. Tyle, Nydiqquer V.E., eds), Academic Press, London, pp. 159–169

172. Haque, K.N. (1992) Immunotherapy in perinatal infection. *Early Hum. Dev.*, **29**, 137–141

173. Weisman, L.E., Cruess, D.F. and Fischer, G.W. (1993) Standard versus hyperimmune intravenous immunoglobulin in preventing or treating neonatal bacterial infections. *Clin. Perinatol.*, **20**, 211–224

174. Weisman, L.E., Anthony, B.F., Hemming, V.G. *et al.* (1993) Comparison of group B streptococcal hyperimmune and standard intravenously administered immune globulin in neonates. *J. Pediatr.*, **122**, 929–937

175. Shigeoka, A.O. (1990) Murine type-specific monoclonal antibodies in experimental group B Streptococcal infection: Interaction with complement components and phagocytes. *Semin. Perinatol.*, **14** (Suppl 1), 30–39

176. Hill, H.R., Gonzales, L.A., Kelsey, D.K. and Raff, H.V. (1992) The potential use of monoclonal antibodies as therapeutic modalities in neonatal infection. *Clin. Rev. Allergy.*, **10**, 29–38

177. Hill, H.R., Gonzales, L.A., Knappe, W.A. *et al.* (1991) Comparative protective activity of human monoclonal and hyperimmune polyclonal antibody against group B Streptococci. *J. Infect. Dis.*, **163**, 792–798

178. Harris, M.C., Douglas, S.D., Kolski, G.B. *et al.* (1982) Functional properties of anti-group B Streptococcal monoclonal antibodies. *Clin. Immunol. Immunopath.*, **24**, 342–350

179. Pincus, S.H., Shigeoka, A.O., Moe, A.A. *et al.* (1988) Protective efficacy of IgM monoclonal antibodies in experimental group B Streptococcal infection is a function of antibody avidity. *J. Immunol.*, **140**, 2779–2785

180. The PREVENT Study Group (1997) Reduction of respiratory syncitial virus hospitalization among premature infants and infants with bronchopulmonary dysplasia using respiratory syncitial virus immune globulin prophylaxis. *Pediatrics,* **99**, 93–99

181. The Impact-RSV Study Group (1998) Palivizumab, a humanized respiratory syncitial virus monoclonal antibody, reduces hospitalization from respiratory syncitial virus infection in high-risk infants. *Pediatrics,* **102**, 531–537

182. Kim, K.S. (1989) High dose intravenous immunoglobulin impairs the antibacterial activity of antibiotics. *J. Allergy Clin. Immunol.,* **84**,,579–588

183. Fukiwara, T., Taniuchi, S., Hattori, K. *et al.* (1997) Effect of immunoglobulin therapy on phagocytosis by polymorphonuclear leucocytes in whole blood of neonates. *Clin. Exp. Immunol.,* **107**, 435–439

184. Krediet, T.G., Beurskens, J.F., van Kijk, H. *et al.* Antibody responses and opsonic activity in sera of preterm neonates with coagulase-negative staphylococcal septicaemia and the effect of the administration of fresh frozen plasma. *Pediatr. Res.,* **43**, 645–651

185. Polin, R.A. (1990) Role of fibronectin in diseases of newborn infants and children. *Rev. Infect. Dis.,* **12** (suppl. 4), 5428–5438

186. Scovill, W.A., Saba, T.M. and Blumenstock, F.A. (1978) Opsonic gamma-2 surface binding glycoprotein therapy during sepsis. *Ann. Surg.,* **188**, 521–529

187. Saba, T.M., Blumenstock, F.A., Shah, D.M. *et al.* (1984) Reversal of fibronectin and opsonic deficiency in patients. *Ann. Surg.,* **199**, 87–96

188. Laurenti, F., Ferro, R., Isacchi, G. *et al.* (1981) Polymorphonuclear leukocyte transfusions for the treatment of sepsis in the newborn infant. *J. Pediatrics,* **98**, 118–122

189. Christensen, R.D., Rothstein, G., Anstall, H. and Bybee, B. (1982) Granulocyte transfusions in neonates with bacterial infection, neutropenia and depletion of mature neutrophils. *Pediatrics,* **70**, 1–6

190. Wheeler, J., Chauvenet, A., Johnson, C. *et al.* (1987) Buffy coat transfusions in neonates with sepsis and neutrophil storage pool depletion. *Pediatrics,* **79**, 422–425

191. Cairo, M.S., Rucker, R., Bennetts, G.A. *et al.* (1984) Improved survival of newborns receiving leukocyte transfusions for sepsis. *Pediatrics,* **74**, 887–892

192. Bailey, J., Stork, E., Warkentin, P. and Shurin, S. (1987) Buffy coat transfusions in neutropaenic neonates with presumed sepsis: a prospective randomized trial. *Pediatrics,* **80**, 712–20

193. Cairo, M.S., Worcester, C., Rucker, R. *et al.* (1992) Randomised trial of granulocyte transfusions versus intravenous immune globulin therapy for neonatal neutropenia and sepsis. *J. Pediatrics,* **120**, 281–285

194. Cairo, M.S., Worcester, C., Rucker, R. *et al.* (1987) Role of circulating complement and polymorphonuclear leukocyte transfusions in treatment and outcome in critically ill neonates with sepsis. *J. Pediatrics,* **110**, 935–41

195. Gillan, E.R., Christensen, R.D., Suen, Y. *et al.* (1994) A randomized, placebo-controlled trial of recombinant human granulocyte colony-stimulating factor administration in newborn infants with presumed sepsis: significant induction of peripheral and bone marrow neutrophilia. *Blood,* **84**, 1427–1433

196. Cairo, M.S., Christensen, R., Sender, L.S. *et al.* (1995) Results of a phase I/II trial of recombinant human granulocyte-macrophage colony stimulating factor in very low birth weight neonates: significant induction of circulating neutrophils, monocytes, platelets and bone marrow neutrophils. *Blood,* **86**, 2509–2515

197. Barak, Y., Leibovitz, E., Mogilner, B. *et al.* (1997) The in vivo effect of recombinant human granulocyte-colony stimulating factor (rbG-CSF) in neutropenic patients with sepsis. *Eur. J. Pediat.,* **156**, 643–6

198. Bedford-Russell, A.R., Graham Davies, E., Ball, S.E. *et al.* (1995) Granulocyte colony stimulating factor treatment for neonatal neutropenia. *Arch. Dis. Child.,* **72**, F53–F54

199. Drossou-Aga Kidou, V., KanaKoudi-TsaKalidou, F., Sarafidis, K. *et al.* (1900) Administration of recombinant human granulocyte-colony stimulating factor to septic neonates induces neutrophilia and enhances the neutrophil respiratory burst and beta 2 integrin expression. Results of a randomized controlled trial. *Eur. J. Pediatr.,* **157**, 583–588

200. Schibler, K.R., Osborne, K.A., Leung, L.Y. *et al.* (1998) A randomized, placebo-controlled trial of granulocyte colony-stimulating factor administration to newborn infants with neutropenia and clinical signs of early-onset sepsis. *Pediatrics,* **102**, 6–13

201. Calhoun, D.A., Rosa, C. and Christensen, R.D. (1996) Transplacental passage of recombinant human granulocyte colony-stimulating factor in women with an imminent preterm delivery. *Am. J. Obstet. Gynecol.,* **174**, 1306–1311

# 16

# Cardiac disorders including ductus arteriosus

**James Wilkinson**

Cyanosis, respiratory distress and other manifestations of congestive cardiac failure are familiar and frequent phenomena in the ELBW infant. Such problems, however, are usually not related to primary cardiac disorders but are more often the consequences of respiratory disease, infection or other early postnatal problems common in this group of infants.

A variety of factors render the severely immature baby vulnerable to cardiac dysfunction. Immaturity of the ductus arteriosus coupled with the relatively high levels of endogenous prostaglandin $E_2$ production, between 20 and 30 weeks' gestation, predispose to prolonged ductal patency and the development of a left-to-right shunt [1]. The heart and lungs of the infant adapt poorly to the development of a significant ductal shunt with its associated high pulmonary blood flow [2,3]. Perinatal hypoxia, respiratory disease perpetuating pulmonary hypertension, metabolic disturbances such as hypoglycaemia or hypocalcaemia, and infection may also have a profoundly adverse effect on cardiac function.

Structural congenital heart disease (other than persistent ductus) does not present a common problem in the ELBW infant. However, such infants are not immune to any of the congenital defects which affect more mature infants and experience in recent years in small preterm babies has included a wide variety of cardiac malformations.

Infective endocarditis, though an uncommon problem in the infant age group generally, has been documented in the small preterm infant with long intravenous catheters (often used for parenteral nutrition) even if the heart is structurally normal.

## Clinical examination

Assessment of cardiovascular signs in the ELBW infant is fraught with problems. Observation is often made difficult by the presence of monitoring equipment and multiple indwelling cannulas, and various tubes. It is frequently difficult to gain access to the infant for physical examination owing to the measures used, in the neonatal intensive care ward, to protect these tiny premature babies from hypothermia and insensible fluid loss. Such obvious signs as cyanosis and respiratory distress are frequently of pulmonary rather than cardiac origin. Pedal oedema (or oedema elsewhere) is a frequent finding in the premature nursery, is not cardiac in origin in most cases and may make assessment of peripheral pulses more difficult.

Palpation of peripheral pulses is extremely important and an assessment of peripheral tissue perfusion along with that of the radial and lower limb pulses is one of the most important initial observations. Bounding pulses are characteristic of the infant with a persistent ductus. Small volume femoral and/or upper limb pulses are common in very sick infants with a variety of non-cardiac problems, though the possibility of coarctation syndrome or hypoplastic left heart syndrome may need to be considered.

The significance of cyanosis is usually best assessed by measuring the response to a period of breathing at increased oxygen concentration. Arterial oxygen saturation is currently measured routinely in many neonatal units using pulse oximetry. A significant improvement in saturation with a period of ventilation in 50% or more oxygen makes major cyanotic heart disease unlikely. However, if doubt persists and if facilities for echocardiography are not readily available, a formal 'hyperoxic test' should be performed. This involves measurement of the arterial oxygen partial pressure $PaO_2$, either directly or transcutaneously, repeating the measurement after a short period of 100% oxygen breathing (either spontaneous or on ventilator). For obvious reasons, high concentrations of oxygen should not be continued beyond 15–20 min unless the arterial oxygen tension remains severely depressed. This test which is also referred to as the 'nitrogen washout' test can be useful in distinguishing between cyanosis of cardiac origin (in which cases the $PaO_2$ will usually remain well below 100 mmHg) and cyanosis due to other causes (where the $PaO_2$ generally rises to levels above 150 mmHg) [4]. However, some infants with severe respiratory problems or with persistent pulmonary hypertension due to pulmonary disease may show depressed arterial oxygen tensions despite high $FiO_2$.

Palpation of the cardiac impulse should be carried out as part of the routine. A forceful parasternal impulse may reflect pulmonary hypertension associated with pulmonary problems or the presence of a left-to-right shunt via a persistent ductus. Auscultation of the heart is mainly limited to the assessment and grading of any systolic or continuous murmur which is present. Such murmurs are often ejection in timing, best heard over the mid or upper precordium and essentially rather non-specific in character. It is usually difficult to reach a definite diagnosis of any specific cardiac pathology unless the coexistence of a murmur with bounding peripheral pulses with or without respiratory symptoms suggests that the murmur is due to a ductus.

## Ancillary investigations

### Chest X-ray

Radiography of the chest is carried out very frequently in the neonatal nursery, but unfortunately the radiographers involved are commonly lacking in expertise in handling tiny preterm infants and for a variety of reasons the quality of films produced is often poor. It is essential that the X-ray be taken with the help of nursing staff who can assist with the positioning and holding the baby. Of necessity, the film will be taken anteroposteriorly with the infant lying supine and with a tube to film distance usually less than 1 m. Furthermore, the lungs are frequently incompletely inflated due to lung disease and the phase of respiration is uncontrolled. All these factors contribute to an exaggeration of heart size and a cardiothoracic ratio of 0.6 or even 0.65 is therefore quite frequent. Assessment of lung vascularity is complicated by the presence of lung disease.

Although chest radiography is clearly an essential part of the investigation of an infant with suspected cardiac problems, in practice clinical findings and echocardiography are usually much more helpful in deciding whether a significant cardiac problem is present.

### Electrocardiogram

The ECG should include the standard 12 leads and a right-sided chest lead. Increased left ventricular forces may be found in the presence of a ductal shunt but are inconstant. The normal right ventricular preponderance which is seen in mature neonates may be rather less pronounced in the small preterm infant [5] and can give way to left ventricular preponderance in the early weeks of life, even in the absence of a large ductal shunt.

### Echocardiography

Echocardiography has become the most useful technique for determining the presence and nature of cardiac defects in infants. Examination of the heart can usually be accomplished simply and rapidly using cross sectional (2D) scanning in a variety of standard views (long axis, four chambers, aortic arch, ductus). The left atrial diameter can be readily measured from 2D or M mode scans and the degree of dilatation of the left atrium in the presence of a persistent ductus is a helpful diagnostic clue. M mode tracings alone can provide an accurate assessment of left atrial diameter but are of very limited value in the preterm infant in other respects as they provide no direct information about ductal patency or shunting through the duct.

Doppler echocardiography, and especially colour flow mapping (if available) will often provide definite diagnostic evidence of a left-to-right ductal shunt even if the ductus itself cannot be imaged satisfactorily. The size of the duct, if adequate imaging can be obtained, and the degree of dilatation of the left atrium and left ventricle, coupled with the Doppler and colour flow mapping information, give a comprehensive picture of the significance of the problem in almost all cases.

Limitations of echocardiography are related to the fact that hyperinflated lungs in a baby who is being ventilated may create considerable difficulties in gaining adequate imaging of the heart. Neonatal complications such as pneumothorax or interstitial emphysema in the mediastinum may provide a further barrier to ultrasound.

A major additional problem, however, pertains to the fact that the technique is heavily operator-dependent. Many paediatricians, radiologists or technicians with a modest amount of training can acquire a clear idea of normal appearances in standard echocardiographic views and of the findings in premature infants with a persistent ductus. However, competence at examining infants with structural congenital heart disease depends on familiarity with a variety of congenital anomalies and the echocardiographic findings to be expected with them. It is unfortunate that some of the more important diagnostic problems with structural cardiac defects (such as transposition of the great vessels, total anomalous pulmonary venous drainage, and coarctation syndrome) tend to present quite substantial challenges and can easily be missed by the less experienced operator, as intracardiac anatomy may appear normal.

## Range of cardiac defects encountered in preterm infants

Whilst the entire range of structural congenital heart disease can occasionally be seen in premature infants, it is clear that persistent ductus arteriosus is the only lesion which presents with any frequency.

Infants of birth weight <1500 g have been seen and treated, by the author, with such lesions as ventricular septal defect, aortic stenosis, coarctation of the aorta, transposition of the great arteries, truncus, aortic arch interruption, pulmonary atresia and total anomalous pulmonary venous drainage. Rarely major cardiac malformations, including transposition, have presented in ELBW infants.

A variety of cardiac problems may arise secondarily in relation to other neonatal problems. These include congestive cardiac failure resulting from lung disease, fluid overload or sepsis. Cor pulmonale may result from bronchopulmonary dysplasia in infants who have required prolonged ventilation. Infective endocarditis in infants who have had long lines may also occur; even in infants without structural cardiac defects as a predisposing factor.

## Management of congestive heart failure

Cardiac failure manifested by respiratory distress, hepatomegaly and oedema may require treatment regardless of its underlying cause. However, it is clearly important that the aetiological factors be identified and if possible treated actively.

Some degree of fluid restriction is desirable in the infant with evidence of congestive failure. This is especially important as fluid overload predisposes to ductal patency [6]. Fluid intake should be limited to 120–150 ml kg$^{-1}$ depending on the severity of symptoms. In some cases fluid restriction alone may ameliorate the symptoms but if significant evidence of congestive failure persists diuretic therapy should be instituted. Traditionally in recent years frusemide (1 mg kg$^{-1}$ once or twice daily orally) has been used as the first choice diuretic but there is some evidence that this drug may stimulate endogenous production of prostaglandin E$_2$ and may thus promote ductal patency [7]. As this would clearly be deleterious in the management of such infants it may be preferable to use chlorothiazide (15 mg kg$^{-1}$ orally) which apparently does not produce the same effect on prostaglandin release. Thus far, however, there appears to be no conclusive evidence that morbidity or mortality are improved by the use of chlorothiazide in preference to frusemide.

Hyponatraemia or hypokalaemia may develop during diuretic therapy. Hypokalaemia can be prevented or corrected by the addition of potassium supplements or of a potassium-sparing diuretic such as Amiloride or Spironolactone.

The use of digitalis in the management of cardiac failure is controversial in premature infants. There is little evidence that digoxin has any useful therapeutic effect and its potential toxicity demands that it be used with considerable caution, if at all [8]. Most neonatologists prefer to avoid its use in the preterm infant.

## Persistent ductus arteriosus

Failure of the ductus to close normally in the newborn period in the ELBW infant is related to a combination of factors. Immaturity of ductal wall structure itself is associated with reduced responsiveness to the increased $PO_2$ of blood perfusing the duct after birth. Secondly, high levels of endogenous prostaglandin $E_2$ further inhibit ductal constriction [1,9]. Thirdly, the presence of pulmonary problems such as hyaline membrane disease tend to result in reduced arterial $PO_2$, which itself prolongs ductal patency.

It has been suggested that delay in closure of the ductus is almost invariable in the ELBW infant and that it is possible to demonstrate a patent ductus on cross-sectional echocardiography in virtually all infants below 32 weeks' gestation [10]. However, echocardiographic studies, with Doppler interrogation of the duct, in infants of more than 30 weeks' gestation suggest that in most the ductus closes spontaneously over 3 to 4 days, even in the presence of respiratory distress syndrome [11]. The incidence of clinically apparent persistent ductus in preterm babies has been reported as being 7–25% of all premature infants and 35% in those below 1500 g. In those below 1000 g the figure is probably greater than 70% [12] and it is clearly in the ELBW infant that the problem is of major and frequent significance.

### Haemodynamics

The appearance of a left-to-right shunt through a persistent ductus arteriosus is dependent on a fall in the level of pulmonary artery pressure and resistance after birth. The presence of severe pulmonary problems and positive pressure ventilation may result in retention of high pulmonary resistance initially and hence a significant shunt may not become apparent for several days.

The development of a large shunt results in substantial volume loading on the left ventricle and, in the small preterm infant in whom left ventricular reserve is very limited, this rapidly results in the appearance of symptoms of left heart failure [2,3]. It has often been suggested that the immature left ventricle responds to volume loading by increased rate rather than increasing stroke volume. This is evidently untrue as evidenced by recent careful echocardiographic studies in which changes in heart rate and stroke volume were measured serially in premature infants. The presence of a significant ductal shunt was universally accompanied by a substantial increase in stroke volume [13,14].

### Symptoms and signs

The appearance of a precordial murmur, often found in the course of routine examination, may be the first manifestation of a ductal shunt; though it should be appreciated that a significant ductal shunt can develop in the absence of any audible murmur [15]. Such murmurs are usually systolic in timing and may be clearly heard along the left sternal border and in the pulmonary area. In some cases the

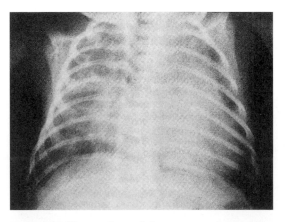

**Figure 16.1** Chest radiograph from preterm infant with large persistent ductus arteriosus. The cardiomegaly and pulmonary congestion are obvious, but most of the features are non-specific in an infant of this age

murmur is more obviously continuous. Commonly the murmur appears and increases in intensity in the latter part of the first week or the second week of life. Characteristically the murmur varies in timing and amplitude from day to day or even hour to hour. Peripheral pulses are often bounding, and this feature in conjunction with murmur is very strongly suggestive of a persistent ductus.

Symptoms of pulmonary congestion include tachypnoea, dyspnoea and in more severe cases the development of respiratory failure with cyanosis and apnoeic attacks. Manifestations of right heart failure with hepatomegaly and oedema are inconstant.

The onset of respiratory symptoms in preterm infants with a persistent ductus often occurs at a time when the infant is beginning to improve after early respiratory difficulties related to hyaline membrane disease. The major indication of a significant ductal shunt may well be an exacerbation of respiratory symptoms in the latter part of the first week or the second week of life and it is often difficult to differentiate between symptomatology related to the initial respiratory disorder and that which results from ductal patency.

## Diagnosis

The presence of a persistent ductus may best be demonstrated by cross-sectional echocardiography with Doppler examination. In the absence of echocardiography the diagnosis rests on clinical findings, but as a highly significant ductal shunt may develop with minimal cardiac

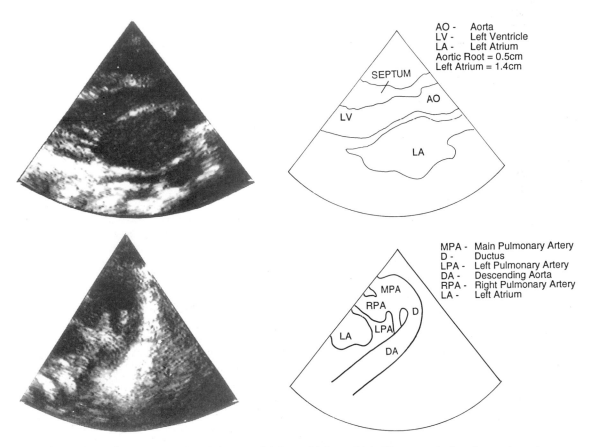

**Figure 16.2** Echocardiograms from 650 g infant, aged 4 days, with large PDA. Upper panels show long axis section through left atrium (LA) and aortic root (AO). The left atrium is markedly dilated, with a ratio of LA:aortic root of more than 2:1. Lower panels show 'ductus cut' with a wide PDA (D) connecting the pulmonary artery (MPA) to the descending aorta (DA). In this view the aortic arch itself is not seen. Doppler interrogation (with continuous wave or pulsed wave sampling) in the ductus or in the pulmonary artery should be used to confirm ductal shunting, which will also be demonstrated by colour flow mapping.

signs the absence of such signs cannot be relied on as a safe means of excluding a persistent ductus [15]. The chest X-ray (Figure 16.1) and ECG findings are frequently non-specific though radiological evidence of cardiomegaly and pulmonary plethora may be found and in some cases left ventricular hypertrophy may be apparent on the ECG after 2–3 weeks.

Cross-sectional echocardiography may show evidence of left atrial and left ventricular dilatation and the ductus arteriosus itself can often be visualized directly (Figure 16.2) [10]. Unfortunately it is not always possible to obtain good imaging of the ductus, especially in the ventilated infant. The left lung if hyperinflated tends to intrude into the path of the ultrasound beam resulting in loss of image.

Dilatation of the left atrium, as indicated by an increased ratio of left atrial diameter to aortic root dimension, has been regarded as a reliable indicator of a significant shunt [16]. This ratio is normally less than one but, in the presence of a ductus, values between 1.1 and 1.5 are usually obtained. These measurements may be made using M mode echocardiography or from cross-sectional images. Unfortunately, a normal left atrial to aortic root ratio does not completely exclude a significant ductus.

Doppler interrogation of the pulmonary artery is the most precise non-invasive means of establishing the diagnosis. Pulsed wave or continuous wave sampling will usually confirm ductal shunting, if present and colour flow mapping will also help to demonstrate the shunt from the aorta to the pulmonary trunk. It is noteworthy that in some premature infants even when the ductus may appear still to be patent on cross-sectional imaging, no flow is demonstrable on Doppler examination, this being usually indicative that the ductus is functionally closed.

Cardiac catheterization should be avoided. It is not usually regarded as being necessary to establish the diagnosis, and carries a significant morbidity and even mortality in small premature infants.

## Treatment

Initial treatment of infants with clinical signs of a persistent ductus follows the lines indicated for the management of congestive heart failure. In the infant who is only mildly symptomatic fluid restriction alone may be sufficient to tide him over until his ductus undergoes spontaneous closure. Those patients with more significant symptoms usually require institution of diuretic therapy.

Infants who remain symptomatic after 24–48 hours of diuretic therapy, combined with fluid restriction, will usually benefit from treatment with prostaglandin synthetase inhibitors, of which indomethacin is the drug which has been used in clinical practice with significant effect [17]. This preparation may be administered orally, rectally or intravenously, and is usually given in a total dose of 0.6 mg $kg^{-1}$ in divided doses. Intravenous administration is simple and effective and is probably preferable to the oral or rectal routes [18]. Traditionally the course of treatment was administered over 24 hours using three doses of 0.2 mg $kg^{-1}$. An alternative is to use prolonged low dose therapy over 6 days giving 0.1 mg $kg^{-1}$ daily [19] and this is now the preferred regime in many institutions.

The policy on the administration of indomethacin has varied widely between different neonatal units. In some centres a very low threshold for drug treatment has been maintained and a high proportion of preterm infants have been given indomethacin treatment in the early days of life [20]. This method of management of persistent ductus in the premature baby has some strong supporters who have reported high rates of spontaneous closure following such therapy. Many other centres have been more cautious in the use of indomethacin, being concerned about such side-effects as gastrointestinal bleeding and renal impairment. In such neonatal units indomethacin treatment is usually withheld until the infant has had a prolonged trial of other and conventional management. Only those infants who are very severely symptomatic and ventilator-dependent have been treated and often not until they are 2–3 weeks old or later. In general, results of such a highly selective approach to indomethacin therapy have been disappointing [21].

A large multicentre trial has suggested that a more appropriate line to pursue is that those infants who have clear-cut manifestations of a ductus (murmur, bounding pulses, respiratory distress) should be managed vigorously with fluid restriction if necessary and subsequent diuretic therapy. If symptoms do not resolve satisfactorily within 48 hours of the institution of such therapy, indomethacin treatment should be started [22]. The recent demonstration, by echocardiography, of infants with significant ductal shunting in the absence of clinical signs raises another issue. It may well prove that optimal management of the ELBW neonate should involve routine echocardiographic screening for a ductal shunt during the early days of life in order that treatment may be initiated if a large left to right shunt is found, notwithstanding that the diagnosis may have been unsuspected previously because of the lack of a murmur or other clinical evidence.

Side-effects of indomethacin treatment are a cause for concern. Gastrointestinal bleeding, intestinal perforation and renal impairment have all been attributed to this drug. These are certainly more frequent in ELBW infants than in those of greater birth weight and as response rates to indomethacin therapy are less good in the ELBW group some authors remain sceptical about the wisdom of employing indomethacin in preference to surgical ligation [23] in these babies. The use of prolonged low dose indomethacin, rather than conventional treatment over 24 hours, was associated with less renal impairment but did not reduce the incidence of other complications of therapy [19].

The employment of prostaglandin synthetase inhibitors in the management of persistent ductus in the preterm neonate has certainly led to a significant increase in the closure rate and a reduction in neonatal morbidity and mortality. The effectiveness of treatment can usually be judged by clinical evidence of a diminution in the ductal shunt. Respiratory symptoms improve and the murmur may well disappear, as also the bounding pulses. Echocardiography will often show a reduction in left atrial dilatation and actual closure of the ductus may be confirmed by cross-sectional imaging or Doppler interrogation.

Unfortunately, a proportion of cases (20–40%) show subsequent re-opening of the ductus and if this leads to a recurrence of symptoms a second course of indomethacin may sometimes be worth considering after an interval of 3–4 days. The relative frequency with which the duct reopens in ELBW infants probably reflects the absence of intimal cushions in the ductal wall [24] (these usually developing in the last ten weeks of gestation). These cushions are implicated in the process by which ductal closure normally becomes 'fixed' within a few hours, so that once closed the mature ductus will not reopen.

Infants who remain severely symptomatic despite these measures and especially those who remain ventilator-dependent and cannot be weaned from respiratory support usually require surgical ligation of their ductus. This procedure can be carried out with low morbidity and mortality even in ELBW infants. In experienced surgical hands ductal ligation is remarkably safe and well tolerated. In some centres surgery is performed in the special care baby unit, the surgeon and his team coming to the patient. Using this approach Coster and colleagues dealt with more than 100 small premature infants, in whom they employed an extrapleural technique applying clips to the ductus, without mortality or significant morbidity [25]. In other institutions the affected infant is transferred to the cardiac surgical department for operation in the cardiac theatre, but in general such infants are transferred back to the neonatal unit after surgery for postoperative care. The diagnosis is confirmed by echocardiography preoperatively and cardiac catheterization is avoided.

## Other structural cardiac defects

Whilst a variety of congenital malformations have been seen in ELBW babies, it would not be appropriate in this chapter to discuss in any detail those problems which are not specific to this group of infants. As in the mature infant, the presentation of serious congenital heart disease in the newborn period is frequently related to ductal closure and its effects on the haemodynamic disturbance produced by the cardiac abnormality. Thus a substantial group of 'ductus-dependent defects' are characterized by presentation in the first week or ten days of life. Such defects include those in which the pulmonary circulation is largely or entirely ductus-dependent, e.g. pulmonary atresia, critical pulmonary stenosis, severe tetralogy of Fallot, tricuspid atresia. Defects of this kind are associated with increasing cyanosis as the ductus constricts. In the small premature infant ductal closure is often delayed for the reasons indicated earlier and infants with these conditions may therefore show little cyanosis in the early days of life, resulting in some cases in delay in diagnosis. It is also noteworthy that as the physical signs may be dominated by the murmur of a ductus and cyanosis may be minimal or absent in the immediate newborn period, therapy to bring about ductal constriction (indomethacin therapy or surgery), which would clearly be harmful to these infants, should not be instituted until the clinical diagnosis has been confirmed by echocardiography.

Another group of ductus-dependent defects are those in which part or all of the systemic circulation is ductus-dependent. Such defects include hypoplastic left heart syndrome, some examples of critical aortic stenosis and conditions in which the lower systemic segment is ductus-dependent postnatally as in aortic arch interruption and particularly infantile coarctation syndrome. Once again in the preterm infant where ductal closure is delayed the clinical signs and symptomatology associated with such defects may appear late and initially at any rate lower limb pulses may be easily palpable, resulting in diagnostic delay.

### Management

Medical treatment of infants with major structural heart defects, who are of very low weight and are considered to be poor surgical candidates, is aimed at controlling heart failure (with anticongestive therapy) or maintaining ductal patency where a ductus-dependent defect is found to be present. The main objective is to get the infant to a stage where surgical palliation or repair is a realistic option. Prolonged intravenous prostaglandin therapy may merit consideration, or alternatively oral PG $E_2$ may be employed. Closed heart procedures including coarctation repair and systemic-to-pulmonary-shunt procedures are applicable to infants at weights down to 1500 g or less, though the prospects of success in the ELBW range are not such as to encourage surgical intervention unless no other option is available. Open heart procedures present almost insuperable barriers in the extremely low birth weight infant as the existing perfusion equipment and cannulae are not designed to cater for this group of patients. However, successful intracardiac repairs have been undertaken, in many centres, for a range of lesions, in infants in the range 1200–1500 g, and in the latter part of 1992 a 900 g infant, from Western Australia, had successful complete repair, on heart/lung bypass, of aortic arch interruption with VSD at the Royal Children's Hospital, Melbourne, this being believed to have been the smallest infant to have had this type of surgery.

## Cardiac problems secondary to non-cardiac disease in the premature

### Cor pulmonale

The development of manifestations of heart failure in infants with chronic respiratory disease (notably bronchopulmonary dysplasia) is an increasingly frequent phenomenon as more tiny preterm infants survive following prolonged and vigorous intensive care.

In such infants manifestations of chronic respiratory disease including dyspnoea, tachypnoea and cyanosis with chronic oxygen dependence are often combined with signs of right heart failure including hepatomegaly and oedema.

The manifestations of cardiac failure tend to develop late, often after the first month of life. It is important to look for evidence of any structural cardiac problem (best excluded by echocardiography) but provided that no such abnormality is present, treatment of cardiac failure follows standard lines and the most important consideration is active management of the underlying lung disease with particular attention to nutrition and to chronic oxygen therapy where indicated. In treating congestive heart failure it is important to bear in mind that the respiratory symptoms are likely to be largely, if not entirely, unrelated to the presence of congestive failure (left heart failure usually being absent in such infants). Treatment should therefore only be aimed at controlling manifestations of right heart failure and diuretic doses should in general be kept to the minimum which will achieve this.

### Endocarditis and sepsis

Whilst infective endocarditis is generally extremely rare in the infant age group, there are now an increasing number of reports of endocarditis occurring in neonates. Most affected infants have suffered from severe bacterial infections (especially septicaemia) associated with the use of long indwelling lines, often used to administer parenteral nutrition [26–29]. Infecting organisms tend to be either *Staphylococcus aureus* or candida, though other pathogens have been implicated. Infection may affect either side of the heart, involving any of the cardiac valves and the two sides have been affected with approximately equal

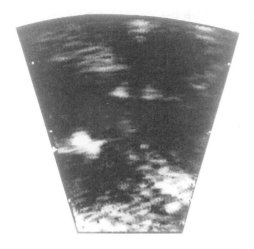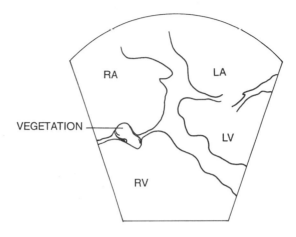

**Figure 16.3** Echocardiogram (four chambers view) from an ELBW infant with endocarditis and vegetation on the tricuspid valve. LA = left atrium. RA = right atrium. LV = left ventricle. RV = right ventricle

frequency [29]. Many patients develop features of disseminated intravascular coagulation [30], though the main characteristics of the disease are the signs of septicaemia associated with the presence of a murmur, with or without manifestations of congestive failure. Signs associated with endocarditis in older children and adults, such as splenomegaly, petechial haemorrhages, Osler nodes, etc. are usually absent. Establishment of a firm diagnosis of endocarditis is dependent on positive blood cultures coupled with identification of vegetations by echocardiography (Figure 16.3), which should be performed routinely in all neonates with long lines who develop evidence of major systemic infection. However, it should be appreciated that endocarditis may occur in the absence of echocardiographically demonstrable vegetations [29]. Effective antimicrobial therapy, which usually necessitates prolonged intravenous therapy with combinations of antibiotics based on bacteriological evidence, may eliminate the infection [30,31], though the disease carries a high mortality.

The indications appear to be that most affected infants have no structural cardiac abnormality prior to the development of endocarditis and in this respect endocarditis in these infants clearly differs from the pattern seen in older children or adults.

Non-bacterial thrombotic endocarditis has been noted at autopsy in neonates dying from a range of causes [29]. The condition occurs predominantly in the right side of the heart and

is again associated with long lines and in some cases evidence of DIC. Other factors implicated have included hypoxia, persistent pulmonary hypertension and respiratory distress syndrome.

---

**Practical points**

1. In the very low birth weight infant 'cardiac' symptoms and signs are often non-cardiac in origin (e.g. cyanosis, oedema, respiratory distress).
2. A significant persistent ductus may be clinically silent (hence the need for routine echocardiography in very low birth weight infants).
3. Indomethacin therapy is more likely to be effective in persistent ductus arteriosus of prematurity if administered early (first 5–10 days).
4. Surgical ligation of persistent ductus arteriosus in the ELBW infant, can be performed safely, often in the neonatal nursery.
5. Septicaemia in the ELBW infant should raise the possibility of endocarditis and makes echocardiography desirable (vegetations?).
6. Ready availability of facilities for echocardiography should be regarded as essential in every neonatal intensive care unit.

# References

1. Clyman, R.I. (1986) Pharmacology of the fetal and neonatal ductus arteriosus. In *Pediatric Cardiology* (E.F. Doyle, M.A. Engle, W.M. Gersony, W.J. Rashkind and N.J. Talner, eds), Springer-Verlag, New York, pp. 871–875
2. Baylen, B., Meyere, R.A., Karfhagen, J., Benzig, G. III, Bubb, M.E. and Kaplan, S. (1977) Left ventricular performance in the critically ill premature infant with patent ductus arteriosus and pulmonary disease. *Circulation*, **55**, 182–188
3. Alverson, D.C., Marlowe, W.E., Johnson, J.D. *et al.* (1983) Effect of patent ductus arteriosus on left ventricular output in premature infants. *J. Pediatr.*, **102**, 754–757
4. Jones, R.W.A., Baumer, J.H., Joseph, M.C. and Shinebourne, E.A. (1976) Arterial oxygenation and response to oxygen breathing in differential diagnosis of congenital heart disease in infancy. *Arch. Dis. Childh.*, **51**, 667–673
5. Thomaidis, C., Varlamis, G. and Karamperis, S. (1988) Comparative study of the electrocardiogram of healthy fullterm and premature newborns. *Acta Paediatr. Scand.*, **77**, 653–657
6. Stevenson, J.G. (1977) Fluid administration in the association of patent ductus arteriosus complicating respiratory distress syndrome. *J. Pediatr.*, **90**, 257–261
7. Green, T.P., Thompson, T.R., Johnson, D.E. and Lock, J.E. (1983) Frusemide promotes patent ductus arteriosus in premature infants with respiratory distress syndrome. *N. Engl. J. Med.*, **308**, 743–748
8. Berman, W., Dubynsky, O., Whitman, V., Friedman, Z. and Maisels, M.J. (1978) Digoxin therapy in low-birth-weight infants with patent ductus arteriosus. *J. Pediatr.*, **93**, 652–655
9. Olley, P.M. and Coceani, F. (1979) Mechanism of closure of the ductus arteriosus. In *Pediatric Cardiology*, Vol. 2 (M.J. Godman and R.M. Marquis, eds), Churchill Livingstone, Edinburgh, pp. 15–24
10. Rigby, M.L., Pickering, D. and Wilkinson, A. (1984) Cross sectional echocardiography in determining persistent patency of the ductus arteriosus in premature infants. *Arch. Dis. Childh.*, **59**, 341–345
11. Reller, M.D., Colasurdo, M.A., Rice, M.J. and McDonald, R.W. (1990) The timing of spontaneous closure of the ductus arteriosus in infants with respiratory distress syndrome. *Am. J. Cardiol.*, **66**, 75–78
12. Siassi, B., Blanco, C., Cabal, L.A. and Coran, A.G. (1976) Incidence and clinical features of patent ductus arteriosus in low birth-weight infants. A prospective analysis of 150 consecutively born infants. *Pediatrics*, **57**, 347–351
13. Lindner, W., Seidel, M., Versmold, H.T., Dohlemann, C. and Riegel, K.P. (1990) Stroke volume and left ventricular output in preterm infants with patent ductus arteriosus. *Pediatr. Res.*, **27**, 278–281
14. Walther, F.M., Kim, D.H., Ebrahimi, M. and Siassi, B. (1989) Pulsed Doppler measurement of left ventricular output as early predictor of symptomatic patent ductus arteriosus in very preterm infants. *Biol. Neonate*, **56**, 121–128
15. Zanardo, V., Milanesi, O., Trevisanuto, D., Rizzo, M., Ronconi, M. and Stellin, G. (1991) Early screening and treatment of 'silent' patent ductus arteriosus in prematures with RDS. *J. Perinatal Med.*, **19**, 291–295
16. Silverman, N.H., Lewis, A.B., Heymann, M.A. and Rudolph, A.M. (1974) Echocardiographic assessment of ductus arteriosus shunt in premature infants. *Circulation*, **50**, 821–825
17. Heymann, M.A., Rudolph, A.M. and Silverman, N.H. (1976) Closure of the ductus arteriosus in premature infants by inhibition of prostaglandin synthesis. *N. Engl. J. Med.*, **295**, 530–533
18. Yeh, T.F., Luken, J.A., Thalji, A., Raval, D., Carr, I. and Pildes, R.C. (1981) Intravenous indomethacin therapy in premature infants with persistent ductus arteriosus, a double blind study. *J. Pediatr.*, **98**, 137–145
19. Rennie, J.M. and Cooke, R.W.I. (1991) Prolonged low dose Indomethacin for persistent ductus arteriosus of prematurity. *Arch. Dis. Childh.*, **66**, 55–58
20. Mahony, L., Carnero, V., Brett, C., Heymann, M.A. and Clyman, R.I. (1982) Prophylactic indomethacin therapy for patent ductus arteriosus in very low birth-weight infants. *N. Engl. J. Med.*, **306**, 506–510
21. Cooke, R.W.I. and Pickering, D. (1979) Poor response to oral indomethacin therapy for persistent ductus arteriosus in very low birth weight babies. *Br. Heart J.*, **41**, 301–303
22. Gersony, W.M., Peckham, G.J., Ellison, R.C., Mieltinen, O.S. and Nadas, A.S. (1983) Effects of indomethacin in premature infants with patent ductus arteriosus: results of a national collaborative study. *J. Pediatr.*, **102**, 895–905
23. Rajadurai, V.S. and Yu, V.S. (1991) Intravenous indomethacin therapy in preterm neonates with patent ductus arteriosus. *J. Paediatr. Child Health*, **27**, 370–375
24. Gittenberger de Groot, A.C., Van Ertenbruggen, I., Moulaert, A.J.M. and Harinck, E. (1980) The ductus arteriosus in the preterm infant: histologic and clinical observations. *J. Pediatr.*, **96**, 88–93
25. Coster, D.D., Gorton, M.E., Grooters, R.K., Thieman, K.C., Schneider, R.F. and Soltanzadeh H. (1989) Surgical closure of the patent ductus in the neonatal intensive care unit. *Ann. Thorac. Surg.*, **48**, 386–389
26. Delberg, D.G., Fisher, D.J., Gross, D.M., Denson, S.E. and Alcock, C.W. (1983) Endocarditis in high risk neonates. *Pediatrics*, **71**, 392–397
27. McGuiness, G.A., Schieken, R.M. and Maguire, G.F. (1980) Endocarditis in the newborn. *Am. J. Dis. Child.*, **134**, 577–580
28. O'Callaghan, C., and McDougall, P. (1988) Infective endocarditis in neonates. *Arch. Dis. Childh.*, **63**, 53–57
29. Millard, D.D. and Shulman, S.T. (1988) The changing spectrum of neonatal endocarditis. *Clin. Perinatol.*, **15**, 587–608
30. Hernandez, I., Arcil, G., Farru, O. and Badner, A. (1990) Neonatal infectious endocarditis. Apropos of 5 cases. *Arch. Mal. Coeur. Vaiss.*, **83**, 627–631
31. Sanchez, P.J., Siegel, J.D. and Fishbein, J. (1991) Candida endocarditis: successful medical management in three preterm infants and review of the literature. *Pediatr. Infect. Dis. J.*, **10**, 239–243

# 17

# Renal function

**Neena Modi and Malcolm Coulthard**

Good clinical practice has to be based on a sound understanding of physiology but unfortunately few studies have been undertaken of renal function in babies weighing less than 1000 g. Further, there is no ideal preterm animal model in which the various aspects of kidney function are known to mature in parallel with that of the human baby. Many of our practices have been based on data extrapolated from larger and mature subjects. There are dangers in this approach, and caution is needed to ensure that data from small babies are not misinterpreted by comparison with inappropriate standards, that investigation techniques for larger subjects really can be applied to these infants, and that what is extrapolation is not regarded as fact.

## Standardizing measurements

In order to compare renal function between very small infants and larger subjects, it is necessary to standardize data by expressing them per unit body size. In older subjects, the glomerular filtration rate (GFR) and the metabolic rate (which largely determines the need for the excretion of waste products) vary closely with body surface area, and this is the most commonly used standard to compare values between individuals. However, this has only been demonstrated to be appropriate after the age of 2 years when the relationship between body surface and body weight alters only slowly. The relationship changes almost

week by week in preterm babies (Figure 17.1) [1,2] so that the standard chosen makes a much greater difference.

Body weight is the best index for standardizing GFR in babies. Variations in GFR between infants of 27–40 weeks' gestation are reduced

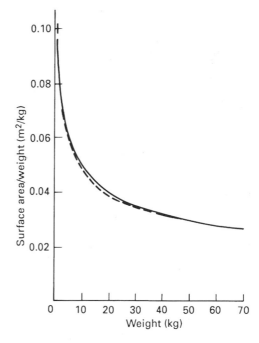

**Figure 17.1** Relation between surface area/weight ratio and body weight, —— calculated from Boyd [1] and --- from Haycock *et al.* [2] using the 50th centile values from national height and weight standards and taken from Coulthard and Hey [3].

more than two-fold by expressing the data as GFR $kg^{-1}$ rather than GFR $m^2$ [3], which is similar to previous findings for metabolic rate [4]. Furthermore, body weight can be accurately and directly measured, whereas values of body surface area can only be estimated from formulae which themselves have been derived from much more mature subjects. The proposal to relate function to the size of the pool over which the kidney exercises control [5] is similarly impractical because, like surface area, fluid volumes would be estimated rather than measured. Furthermore, no single fluid volume would be appropriate; total body water would be best for considering urea and water handling, whereas extracellular fluid volume would be best for creatinine or gentamicin handling. Clinical management decisions such as fluid and electrolyte requirements and drug dosages are all based on body weight, and the use of a different system to describe kidney function does nothing to help incorporate information derived from renal research into routine practice. Clearly body weight is the best practical standard, but as has been observed in the past, it has proved difficult to change established practice.

## Developmental changes and implications for clinical management

### Glomerular filtration

The development of new glomeruli occurs only slowly in the last trimester and stops by about 36 weeks [6]. Renal growth thereafter depends on an increase in the size and number of cells of the existing nephrons. The earliest glomeruli to mature are the deep (corticomedullary) ones which are associated with the longest loops of Henle and have the greatest role in sodium conservation [7]. The glomeruli are relatively larger than the tubules, with a glomerular surface area:proximal tubular volume ratio about ten times that seen in adults [8]. Despite this anatomical glomerulo-tubular imbalance, it is clear that glomerular and tubular functions must be linked and develop in parallel for physiological balance to be achieved.

The GFR has been described as increasing from 32 weeks [9] and 34 weeks [10] and even as slowing from 35 weeks' gestation [11]. For

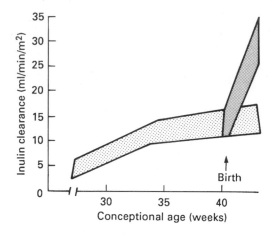

**Figure 17.2** Diagram from Fawer *et al.* [11] showing how glomerular filtration rate $m^2$ was considered to develop with post-conceptional age and illustrating how birth was considered to be 'the signal to a striking increase in glomerular filtration rate'

some time it was thought that GFR was extremely low *in utero* while the baby was effectively dialysed through the placenta, and that it rose steeply 'in response to need after birth' [11] (Figure 17.2). However, more recently it has been shown that GFR rises logarithmically in a 'programmed' fashion with increasing post-conceptional age and is independent of postnatal age [9,10,12]. Apparent contradictions between studies have been shown to be the result of the way in which the data have been expressed. On recalculation, all studies show the same logarithmic rise of absolute GFR which is uninfluenced by the timing of birth. This includes the data from which Figure 17.2 was derived (Figure 17.3) [12]. It is almost universally assumed that GFR is especially low in the first 2 days after birth, but very few measurements have been made [12].

The efficiency of elimination of a substance that is removed mainly by glomerular filtration (such as gentamicin) is best defined by the half life; the time taken for its plasma concentration to fall to half of its original value. This is dependent on both the absolute GFR and the volume of the pool into which the substance is distributed, which in the case of gentamicin is the extracellular fluid (ECF). Since GFR increases with conceptional age and ECF is determined primarily by body weight, it follows that the efficiency of the infant kidney

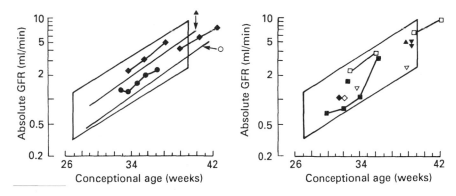

**Figure 17.3** Graphs of the effects of absolute GFR (note the logarithmic scale) on post-conceptional age taken from Coulthard [12]. The boxes represent the confidence limits for data from that study and the other lines and symbols show the results in 12 other studies. Where necessary data were recalculated to be presented in this format. Note that (▲) is the regression line calculated from the data of Fawer *et al.* [11] (see Figure 17.2)

to clear substances such as gentamicin depends upon the relationship between body weight and conceptional age. As growth rates may show tremendous variation, clinical decisions dependent on renal clearance, such as gentamicin dosage, should be based on maturity rather than weight. For example, a newborn 1000 g baby of 26 weeks' gestation will demonstrate much poorer gentamicin clearance than a baby born small for dates at 30 weeks, and who still weighs only 1000 g a month later.

There are problems associated with the estimation of GFR in very small infants [13] in the context of both research and clinical practice. It is difficult to obtain accurately timed and complete urine collections. It is possible to measure GFR by methods which do not rely on urine collection, such as the constant inulin infusion and single-shot inulin techniques. However, these must be greatly modified in babies because of the much slower equilibration of glomerular markers [14], or their application will lead to invalid results [15].

In clinical practice the plasma creatinine concentration is the most widely used index of GFR; urea is a very poor marker [16]. It was predicted [17] and confirmed [17–20] that the accuracy of estimating GFR from plasma creatinine concentration in older children could be increased by factoring for body length, and attempts have therefore been made to apply this to babies. However, it was argued that because their GFR does not vary with surface area there would be no benefit for neonatal data [16,20], and little [21] or none [16] has been reported. Since the production of creati-

ninc in babies varies closely with body weight [16,22], and its clearance depends on absolute GFR which varies with post-conceptional age, the normal range for plasma creatinine concentration for a particular baby will be determined both by weight and post-conceptional age. The wide range of values seen for serum creatinine against postnatal age [23] is probably largely due to the wide variations in weight for post-conceptional age in these babies. A single measure of plasma creatinine provides no more than a crude estimate of renal function. In the first weeks after birth, plasma creatinine falls, initially exponentially, then more gradually. Following the trend in plasma creatinine over time is likely to be more rewarding than attempts to interpret a single measurement.

## Tubular function

### Sodium

Na+, K+-ATPase is the enzyme responsible for active sodium transport in all eukaryotic cells. It is a transmembrane protein, made up of two subunits. There are many forms of Na+, K+-ATPase, each encoded by specific groups of Na+, K+-ATPase genes. In renal tubular cells Na+, K+-ATPase creates an electrochemical gradient which is the energy source for the cotransport, involving specific transporter proteins, of Na+ and glucose and Na+ and amino acids and the countertransport of Na+ and H+. These transporters are also transmembrane proteins. There is a postnatal, maturational increase in abundance of Na+, K+-ATPase and other transporter proteins [24]. This postnatal increase is accompanied by an increase in Na+, K+-ATPase mRNA [25,26]. There are tissue specific differences in the time scale of such maturational changes [26].

Sodium balance is subject to both long- and short-term regulation [27]. Changes in the abundance of sodium transporters are responsible for long-term regulation. Glucocorticoids, for example, lead to an increased abundance of Na+, K+-ATPase. Short-term regulation of sodium balance is brought about by increases or decreases in the activity of the sodium transporters. Downregulatory factors, which cause natriuresis, include atrial natriuretic peptide, dopamine and diuretics. Noradrenaline is an upregulatory factor, which results in sodium retention. Dopamine inhibits and noradrenaline stimulates, Na+, K+-ATPase activity. Under conditions of stress, very preterm babies appear able to conserve sodium more avidly. We have seen a 28-week gestation, 960 g baby, reduce his sodium excretion to only 1% of the filtered loan, under conditions of dehydration by 3 days after birth (unpublished observation).

Regulatory factors exert their effects via a cascade of intracellular messengers. These intracellular signal systems also undergo postnatal maturation. End organ responsiveness increases with postnatal maturation of cellular signal systems [26,28,29]. For example, atrial natriuretic peptide (ANP) stimulates membrane bound guanylate cyclase, which leads to an increase in the intracellular second messenger, cyclic guanosine monophosphate (cGMP), generated from endogenous GTP. Cyclic GMP interacts with specific protein kinases which in turn catalyse the phosphorylation of several protein substrates and finally leads to a biological effect such as inhibition of sodium reabsorption. Each step in such a cascade is subject to developmental regulation. In a study of preterm babies, the ratio of cGMP to ANP was found to increase exponentially in the first 3 days after birth, then reaching a plateau. The ratio of sodium excretion to cGMP continued to increase over the 10 days of the study [29]. This suggests a postnatal increase in the ANP/cGMP/sodium excretion cascade and thus an increasing postnatal ability to excrete sodium.

Age-dependent differences in the ability of glucocorticoids to induce Na+, K+-ATPase have been shown [25]. In rats, betamethasone will increase Na+, K+-ATPase mRNA in the kidney during infancy, but not during fetal life, nor in adults. In contrast, lung tissue Na+, K+-ATPase is maximally induced by glucocorticoids during the perinatal period. The inference is that glucocorticoids interact with other transcriptional factors, expressed in an age dependent fashion, to activate the genes for Na+, K+-ATPase so that different tissues have different periods of sensitivity to glucocorticoid regulation. In the future, the therapeutic activation of transcriptional factors determining tissue maturation may be possible.

Neonates conserve the sodium they need for growth, in a different way from older subjects. A smaller fraction of the filtered sodium is reabsorbed in the proximal tubule [30,31]. While mature babies are able to reabsorb most of the filtered sodium load, under the influence of very high renin-angiotensin-aldosterine system (RAAS) activity [32], a 1000 g baby usually does not manage this. Renal salt wasting is common in babies below 32 weeks' gestation and is due to impaired reabsorption at both proximal and distal tubule. Intestinal absorption is also limited [33]. Rapid postnatal maturation occurs by an increase in Na+, K+-ATPase [24,34] and by increasing responsiveness of distal tubule to aldosterone [9,35].

## Bicarbonate

The plasma bicarbonate concentrations in preterm babies are lower than in older children [36]. However, like fetal lambs [37], this appears to be due to the bicarbonate threshold being set lower [38,39] and not to an inability to reabsorb the filtered loan. Babies of less than 1000 g reabsorb virtually all their filtered bicarbonate when the blood pH falls to 7.22 [40]. Possibly other factors such as a limited excretion of buffers and ammonia [38] may be responsible for the metabolic acidosis described in these babies.

## Water

As nutrition can only be provided to babies in liquid form, a high fluid intake is mandatory and the baby must have a high urine flow in order to maintain water balance. GFR is relatively lower in very immature babies and in addition, the reabsorption of sodium and water by the proximal tubules is isotonic. A greater proportion of filtered water is therefore delivered distally in preterm babies compared to older subjects and a high urine flow rate is achieved by a much greater fractional excretion of glomerular filtrate ($Fe_{H_2O}$). A mean value of 13.1% has been reported in babies with an average weight of 1600 g and a daily fluid intake of 200 ml $kg^{-1}$ [41]. Similar $Fe_{H_2O}$ values in adults would result in a daily urine volume of over 20 litres. Indeed, normal values of values $Fe_{H_2O}$ in babies have previously been interpreted as evidence of a harmful osmotic diuresis because they were inappropriately compared to adult normal ranges [42].

Healthy preterm babies have been shown to be able to adjust their water excretion appropriately from the second day after birth, when their daily intakes were varied between 95 and 200 ml $kg^{-1}$, sodium intake remaining constant [41]. This was achieved by altering the $Fe_{H_2O}$ from a mean of 7.4% to 13.1% of the filtered volume, and occurred without causing any alteration to the amount of sodium lost in the urine. The widely held view that babies are unable to sustain a high urine flow without an increased loss of sodium [43,44] was suggested by a study [15] in which the design [41] and measurement techniques [14] have been questioned.

Neonates can achieve a maximum urine osmolality of about 500–600 mosmol $kg^{-1}$, compared to two or three times this in older subjects, a difference due in part to their lower urea concentrations and in part to their shorter loops of Henle. Fetal animals [45] and preterm babies are sensitive to antidiuretic hormone (arginine vasopressin, AVP) and can achieve these maximum osmolalities from birth. Babies born after fetal distress or after difficult delivery have higher circulating AVP levels than those born uneventfully [46]. Rees *et al.* [47] have shown peaks of AVP occurring during acute clinical events such as the development of a pneumothorax and cite this as evidence for the frequent occurrence of inappropriate ADH secretion in preterm neonates. However, the secretion of ADH can only be said to be 'inappropriate' if it occurs in the absence of osmotic or volume stimuli. In addition to its role in water homeostasis, AVP is a potent vasoconstrictor which is released in very large amounts (even in fetuses) in the face of hypotension [48],

hypoxia [49], or hypovolaemia [50] and contributes to maintenance of blood pressure [51–54].

Hypovolaemia probably occurs more frequently than is recognized in neonates receiving intensive care and in the postoperative period [55]. More attention should be paid to assessment of the circulation using invasive arterial blood pressure and central venous pressure monitoring [56] and, non-invasively, core–peripheral temperature gradient, aiming to maintain this below 1–1.5°C. The latter parameter is an extremely useful index of volume depletion as shown by its strong correlation with circulating AVP [57]. Failure to provide adequate volume support in the form of salt containing solutions will lead to an appropriate stimulus to AVP release, water retention and hyponatraemia. Once this has occurred water restriction will be necessary to correct the hyponatraemia safely.

Preterm babies are able to achieve similar minimal urine osmolalities to adults, with values of 50 mosmol $kg^{-1}$ or less [41,58]. Using these values and the measured renal solute loads of about 10–15 mosmol $kg^{-1}$ in healthy preterm infants [58], it is possible to estimate the appropriate minimum and maximum urine flow rates that these infants can achieve and still remain in solute and water balance. Thus, a typical 1000 g baby who can produce urine with an osmolality of 600 would need to pass at least 22 ml urine in order to excrete 13 mmol solute daily. This compared closely to the 1 ml $kg^{-1}$ $hour^{-1}$ widely used as a clinical indication of renal failure.

On the other hand, the largest daily volume of urine such a baby could pass with a minimum osmolality of 50 and without passing more than 13 mosmol of solute would be 260 ml. This volume is probably greater than the amount available from glomerular filtration in many preterm babies, so that diluting ability is unlikely to limit water excretion. For example, a typical 26-week gestation baby weighing 700 g would have a GFR of 0.8 ml $kg^{-1}$ $min^{-1}$ [12], so that with 20% of the filtrate delivered distally, the maximum available for excretion would be 230 ml $kg^{-1}$ daily. Certainly most preterm babies are able to achieve a urine flow rate of around 7 ml $kg^{-1}$ $hour^{-1}$. Leake *et al.* [15] found a group of babies of 28–34 weeks' gestation to increase urine flow rate to a mean of 12 ml $kg^{-1}$ $hour^{-1}$

during acute increases in infusion rate to 250 ml kg$^{-1}$ day$^{-1}$.

## Postnatal adaptation and respiratory distress syndrome

After birth, several adaptive processes take place. These are necessary for successful transition from the aqueous intrauterine to the gaseous postnatal environment. The extracellular compartment contracts, due to loss of interstitial fluid [59–63]. This accounts, at least in part, for early postnatal weight loss. This change appears to be closely interrelated with cardiopulmonary adaptation. Several studies now suggest that the postnatal extracellular volume contraction is triggered by a surge in atrial natriuretic peptide release brought about by increased atrial stretch as pulmonary vascular resistance falls [64–69]. Extracellular fluid loss is marked clinically by a postnatal diuresis, well recognized in babies with respiratory distress syndrome, but which also occurs in healthy neonates [41,70]. As the diuresis/natriuresis is only a consequence of a fall in pulmonary vascular resistance, this explains the failure of furosemide therapy to improve respiratory distress syndrome [71].

The intravascular compartment may also be acutely expanded during birth, because of reabsorption of lung liquid and a variable placental transfusion. It has been suggested that there is movement of water from the intracellular to the extracellular compartment immediately after birth, though the evidence for this is not conclusive as the study in question drew conclusions from cross-sectional data from dehydrated subjects [72].

If isotonic contraction of the extracellular compartment is to occur, net water and sodium balance in the first days after birth must be negative and should be regarded as physiological. That early negative sodium balance is physiological is borne out by the observation that, in healthy newborn babies, an increase in early sodium intake leads to an increase in sodium excretion [63,73,57]. However all preterm babies have a limited (but variable) capacity to excrete a sodium load so that, despite increasing excretion in response to an increase in intake, sodium retention readily occurs [74,75]. Acute sodium loading in neonates results in only a blunted fall in RAAS activity and limited natriuretic response [76].

Shaffer and Meade [63] studied sodium balance and extracellular volume regulation in a group of babies of 25–31 weeks' gestation in the first 10 days after birth. In the group given a sodium intake of 3 mmol kg$^{-1}$ day$^{-1}$, 50% became hypernatraemic, as did 20% in the group given 1 mmol kg$^{-1}$ day$^{-1}$. In this study, water intake began at 75 ml kg$^{-1}$ day$^{-1}$ on the first day, increasing by 10 ml kg$^{-1}$ day$^{-1}$ until day 5. If a more liberal water intake is allowed in conjunction with sodium intake, extracellular tonicity is maintained by expansion of the extracellular compartment. This is a common occurrence in neonatal intensive care units; many babies gain weight in the first days after birth, when nutritional intake is clearly insufficient to sustain growth and have a positive sodium balance with a normal serum sodium concentration [75,77]. In the majority of babies this cumulative positive balance is subsequently lost; in other words, the normal postnatal changes in both water distribution occur, but are delayed [75]. Costarino *et al.* [74] confirmed some of these observations in a blind trial comparing sodium restriction in the first 5 days after birth with sodium supplementation of 3–4 mmol kg$^{-1}$ day$^{-1}$ from birth. Water intake was administered independently. Unfortunately extracellular volume was not measured in this study, nor were the babies weighed. However, sodium balance was positive in the sodium supplemented group on the first day after birth and this group had a significantly higher incidence of bronchopulmonary dysplasia.

It is widely assumed that babies with respiratory distress syndrome or requiring ventilation have an impaired GFR, but evidence for this is far from definite. While it is not surprising that babies who are hypoxaemic and hypovolaemic are likely to have a reduced GFR, there is no evidence that this is true for those infants whose clinical and biochemical status has been stabilized by therapy [78]. Furthermore, reports that continuous positive airway pressure causes a fall in GFR [79] or that intermittent positive pressure ventilation alters intrarenal blood flow [80] should be considered with caution. These observations were made in newborn animals with normal lungs, capable of transmitting inflation pressures to the rest of the intrathoracic contents and thereby altering factors such as venous return; the situation is probably very different in the baby with non-compliant lungs.

## Clinical implications of developmental changes

Early management of fluid balance should permit an isotonic contraction of the extracellular compartment. In order to allow the reduction in extracellular fluid volume which is the basis for weight loss, the primary necessity is to avoid an early intake of sodium. Early water intake should be sufficient to maintain glomerular filtration to allow the excretion of the relatively small renal solute load [81] and to maintain tonicity in the face of high, but rapidly changing, transepidermal losses [82]. A reasonable 'best guess' of the volume at which to start is therefore 30–60 ml kg$^{-1}$ day$^{-1}$ *plus* estimated insensible water loss. Subsequently, the appropriate volume of intake will be determined by the nutritional content of the fluid used. Early physiological weight loss should be of the order of 7% of birth weight [59,60], but this is only an approximation as hydration at birth is variable and birth weight does not correlate closely with extracellular water volume [61].

Neonatal paediatricians have long been concerned about 'excessive' fluid intake. Associations have been described between high fluid intakes and increased risk of symptomatic patent ductus arteriosus, necrotizing enterocolitis and bronchopulmonary dysplasia [74,83–87]. In the former condition an expanded intravascular compartment might exacerbate left to right shunting and in the latter conditions, interstitial oedema has been implicated in pathogenesis. Regrettably, these studies have, without exception, failed to standardize sodium intake, so that increased 'fluid' has meant an increased intake of both sodium and water.

Further, as mature babies ingest relatively small volumes of milk initially, and preterm babies are usually intolerant of full volume feeds soon after birth, it has been traditional to increase fluid volumes slowly, even when much or all of the volume is administered parenterally. Since healthy preterm babies have been shown to be capable of excreting large volumes of water from the third day [41] there seems to be no logic behind this gradualistic approach. Once postnatal weight loss has been achieved, a parenteral intake of 200 ml kg$^{-1}$ may be given, without stepwise increments.

The principles of management of sodium balance during the period of postnatal adaptation should be clearly distinguished from those pertaining subsequently. An early intake of sodium is unnecessary and possibly harmful and therefore should be avoided or at least minimized until the physiological postnatal diuresis/natriuresis [64,69]. If this point is indeterminate, supplementation should be deferred until a steady weight loss of at least 7% of birth weight has occurred. Inappropriate early sodium supplementation may lead to delay or failure to lose weight after birth. Weight loss in preterm babies in the first days after birth is associated with a reduced morbidity from symptomatic patent ductus arteriosus [83,84], necrotizing enterocolitis [85] and bronchopulmonary dysplasia [74,86,87]. Once the phase of immediate postnatal adaptation is over, growth becomes of paramount importance. Chronic limitation of sodium intake is associated with poor growth [24,88–90] and adverse neurodevelopmental outcome. There is increasing evidence that sodium is a permissive factor for growth [91]. Sodium deficiency inhibits DNA synthesis in the most immature cells [91]. Human milk contains an inadequate quantity of sodium to support growth in preterm babies who frequently develop hyponatraemia if fed unsupplemented or unfortified breast milk, in contrast to full term babies. Therefore, once nutritional intake is sufficient to support growth, extremely immature babies require a sodium intake of at least 4 mmol kg$^{-1}$ day$^{-1}$, or more if on treatment with xanthines or other diuretics. This will ensure the retention of the 1 mmol kg$^{-1}$ day$^{-1}$ necessary for growth [24] and will abolish late hyponatraemia. For babies of less than 32 weeks' gestation sodium supplementation should continue for around 2–4 weeks, by which time postnatal maturation of sodium conservation should have occurred [89,92]. It is not known whether supplementation beyond this time is harmful, for example, in terms of chronic sodium retention and the development of hypertension.

## Indomethacin

Indomethacin is a prostaglandin synthetase inhibitor which is commonly used to facilitate the closure of a symptomatic patent ductus arteriosus. It is also administered antenatally as a tocolytic, and to reduce liquor volume in polyhydramnios. In older subjects it is known to reduce sodium excretion and urine flow by enhancing tubular reabsorption, but in addition to this there have been anxieties that it may lower GFR in preterm infants. This difference may reflect the dependence of these subjects on renal prostaglandins to maintain an adequate renal blood flow in the face of high RAAS activity; a parallel can be seen in the study of dogs where indomethacin was shown to induce a fall in GFR only when the RAAS activity was increased by sodium depletion [93].

A temporary reduction of sodium and water excretion is described in all reports of babies given indomethacin for duct closure. The simultaneous administration of $1 \, mg \, kg^{-1}$ of frusemide has been shown to eliminate the renal side-effects of $0.3 \, mg$ indomethacin without reducing its efficacy in duct closure [94]. In a randomized, controlled trial, similar claims for concurrent dopamine therapy were found to be unsubstantiated [95].

## Inotropes

Dopamine and dobutamine are now frequently used in neonatal intensive care, to support blood pressure and cardiac output, and also for their purported renal effects at low dose. Three randomized studies [96–98], comparing the efficacy of dopamine and dobutamine, all showed that dopamine is more effective at raising and maintaining blood pressure than dobutamine. However, in only one of these studies was left ventricular output measured as well and this showed that dopamine did not increase cardiac output in contrast to dobutamine, which produced a mean increase in left ventricular output of 21% [98]. Seri *et al.* [99] showed that dopamine at a dose of $2 \, \mu g \, kg^{-1} \, min^{-1}$, induced maximal diuresis and natriuresis in sick preterm neonates, if systemic blood pressure was within the normal range. An increase to $4 \, \mu g \, kg^{-1} \, min^{-1}$ resulted in a further increase in blood pressure, but no change in urine output and sodium excretion.

## Management of acute renal failure

Renal impairment is common in very small infants. The majority of babies who weigh less than $1000 \, g$ and have renal failure will not have a primary kidney disease but will have developed pre-renal failure progressing to established renal failure, secondary to factors such as hypotension, hypoxia and cardiac failure.

It is, nevertheless, important to exclude congenital abnormalities of the kidneys such as agenesis, dysplasia and infantile-type polycystic disease, and to diagnose renal vein thrombosis or treatable obstructive lesions such as posterior urethral values. These can all be identified using ultrasound; the intravenous urogram produces poor images in normal preterm babies and has no role in those with renal impairment. As in older patients, the best indicator to distinguish pre-renal from established renal failure is the fractional excretion of sodium ($Fe_{Na}$). This is readily calculated from the sodium and creatinine concentrations of plasma (P) and a spot urine (U) sample:

$$Fe_{Na} = (U/P) \, sodium \times (P/U) \, creatinine \, (\times 100\%)$$

If the tubules are still functioning and the infant is in oliguric pre-renal failure then the $Fe_{Na}$ will be less than 2.5% [100] or 3% [101]. Once tubular necrosis has occurred the $Fe_{Na}$ is usually considerably higher, and often about 10% [100,101].

The management of a baby with pre-renal failure is to ensure that the vascular compartment is adequately filled, usually by the administration of up to $20 \, ml \, kg^{-1}$ saline, and then to administer frusemide. The latter not only increases the flow of tubular fluid, but also stimulates prostaglandin release and reduces renal metabolic requirements by inhibiting the sodium pump. Doses of $1 \, mg \, kg^{-1}$ [102] or up to $3 \, mg \, kg^{-1}$ [101] have been recommended. Because frusemide exerts its effects on the loop of Henle only after glomerular filtration, high plasma levels are necessary when the GFR is low, and we use $5 \, mg \, kg^{-1}$. However, because the half life of frusemide clearance is almost 24 hours in healthy preterm infants that are not in renal failure [103], clearance will almost certainly be several days in babies remaining in renal failure, and there is no rationale for repeating the dose; this would only lead to accumulation. If this therapy does not produce a diuresis then the baby needs to be managed like an infant in established renal failure. Although dopamine has been reported to enhance the action of frusemide in this situation [102], the diuresis produced may equally have been due to the simultaneous administration of a second 1 mg kg$^{-1}$ dose of frusemide.

The management of the tiny infant who is in established renal failure or has failed to respond to volume repletion and frusemide is difficult. Efforts should be directed towards full support of physiological variables. Conservative management remains the mainstay of treatment. Careful attention should be paid to reduce total intake volume to no more than insensible losses plus urine output, as water overload very readily occurs. Sodium intake should similarly be limited to the replacement of losses, bearing in mind the frequent need for base in the form of sodium bicarbonate and that substantial inadvertent sodium administration frequently occurs, for example from saline flushes, drugs and colloid. Clinical fluid management is best regulated in oligoanuric patients by distinguishing clearly between three categories of fluid replacement: that needed to replace insensible losses, that to replace measured losses, and any extras, to administer drugs, etc. Insensible water should be replaced without sodium, but at a relatively high glucose concentration to supply calories. Replacements for gut and urine losses should be administered in equivalent volumes to the measured (or weighed) losses, using fluids with a similar sodium concentration (electrolytes must be measured in vomitus and stool supernatant as well as urine). Fine tuning of the replacement fluid electrolytes can be guided by the plasma sodium concentration. Frequently, a commercially available intravenous fluid is suitable, but adjustments can be made to these by adding 30% sodium chloride (5 mmol/ml) or 8.4% sodium bicarbonate (1 mmol/ml) solutions, as appropriate. Any extra fluid should be provided at a sodium concentration of approximately 140 mmol/L. This is because the extra volume will be retained until the baby has a diuresis or is dialysed. It is very common for oligoanuric babies to develop profound dilutional hyponatraemia after hypotonic fluid administration. To help determine prognosis in an anuric baby, radionuclide scans such as $^{99}$Tc-DTPA may be used to assess whether the kidneys are still perfused, but a false negative has been reported [103]. If it is felt that the baby would be likely to survive but for renal failure, then dialysis should be considered.

## Peritoneal dialysis

At present peritoneal dialysis is the preferred practical technique for dialysing babies that weigh less than 1000 g, and the only method feasible outside a specialised paediatric nephrology unit. It is now possible to haemodialyse using a very small extracorporeal circuit and freshly obtained heparinised blood for priming [104], and a novel circuit has been described for very small pre-term infants which requires a circuit blood volume of only 11 ml [105]. Presently this is a manual technique which is very tedious, but is being mechanised. The indications for peritoneal dialysis are severe water overload, an intractable metabolic acidosis and electrolyte disturbance. A rising serum creatinine is not, on its own, an indication and dialysis may often be avoided if meticulous attention is paid to medical management.

Standard peritoneal dialysis catheters are unsuitable for extremely small babies; they are too rigid and the side holes extend too far. Very soft chest drain tubes, with side holes, inserted in the left upper quadrant so that they can curl up in the peritoneal space, may be used. Hourly cycles of up to 35 ml kg$^{-1}$ are used initially provided they do not cause respiratory difficulty, and the cycle times are lengthened as dictated by the biochemical response. Once a child has been stabilized on bicarbonate based dialysis, it is reasonable to change them to lactate based dialysate whilst monitoring pH closely – this is likely to be successful in the majority of cases. Intravenous calcium supplements are usually necessary and in some cases, insulin infusions to control the hyperglycaemia resulting from glucose absorbed from the dialysis fluid. Heparin (1 unit ml$^{-1}$) may be added to the dialysis fluid, particularly if the effluent is blood-stained, to prevent clots forming in the catheter holes. If an aminoglycoside is indicated this may be added to the dialysis fluid at the appropriate concentration to be achieved in the plasma (10 mg l$^{-1}$ for gentamicin) and one loading dose given parenterally if it had not previously been started. The dose of systemically admin-

> **Practical points**
>
> 1. Maturity is more important than weight, when considering renal function.
> 2. A very immature baby may have a high initial water requirement because of high transepidermal loss. However the skin matures rapidly and transepidermal losses fall. This is a function of postnatal age.
> 3. When prescribing water, sodium and dextrose, consider requirements independently. Avoid the use of fixed formula solutions if possible.
> 4. Assessment of daily weight, plasma creatinine, sodium and potassium and urine output, are mandatory requirements for basic monitoring of renal function during intensive care.
> 5. In extremely immature neonates, early hyponatraemia is usually due to water overload, and late hyponatraemia, to sodium depletion.

istered penicillins should be halved during dialysis, and other renally excreted drugs individually adjusted.

Peritonitis is a major hazard of peritoneal dialysis at all ages. The risks can be minimized by using a complete neonatal administration set rather than making one up from separate components, and by obsessional nursing care. Microscopy and culture of the effluent fluid should be carried out daily and antibiotics added to the dialysis fluid at the earliest suspicion of an infection.

## Conclusions

The neonatal paediatrician should bear in mind the differing needs of the preterm baby. Immediately after birth, optimal management should promote normal postnatal adaptation; subsequently, the demands of growth become paramount. Other organ systems, such as the skin, influence fluid balance. Immediately after birth, the immature skin is the major route of water loss. It is our impression that neonatal renal impairment has become less common over the last decade. This is no doubt attributable to better basic care, with improved monitoring and support of blood pressure and other physiological variables. It is to be hoped that continued improvements in neonatal intensive care, with, for example, central venous pressure monitoring, longitudinal, non-invasive assessment of cardiac output assessment and regional tissue perfusion, will continue this trend.

## References

1. Boyd, E. (1935) *The Growth of the Surface Area of the Human Body*. University of Minnesota Press, Minneapolis
2. Haycock, G.B., Schwartz, G.J. and Wisotsky, D.H. (1978) Geometric method for measuring body surface area: a height–weight formula validated in infants, children and adults. *J. Pediatr.*, **93**, 62–66
3. Coulthard, M.G. and Hey, E.N. (1984) Weight as the best standard for glomerular filtration in the newborn. *Arch. Dis. Childh.*, **59**, 373–375
4. Hey, E.N. (1969) The relation between environmental temperature and oxygen consumption in the newborn baby. *J. Physiol.*, **200**, 589–603
5. McCance, R. and Widdowson, E.M. (1952) The correct physiological basis on which to compare infant and adult renal function. *Lancet*, **ii**, 860–862
6. McDonald, M.S. and Emery, J.L. (1959) The late intrauterine and postnatal development of human renal glomeruli. *J. Anat.*, **93**, 331
7. Aschinberg, L.G., Goldsmith, D.I., Olbing, H., Spitzer, A., Edelmann, C.M. Jr and Blaufox, M.D. (1975) Neonatal changes in renal blood flow distribution in puppies. *Am. J. Physiol.*, **228**, 1453–1461
8. Fetterman, G.F., Shuplock, N.A., Philipp, F.G. and Gregg, H.S. (1965) The growth and maturation of human glomeruli and proximal convolutions from term to adulthood. Studies by microdissection. *Pediatrics*, **35**, 601
9. Al-Dahhan, J., Haycock, G.B., Chantler, C. and Stimmler, L. (1983) Sodium homeostasis in term and preterm neonates. I. Renal aspects. *Arch. Dis. Childh.*, **58**, 335–345
10. Arant, B.S. Jr (1978) Developmental patterns of renal function maturation compared in the human neonate. *J. Pediatr.*, **92**, 705–712
11. Fawer, C.L., Torrado, A. and Guignard, J.P. (1979) Maturation of renal function in full-term and premature neonates. *Helv. Paediatr. Acta.*, **34**, 11–21
12. Coulthard, M.G. (1985) Maturation of glomerular filtration in preterm and mature babies. *Early Hum. Dev.*, **11**, 281–292
13. Arant, B.S., Jr. (1984) Estimation glomerular filtration rate in infants. *J. Pediatr.*, **104**, 890–893
14. Coulthard, M.G. (1983) Comparison of methods of measuring renal function in preterm babies using inulin. *J. Pediatr.*, **102**, 923–930

15. Leake, R.D., Zakauddin, S., Trygstad, C.W., Fu, P. and Oh, W. (1976) The effect of large volume intravenous fluid infusion on neonatal renal function. *J. Pediatr.*, **89**, 968–972

16. Coulthard, M.G., Hey, E.N. and Ruddock, V. (1985) Creatinine and urea clearances compared to inulin clearance in preterm and mature babies. *Early Hum. Dev.*, **11**, 11–19

17. Counahan, R., Chantler, C., Ghazali, S., Kirkwood, B., Rose, F. and Barratt, T.M. (1976) Estimation of glomerular filtration rate from plasma creatinine concentration in children. *Arch. Dis. Childh.*, **51**, 875–878

18. Davies, J.G., Taylor, C.M., White, R.H.R. and Marshall, T. (1982) Clinical limitations of the estimation of glomerular filtration rate from height/plasma creatinine ratio: a comparison with simultaneous ⁵¹Cr-edetic acid slope clearance. *Arch. Dis. Childh.*, **57**, 607–610

19. Morris, M.C., Allanby, C.W., Toseland, P., Haycock, G.B. and Chantler, C. (1982) Evaluation of height/plasma creatinine formula in the measurement of glomerular filtration rate. *Arch. Dis. Childh.*, **57**, 611–615

20. Schwartz, G.J., Haycock, G.B., Edelmann, C.M. Jr and Spitzer, A. (1976) A simple estimate of glomerular filtration rate in children derived from body length and plasma creatinine. *Pediatrics*, **58**, 259–263

21. Zachello, G., Bondio, M., Saia, O.S., Largaiolli, G., Vedaldi, R. and Rubaltelli, F.F. (1982) Simple estimate of creatinine clearance from plasma creatinine in neonates. *Arch. Dis. Childh.*, **57**, 297–300

22. Modi, N. and Hutton, J.L. (1990) Urinary creatinine excretion and estimation of muscle mass in infants of 25–34 weeks' gestation. *Acta Paediatr. Scand.*, **79**, 1156–1162

23. Stonestreet, B.S. and Oh, W. (1978) Plasma creatinine levels in low-birth-weight infants during the first three months of life. *Pediatrics*, **61**, 788–789

24. Haycock, G.B. and Aperia, A. (1991) Salt and the newborn kidney. *Pediatr. Nephrol.*, **5**, 65–70

25. Celsi, G., Wang, Z.M., Akusjarvi, G. and Aperia, A. (1993) Sensitive periods for glucocorticoid regulation of Na⁺,K⁺-ATPase mRNA in the developing lung and kidney. *Pediatr. Res.*, **33**, 5–9

26. Orlowski and Lingrel, J.B. (1988) Tissue-specific and developmental regulation of rat Na, K-ATPase catalytic α isoform and β subunit mRNAs. *J. Biol. Chem.*, **263**, 10436–10442

27. Modi, N. Sodium intake and preterm babies. *Arch. Dis. Childh.*, **69**, 87–91

28. Fukuda, Y., Bertorelli, A. and Aperia, A. (1991) Ontogeny of the regulation of Na⁺,K⁺-ATPase activity in the renal proximal tubule cell. *Pediatr. Res.*, **30**, 131–134

29. Midgley, J.P., Modi, N., Littleton, P., Carter, N., Royston, P. and Smith, A. (1992) Atrial natriuretic peptide, cyclic guanosine monophosphate and sodium excretion during postnatal adaptation in male infants below 34 weeks' gestation with severe respiratory distress syndrome. *Early Hum. Dev.*, **28**, 145–154

30. Horster, M. and Valtin, H. (1971) Postnatal development of renal function: micropuncture and clearance studies in the dog. *J. Clin. Invest.*, **50**, 779–795

31. Spitzer, A. and Brandis, M. (1974) Functional and morphologic maturation of the superficial nephrons. Relationship to total kidney function. *J. Clin. Invest.*, **53**, 279–287

32. Kotchen, T.A., Strickland, A.L., Rice, T.W. and Walters, D.R. (1972) A study of the renin-angiotensin system in the newborn infant. *J. Pediatr.*, **80**, 938–946

33. Al-Dahhan, Haycock, G.B., Chantler, C. and Stimmler, L. (1983) Sodium homeostasis in term and preterm neonates. II. Gastrointestinal aspects. *Arch. Dis. Childh.*, **58**, 343–345

34. Herin, P. and Aperia, A. (1994) Neonatal kidney, fluids and electrolytes. *Curr. Opin. Pediatr.*, **6**, 154–157

35. Sulyok, E., Nemeth, M., Tenyi, I. *et al.* (1979) Postnatal development of renin-angiotensin-aldoesterone system, RAAS, in relation to electrolyte balance in premature infants. *Pediatr. Res.*, **13**, 817–820

36. Sulyok, E., Heim, T., Soltesz, G. and Jaszai, V. (1972) The influence of maturity on renal control of acidosis in newborn infants. *Biol. Neonate*, **21**, 418–435

37. Robillard, J.E., Sessious, C., Burmeister, L. and Smith, F.G., Jr. (1977) Influence of fetal extracellular volume contraction on renal reabsorption of bicarbonate in fetal lambs. *Pediatr. Res.*, **11**, 649–655

38. Svenningsen, N.W. (1974) Renal acid–base titration studies in infants with and without metabolic acidosis in the postneonatal period. *Pediatr. Res.*, **8**, 659–672

39. Schwartz, G.J., Haycock, G.B., Edelmann, C.M. Jr. and Spitzer, A. (1979) Late metabolic acidosis: a reassessment of the definition. *J. Pediatr.*, **95**, 102–107

40. Zilleruelo, G., Sultan, S., Bancalari, E., Steele, B. and Strauss, J. (1986) Renal bicarbonate handling in low-birth-weight infants during metabolic acidosis. *Biol. Neonate*, **49**, 132–139

41. Coulthard, M.G. and Hey, E.N. (1985) Effect of varying water intake on renal function in healthy preterm babies. *Arch. Dis. Childh.*, **60**, 614–620

42. Stonestreet, B.S., Rubin, L., Pollak, A., Cowett, R.M. and Oh, W. (1980) Renal functions of low birth weight infants with hyperglycaemia and glucosuria produced by glucose infusions. *Pediatrics*, **66**, 561–567

43. Leake, R.D. (1977) Perinatal nephrobiology: a developmental perspective. *Clin. Perinatol.*, **4**, 321–349

44. Engle, W.D. (1986) Evaluation of renal function and acute renal failure in the neonates. *Pediatr. Clin. N. Am.*, **33**, 129–151

45. Alexander, D.P., Bashore, R.A., Britton, H.G. and Forsling, M.L. (1976) Antidiuretic hormone and oxytocin release and antidiuretic hormone turnover in the fetus, lamb and ewe. *Biol. Neonate*, **30**, 80–87

46. Leung, A.K.C., McArthur, R.G., McMillan, D.D. *et al.* (1980) Circulating antidiuretic hormone during labour and in the newborn. *Acta Paediatr. Scand.*, **69**, 505–510

47. Rees, L., Brook, C.D.G., Shaw, J.C.L. and Forsling, M.L. (1984) Hyponatraemia in the first week of life in preterm infants. I. Arginine vasopressin secretion. *Arch. Dis. Childh.*, **59**, 414–422

48. Daniel, S.S., Stark, R.I., Zubrow, A.B., Tropper, P.J. and James, L.S. (1985) Vasopressin and plasma renin activity following disturbances in blood pressure, osmolality and/or blood volume in the fetus. In *The Physiological Development of the Fetus and Newborn* (C.T. Jones and P.W. Natriandiez, eds), Academic Press, London, pp. 331–334

49. Alexander, D.P., Forsling, M.L., Martin, M.J. *et al.* (1972) The effect of maternal hypoxia on fetal pituitary hormone release in the sheep. *Biol. Neonate*, **21**, 219–228

50. Alexander, D.P., Britton, H.G., Forsling, M.L., Nixon, D.A. and Ratcliffe, J.G. (1974) Pituitary and plasma concentrations of adrenocorticotrophin, growth hormone, vasopressin and oxytocin in fetal and maternal sheep during the latter half of gestation and the response to haemorrhage. *Biol. Neonate*, **24**, 206–219

51. Aisenbrey, G.A., Handelman, W.A., Arnold, P., Manning, M. and Schrier, R.W. (1981) Vascular effects of arginine vasopressin during fluid deprivation in the rat. *J. Clin. Invest.*, **67**, 961–968

52. Gardiner, S.M. and Bennett, T. (1985) Interactions between neural mechanisms, the renin–angiotensin system and vasopressin in the maintenance of blood pressure during water deprivation: studies in Long Evans and Brattleboro rats. *Clin. Sci.*, **68**, 647–757

53. Cowley, A.W. Jr, Switzer, S.J. and Guinn, M.M. (1980) Evidence and quantifications of the vasopressin arterial pressure control system in the dog. *Circ. Res.*, **46**, 58–67

54. Gardiner, S.M. and Bennett, T. (1983) Effects of haemorrhage in rats lacking vasopressin (Brattleboro strain): influence of naloxone. *Clin. Sci.*, **65**, 19–25

55. Judd, B.A., Haycock, G.B., Dalton, N. and Chantler, C. (1987) Hyponatraemia in premature babies and following surgery in older children. *Acta Paediatr. Scand.*, **76**, 385–393

56. Skinner, J.R., Milligan, D.W.A., Hunter, S. and Hey, E. (1992) Central venous pressure in the ventilated neonate. *Arch. Dis. Childh.*, **67**, 374–377

57. Lambert, H.J., Coulthard, M.G., Palmer, J.M., Baylis, P.H. and Matthews, J.N.S. (1990) Control of sodium and water balance in the preterm neonate. *Pediatr. Nephrol.*, **4**, C53

58. Ekhard, E., Ziegler, M.D. and Ryu, J.E. (1976) Renal solute load and diet in growing premature infants. *J. Pediatr.*, **89**, 609–611

59. Bauer, K., Bovermann, G., Roithmaier, A., Gotz, M., Proiss, A. and Vermold, H. (1991) Body composition, nutrition and fluid balance during the first two weeks of life in preterm neonates weighing less than 1500 g. *J. Pediatr.*, **118**, 615–620

60. Bauer, K. and Versmold, H. (1989) Postnatal weight loss in preterm neonates less than 1500 g is isotonic dehydration of the extracellular volume. *Acta Paediatrica Scand.*, **360**, (Suppl.), 37–42

61. Shaffer, S.G., Bradt, S.K. and Hall, R.T. (1986) Postnatal changes in total body water and extracellular volume in the preterm infant with respiratory distress syndrome. *J. Pediatr.*, **109**, 509–514

62. Stonestreet, B.S., Bell, E.F., Warburton, D. and Oh, W. (1983) Renal responses in low birth weight neonates; results of prolonged intake of two different amounts of fluid and sodium. *Am. J. Dis. Child.*, **137**, 215–219

63. Shaffer, S.G. and Meade, V.M. (1989) Sodium balance and extracellular volume regulation in very low birth weight infants. *J. Pediatr.*, **115**, 285–290

64. Modi, N. and Hutton, J.L. (1990) The influence of postnatal respiratory adaptation on sodium handling in preterm neonates. *Early Hum. Dev.*, **21**, 11–20

65. Rozycki, J.H. and Baumgart, S. (1991) Atrial natriuretic factor and postnatal diuresis in respiratory distress syndrome. *Arch. Dis. Childh.*, **66**, 43–47

66. Midgley, J.P., Modi, N., Smith, A., Littleton, P. and Carter, N. (1991) Changes in circulating atrial natriuretic peptide during cardiopulmonary adaptation in preterm neonates. *Early Hum. Dev.*, **25**, 56

67. Kojima, T., Hirata, Y., Fukuda, Y., Iwase, S. and Koboyashi, Y. (1987) Plasma atrial natriuretic peptide and spontaneous diuresis in sick neonates. *Arch. Dis. Childh.*, **62**, 667–670

68. Tulassay, T., Seri, I. and Rascher, W. (1987) Atrial natriuretic peptide and extracellular volume control after birth. *Acta Paediatr. Scand.*, **76**, 444–446

69. Modi, N. and Bétrémieux, P. (1995) Longitudinal changes in extracellular fluid volume, sodium excretion and atrial natriuretic peptide, in preterm neonates with hyaline membrane disease. *Earl. Hum. Dev.*, **41**, 221

70. Lorenz, J.M., Kleinman, L.I., Kotagal, U.R. and Reller, M.D. (1982) Water balance in very-low-birth-weight infants: relationship to water and sodium intake and effect on outcome. *J. Pediatr.*, **101**, 423–432

71. Aranda, J.V., Chemtob, S., Laudignon, N. and Sasyniuk, B.I. (1986) Furosemide and vitamin E: two problem drugs in neonatology. *Pediatr. Clin. N. Am.*, **33**, 583–599

72. MacLaurin, J.C. (1966) Changes in body water distribution during the first two weeks of life. *Arch. Dis. Childh.*, **41**, 286–291

73. Rees, L., Shaw, J.C.L., Brook, C.G.D. and Forsling, M.L. (1984) Hyponatraemia in the first week of life in preterm infants. Part II. Sodium and water balance. *Arch. Dis. Childh.*, **59**, 423–429

74. Costarino, A.T., Gruskay, J.A., Corcoran, L., Pollin, R.A. and Baumgart, S. (1992) Sodium restriction versus daily maintenance replacement in very low birth weight premature neonates: a randomised, blind therapeutic trial. *J. Pediatr.*, **120**, 99–106

75. Modk, N. (1991) Aspects of renal function in infants between 25–34 weeks' gestation. MD Thesis. University of Edinburgh.

76. Drukker, A., Goldsmith, D.I., Spitzer, A., Edelmann, C.M. and Blaufox, M.D. (1980) The renin angiotensin system in newborn dogs: developmental patterns and response to acute saline loading. *Pediatr. Res.*, **14**, 304

77. Tang, W., Modi, N. and Clark, P. (1994) Dilution kinetics of $H_2^{18}O$ for the measurement of total body water in preterm babies in the first week after birth. *Arch. Dis. Childh.*, **69**, 28–31

78. Siegel, S.R., Fisher, D.A. and Oh, W. (1973) Renal function and serum aldosterone levels in infants with respiratory distress syndrome. *J. Pediatr.*, **83**, 854–858

79. Fewell, J.E. and Norton, J.B. (1980) Continuous positive airway pressure impairs renal function in newborn goats. *Pediatr. Res.*, **14**, 1132–1134

80. Moore, E.S., Galvez, M.B., Paton, J.B., Fisher, D.E. and Behrman, R.E. (1974) Effects of positive pressure ventilation on intrarenal blood flow in infant primates. *Pediatr. Res.*, **8**, 792–796

81. Ziegler, E. and Fomon, S.J. (1971) Fluid intake, renal solute load and water balance in infancy. *J. Pediatr.*, **78**, 561 568

82. Rutter, N. (1988) The immature skin. *Br. Med. Bull.*, **44**, 957–956

83. Bell, E.F., Warburton, D., Stonestreet, B. and Oh, W. (1980) Effect of fluid administration on the development of symptomatic ductus arteriosis and congestive heart failure in premature infants. *N. Engl. J. Med.*, **302**, 598–604

84. Stevenson, J.G. (1977) Fluid administration in the association of patent ductus arteriosus complicating respiratory distress syndrome. *J. Pediatr.*, **90**, 257–261

85. Bell, E.F., Warburton, D., Stonestreet, B. and Oh, W. (1979) High volume fluid intake predisposes premature infants to necrotising enterocolitis. *Lancet*, **2**, 90

86. Brown, E.R., Stark, A., Sosneko, I., Lawson, E.F. and Avery, M.E. (1978) Bronchopulmonary dysplasia: possible relationship to pulmonary oedema. *J. Pediatr.*, **92**, 982–984

87. Van Marter, L.J., Leviton, A., Allred, E.N., Pagano, M. and Kuban, K.C. (1990) Hydration during the first days of life and the risk of bronchopulmonary dysplasia in low birth weight infants. *J. Pediatr.*, **116**, 942–949

88. Chance, G.W., Radde, I.C., Willis, D.M., Roy, R.N., Park, E. and Ackerman, J. (1977) Postnatal growth of infants of <1.3 kg birth weight; effects of metabolic acidosis, of caloric intake and of calcium, sodium and phosphate supplementation. *J. Pediatr.*, **91**, 787–793

89. Al-Dahhan, J., Haycock, G.B., Nichol, B., Chantler, C. and Stimmler, L. (1984) Sodium homeostasis in term and preterm neonates. III. Effect of salt supplementation. *Arch. Dis. Childh.*, **59**, 945–950

90. Wassner, S.J. (1989) Altered growth and protein turnover in rats fed sodium-deficient diets. *Pediatr. Res.*, **26**, 608–613

91. Ostlund, E.V., Eklof, A.C. and Aperia, A. (1993) Salt deficient diet and early weaning inhibit DNA synthesis in immature rat proximal tubular cells. *Pediatr. Nephrol.*, **7**, 41–44

92. Roy, R.N., Chance, G.W., Radde, I.C., Hill, D.E., Willis, D.M. and Sheepers, J. (1976) Late hyponatraemia in very low birthweight infants (<1.3 kg). *Pediatr. Res.*, **10**, 526–531

93. Oliver, J.A., Pinto, J., Sciacca, R.R. and Cannon, P.J. (1980) Increased renal secretion of norepinephrine and prostaglandin $E_2$ during sodium depletion in the dog. *J. Clin. Invest.*, **66**, 748–756

94. Yeh, T.F., Wilks, A., Singh, J., Bethkerur, M., Lilien, L. and Pildes, R.S. (1982) Furosemide prevents the renal side effects of indomethacin therapy in premature infants with patent ductus arteriosus. *J. Pediatr.*, **101**, 433–437

95. Fajardo, C.A., Whyte, R.K. and Steele, B.T. (1992) Effect of dopamine on failure of indomethacin to close the patent ductus arteriosus. *J. Pediatr.*, **121**, 771–775

96. Klarr, J.M., Raix, R.G., Pryce, C.J. and Bhatt, M.V. (1994) Randomised blind trial of dopamine versus dobutamine for treatment of hypotension in preterm infants with respiratory distress syndrome. *J. Pediatr.*, **125**, 117–122

97. Greenough, A. and Emery, E.F. (1993) Randomised trial comparing dopamine and dobutamine in preterm infants. *Eur. J. Pediatr.*, **152**, 925–927

98. Roze, J.C., Tohier, C., Maingueneau, C., Lefevre, M. and Mouzard, A. (1993) Response to dobutamine and dopamine in the hypotensive, very preterm infant. *Arch. Dis. Childh.*, **69**, 59–63

99. Seri, I., Rudas, G., Bors, Z., Kanyicska, B. and Tulassay, T. (1993) Effects of low dose dopamine infusion on cardiovascular and renal functions, cerebral blood flow and plasma catecholamine levels in sick, preterm neonates. *Pediatr. Res.*, **34**, 742–749

100. Matthew, O.P., Jones, A.S., James, E., Bland, H. and Groshong, T. (1980) Neonatal renal failure: usefulness of diagnostic indices. *Pediatrics*, **65**, 57–60

101. Norman, M.E. and Asadi, F.K. (1979) A prospective study of acute renal failure in the newborn infant. *Pediatrics*, **63**, 475–479

102. Tulassay, T. and Seri, I. (1986) Acute oliguria in preterm infants with hyaline membrane disease: interaction of dopamine and furosemide. *Acta Paediatr. Scand.*, **75**, 420–424

103. Chevalier, R.L., Campbell, F. and Brenbridge, A.N.A.G. (1984) Prognostic factors in neonatal acute renal failure. *Pediatrics*, **74**, 265–272

104. Coulthard, M.G. and Vernon, B. (1995) Managing acute renal failure in very low birthweight infants. *Arch. Dis. Child, Fetal Neonatal Ed.*, **73**, F187–192

105. Coulthard, M.G. and Sharp, J. (1995) Haemodialysis and ultrafiltration in babies weighing under 1000 g. *Arch. Dis. Child, Fetal Neonatal Ed.*, **73**, F162–165

# 18

# Neurological abnormalities

## I. AETIOLOGY

### Richard Cooke

During the perinatal period the human brain is exceptionally vulnerable to a variety of insults which may produce lifelong consequences in survivors. The ELBW infant is more vulnerable than most, with the highest incidence and severity of neurological sequelae. Although the disease processes involved in the aetiology of neurological lesions are similar to those in larger infants, the frequency of physiological disturbances due to respiratory distress and intrapartum hypoxia is greater, and the size and maturity of the brain different, even from that of a larger preterm infant.

Most ELBW infants will be of 28 weeks' gestation or less, although a few very growth regarded ones will be up to 34 weeks. The maturity determines which parts of the brain have developed and which are yet to form, the distribution and responsiveness of the cerebral circulation, the stage of calcification and resilience of the skull, and capillary function. Irrespective of maturity, the relative size of the brain to body weight is very large in the ELBW, at 16–20% of body weight [1]. Although the cerebral blood flow in the very preterm is lower than in the mature brain [2], a relatively large proportion of the cardiac output will still be required for normal function. While this is easily achieved in the well infant, supply may well be compromised in the sick infant. Such problems may account for the frequency with which ischaemic and haemorrhagic injury is seen in the ELBW brain.

## Development of the cerebral circulation

In the early embryo the arterial supply to the developing brain consists of two systems, one ventriculopetal and the other ventriculofugal [3]. Both systems originate on the surface of the brain, but the latter on reaching the periventricular area recurves to flow outwards. The arterial supply does not extensively anastomose and thus acts as an end arterial system with a series of vulnerable boundary zones between ventriculopetal arteries in the cortex, and between the ventriculopetal and ventriculofugal arteries in the periventricular area. The arterial system supplying the brain is established at least externally by about 7 weeks of embryonic life, although there is extensive branching later as the cerebrum greatly increases in size during fetal life [4]. Penetration of the cerebrum and internal vascularization proceeds from 7 weeks with the development of a superficial capillary network and later deep branches to the subependymal bed at 12 weeks of age [5]. For a period between the sixth and seventh month of gestation the basal branches of the anterior and middle cerebral arteries which supply the basal ganglia are relatively larger reflecting their phylogenetic importance [6].

The subependymal layer or germinal matrix is the source of 80% of intraventricular haemorrhages, and consists of a mass of glioblastic cells supplied by a vascular network. This has been described as a 'primitive vascular rete', whose peculiar structure made it more vulnerable to haemorrhage [7]. These observations were made using injection techniques. More recent studies using alkaline phosphatase stains to identify arteries and veins, suggest that the vascular structure of the germinal matrix is conventional, with arteries connecting with veins only through a capillary network. The source of haemorrhage appeared to be from the venous side of the network [8].

The germinal matrix thins out after 30 weeks and becomes vestigial in the more mature brain. The arterial supply is by Heubner's artery, branches of the lateral striate arteries and the anterior choroidal artery. The capillary network in the germinal matrix supplies the superficial and deep parts leaving the centre relatively avascular [7]. The developing cortex is supplied at 24 weeks by spiral perforating medullary arteries. By 28 weeks cell migration to the cortex has largely ceased and dendritic proliferation begins [9]. The short cortical arteries increase in number and the longer perforating arteries increase in calibre to meet the increasing needs of the expanding cerebrum. By 32 weeks differentiation of white matter from the cortex begins.

The cerebral venous system develops from a number of venous plexuses which extensively communicate and are remodelled greatly during fetal development. Eventually the thin walled dural sinuses and the deep or Galenic system remain. The cortex is drained by regularly branching veins which develop in parallel to the cortical arteries but are fewer in number. The white matter of the cerebral hemispheres is drained almost entirely by the thalamostriate or terminal veins, the septal veins, and the basal veins into the Galenic system. Although anastomoses do exist between the deep and superficial venous systems, obstruction of the deep venous system frequently leads to venous infarction of the white matter suggesting that in the immature brain these alternative pathways are unable to cope, as a much greater proportion of the brain is drained by the deep system than later in development [10].

The maturation of the capillary at an ultrastructural level is poorly documented. Animal studies are difficult to extrapolate to the human fetus and newborn. Human studies seem to indicate that a wide variety of stages of development of capillaries may be seen in the same embryo or fetus, and that the appearance of structures such as the basement membrane, important for the function of the 'blood–brain barrier', is more related to the age of the capillary than to the age of the fetus, at least in the first half of gestation [11]. Another study suggests that the structure of the capillaries is mature at 22 weeks, although no functional information is available [12].

Capillary permeability in newborn rabbits as measured by fluorescein-labelled dextran of differing molecular weights was increased in preterm offspring, but more markedly so in rabbits of all gestational ages when exposed to hypoxia or an increase in venous pressure [13]. Grontoft showed in the human fetus that the blood–brain barrier was impermeable to Trypan blue in fetuses of 5–30 cm in length, but that hypoxia readily increased their permeability [14]. The resistance to hypoxia appeared to increase with the maturity of the fetus. Increased capillary permeability is usually considered in relation to hypoxia or venous pressure but a variety of other variables such as hypercarbia, acidosis, arterial hypertension and hyperosmolality of the plasma may be of equal importance. Various prostaglandins, in particular prostacyclin, increase capillary leakage. High circulating levels of prostacyclin have been demonstrated in preterm infants suffering from hyaline membrane disease, and especially in those going on to show evidence of cerebral haemorrhage [15]. The source of these prostanoids is likely to be the lungs, and their release to be associated with mechanical ventilation [16]. There seems to be little evidence that the capillaries of the ELBW infant are functionally immature, but that perhaps they are more vulnerable to the frequent insults to which they are liable.

## Causes of perinatal brain injury

Although it is generally agreed that the cerebral blood supply is critical for the support of cerebral function, the lack of reliable methods for measurement in the preterm infant makes many of our ideas on the role of the cerebral circulation in the aetiology of perinatal brain injury speculative. Such attempts as have been made to measure cerebral blood flow in preterm infants suggest that it is similar to or lower than in older infants when related to brain weight [2,17]. Unstable flow patterns have been associated with an increased likelihood of later haemorrhage and to be related to unstable systemic blood pressure, usually as the result of the infant struggling against mechanical ventilation [18,19].

The cerebral circulation is likely to be affected by the birth process. Both a fall and a rise in cerebral blood flow after birth in the first 48 hours have been reported by investigators using different techniques. Using volumetric Doppler techniques, the flow to the brain has been shown to be relatively stable following birth, but with the velocity in the cerebral arteries increasing over the first 3 days [20]. These findings imply that cerebral artery reactivity and autoregulatory control develop over this period. They also suggest that for this early period in preterm infants there may be an increased vulnerability of the cerebral circulation to exposure to surges in flow related to the unstable systemic circulation. This is supported by the known high incidence of haemorrhagic lesions in the periventricular region at this time.

Mean arterial blood pressure shows a consistent rise over the first 48 hours after birth with a coefficient of variation of around 8%. Pressures are lower in ELBW infants, but show similar variation [21]. Continuous arterial pressure monitoring in ELBW infants has shown that routine clinical procedures may result in brief high peaks of blood pressure which are associated with cerebral haemorrhage particularly in ELBW infants [22]. However, a controlled trial in which infants were randomized to standard or reduced manipulation was unable to demonstrate a reduction in intraventricular haemorrhage or other adverse outcomes [23].

Hypotension in ELBW infants during the first 48 hours relates closely to periventricular haemorrhage (PVH), especially of severer degree [21,24,25]. The cause of the hypotension is not certain, but likely to be related to poor cardiac output or to hypovolaemia. The latter may relate to fluid losses from the vascular space due to increased capillary permeability, or to cord clamping at birth before lung expansion has occurred and the placental transfer of blood completed. The perinatal circulation may also be affected by maternal factors such as antepartum haemorrhage. This often precedes major parenchymal lesions, and has its effect through a reduction in placental perfusion leading to fetal ischaemia or hypovolaemia [26].

Factors such as birth asphyxia and hyaline membrane disease are related to an increase in cerebral injury [27], and both are common in ELBW infants. If causal, the influence of these factors is likely to be through their action in changing capillary permeability, hypotension and circulatory instability. However, the use of exogenous pulmonary surfactants, particularly prophylactically, results in a reduction in morbidity and mortality from hyaline membrane disease, but does not reduce the risk of periventricular haemorrhage [28]. Ante-natal prophylaxis with corticosteroids results in substantial reductions in both respiratory morbidity and cerebral haemorrhage [29]. The association between periventricular haemorrhage and respiratory distress may simply be through a common factor of immaturity.

Other physical factors which may be relevant include the properties of the ELBW infant's skull. This is very soft and may allow considerable deformation to occur during delivery. In a few cases this may cause direct brain trauma from fracture and displacement of the occipital bone [30]. In larger infants venous infarction from prolonged brain compression during long labours has been described [31]. It is possible that such a process may at least contribute to cerebral ischaemia in ELBW infants. If this were so, the mode of delivery would be relevant. There are no randomized trials studying the effect of Caesarean section on the incidence of intraventricular haemorrhage, but a number of epidemiological studies suggest a protective role [32].

Apart from direct trauma, malformations, infections, and the effects of toxins such as aminoglycosides and bilirubin, lesions of the very preterm brain may be considered under three main groupings:

(1)  Germinal matrix and intraventricular haemorrhage.
(2)  Parenchymal haemorrhage and infarction.
(3)  Periventricular leucomalacia.

These groups are not mutually exclusive and may coexist and be related by the mechanisms already discussed.

## Germinal layer haemorrhage (GLH) and intraventricular haemorrhage (IVH)

The reported rate for periventricular haemorrhage in ELBW infants varies, but probably lies in the range of 50–60%. More recent publications appear to indicate a falling incidence, although mainly in larger infants [33,34]. ELBW infants not only have a higher rate of haemorrhage, but also suffer severer grades of bleeding [35,36]. It is now generally recognized that haemorrhage can broadly be divided into early and late onset; 50% of all bleeds may be detected in the first 12 hours after birth. Such early bleeds occur more often in infants with lower gestational age and birth weight, and appear to be closely related to evidence of fetal distress, acidosis, and mode of delivery. Premature rupture of the amniotic membranes and maternal pregnancy-induced hypertension appear to protect against early haemorrhage [36]. Late onset of periventricular haemorrhage is seen in rather more mature preterm infants and is more clearly related to postnatal events such as respiratory distress syndrome, derangement of blood gases, pneumothorax, endotracheal tube suctioning, hypothermia and excessive use of heparin. Periventricular haemorrhage is rarely seen as an initial event more than 4 or 5 days after birth [37]. The reason for this remains unclear. Immediately after birth the cerebral vasculature is relatively dilated and unreactive. Changes in vascular permeability occur, possibly related to circulating prostacyclin levels which are high immediately after birth, but fall to low levels within 2–3 days, even in sick infants [15]. Early haemorrhage may progress and when this occurs the final grade of the bleed is often more extensive than that in later bleeds.

Periventricular haemorrhage begins in the great majority of cases in the germinal matrix, although a small proportion originate in the choroid plexus, particularly in more mature infants. It appears to originate from the venous side of the capillary bed, is often multifocal, and may be confined to the germinal layer or extend to rupture into and even fill the ventricular system [38]. It has been proposed that the anatomy of the germinal matrix makes it vulnerable in that it is a primitive vascular rete, an irregular network of thin and poorly supported vessels, with some vascular shunts [7]. Recent work has challenged this by demonstrating that the germinal matrix has a normal vascular configuration [8]. There is a relatively avascular central area in the germinal matrix which may render it more liable to infarction, and the arterial supply to this area is a boundary zone. Although the germinal layer is a low flow area in the beagle puppy model of preterm cerebral haemorrhage, it is generally an area of high flow and metabolic activity in the human fetus in the midtrimester [39]. Early systemic hypotension has been observed in several studies, leading to the suggestion that it is the restoration of blood pressure and consequent blood flow that causes haemorrhage [21,25]. Such a process could be simply mechanical, or involve an ischaemia/reperfusion phenomenon with the generation of oxygen derived free radicals and consequent injury. The association of germinal layer haemorrhage (GLH) with an extended capillary bleeding time in the first 6 hours after birth suggests that a platelet/capillary function disorder may be important [40]. Prostacyclin has an important influence in this area and the high levels of prostacyclin metabolites reported prior to haemorrhage may be relevant [15]. Free radical damage to capillary endothelium subsequent to ischaemia/reperfusion may be the source, or they may originate from ventilated lung. Evidence for a role for major coagulation defects in GLH is lacking, and early studies reporting such associations were probably observing coagulation disorders occurring as the result of major haemorrhage rather than being its cause [40].

Post-haemorrhagic hydrocephalus is commonly seen in ELBW infants following GLH/IVH and relates to the extent of the lesion, being uncommon with minor bleeds, but almost invariable when both cerebral ventricles are entirely filled with blood clot [41]. Some degree of ventricular enlargement almost always occurs after IVH, but is usually transient and is resolving by 3–4 weeks of age [27]. This probably relates to a temporary abnormality in cerebrospinal fluid production or absorption induced by fibrin deposition. The majority of infants with post-haemorrhagic hydrocephalus also have some degree of parenchymal involvement and the outcome in these infants following surgical treatment appears to relate to the extent of cystic changes in the parenchyma. There is, however, some evidence to suggest that the degree of ventricular enlargement alone may also relate to outcome, although this is probably because many of these infants have a degree of cerebral atrophy contributing to the enlargement. In ELBW infants the outcome of post-haemorrhagic hydrocephalus is particularly poor [42].

## Parenchymal haemorrhage and infarction

The extent of parenchymal brain injury, whether due to haemorrhage or infarction, is the most important determinant of outcome in follow-up studies of ELBW survivors [43]. There is debate as to the origin and nature of the pathological lesion responsible for the cranial ultrasound scan appearance of 'intraparenchymal echodense lesion' (IPL) [44]. Such lesions have been assumed to be simply extensions of smaller GLH/IVH. Grading systems for periventricular haemorrhage present an apparent sequence from one to the other, but pathological studies suggest that this is most unlikely, as often the lesions are not in direct continuity with each other. IPL is nevertheless strongly associated with GLH/IVH both in timing and laterality [45]. IPL usually occurs after GLH/IVH and is more often unilateral. Various explanations for this have been offered. Firstly, there may be a common antecedent to both lesions such as ischaemia followed by reperfusion causing haemorrhage into the infarcted germinal layer, and into an infarcted area of white matter in a watershed zone adjacent to the lateral ventricle [46]. Alternatively, the GLH/IVH may be the initiating factor for the IPL. Mechanisms suggested have been the induction of venous thrombosis in the terminal vein as it passes through the germinal matrix, with subsequent retrograde venous infarction of the parenchyma [47], or

the release of vasoactive substances from the GLH/IVH producing local ischaemia and infarction [48].

## Periventricular leucomalacia (PVL)

Perinatal pathologists have long recognized neuronal loss and gliosis in the periventricular regions of the brains of small infants dying following perinatal difficulties, and have speculated about their possible significance in the aetiology of neurological deficits in survivors [49]. The aetiology of PVL has always been assumed to be ischaemic, at least in recent years. The extensive use of neonatal cranial ultrasound scanning has revealed how common the lesion is in surviving infants [45,50]. The ischaemia may result from hypotension leading to poor perfusion of the boundary zone between the ventriculopetal and ventriculofugal arteries supplying the periventricular region, or to venous stasis within the white matter induced by thrombosis of veins from the deep system as they pass through the germinal matrix [51]. The clinical antecedents of PVL and 'parenchymal' periventricular haemorrhage are essentially similar, except that the latter has been preceded by a GLH/IVH, and that PVL has often been described as occurring later in association with an episode of necrotizing enterocolitis or septicaemia. Both lesions probably represent a common end-point. PVL has been put forward as the pathological lesion which in survivors leads to spastic cerebral diplegia, although there is little evidence that this is the only disability associated with such an ultrasound scan appearance. In recent studies, PVL of more than a minor extent has been associated with a poor clinical outcome, with severe degree of cerebral palsy, mental retardation or cortical blindness [45,50].

## Prevention of periventricular haemorrhage

Periventricular haemorrhage has been the outcome variable for a wide range of therapeutic interventions in both obstetrics and neonatal medicine. Although the populations studied were usually of infants or fetuses of 1500 g and below, ELBW subgroups are often identified separately.

The most obvious intervention for reducing PVH is often supposed to be one which would reduce the rate of premature delivery. Trials of tocolytics such as ritodrine and indomethacin, have not shown a consistent benefit in terms of reduction in PVH, and some have shown an increase in adverse side-effects in the preterm infant such as necrotizing enterocolitis, PVH and chronic lung disease [52].

Epidemiological studies have suggested that the mode of delivery is important, at least in determining the incidence of early GLH/IVH, and that delivery by Caesarean section was protective [53]. Others have suggested that it is the presence of active labour irrespective of the final route of delivery that is the main determinant of outcome [54,55]. In none of these studies had the mothers been randomized with respect to mode of delivery. Antenatal prophylaxis with corticosteroids is an effective method of reducing pulmonary pathology at all gestations. Meta-analysis of those studies recording PVH as an outcome also showed a significant reduction of about 50% in the likelihood of cerebral haemorrhage [29]. While it is possible that the reduction in PVH attributable to steroids is caused by a reduction in respiratory distress, there is evidence to suggest that the effect is independent of this, and may relate to maturational effects on the central nervous system. Whatever the mechanism, antenatal steroids confer as great a protection against PVH as any other pharmacological intervention. Concerns about the effects of steroids on brain growth and development do not appear to have been substantiated in follow-up studies [56].

While there is no convincing evidence that treatment with exogenous surfactants alone for respiratory distress syndrome reduces PVH, both epidemiological and controlled trial evidence suggest a protective effect with combined therapy with antenatal steroids [57,58].

Various other pharmacological interventions for prophylaxis of PVH have been investigated by means of controlled trials during the past decade, although none has proved entirely satisfactory.

Vitamin E was first suggested as a prophylactic for PVH over 40 years ago because its deficiency was observed to cause cerebral haemorrhage in chicks. Chiswick and Speer have both shown a reduction in incidence of some grades of PVH [59,60]. A subsequent study showed an increase in incidence of major haemorrhage with vitamin E given intravenously [61]. Fish *et al.* undertook a randomized controlled trial of intramuscular vitamin E in ELBW infants which showed a reduction of incidence and severity of haemorrhage in infants weighing less than 501–750 g [62]. Ethamsylate is a water soluble, non-steroidal drug which reduces capillary bleeding time. Three randomized controlled trials involving VLBW infants showed reductions in incidence and severity of PVH [63–65], although a recent randomized study in Europe involving infants under 32 weeks' gestation did not show a difference between treated and control infants [66].

Phenobarbitone has been used both antenatally and postnatally to prevent PVH in clinical trials. Postnatal administration was initially shown in small studies to be protective but subsequently larger studies showed adverse effects [67]. Antenatal prophylaxis has similarly shown conflicting results, together with evidence for an increase in need for respiratory support in treated infants [68].

Indomethacin given postnatally has been evaluated in seven controlled trials. Again the earlier studies have proved inconclusive mainly because of small trial size. Most recently a large study of infants of 600–1250 g birth weight demonstrated a marked reduction in the incidence of severe PVH, with no apparent adverse effects attributable to indomethacin [69]. Use of indomethacin to close a persistent duct has not been shown to cause or prevent progression of GLH/IVH already present [70,71].

## Toxic neuronal damage

In the mature and intact human brain the neurones are protected from the effect of toxins by the integrity and selective behaviour of the blood–brain barrier (BBB). While it is unlikely that the BBB is functionally immature even in the ELBW infant, it is certainly vulnerable to the insults associated with neonatal diseases which are more frequent in the ELBW. Toxins may take the form of natural metabolites such as bilirubin or administered drugs such as gentamicin. Damage to the basal ganglia from the entry of bilirubin (kernicterus) has long been recognized in term infants with rhesus isoimmunization. Although the emphasis in prevention was always on keeping bilirubin levels low, more recent work suggests that the loss of integrity of the BBB due to intercurrent illness was probably more important in its causation. This is in keeping with the pathological findings of yellow staining of the basal ganglia in very preterm infants who had never experienced very high bilirubin levels [72].

The nature of the clinical presentation of such bilirubin-induced injury in the very preterm survivor is uncertain. Classical choreoathetosis is uncommon in ELBW survivors, and it has been suggested that other forms of cerebral palsy or the high incidence of nerve deafness in ELBW infants is due to bilirubin toxicity. The occurrence of abnormalities of cortical evoked potentials in association with hyperbilirubinaemia might be seen as supportive evidence, although these changes are reversible [73].

The case for neurotoxicity of drugs such as gentamicin is even less clear. Streptomycin certainly caused deafness in babies in the early days of its use, but is no longer used in preterm infants. Gentamicin is frequently used, but any association between its use and subsequent neurological deficit such as deafness is confounded by the presence of other factors such as acidosis or meningitis. Other possible toxic substances include aminoacids infused as part of total intravenous nutrition, some of which may reach potentially toxic levels in sick infants.

---

**Practical points**

1. ELBW infants are at greatest risk for acquiring cerebral injury in the perinatal period mainly as the result of immaturity of respiratory and other systems.
2. GLH/IVH and parenchymal haemorrhage and infarction are related but may occur independently of each other.
3. Prevention of cerebral injury in ELBW infants depends upon avoidance of preterm birth, intrapartum hypoxia, and cardiorespiratory instability. The role of pharmacological prophylaxis remains unclear, although antenatal corticosteroids and postnatal low-dose indomethacin appear the most promising agents.

---

# References

1. Cooke, R.W.I., Lucas, A., Pryse-Davies, J. and Yudkin, P.L.N. (1977) Head circumference as an index of brain weight in the fetus and newborn infant. *Early Hum. Dev.*, **1**, 145–149
2. Volpe, J.J., Herescovitch, P., Perlman, J.M. and Raichle, M.E. (1983) Positron emission tomography in the newborn; extensive impairment of regional cerebral bloodflow with intraventricular hemorrhage and hemorrhagic cerebral involvement. *Pediatrics*, **72**, 589–601
3. Van den Bergh, R. (1967) The periventricular intracerebral blood supply. In *Research on the Cerebral Circulation (3rd International Salzburg Conference)*, (J.S. Meyer, M. Lechner and O. Eickhorn, eds), Thomas, Springfield, Illinois, pp. 52–63
4. Dorovini-Zis, K. and Dolman, C.L. (1977) Gestational development of the brain. *Arch. Pathol. Lab. Med.*, **101**, 192–195
5. Duckett, S. (1971) The establishment of internal vascularisation in the human telencephalon. *Acta Anat.*, **80**, 107–113
6. Keir, E.L. (1974) Fetal cerebral arteries; a phylogenetic and ontogenetic study. In *Radiology of the Skull and Brain, Vol. 2, Book 1* (T.H. Newton and D.G. Potts, eds), Mosby, St. Louis, pp. 1089–1130
7. Pape, K.E. and Wigglesworth, J.S. (1979) Blood supply to the developing brain. In *Haemorrhage, Ischaemia and the Perinatal Brain, Clin. Dev. Med.*, **69/70**, pp. 16–17, SIMS, Heinemann, London
8. Moody, D.M., Brown, W.R., Challa, V.R. and Block, S.M. (1994) Alkaline phosphatase histochemical staining of germinal matrix hemorrhage and brain vascular morphology in a very low birth weight neonate. *Pediatr. Res.*, **35**, 424–430
9. Dobbing, J. and Sands, J. (1970) Timing of neuroblast multiplication in developing human brain. *Nature*, **226**, 639–640
10. Pape, K.E. and Wigglesworth, J.S. (1979) Blood supply to the developing brain. In *Haemorrhage, Ischaemia and the Perinatal Brain, Clin. Dev. Med.*, **69/70**, pp. 26–27, SIMS, Heinemann, London
11. Hauw, J.J., Berger, B. and Escourolle, R. (1975) Electron microscopic study of the developing capillaries of human brain. *Acta Neuropathol.*, **31**, 229–242
12. Gruner, J.E. (1970) The maturation of human cerebral cortex in electron microscopy study of post-mortem punctures in premature infants. *Biol. Neonate*, **16**, 243–255
13. Takashima, S. and Tanaka, K. (1978) Microangiography and vascular permeability of the subependymal matrix in the premature infant. *Can. J. Neurosci.*, **5**, 45–50

14. Grontoft, O. (1958) Intracerebral and meningeal haemorrhages in perinatally distressed infants; intracerebral haemorrhages, pathologic-anatomical and obstetrical study. *Acta Obstet. Gynecol. Scand.*, **3**, 308–334

15. Rennie, J.M., Doyle, J. and Cooke, R.W.I. (1987) Elevated levels of immunoreactive prostacyclin metabolite in babies who develop intraventricular haemorrhage. *Acta Paediatr. Scand.*, **76**, 19–23

16. Elund, A., Bomfim, W., Kaiser, L. *et al.* (1981) Pulmonary formation of prostacyclin in man. *Prostaglandins*, **22**, 323–331

17. Ment, L.R., Duncan, C.C., Ehrenkranz, R.A. *et al.* (1984) Intraventricular haemorrhage in the preterm neonate: timing and cerebral bloodflow changes. *J. Pediatr.*, **104**, 419–425

18. Perlman, J.M., McMenamin, J.B. and Volpe, J.J. (1983) Fluctuating cerebral blood flow velocity in respiratory distress syndrome. *N. Engl. J. Med.*, **309**, 204–209

19. Perlman, J.M., Goodman, S., Kreusser, K.L., Volpe, J.J. (1985) Reduction in intraventricular hemorrhage by elimination of fluctuating cerebral bloodflow velocity in preterm infants with respiratory distress syndrome. *N. Engl. J. Med.*, **312**, 1353–1357

20. Drayton, M.R. and Skidmore, R. (1987) Vasoactivity of the major intracranial arteries in newborn infants. *Arch. Dis. Childh.*, **62**, 236–240

21. Bada, H.S., Korones, S.B., Perry, E.H. *et al.* (1990) Mean arterial blood pressure changes in premature infants and those at risk for intraventricular hemorrhage. *J. Pediatr.*, **117**, 607–614

22. Perry, E.H., Bada, H.S., Ray, J.D. *et al.* (1990) Blood pressure increases, birth weight-dependent stability boundary, and intraventricular hemorrhage. *Pediatrics*, **85**, 727–732

23. Bada, H.S., Korones, S.B., Perry, E.H. *et al.* (1990) Frequent handling in the neonatal intensive care unit and intraventricular hemorrhage. *J. Pediatr.*, **117**, 126–131

24. Fujimura, M., Salisbury, D.M., Robinson, R.O. *et al.* (1979) Clinical events relating to intraventricular haemorrhage in the newborn. *Arch. Dis. Childh.*, **54**, 409–414

25. Watkins, A., West, C. and Cooke, R.W.I. (1987) Blood pressure and cerebral injury in sick very low birthweight infants. *Arch. Dis. Childh.*, **62**, 648–649

26. Weindling, A.M., Rochfort, M.J., Calvert, S.A., Fok, T.F. and Wilkinson, A. (1985) Development of cerebral palsy after ultrasonographic detection of periventricular cysts in the newborn. *Dev. Med. Child. Neurol.*, **27**, 800–806

27. Cooke, R.W.I. (1981) Factors associated with periventricular haemorrhage in very low birthweight infants. *Arch. Dis. Childh.*, **56**, 425–431

28. Leviton, A., VanMarter, L. and Kuban, K.C.K. (1989) Respiratory distress syndrome and intracranial hemorrhage: cause or association? Inferences from surfactant clinical trials. *Pediatrics*, **84**, 915–920

29. Crowley, P., Chalmers, I. and Keirse, M.J.N.C. (1990) The effects of corticosteroid administration before preterm delivery: an overview of the evidence from controlled trials. *Br. J. Obstet. Gynaecol.*, **97**, 11–26

30. Wigglesworth, J.S. and Husemeyer, R.P. (1977) Intracranial birth trauma in vaginal breech delivery: the continued importance of injury to the occipital bone. *Br. J. Obstet. Gynaecol.*, **84**, 684–691

31. Schwartz, P. (1961) *Birth Injuries in the Newborn*, Karger, Basel.

32. Philip, A.G.S. and Allan, W.C. (1991) Does caesarian section protect against intraventricular hemorrhage in preterm infants? *J. Perinatol.*, **11**, 3–94

33. Strand, C., Laptook, A.R., Dowling, S. *et al.* (1990) Neonatal intracranial hemorrhage: 1. Changing pattern in inborn low birthweight infants. *Early Hum. Dev.*, **23**, 117–128

34. Philip, A.G.S., Allan, W.A., Tito, A.M. and Wheeler, L.R. (1989) Intraventricular hemorrhage in preterm infants: declining incidence in the 1980's. *Pediatrics*, **84**, 797–801

35. Perlman, J.M. and Volpe, J.J. (1986) Intraventricular hemorrhage in extremely small premature infants. *Am. J. Dis. Child.*, **140**, 1122–1124

36. Ment, L.R., Oh, W., Philip, A.G.S. *et al.* (1992) Risk factors for early intraventricular hemorrhage in low birth weight infants. *J. Pediatr.*, **121**, 776–783

37. Ment, L.R., Oh, W., Ehrenkrantz, R.A. *et al.* (1993) Risk period for intraventricular hemorrhage of the preterm neonate is independent of gestational age. *Semin. Perinatol.*, **17**, 338–341

38. Hambleton, G. and Wigglesworth, J.S. (1976) Origin of intraventricular haemorrhage in the preterm infant. *Arch. Dis. Childh.*, **51**, 651–659

39. Pasternak, J.F., Groothuis, D.R., Fischer, J.M. and Fischer, D.P. (1982) Regional cerebral blood flow in the beagle pup: the germinal matrix is a low-flow structure. *Pediatr. Res.*, **16**, 499–503

40. Setzer, E.S., Webb, L.B., Wassenaar, J.W. *et al.* (1982) Platelet dysfunction and coagulopathy in intraventricular hemorrhage in the premature infant. *J. Pediatr.*, **100**, 599–605

41. Hill, A. and Volpe, J.J. (1981) Normal pressure hydrocephalus in the newborn. *Pediatrics*, **68**, 623–629

42. Cooke, R.W.I. (1987) Determinants of major handicap in post-haemorrhagic hydrocephalus. *Arch. Dis. Childh.*, **62**, 504–506

43. Cooke, R.W.I. (1994) Factors affecting survival and outcome at 3 years in extremely preterm infants. *Arch. Dis. Childh.*, **71**, F28–31

44. Perlman, J.M., Rollins, N., Burns, D. and Risser, R. (1993) Relationship between periventricular intraparenchymal echodensities and germinal matrix-intraventricular hemorrhage in the very low birthweight neonate. *Pediatrics*, **91**, 474–480

45. Cooke, R.W.I. (1987) Early and late ultrasound appearances and outcome in very low birthweight infants. *Arch. Dis. Childh.*, **62**, 931–937

46. Rushton, D.I., Preston, P.R. and Durbin, G.M. (1985)

Structure and evolution of echodense lesions in the neonatal brain. A combined ultrasound and necropsy study. *Arch. Dis. Childh.*, **60**, 798–808

47. Gould, S.J., Howard, S., Hope, P.L. and Reynolds, E.O.R. (1987) Periventricular intraparenchymal cerebral haemorrhage in preterm infants: the role of infarction. *J. Pathol.*, **151**, 197–202

48. Stutchfield, P.R. and Cooke, R.W.I. (1989) Electrolytes and glucose in cerebrospinal fluid of premature infants with IVH: role of potassium in cerebral infarction. *Arch. Dis. Childh.*, **64**, 470–475

49. Banker, B.Q. and Larroche, J.C. (1962) Periventricular leukomalacia in infancy. *Arch. Neurol.*, **7**, 386–410

50. de Vries, L.S., Dubowitz, L.M.S., Dubowitz, V. *et al.* (1985) Predictive value of cranial ultrasound in the newborn baby: a reappraisal. *Lancet*, **ii**, 137–140

51. Armstrong, D. and Norman, M.G. (1974) Periventricular leucomalacia in neonates: complications and sequelae. *Arch. Dis. Childh.*, **49**, 367–375

52. Norton, M.E., Merrill, J., Cooper, B.A. *et al.* (1993) Neonatal complications after administration of indomethacin for preterm labor. *N. Engl. J. Med.*, **329**, 1602–1607

53. Anderson, G.D., Bada, H.S., Sibai, B.M. *et al.* (1988) The relationship between labor and route of delivery in the preterm infant. *Am. J. Obstet. Gynecol.*, **158**, 1382–1390

54. Anderson, G.D., Bada, H.S., Shaver, D.C. *et al.* (1992) The effect of cesarean section on intraventricular hemorrhage in the preterm infant. *Am. J. Obstet. Gynecol.*, **166**, 1091–1101

55. Tejani, N., Rebold, B., Tuck, S. *et al.* (1984) Obstetric factors in the causation of early periventricular–intraventricular hemorrhage. *Obstet. Gynecol.*, **64**, 510–515

56. Doyle, L.W., Kitchen, W.H., Ford, G.W. *et al.* (1989) Antenatal steroid therapy and 5-year outcome of extremely low birth weight infants. *Obstet. Gynecol.*, **73**, 743–746

57. Farrell, E.E., Silver, R.K., Kimberlin, L.V. *et al.* (1989) Impact of antenatal dexamethasone administration on respiratory distress syndrome in surfactant-treated infants. *Am. J. Obstet. Gynecol.*, **161**, 628–633

58. Kari, M.A., Hallman, M., Eronen, M. *et al.* (1994) Prenatal dexamethasone treatment in conjunction with rescue therapy of human surfactant: a randomised placebo-controlled multicentre study. *Pediatrics*, **93**, 730–736

59. Chiswick, M.L., Johnson, M., Woodhall, C. *et al.* (1983) Protective effect of Vitamin E against intraventricular haemorrhage in premature babies. *Br. Med. J.*, **287**, 81–84

60. Speer, M.E., Blifield, C., Rudolph, A.J. *et al.* (1984) Intraventricular hemorrhage and Vitamin E in the very low birthweight infant: evidence for efficacy of early intramuscular Vitamin E administration. *Pediatrics*, **74**, 1107–1112

61. Phelps, D.L. (1984) Vitamin E and CNS hemorrhage. *Pediatrics*, **74**, 1113–1114

62. Fish, W.H., Cohen, M., Franzek, D. *et al.* (1990) Effect of intramuscular vitamin E on mortality and intracranial hemorrhage in neonates of 1000 grams or less. *Pediatrics*, **85**, 578–584

63. Morgan, M.E.I., Benson, J.W.T. and Cooke, R.W.I. (1981) Ethamsylate reduces the incidence of periventricular haemorrhage in very low birthweight babies. *Lancet*, **ii**, 830–831

64. Benson, J.W.T., Drayton, M.R., Hayward, C. *et al.* (1986) Multicentre trial of ethamsylate for prevention of periventricular haemorrhage in very low birth weight infants. *Lancet*, **ii**, 1297–1300

65. Chen, J. (1983) Ethamsylate in the prevention of periventricular-intraventricular hemorrhage in premature infants. *J. Formos. Med. Assoc.*, **92**, 889–893

66. The EC Ethamsylate Trial Group (1994) The EC randomised controlled trial of prophylactic ethamsylate for very preterm neonates: early mortality and morbidity. *Arch. Dis. Childh.*, **70**, F201–205

67. Kuban, R.C.K., Leviton, A., Pagano, M. *et al.* (1986) Neonatal intracranial hemorrhage and phenobarbital. *Pediatrics*, **77**, 4543–450

68. Kaempf, J., Porreco, R., Molina, R. *et al.* (1990) Antenatal phenobarbital for the prevention of periventricular and intraventricular hemorrhage: a double-blind, randomised, placebo controlled, multi-hospital trial. *J. Pediatr.*, **117**, 933–938

69. Ment, L.R., Oh, W., Ehrenkranz, R.A. *et al.* (1994) Low-dose indomethacin and prevention of intraventricular hemorrhage: a multicentre randomised trial. *Pediatrics*, **93**, 543–550

70. Maher, P., Lane, B., Ballard, R. *et al.* (1985) Does indomethacin cause extension of intracranial hemorrhages: a preliminary study. *Pediatrics*, **75**, 497–500

71. Ment, L.R., Oh, W., Ehrenkranz, R.A. *et al.* (1994) Low-dose indomethacin therapy and extension of intraventricular hemorrhage: a multicentre randomised trial. *J. Pediatr.*, **124**, 951–955

72. Levine, R.L., Fredericks, W.R., Rapoport, S.I. (1982) Entry of bilirubin into the brain due to opening of the blood–brain barrier. *Pediatrics*, **69**, 255–259

73. Wennberg, R.P., Ahlfors, C.E., Bickers, R.G. *et al.* (1982) Abnormal auditory brain stem response in a newborn infant with hyperbilirubinaemia: improvement with exchange transfusion. *J. Pediatr.*, **100**, 624–626

## II. CLINICAL EVALUATION

### Lilly Dubowitz and Eugenio Mercuri

With the improvement in perinatal and neo-natal care there has been a dramatic increase in the survival of ELBW infants in the last decade. This great improvement, unfortunately, has not been paralleled by a reduction in the rate of neuro-developmental handicap in the survivors. The management of these infants has posed hitherto unknown problems to the neonatologists in intensive care units. There are differences both in nutrition and environment for these infants who are reared for 12–16 weeks outside the uterus during a very critical period of neural development compared to a fetus at that gestation. It is to be expected that these differences will affect neural maturation. However, whether this artificial environment will produce deviant or delayed maturation by not providing the natural balance of nutrients or possibly accelerate it by earlier stimulation has not yet been established. In order to appreciate what represents abnormal development much more must be known about the maturational process of ELBW infants who had an optimal perinatal period and it will be necessary to document any changes which occur following a complication.

The aim of this section is to describe:

(1) The tools which are available for the neurological evaluation of the ELBW infant.
(2) What is now known of the similarity or differences in neurological maturation of extremely premature infants outside the uterus compared to the fetus *in utero*.
(3) The neurological findings in some of the more commonly encountered pathological conditions in these infants.

## Neurological assessment

### Estimation of gestational age

The relevance of gestational age (GA) for neonatal or follow-up studies cannot be sufficiently stressed. Not only will perinatal pathology differ according to the maturity of the neonate but various aspects of the early neuro-logical examination and of later growth and development can only be correctly evaluated if gestational age is taken into account. The findings will be very different in an infant weighing 900 g at 25 weeks from one with similar weight but a GA of 35 weeks or more. In women with regular periods gestational age can be estimated from the date of the last menstrual period, but this is often uncertain. Thus a number of indirect methods have been utilized to estimate gestational age.

Ultrasound estimation of fetal size, when used before 16 weeks' gestation, such as the fetal crown–rump measurement [1] and the biparietal diameter [2] are probably the most accurate guides for gestational age. After 16 weeks' gestation the latter becomes increasingly inaccurate [3]. Since nervous system and skin maturation are relatively spared in intrauterine growth retardation, the development of these has been employed in various schemes to estimate gestational age [4–10]. The argument in favour of neurological criteria is that they are least affected by fetal growth retardation even if it is very severe, while the argument against their use is that they might be difficult to elicit in ill infants and can be influenced by neurological abnormality [11]. Physical characteristics can be easily observed, but they are influenced by fetal growth failure [12], particularly if severe. Many also change rapidly in the extrauterine environment especially with the use of radiant heaters. In the authors' experience, the best estimate of gestational age can be obtained when a combination of neurological and physical criteria are used [13,14]. The error is least when many types of observations are added together. However, in infants below 28–29 weeks' gestation little change can be noted in either neurological or physical characteristics with decreasing gestational age, thus there will be a tendency to overestimate maturity. The only suitable and reliable estimate of gestational age in ELBW babies is the measurement of nerve conduction velocity [15–18]. This is a relatively simple technique which can be taught to ancillary staff and will give a reliable estimate of gestational age if performed within the first 3 weeks of life [19].

NAME:_____.    CODE:_____.  SEX:_____.  RACE_____

D.O.B.:_____.    D.O.E.:_____.    AGE:_____.    G.A.:_____.  BW:_____.

| | | | S T A T E | A S Y M M . |
|---|---|---|---|---|

## Tone

| | | | | | | |
|---|---|---|---|---|---|---|
| **POSTURE** Infant supine, look mainly at position of legs but also note arms. *score predominant posture* | arms and legs extended or very slightly flexed | legs slightly flexed | leg well-flexed but not adducted | legs well flexed and adducted near abdomen | abnormal posture: a) opistotonus b) | | |
| **ARM RECOIL** Take both hands, quickly extend arms parallel to the body, Count to three. Release. Repeat X 3 | arms do not flex | arms flex slowly, not always; not completely | arms flex slowly; more complete | arms flex quickly and completely | arms difficult to extend; snap back forcefully | | |
| **ARM TRACTION** Hold wrist and pull arm upwards. Note flexion at elbow and resistance while shoulder lifts off table. *Test each side separately* | arms remain straight; no resistance | arms flex slightly or some resistance felt | arms flex well till shoulder lifts, then straighten | arms flex at approx 100° & mantained as shoulder lifts | flexion of arms <100°; mantained when body lifts up | | |
| **LEG RECOIL** Take *both* ankles in one hand, flex hip+knees. Quickly extend. Release. Repeat X3 | No flexion | incomplete or variable flexion | complete but slow flexion | complete fast flexion | legs difficult to extend; snap back forcefully | | |
| **LEG TRACTION** Grasp ankle and slowly pull leg upwards. Note flexion at knees and resistance as buttocks lift. *Test each side separately* | legs straight - no resistance | legs flex slightly or some resistance felt | legs flex well till bottom lifts up | knee flexes remains flexed when bottom up | flexion stays when back+bottom up | | |
| **POPLITEAL ANGLE** Fix knee on abdomen, extend leg by gentle pressure with index finger behind the ankle. Note angle at knee. *Test each side separately* | 180° | ≈ 150° | ≈110° | ≈90° | <90° | | |
| **HEAD CONTROL (1)** **(extensor tone)** Infant sitting upright; Hold at shoulder. Let head drop forward. | no attempt to raise head | infant tries: effort better felt than seen | raises head but drops forward or back | raises head: remains vertical; it may wobble | | | |
| **HEAD CONTROL (2)** **(flexor tone)** Infant sitting upright; Hold at shoulder. Let head drop backward. | no attempt to raise head | infant tries: effort better felt than seen | raises head but drops forward or back | raises head: remains vertical; it may wobble | head upright or extended; cannot be passively flexed | | |
| **HEAD LAG** Pull infant to towards sitting posture by traction on both wrists and support head slightly. Also note arm flexion | head drops and stays back | tries to lift head but it drops back | able to lift head slightly | lifts head in line with body | head in front of body | | |
| **VENTRAL SUSPENSION** Hold infant in ventral suspension; observe curvature of back, flexion of limbs and relation of head to trunk. | back curved, head and limbs hang straight | back curved, head ↓, limbs slightly flexed | back slightly curved, limbs flexed | back straight, head in line, limbs flexed | back straight, limbs above body | | |

**Figure 18.1** Neurological form for examination (*continued*)

## Tone patterns

| | | | | | | |
|---|---|---|---|---|---|---|
| **FLEXOR TONE**<br>**(arm versus leg 1)**<br>compare scores of arm traction with leg traction | | arm flexion less than leg flexion | arm flexion equal to leg flexion | arm flexion more than leg flexion but difference 1 column or less | arm flexion more than leg flexion but difference more than 1 column | |
| **FLEXOR TONE**<br>**(arm versus leg 2)**<br>posture in supine | | | arms and legs flexed | strong arm flexion with strong leg extension<br>*intermittent* | strong arm flexion with strong leg extension<br>*continuous* | |
| **LEG EXTENSOR TONE**<br>compare scores of popliteal angle and leg traction | | leg traction less than popliteal angle | leg traction equal to popliteal angle | leg traction more than popliteal angle but difference 1 column or less | leg traction more than popliteal angle but difference more than 1 column | |
| **NECK EXTENSOR TONE**<br>**(SITTING)**<br>compare head control 1 and 2 | | head extension less than head flexion | head extension equal to head flexion | head extension more than head flexion. but difference 1 column or less | head extension more than head flexion but difference more than 1 column | |
| **INCREASED EXTENSOR TONE (HORIZONTAL)**<br>compare scores of head lag and ventral suspension | | ventral suspension less than head lag | ventral suspension equal to head lag | ventr suspension more than head lag but difference 1 column or less | ventr suspension more than head lag but difference more than 1 column | |

## Reflexes

| | | | | | | | |
|---|---|---|---|---|---|---|---|
| **TENDON REFLEX**<br>test biceps, knee and ankle jerks. | absent | felt, not seen | seen | ' exaggerated' | clonus | | |
| **SUCK / GAG**<br>Little finger into mouth with pulp of finger upwards. | no gag / no suck | weak irregular suck only:<br><br>No stripping | weak regular suck<br><br>Some stripping | strong suck:<br>(a) irregular<br>(b) regular<br>Good stripping | no suck<br>but strong clenching | | |
| **PALMAR GRASP**<br>Put index finger into the hand and gently press palmar surface. Do not touch dorsal surface.<br>*Test each side separately* | no response<br><br>R    L | short, weak flexion of fingers<br><br>R    L | strong flexion of fingers<br><br>R    L | strong finger flexion, shoulder ↑<br><br>R    L | very strong grasp; infant can be lifted off couch<br><br>R    L | | |
| **PLANTAR GRASP**<br>Press thumb on the sole below the toes.<br><br>*Test each side separately* | no response<br><br><br>R    L | partial plantar flexion of toes<br><br>R    L | toes curve around the examiner's finger<br><br>R    L | | | | |
| **PLACING**<br>Lift infant in an upright position and stroke the dorsum of the foot against a protruding edge of a flat surface.<br>*Test each side separately* | No response<br><br><br><br><br>R    L | dorsiflexion of ankle only<br><br><br><br><br>R    L | full placing response with flexion of hip, knee & placing sole on surface<br>R    L | | | | |
| **MORO**<br>One hand supports infant's head in midline, the other the back. Raise infant to 45° and when relaxed let his head fall through 10° . Note if jerky. Repeat 3 times | no response or opening of hands only | full abduction at shoulder and extension of the arms; no adduction | full abduction but only delayed or partial adduction | partial abduction at shoulder and extension of arms followed by smooth adduction | • no abduction or adduction;<br>• only forward extension of arms from the shoulders<br>• marked adduction only | | |

## Systematic neurological evaluation

Until fairly recently there have been no adequate tools for the assessment of the neonatal nervous system. The impetus for standardized neurological examination for the newborn and particularly for the preterm infant came originally from André-Thomas and Saint-Anne Dargassies and their associates in Paris [20–24]. They mapped out the maturation of active and passive tone and primitive reflexes and developed an examination based

## Movements

| | | | | | | | |
|---|---|---|---|---|---|---|---|
| **SPONTANEOUS MOVEMENT (quantity)** Watch infant lying supine | no movement | sporadic and short isolated movements | frequent isolated movements | frequent generalised movements | continuous exaggerated movements | | |
| **SPONTANEOUS MOVEMENT (quality)** Watch infant lying supine | only stretches | stretches and random abrupt movements; some smooth movements | fluent movements but monotonous | fluent alternating movements of arms + legs; good variability | • cramped synchronised; • mouthing • jerky or other abn. mov. | | |
| **HEAD RAISING PRONE** Infant in prone, head in midline | no response | infant rolls head over, chin not raised | infant raises chin, rolls head over | infant brings head and chin up | infant brings head up and keeps it up | | |

## Abnormal signs/patterns

| | | | | | | | |
|---|---|---|---|---|---|---|---|
| **ABNORMAL HAND OR TOE POSTURES** | | hands open, toes straight most of the time | intermittent fisting or thumb adduction | continuous fisting or thumb adduction; index finger flexion, thumb opposition | continuous big toe extension or flexion of all toes | | |
| **TREMOR** | | no tremor or tremor only when crying | tremor only after Moro or occasionally when awake | frequent tremors when awake | continuous tremors | | |
| **STARTLE** | no startle even to sudden noise | no spontaneous startle but react to sudden noise | 2-3 spontaneous startles | more than 3 spontaneous startles | continuous startles | | |

## Orientation and behaviour

| | | | | | | | |
|---|---|---|---|---|---|---|---|
| **EYE APPEARANCES** | does not open eyes | | full conjugated eye movements | *transient* • nystagmus • strabismus • roving eye movements • sunset sign | *persistent* • nystagmus • strabismus • roving eye movements abnormal pupils | | |
| **AUDITORY ORIENTATION** Infant awake. Wrap infant. Hold rattle 10 - 15 cms from ear. | no reaction | auditory startle; brightens and stills; no true orientation | shifting of eyes, head might turn towards source | prolonged head turn to stimulus; search with eyes; smooth | turns head and eyes towards noise every time; jerky abrupt | | |
| **VISUAL ORIENTATION** Wrap infant, wake up with rattle if needed or rock gently.Note if baby can see and follow red ball (B)or target (T) | does not follow or focus on stimuli B        T | stills, focuses, follows briefly to the side but loses stimuli B        T | follows horizontally vertically; no head turn B        T | follows horizontally and vertically; turns head B        T | follows in a circle B        T | | |
| **ALERTNESS** *Tested as response to visual stimuli* (B or T) | will not respond to stimuli | when awake, looks only briefly | when awake, looks at stimuli but loses them | keeps interest in stimuli | does not tire (hyper-reactive) | | |
| **IRRITABILITY** in response to stimuli | quiet all the time, not irritable to any stimuli | awakes, cries sometimes when handled | cries often when handled | cries always when handled | cries even when not handled | | |
| **CONSOLABILITY** Ease to quiet infant | not crying consoling not needed | cries briefly; consoling not needed | cries; becomes quiet when talked to | cries; needs picking up to console | cries cannot be consoled | | |
| **CRY** | no cry at all | whimpering cry only | cries to stimuli but normal pitch | | High pitched cry; often continuous | | |

**SUMMARY OF EXAMINATION:**

HEAD AND TRUNK TONE:                          LIMB TONE:

MOTILITY:                                     REFLEXES:

ORIENTATION AND ALERTNESS:                    IRRITABILITY:

CONSOLABILITY:                                LIST DEVIANT SIGNS:

mainly on these items. The more recent schemes included the assessment of hearing and vision as well [25]. The other main contribution came from Prechtl [26] in Holland who developed an examination geared for the full term infant. He particularly stressed the importance of age-specific techniques for any neonatal neurological examination and the impact the behavioural states have on nervous system functioning. He also suggested the use of the optimality concept to achieve objective scoring [27].

In the last two decades, interest has also developed in the behaviour of newborn babies. Brazelton [28] introduced a neurobehavioural scale to evaluate this. Although the examination has been frequently used as a neurological evaluation it is not suitable for that purpose as it is much more global and thus a less specific way of assessing neurological integrity [11].

The above examinations are not suitable for early or frequent monitoring of ELBW infants who often require life-support equipment or oxygen therapy. None has been developed for the ill infant as they require considerable expertise and are time consuming. In addition, some have only been standardized for full term infants [26–28]. Thus preterm infants can only be assessed when they have reached 40 weeks post-menstrual age (PMA). The validity of applying standards evolved for full term infants to preterm infants who might have spent as much as 10–16 weeks in an extrauterine, rather than an intrauterine, environment can also be questioned, particularly if the optimality scores developed for full term infants are applied to preterm infants at 40 weeks PMA [29].

A neurological examination suitable for ELBW infants must have as many items as possible which can be applied at birth, even to infants on ventilators, and must be suitable for longitudinal assessment. Good inter-observer correlation should be possible even when the examination is performed by relatively inexperienced staff, and it should take no longer than 10–15 min. By having a proforma with well defined instructions of how to elicit the requested items and aiding the recording with diagrams this can be achieved (Figure 18.1). The examination should include the assessment of behavioural states, tone and motility, some of the primitive reflexes and aspects of behaviour such as hearing, vision and consolability [30].

## Items to be evaluated

### Behavioural state

The definition of behavioural states is important as they represent a centrally coordinated neural activity, which expresses itself in a variety of ways [31]. Thus the cause of the lower $Po_2$ in state 2 is not only due to the cardiorespiratory changes but also to different control of respiratory muscle activity and possibly to different reactivity to changes in arterial $Po_2$ and $Pco_2$. Behavioural state should be recorded for all items elicited. In infants above 36 weeks PMA this can be achieved easily by observing eye movements and alertness. At this age these show good correlation with other physiological variables such as electroencephalogram (EEG) pattern, respiratory rate and heart rate. In the younger preterm infants the well defined coordinated states do not exist but there are cycles of EEG activity, motility, regular and irregular breathing with or without eye movements. These may alternate independently or overlap. To what extent these rudimentary state cycles are responsible for the variability of heart rate, respiration, blood pressure and muscle tone in the extremely premature infant is not known. It is important to realize, however, that the cyclical variations in the cardiorespiratory status might be more a sign of good health than disease even in the most immature infant [11]. Examining infants halfway between feeds and following a set sequence through the examination will achieve a comparable state for the same items.

### Assessment of tone and posture

Observation of the infant in supine and prone positions (Figure 18.2), in sitting and ventral suspension, will give a good assessment of the tone of the muscles controlling the head and trunk, and also of the limbs. Further evaluation can be made by recording resistance to passive movement, but the objective recording of this requires familiarity of the norms for various gestational ages. Other methods used are the measurement of the power of recoil when the limbs are stretched or the angle of resistance either during passive movement or when traction is applied to the limbs (Figure 18.3a and b).

In infants who have been examined repeatedly longitudinally or at various gestational ages, it can be shown that with increasing

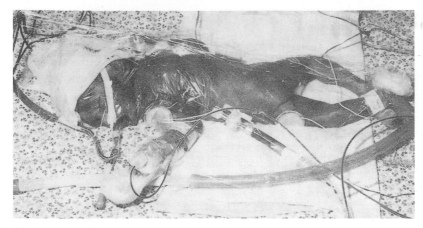

*(a)*

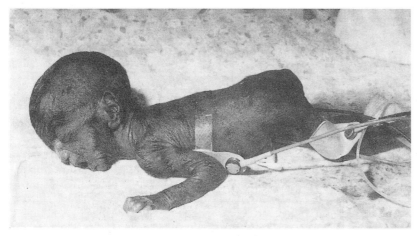

*(b)*

**Figure 18.2** *(a)* Infant born at 26 weeks' gestation, weight 860 g, aged 6 days. *(b)* Infant born at 28 weeks' gestation, weight 750 g, aged 8 days. Note elevated hip in infant *(b)* who is small for gestational age and well, indicating better tone

maturity there is an increase in muscle tone [32,33]. In a normal infant this follows a predetermined pattern. Tone can be documented in the lower limbs before the upper limbs, and in the neck flexor muscles before the neck extensors. Limb tone can be assessed at birth even on infants on ventilators; some flexor tone in the lower limbs is found even at 25 weeks PMA, but is rarely observed in the upper limbs in well appropriate for gestational age (AGA) infants before 30 weeks' gestation [32]. Increase in flexor tone in the arms is, however, common in all hyperexcitable infants; thus, it can be frequently observed in small for gestational age (SGA) infants under 1000 g, even before 29 weeks PMA. Longitudinal documentation allows the comparison in the pattern of development inside and outside the uterus in well and ill infants (Figure 18.4).

*Assessment of movement*

The quality, quantity and symmetry of spontaneous movements can be easily observed even in the smallest and most ill infants. Both quantity and quality can be noted to change with increasing maturity. The movements of the very immature infants often consist of slow asymmetrical twisting and stretching movements of the trunk and limbs, which is often termed athetoid. This may be accompanied by rapid repetitive wide amplitude movements of the limbs resembling myoclonus. With increasing maturity there is a gradual change to smooth alternating movements with medium speed and intensity. The quantity of motor activity changes little from approximately 28–35 weeks PMA, but decreases rapidly thereafter [34].

Abnormality of motor function may also be manifested by inappropriate quality and

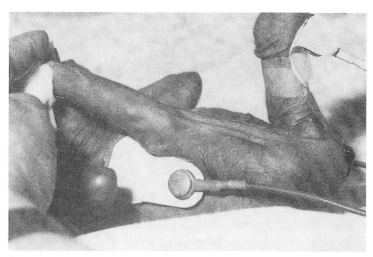

*(a)*

quantity of movement for the infant's maturity or by asymmetries. The norms for these are poorly defined for ELBW infants, thus the differentiation of abnormal movement and even convulsions can be difficult. The normal myoclonic movements can be interpreted as convulsions, while twitches representing seizures may be overlooked.

### Neonatal 'reflexes'

A number of transitory 'reflexes' which are unique to the neonate have been described. Many of them are already present at a very early gestation and show a distinctive developmental profile. In spite of the extensive literature on their description and development, little is known about the mechanisms which produce them. They tend to show certain common features in relation to neurological insults, similar to those in heavier infants. Absent and high threshold responses will be found in apathetic non-alert infants. Newborn infants who are hyperexcitable because of biochemical or central nervous system disturbances will have a low threshold or inappropriately mature responses for their PMA. These will therefore be common in otherwise well SGA infants at birth. Cortical injuries have no apparent effect on most of these reflexes. There are two notable exceptions. Poor plantar and placing reactions may be observed on the contralateral side of a large parenchymal haemorrhage. The probable mechanism is reduced afferent input so that the response is not elicited. In ELBW

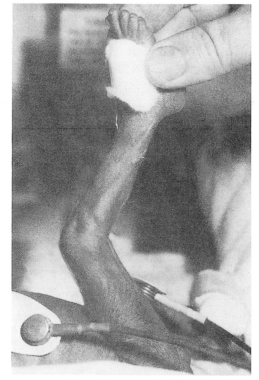

*(b)*

infants asymmetry of the plantar grasp is commonly the earliest sign of a future hemiplegia.

### Sucking and feeding

Feeding requires the coordinated action of sucking, swallowing and breathing. Adequate

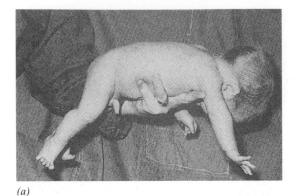

*(a)*

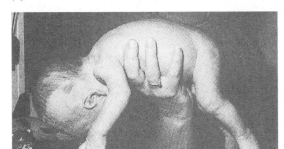

*(b)*

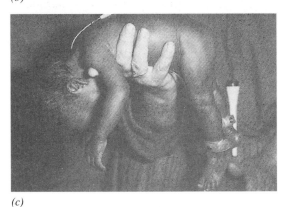

*(c)*

**Figure 18.4** Ventral suspension at 40 weeks PMA. *(a)* Normal infant born at 29 weeks' gestation, weight 1100 g. *(b)* Normal infant born at 26 weeks' gestation, weight 780 g. *(c)* Infant with large PVH born at 28 weeks' gestation, weight 850 g. Note poorer head control in infant born at 26 weeks and even poorer in infant with PVH

coordination already exists for this at 28 weeks' gestation; but at this stage the sucking is neither powerful enough nor is there sufficient synchrony with swallowing to allow adequate feeding. With increasing maturity, sucking becomes more coordinated and a characteristic feeding posture develops [35].

*Assessment of visual function and alertness*
This function can and should be tested as part of the routine neurological assessment. A red woollen ball is an excellent stimulus which can be presented at a distance of 15–20 cm. Starting at the midline the ball is moved laterally in either direction, then vertically and finally in an arc (Figure 18.5). The infant's ability to focus and track this object is assessed [36]. From 29–30 weeks PMA, infants are able to focus and track briefly horizontally and vertically. The function is more consistent in SGA infants. With increasing maturity they can track the ball more smoothly and in an arc.

The integrity of the visual pathway can also be assessed by visually evoked potentials (VEP). VEP to flash stimulation can be consistently recorded from 27 weeks PMA [37] and again a maturational profile can be demonstrated. While studies of VEP maturation are of interest, their relevance to clinical diagnoses in the early neonatal period is doubtful.

Alertness should not be assessed from the infant's appearance but from the ability to respond to visual stimulation. In some ELBW infants treated with theophylline, staring eyes

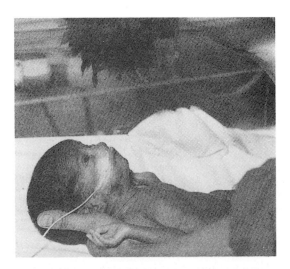

**Figure 18.5** Visual tracking of a red woollen ball in an infant born at 29 weeks' gestation and weight 940 g, assessed at 2 weeks of age. Note infant is able to track vertically

with retracted lids may give the appearance of alertness, yet they may have very poor responsiveness to stimuli.

### Assessment of hearing

This should be part of a routine neurological examination. It can be tested either with a rattle producing a broad band of frequencies [30], an auditory cradle [38], or with auditory brainstem response (ABR) [39]. The former has the advantage that it is cheap, can be performed during the routine examination of the infant, and can be used with even the smallest infant from the moment of birth. Compared to the cradle, it has the disadvantage that a higher number of infants will fail the test even when the presence of good auditory evoked responses can be demonstrated at a 60 dB level. At present the cradle has not been evaluated for testing infants under 1500 g. Its advantage is that it is fully automated, thus is also free of any possible observer bias.

Our routine is to test infants with a rattle weekly from birth. The head is elevated about 20° and supported in the midline by the examiner's hand, leaving it free to rotate (Figure 18.6). The stimulus is presented on each side in turn with the hand and rattle out of sight. Infants in incubators and on ventilators can also be tested. Those who fail this test on repeated occasions are tested with an ABR before discharge or at 36 weeks PMA. At present, the ABR is the most reliable method for testing hearing in very small infants. The type of loss can be established and it can also test the hearing threshold [40].

The response to the rattle can be persistently elicited in neurologically normal infants from 27–28 weeks PMA. Asymmetrical responses correspond with asymmetrical ABRs. Regular assessment of hearing in the neonatal period has been able to demonstrate that infants with periventricular haemorrhage (PVH) tend to have a poor auditory response at the time of the bleed; this tends to recover quickly and permanent hearing loss does not follow unless there is another complication. Jaundice, on the other hand, even at relatively low levels when it is persistent and associated with acidosis may cause permanent damage [41].

The incidence of mild hearing loss in ELBW infants in the early weeks of postnatal life is very common, even in the absence of PVH and jaundice. Most recover completely, often

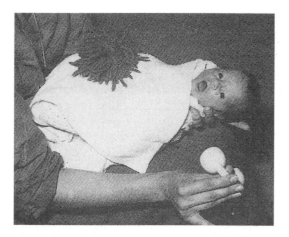

**Figure 18.6** Assessment of hearing with a rattle. Infant assessed at 36 weeks PMA. Born at 28 weeks' gestation and 950 g. Note that the baby becomes alert and the head turns to the side of the rattle

before their discharge from the unit. Although ABRs can be performed early they are time consuming; in view of the common but transient hearing loss, we recommend that ABRs should be performed later – at 36 weeks PMA. An exception to this is a persistent hearing loss in an otherwise well infant with marked growth retardation. This should raise the suspicion of cytomegalovirus infection, and in these babies the hearing loss should be confirmed with an ABR. In our experience hearing loss recovering by 36 weeks has no permanent effect but there is a higher incidence of neurodevelopmental abnormalities, including language delay, in infants where it persists beyond 40 weeks PMA, even if it recovers later.

## Neurological profile of well infants and those with specific neurological insults

### Neurological development in ELBW babies

#### Developmental profiles

Early reports claimed that neurological development is similar inside and outside the uterus [22]. More recently differences in the pattern of development have been noted and their variation with postnatal age [29,32,33,42,43]. The reports have not shown consistent findings. They probably reflect not only differences in the population studied and the criteria used for assessment, but also differences in the environment of these infants, such as nutrition, position of nursing and exposure to stimulation. These factors also interact in the same nursery, and norms are thus difficult to establish. We found that, in infants born between 28 and 35 weeks' gestation, at 40 weeks PMA there is increasingly better head control with increasing postnatal age. The difference may be the result of placing very preterm infants in a prone position, thus promoting head control, however even well infants below 28 weeks' gestation have much poorer development of head control. In this case it is possible that their nutritional state was less satisfactory, affecting both neuronal and muscle maturation.

There are also a number of other neurological functions which show definite acceleration in development in the extrauterine environment. Thus in well infants the development of sucking and sucking posture relates more to postnatal age than PMA [35]. The same may be observed for visual tracking responses [30]. Thus a visual performance in a preterm infant at 40 weeks PMA which is similar to that of the full term infant during the first few days of life, represented delayed development and is observed in infants who have suffered a neurological insult, particularly PVH/IVH [44]. This delay does not appear to be a marker for later abnormality in neurological or visual development. Similar delay in development may be observed in the maturation of VEP under these circumstances; again this does not seem to have a prognostic significance [45]. However, absent or deviant VEPs do seem to be associated with future abnormalities [46].

We have found that repeated neurological examination can also document deviant patterns in the development outside the uterus compared to that within, both in well and ill infants. By correlating these with early cranial ultrasound and electrophysiological findings, and also with later neuro-developmental outcome, one might identify those differences which are normal for ELBW babies and need no intervention, from those which are abnormal and need attention.

Marked arm and leg extension in ventral suspension is normal in preterm infants born at less than 35 weeks' gestational age when they reach 40 weeks PMA [32] (Figure 18.4a). A similar posture in a full term infant would suggest later spasticity. Flexor tone in the arm equal to that in the legs is normal in full term infants, but in the preterm infant at 40 weeks PMA it is usually associated with later shoulder retraction and this will need attention. Although in the absence of other neurological abnormality this rectifies itself, it interferes with early bimanual manipulation [47] and produces a rather frustrated infant (Figure 18.7a and b).

High frequency, low amplitude tremors and startles were commonly noted in apparently well premature infants reaching 40 weeks PMA, particularly in those with extreme prematurity, by Piper *et al.* [29]. In our experience they are frequently associated with other abnormal signs or cranial ultrasound abnormalities and thus should not be regarded as normal.

When abnormal signs are present their significance is generally quite different from those in a full term infant. Thus hypotonia and weak responses are common in infants with prolonged illness such as bronchopulmonary dysplasia (BPD) [29], even in the absence of a neurological insult. In these infants they represent a delay in maturation rather than loss of function and thus they carry a more favourable prognosis than in a full term infant. Deviant patterns of development and the persistence of deviant signs appear to be prognostically much more significant.

## Neurological profiles of specific insults

Repeated neurological examinations also allow the documentation of the signs associated with some specific insults.

### *Periventricular and intraventricular haemorrhage*

This is by far the commonest neurological insult seen in ELBW infants. Although many of these lesions have been 'clinically silent' [48], careful examination reveals abnormal neurological signs in nearly all cases.

Volpe [49] described two characteristic syndromes associated with the larger intraventricular haemorrhages. The first was the characteristic deterioration which occurs in the infants that usually do not survive. They passed

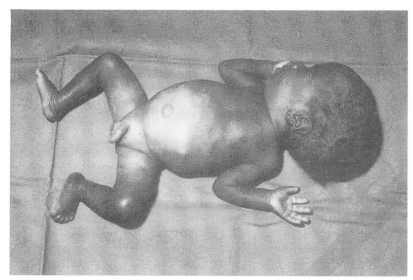

*(a)*

**Figure 18.7** Marked arm flexor tone at 40 weeks PMA. *(a)* Compared with normal for premature infants at this age. *(b)* This is often associated with shoulder retraction in infancy

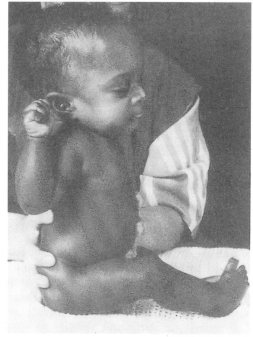

*(b)*

from stupor to coma, developed apnoea, generalized tonic seizures, fixed pupils and flaccid quadriplegia. With the advent of cranial ultrasonography it has been possible to study the evolution of these haemorrhages. It has been noted that while the above findings do accompany some of the larger bleeds, they can also be noted in their absence. The second syndrome he described was the saltatory syndrome, which consisted of alteration of levels of consciousness, change in the quality and quantity of movement. Deterioration and improvement occurred for many hours.

By closely correlating ultrasound findings with repeated clinical examinations, we were able to identify most haemorrhages clinically [50] and map out the signs related to their evolution [51]. Preceding the haemorrhage or at the time of onset, hypertonicity is more marked in the arms and excessive motility with tremors and startles may be noted. Tendon reflexes are brisk, the Moro response is abnormal, and visual and auditory orientation is absent. The infant is usually irritable. Stage 2 occurs after the haemorrhage has occurred. Tone and motility are decreased but the popliteal angle is relatively tight. There is poor reactivity and visual orientation is absent. Stage 3 is the phase of recovery. Limb tone becomes normal first, including the popliteal angle, and motility improves next. First auditory then visual orientation recovers, and head and trunk control are the last to become

normal. During this phase, roving eye movements are often noted. Also at this stage, a number of deviant signs become apparent in infants who later show an abnormal outcome. These include persistent asymmetry of tone, spontaneously up-going toes (Figure 18.8a and b), adducted thumbs (Figure 18.9) and primitive reflexes.

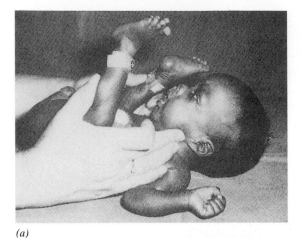

*(a)*

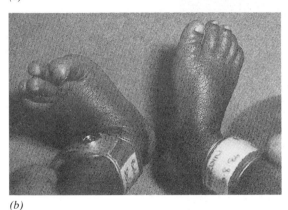

*(b)*

**Figure 18.8** Infant born at 28 weeks' gestation and 880 g. Large PVH on the right on day 2. Examined at 36 weeks PMA. Note *(a)* asymmetric popliteal angle tighter on the left and *(b)* spontaneously up-going toe on the left

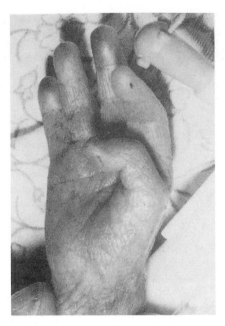

**Figure 18.9** Adducted thumb in neurologically abnormal preterm infant not associated with fisting which would be common in the more mature infant

It is interesting that the severity of the signs in the early stages do not necessarily correlate either with the size of the lesion or with later outcome. There is, however, a good correlation between the speed of recovery and later outcome, and the number of deviant signs as opposed to delayed maturation are also good markers [52]. Post-haemorrhagic ventricular dilatation produces practically no abnormal signs even when there is considerable increase in the head size provided intracranial pressure is not markedly elevated. The only abnormal sign related to the hydrocephalus is poor head control, the severity of which correlates with head size. The hydrocephalus only rarely produces deterioration in either visual or auditory evoked potential. They may even become normal when there is progressive ventricular dilatation. With rising pressure the infant often becomes irritable and tremulous; increased arm flexor tone and neck extensor hypertonia may also be noted. Auditory and visually evoked potentials may remain remarkably normal during the neonatal period despite considerably elevated intracranial pressure. If the potentials are abnormal, they may not revert to normal after ventricular drainage. Thus, in contrast to older infants, they are of little use in monitoring the effect of ventricular dilatation in this population.

### Cystic periventricular leucomalacia (PVL)

Generalized severe ischaemia in the absence of a significant PVH does not seem to produce cystic leucomalacia in the very immature infant. Thus, in these babies the lesions are not usually seen at the time of birth or soon after. However, if they suffer a severe collapse, repeated prolonged bradycardia or, particularly, necrotizing enterocolitis, the lesion may develop even at several weeks of age [53]. This is in marked contrast to PVH which rarely develops after the first week of life. The early signs of the lesion are hypotonia and lethargy which may be masked by the

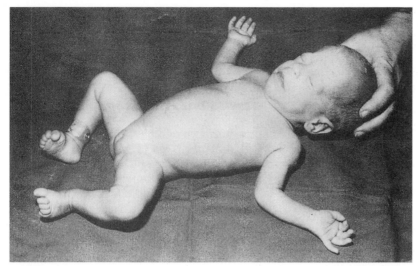

(a)

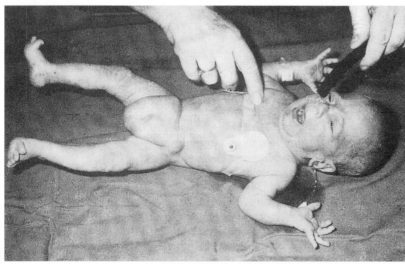

(b)

**Figure 18.10** Twins born at 28 weeks' gestation. Twin *(a)* weighed 950 g, small PVH on day 2. Twin *(b)* weighed 720 g, periventricular cystic leucomalacia. Note normal supine posture appropriate for age (40 weeks PMA) in twin *(a)*, extended posture with flexed arms and up-going toes in twin *(b)*

illness which actually produces the lesions. Auditory and visual responses tend to be appropriate.

The infants then improve and for a period in fact may appear normal; however, between six and ten weeks after the insult a characteristic picture emerges. They gradually become more irritable and although they can be pacified with feeding, very little else is of use. Abnormal tone pattern with an increase in flexor tone in the arms and extensor tone in the legs and marked neck extensor hypertonia may be observed (Figure 18.10). This abnormal tone pattern is much less marked in infants with

BPD. Movement may be abnormal or stereotyped. Tongue protrusion is often present giving the appearance of hypothyroidism. Fisting and adducted thumbs are usually rare at this stage, but abnormal finger and toe posture are common. This includes flexion of the index finger with other fingers extended and spontaneously up-going toes in a supine infant lying quietly (Figure 18.11). The placing reaction is poor. The Moro response is abnormal, consisting of extension at the elbow only without any abduction or adduction of the arms. At this stage visual and auditory functions are normal [54]. In the neonatal

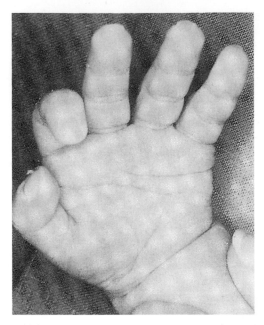

**Figure 18.11** Abnormal finger posture consisting of flexion in index finger and thumb with other fingers extended. This sign is frequently noted in infants with PVL even when quiet. It may be seen in normal infants when crying

period there is no difference in the clinical signs between the infants with periventricular and subcortical leucomalacia, but the EEG and VEPs are always abnormal in the latter while they are usually normal at this stage in the former.

If these infants are evaluated only at the time of discharge, the abnormal neurological signs may be minimal and thus easily missed. At 40 weeks PMA the cysts are often no longer visible while the clinical signs are prominent. At this stage there is clinically no difference in visual function between the infants who maintain their vision and those who are later cortically blind, but there is a marked difference in the appearance of the VEPs. This condition illustrates not only the importance of repeated evaluations but also the value of an integrated approach.

## Conclusion

The neurological evaluation of ELBW infants is not only feasible but essential. It provides a means of studying the effect of the environ-

ment – both stimulation and deprivation – on the maturing nervous system. Manipulation of this environment might show us to what extent this neurological development can be altered through the plasticity of the nervous system in normal and abnormal infants. Regular assessments will also allow earlier recognition of disability. By instituting treatment early, the impact of these could be reduced. Finally, a knowledge of the normal for the infants reared outside the uterus can also help the paediatrician to reassure parents about some of their anxieties and thus promote better parent and infant relationships.

---

**Practical points**

1. The assessment of the gestational age is essential, as abnormal neurological signs can be interpreted only in the context of the maturity of the babies.
2. Areas of neurological function evaluated should include: behavioural states, posture and tone, movements, primitive reflexes, auditory and visual orientation, irritability and consolability.
3. The evolution of neurological signs is more important than the isolated neurological findings, therefore longitudinal neurological examinations are essential.
4. The possibility of the effect of environmental factors on maturation must be taken into account as this may accelerate or retard some aspects of the neurological development.
5. Neurological examination by itself can only elicit whether the neurological status of the newborn is normal or abnormal and whether the abnormalities are permanent or transitory over the period of study. This can be used as a guide to prognosis but it is not always a reliable prognostic index for individual cases.
6. An integrated approach coupling clinical and radiological investigations will help to elucidate the effect of physiological disturbances or pathological lesions on the neurological status and to establish a clinical pattern for various types of pathological injuries (e.g. IVH, PVL).

# References

1. Robinson, H.P. and Fleming, J.E.E. (1975) A critical evaluation of sonar crown–rump length measurements. *Br. J. Obstet. Gynaecol.*, **82**, 702–710
2. Campbell, S. (1969) The prediction of fetal maturity by ultrasonic measurement of the biparietal diameter. *J. Obstet. Gynecol.*, **76**, 603–609
3. Dubowitz, L.M.S. and Goldberg, G. (1976) Assessment of gestational age in various stages of pregnancy in infants differing in size and ethnic origin. *Br. J. Obstet. Gynaecol.*, **83**, 255–259
4. Brett, E. (1963) The estimation of foetal maturity by the neurological examination of the neonate. In *Gestational Age, Size and Maturity* (M. Dawkins and B. MacGregor, eds), *Clin. Dev. Med.*, **19**, SSMEIU/Heinemann, London
5. Robinson, R.J. (1966) Assessment of gestational age by neurological examination. *Arch. Dis. Childh.*, **41**, 437–447
6. Mitchell, R.G. and Farr, V. (1965) The meaning of maturity and the assessment of maturity at birth. In *Gestational Age, Size and Maturity* (M. Dawkins and B. MacGregor, eds), *Clin. Dev. Med.*, **19**, 83–99, SSMEIU/Heinemann, London
7. Farr, V., Mitchell, R.G., Nelligan, G.A. and Parkins, J.M. (1966) The definition of some external characteristics used in the assessment of gestational age in newborn infants. *Dev. Med. Child Neurol.*, **8**, 657
8. Usher, R., McLean, F. and Scott, K.E. (1966) Clinical significance of gestational age and an objective method for its assessment. *Pediatr. Clin. N. Am.*, **13**, 835–848
9. Amiel-Tison, C. (1968) Neurological evaluation of the maturity of newborn infants. *Arch. Dis. Childh.*, **43**, 89–93
10. Hittner, H.M., Hirsh, N.J. and Rudolph, A.J. (1977) The lens in the assessment of gestational age. *J. Pediatr.*, **91**, 455–460
11. Casaer, P., Eggermont, E. and Volpe, P.J. (1986) Neurological problems in the newborn. In *Textbook of Neonatology* (N.R.C. Roberton, ed.), Churchill Livingstone, Edinburgh, pp. 527–537
12. Farr, V. and Mitchell, R.G. (1967) The effect of birthweight on maturity scoring. *Dev. Med. Child Neurol.*, **9**, 745
13. Dubowitz, L.M.S., Dubowitz, V. and Goldberg, C. (1970) Clinical assessment of gestational age in the newborn infant. *J. Pediatr.*, **77**, 1–10
14. Dubowitz, L.M.S. and Dubowitz, V. (1977) *Gestational Age of the Newborn: A Clinical Manual*, Addison-Wesley, London
15. Dubowitz, V., Whittaker, G.F., Brown, B.H. and Robinson, A. (1968) Nerve conduction velocity: an index of neurological maturity of the newborn infant. *Dev. Med. Child Neurol.*, **10**, 741–749
16. Schulte, F.J., Michaelis, R., Linke, I. and Nolter, R. (1968) Motor nerve conduction velocity in term, preterm and small for date infants. *Pediatrics*, **42**, 17–21
17. Moosa, A. and Dubowitz, V. (1971) Postnatal maturation of peripheral nerves in preterm and full term infants. *J. Pediatr.*, **79**, 915–922
18. Miller, G., Heckmatt, J.Z., Dubowitz, L.M.S. and Dubowitz, V. (1983) Use of nerve conduction velocity to determine gestational age in infants at risk and in very low birth weight infants. *J. Pediatr.*, **103**, 109–112
19. De Vries, L.S., Heckmatt, J.Z., Burrin, J.M., Dubowitz, L.M.S. and Dubowitz, V. (1986) Low serum thyroxine concentrations and neural maturation in preterm infants. *Arch. Dis. Childh.*, **61**, 862–866
20. André Thomas and Saint-Anne Dargassies, S. (1952) *Etudes Neurologiques sur le Nouveau-né et la Jeune Nourisson*, Masson, Paris
21. André Thomas, Chesni, Y. and Saint-Anne Dargassies, S. (1960) The neurological examination of the infant. *Little Club Clinics in Developmental Medicine*, No. 1, National Spastics Society, London
22. Amiel-Tison, C. and Grenier, A. (1980) *Evaluation Neurologique du Nouveau-né et du Nourisson*, Masson, Paris
23. Amiel-Tison, C., Barrier, G., Shnider, S.M., Levinson, S.C. and Stefani, S.J. (1982) A new neurologic and adaptive scoring system for evaluating obstetric medications in full term newborn infants. *Anesthesiology* **56**, 340–350
24. Saint-Anne Dargassies, S. (1966) Neurological maturation of the premature infant of 28 to 41 weeks gestational age. In *Human Development* (F. Falkner, ed.), Saunders, Philadelphia, pp. 302–325
25. Saint-Anne Dargassies, S. (1977) *Neurological Development in Full Term and Premature Neonates*, Elsevier/North Holland/Excerpta Medica, Amsterdam
26. Prechtl, H.F.R. (1977) *The Neurological Examination of the Full Term Newborn Infant*, 2nd edn, *Clin. Dev. Med.*, **63**, SIMP/Heinemann, London
27. Prechtl, H.F.R. (1980) The optimality concept. *Early Hum. Dev.*, **4**, 201–206
28. Brazelton, T.B. (1973) Neonatal behavioural assessment scale. *Clin. Dev. Med.*, **50**, SIMP/Heinemann, London
29. Piper, M.C., Kunos, I., Willis, D.M. and Mazer, B. (1975) Effect of gestational age on neurological functioning of the very low birthweight infant at 40 weeks. *Dev. Med. Child Neurol.*, **27**, 596–605
30. Dubowitz, L., Dubowitz, V. and Mercuri, E. (1998) The neurological assessment of the preterm and full term newborn infant. *Clin. Dev. Med.*, McKeith Press, Cambridge University Press, London
31. Prechtl, H.F.R. and O'Brien, M.J. (1982) Behavioural states of the full term newborn: the emergence of a concept. In *Psychobiology of the Human Newborn* (P. Statton, ed.), Wiley, New York, pp. 53–73
32. Palmer, P.G., Dubowitz, L.M.S., Verghote, M. and Dubowitz, V. (1982) Neurological and neurobehavioural differences between preterm infants at term and full term newborn infants. *Neuropediatrics*, **13**, 183–189

33. Lacey, J.L., Henderson-Smart, D.J., Edwards, D.A. and Storey, B. (1985) The early development of head control in preterm infants. *Early Hum. Dev.*, **ii**, 199–212

34. Prechtl, H.F.R., Fargel, J.W., Weinmann, H.M. and Bakker, H.H. (1979) Postures, motility and respiration of low risk preterm infants. *Dev. Med. Child Neurol.*, **21**, 3–27

35. Casaer, P., Daniels, H., Devlieger, H., de Cock, P. and Eggermont, E. (1982) Feeding behaviour in preterm neonates. *Early Hum. Dev.*, **7**, 331–346

36. Dubowitz, L.M.S., Dubowitz, V., Morante, A. and Verghote, M. (1980) Visual function in the premature and full term newborn infant. *Dev. Med. Child Neurol.*, **22**, 465–475

37. Hrbek, A., Karlberg, P. and Olsson, T. (1973) Development of visual and somatosensory evoked responses in low birthweight infants. *Electroencephalogr. Clin. Neurophysiol.*, **34**, 225–232

38. Bhaitacharia, J., Beneh, M.J. and Tucker, S.M. (1984) Long term follow up of newborns tested with the auditory response cradle. *Arch. Dis. Childh.*, **59**, 504–511

39. Stockard, J.E. and Stockard, J.J. (1981) Brainstem auditory evoked potentials in normal and otoneurologically impaired newborns and infants. In *Current Clinical Neurophysiology: Update on EEG and Evoked Potentials* (C.E. Henry, ed.), Elsevier/North Holland, Amsterdam, pp. 9–71

40. Lary, S., Briassoulis, G., de Vries, L., Dubowitz, L.M.S. and Dubowitz, V. (1985) Hearing threshold in preterm and term infants by auditory brainstem response. *J. Pediatr.*, **107**, 593–599

41. De Vries, L.S., Lary, S. and Dubowitz, L.M.S. (1985) Relationship of serum bilirubin levels to ototoxicity and deafness in high risk low birthweight infants. *Pediatrics*, **76**, 415–417

42. Howard, J., Parmelee, A.H., Kopp, C.B. and Littman, B. (1976) A neurological comparison of preterm and full term infants at term conceptual age. *J. Pediatr.*, **88**, 995–1002

43. Kutzberg, D., Vaughan, H.G., Dau, M.C., Grellong, B.A., Albin, S. and Rotkin, L. (1979) Neurobehavioural performances of low birthweight infants at 40 weeks conceptional age. Comparison with full term infants. *Dev. Med. Child Neurol.*, **21**, 596–607

44. Morante, A., Dubowitz, L.M.S., Levene, M. and Dubowitz, V. (1982) The development of visual function in normal and neurologically abnormal preterm and full term infants. *Dev. Med. Child Neurol.*, **24**, 771–784

45. Placzek, M., Mushin, J. and Dubowitz, L.M.S. (1985) Maturation of the visual evoked response and its correlation with visual acuity in preterm infants. *Dev. Med. Child Neurol.*, **27**, 448–454

46. Kutzberg, D. and Vaughan, H.G. (1985) Electrophysiological assessment of auditory and visual function in the newborn. *Clin. Perinatol.*, **12**, 277–298

47. Touwen, B.C.L. and Hadders Algra, M. (1983) Hyperextension of the neck and trunk and shoulder retraction in infancy: a prognostic study. *Neuropediatrics*, **14**, 202

48. Papile, L., Burnstein, J., Burnstein, R. and Koffler, H. (1978) Incidence and evolution of subependymal and intraventricular haemorrhage: a study of infants with birthweight less than 1500 g. *J. Pediatr.*, **92**, 529–534

49. Volpe, J.J. (1978) Neonatal periventricular hemorrhage, past, present and future. *Pediatrics*, **92**, 693–696

50. Dubowitz, L.M.S., Levene, M.I., Morante, A., Palmer, P. and Dubowitz, V. (1981) Neurological signs in neonatal intraventricular hemorrhage: correlation with real-time ultrasound. *J. Pediatr.*, **99**, 127–133

51. Dubowitz, L.M.S. (1985) Neurological assessment of the full term and preterm newborn infant. In *The At-Risk Infant: Psycho/Social/Medical Aspects* (S. Harel and N.Y. Anastolsiow, eds), Paul H. Brooks, Baltimore, pp. 185–196

52. Dubowitz, L.M.S., Dubowitz, V., Palmer, P.G., Miller, G., Fawer, C.L. and Levene, M.I. (1984) Correlation of neurological assessment in the preterm newborn infant with outcome at one year. *J. Pediatr.*, **105**, 452–456

53. De Vries, L.S., Regev, R. and Dubowitz, L.M.S. (1986) Late onset cystic leukomalacia. *Arch. Dis. Childh.*, **61**, 298–299

54. De Vries, L.S., Dubowitz, L.M.S., Dubowitz, V. *et al.* (1985) Predictive value of cranial ultrasound in the newborn baby: a reappraisal. *Lancet*, **ii**, 137–140

# III. THE NORMAL ELECTROENCEPHALOGRAM

## Janet Eyre

The period from 24 weeks' gestation to term is a critical time for maturation and organization of the cerebral cortex; those born very prematurely are at greatest risk of a disturbance in this process. It has been known for many years that there are striking changes in the electroencephalogram (EEG) of the preterm infant with increasing post-conceptional age. These changes are a reflection of the progressive maturation of the central nervous system. Repeated recording of the EEG can provide a simple and non-invasive means to monitor cerebrocortical maturation but only if the ontogenesis of the EEG is well understood.

The pattern of the EEG in a healthy baby is dependent upon the baby's gestational age and so is related only indirectly to birth weight. In this section, therefore, the EEG of babies of less than 32 weeks' gestational age will be discussed because 1000 g is the third centile for the birth weight of girls at 32 weeks of gestation [1].

## Development of the cerebral cortex

The ontogenesis of the human central nervous system begins during embryogenesis. In these first 30 days of life the neural plate and groove are formed to be followed by the development of the primitive neural tube [2]. In the second month of life the rostral end of the neural tube (the prosencephalon) differentiates into the diencephalon, from which the thalmi and the hypothalamus are formed, and the telencephalon, which gives rise to the basal ganglia, the lateral ventricles and the cerebral hemispheres [2,3]. It is during this period of ventral induction that neural proliferation and migration begins. The neurones are derived from cells lying in the subependymal region and migrate from there to their ultimate position. The cerebral cortex is derived therefore from cells arising in the periventricular region, with the earliest cells forming the deepest layer of the cortex (layer six) and the later neurones passing through these cells to form the more superficial layers [4,5]. The peak period for neural proliferation is 2–4 months of gestation and for neural migration is 3–5 months. It is not completely clear when neuronal proliferation ceases in the cerebral cortex; however, by the end of the sixth month mitotic figures are no longer observed and the cortex presumably has acquired its full complement of nerve cells [6].

The differentiation and the organization of the cerebral cortex occurs between 24 and 40 weeks of gestational age. At 24 weeks a rapid multiplication of glial cells commences. This is accompanied by the differentiation, alignment and orientation of cortical neurones into identifiable layers. In addition there is the elaboration of neuronal dendritic processes, the formation of synapses between cortical neurones and the establishment of thalamocortical connections [7–9]. The arborization of dendrites is perhaps the most critical factor in the development of the central nervous system since dendrites provide the major part of the membrane surface area for the integration of both excitatory and inhibitory synaptic activity.

It is assumed from animal studies and from detailed recordings in adults that the EEG recorded from scalp electrodes represents the summation of excitatory and inhibitory postsynaptic potentials generated in the superficial cortical neurones. The rhythmicity and the rate of firing of the neurones, however, is influenced by subcortical centres, primarily in the thalamus [10]. It is not surprising therefore to find that there are striking changes in the EEG over this period of rapid differentiation and maturation of the cortical neurones. The changes in the pattern of the EEG in the preterm newborn baby with increasing gestational age reflect the differentiation of cortical neurones and the development of dendrites and dendritic spines. The appearance of cyclical changes in the pattern of the EEG with sleep and wakefulness, and the synchronization of these rhythms with changes in the pattern of other physiological parameters are thought to correspond with the development of thalamocortical connections. A knowledge of the age-related changes in the EEG and repeated recordings in individual babies will allow the process of cortical maturation to be monitored during this critical period of development.

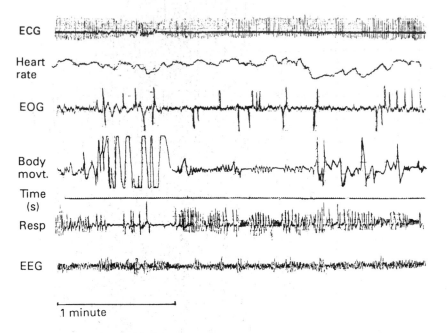

ECG

Heart
rate

EOG

Body
movt.

Time
(s)

Resp

EEG

|—————| 1 minute

**Figure 18.12** A polygraphic
record during active sleep
or wakefulness in a term
baby. It shows an irregular
heart rate, frequent eye
movements, body
movements, an irregular
respiration rate and a fast,
mixed voltage EEG

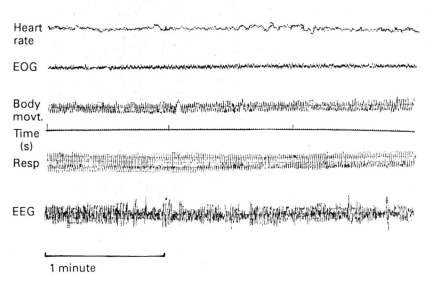

Heart
rate

EOG

Body
movt.

Time
(s)

Resp

EEG

|—————| 1 minute

**Figure 18.13** A polygraphic
record during quiet sleep in
a term baby. It shows a
regular heart rate, an
absence of eye movements,
no body movements, a
regular respiration rate and
a slow high voltage EEG

## Maturation of the EEG from 24 to 32 weeks' gestational age

The systematic study of the EEG of newly born babies began with the pioneering descriptions of Gibbs and Gibbs in 1950 [11]. The description by Askerinsky and his colleagues [12,13] of the cyclical organization of sleep by the use of polygraphic studies aroused interest in studies of the EEG in the neonate and in the premature infant in relationship to sleep and

wakefulness. The healthy full term infant has since been shown to have well developed and easily recognizable sleep–wake cycles [14]. These states can be identified by the EEG, the polygraphic and the behavioural criteria defined by Prechtl [15], and by Anders and colleagues [16] (Figures 18.12, 18.13 and 18.14). Unlike the term baby, the very preterm baby does not have clearly defined sleep states. This is because there are no consistent temporal relationships between the eye movements,

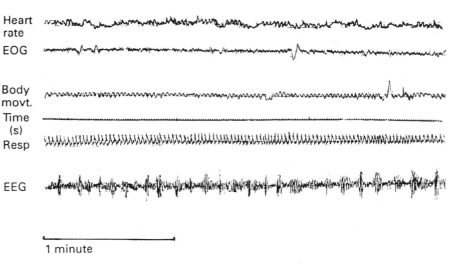

Heart
rate

EOG

Body
movt.

Time
(s)

Resp

EEG

1 minute

**Figure 18.14** A polygraphic record during sleep in a term baby. It shows a regular heart rate, an absence of eye movements, no body movements, a regular respiration rate and a discontinuous, *tracé alternant*, pattern of the EEG

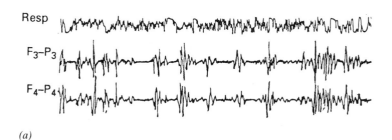

Resp

F₃–P₃

F₄–P₄

*(a)*

**Figure 18.15** EEG recorded from a 24-week gestation healthy preterm infant showing the two patterns of the EEG: *(a)* a discontinuous *tracé alternant* pattern and *(b)* a continuous EEG

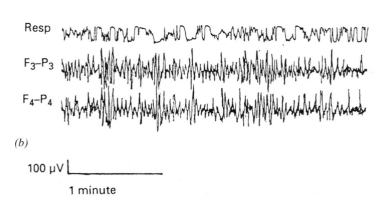

Resp

F₃–P₃

F₄–P₄

*(b)*

100 μV

1 minute

body motility, the pattern of respiration, the variability of the heart rate and the EEG which together define sleep states.

The first signs of behavioural state organization do begin, however, well before 24 weeks of gestational age with the emergence of two distinct patterns of EEG (Figure 18.15). The first pattern, comprising clusters of bursts of high voltage slow wave activity interspersed between periods of suppressed EEG activity, is called *tracé alternant* or burst suppression pattern, and is characteristic of the EEG during quiet sleep in the term baby (Figure 18.14). The second, a continuous EEG of

**Table 18.1.** The duration of continuous and *tracé alternant* (discontinuous) EEG activity in relation to gestational age

| Gestation (weeks) | Total CA/24 h (h) | | Duration of epochs of CA (min) | | Duration of epochs of TA (min) | |
|---|---|---|---|---|---|---|
| | Median | Range | Median | Range | Mean | SD |
| 26 | 10.5 | 8.9–11.5 | 13 | 10–36 | 21 | 1.5 |
| 28 | 16.7 | 8.3–16.9 | 17 | 12–36 | 19 | 1.1 |
| 30 | 18.5 | 18.1–20.0 | 25 | 15–38 | 15 | 0.9 |
| 32 | 19.4 | 18.0–21.2 | 38 | 25–52 | 12 | 0.75 |

CA = continuous activity; TA = *tracé alternant*.
Table adapted from Eyre, Nanei and Wilkinson [21]

mixed frequencies with a predominance of slow wave activity, is the precursor of the EEG patterns later associated with wakefulness and active sleep in more mature babies (Figure 18.12).

It is often stated that the EEG of the very preterm baby comprises almost entirely the second, discontinuous, pattern with little or no continuous activity [17,18]. This conclusion, however, has been based either on the findings of early studies of the EEG when such preterm babies were previable and the subjects were very ill and subsequently died, or from recordings made from sleeping infants. Continuous electrical activity has in fact been recorded in the pons of human fetuses from as early as 10 weeks. A second, intermittent pattern of EEG was recorded from 17 weeks' gestational age in the rostral part of the brainstem and from the hippocampus [19]. Thus the two distinct patterns of the EEG can be recorded from fetuses well before 24 weeks' gestational age.

Recently it has become possible to make continuous recordings of the EEG over many days [20] in healthy preterm babies. These studies have demonstrated that although the EEG of babies born as prematurely as 24 weeks' gestational age is predominantly discontinuous, there are periods of continuous activity particularly during wakefulness [21]. The duration of individual epochs of continuous activity and the percentage of the total EEG which is continuous increase progressively as the baby matures and there is a reciprocal reduction in the duration of the discontinuous activity so that the EEG changes rapidly from being predominantly discontinuous at 24 weeks to predominantly continuous by 28 weeks (Table 18.1).

While the two basic patterns of EEG exist in very preterm babies there is little synchroniza-tion of the EEG with the other parameters which together define sleep states in the older baby. Thus eye movements, body movements, irregularity of the respiratory pattern and spontaneous fluctuations of the skin resistance can and do occur independently and with either pattern of the EEG. It is not until 32 weeks of gestation that organization of these parameters into recognizable sleep states begins; from then until 40 weeks' post-conceptional age the interrelations between different elements become more clearly defined and organized into the two sleep states termed active and quiet sleep. The two sleep states appear to mature independently and studies by Dreyfus-Brisac [22] show that active sleep is seen in its typical form by 35 weeks and quiet sleep by 37 weeks' gestational age.

The measurement of the relative durations of continuous and discontinuous EEG activity in any individual baby requires continuous recording of the EEG for at least 24 hours and this may not be practical for the clinical assessment of very preterm babies. There are, however, changes in the background activity of the EEG which are age dependent and which also reflect the increasing maturity of the cerebral cortex. Two variables, the progressive changes in the *tracé alternant* pattern and the incidence of delta brush, can easily be quantified from short recordings of the EEG and these provide useful indices of cortical maturity.

## Changes in the background activity of the discontinuous EEG with increasing gestational age

There are progressive changes in the discontinuous or *tracé alternant* pattern of the EEG with

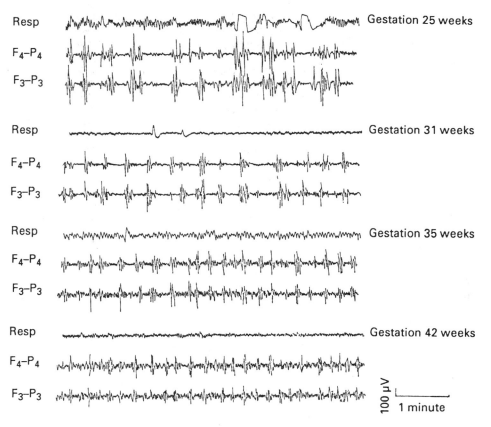

Resp                                 Gestation 25 weeks

$F_4$–$P_4$

$F_3$–$P_3$

Resp                                 Gestation 31 weeks

$F_4$–$P_4$

$F_3$–$P_3$

Resp                                 Gestation 35 weeks

$F_4$–$P_4$

$F_3$–$P_3$

Resp                                 Gestation 42 weeks

$F_4$–$P_4$

$F_3$–$P_3$

100 μV
1 minute

**Figure 18.16** Discontinuous or *tracé alternant* EEG recorded from healthy preterm babies illustrating the progressive changes with increasing maturity

increasing gestational age (Figure 18.16). Perhaps the most striking change is a progressive reduction in the duration of the individual periods of suppression between the bursts of the high voltage slow waves [21,23]. The mean durations of these intervals in relation to gestational age can be calculated and are tabulated in Table 18.2. In addition to the longer mean duration of suppression between bursts, a much greater variability of this duration about the mean is found in very preterm babies, and this too decreases markedly with increasing maturity.

In contrast to the duration of suppression, the duration of each burst of high voltage slow waves does not change with increasing gestation and remains between 2 and 5 s [21,23]. The amplitude of the high voltage slow wave activity during bursts does, however, change with gestational age; it is significantly greater in very preterm babies in comparison to more mature

babies (Table 18.2). The mean voltage does not change, however, until 31 weeks' gestation and, from then until term, there is a progressive decrease from a mean of 440 μV at 31 weeks to 130 μV at 42 weeks. The variability of the maximum voltage is much greater in very preterm babies and this variability decreases significantly over the same period.

To summarize these data: with increasing maturity the duration of the suppressed intervals becomes shorter, the difference between the amplitude of the activity in the suppressed periods and the bursts becomes less marked and the minute to variability of the pattern becomes less pronounced. The overall tendency is for the *discontinuous* pattern to become essentially more *continuous* in nature with increasing gestational age; in fact this discontinuous pattern of EEG is no longer seen in the EEG of a normal baby from 3 months after term.

**Table 18.2.** The characteristics of the *tracé alternant* in relation to gestational age

| Gestation (weeks) | Interval of suppression (s) | | Duration of bursts (s) | | Maximum voltage in bursts (µV) | |
| --- | --- | --- | --- | --- | --- | --- |
| | Mean | SD | Mean | SD | Mean | SD |
| 26 | 26 | 7.3 | 3.3 | 0.7 | 420 | 75 |
| 28 | 24 | 6.5 | 2.9 | 0.5 | 432 | 80 |
| 30 | 16 | 4.1 | 3.0 | 0.4 | 435 | 70 |
| 32 | 13 | 3.1 | 2.5 | 0.6 | 300 | 65 |

Table adapted from Eyre, Nanei and Wilkinson [21]

## Delta brush

Delta brush is the name given to high frequency spindle-like activity which is superimposed on slow wave delta activity (Figure 18.17). While the origin of this activity is unknown, this pattern of activity is recognized to be one of the characteristic signatures of the EEG of very preterm babies [24,25]. The presence and the frequency of the occurrence of the delta brush is highly dependent upon gestational age and so it provides a useful index of the degree of cortical maturity. Delta brush is seen only very infrequently, less than once in 5 min of EEG recording in babies of 27 or less weeks' gestation [23]; from 27–31 weeks the frequency of its occurrence increases rapidly so that by 31 weeks it occurs as often as 30–50 times in a 5 min period of EEG recording [25]. The incidence of delta brush then becomes progressively smaller and it is rarely seen in the EEG of a baby of greater than 36 weeks' gestation (1–2 delta brushes in 5 min).

The data presented concerning the pattern of the normal EEG in relation to gestational age clearly show that there are progressive changes which are a reflection of increasing cerebral maturity. There is a wide normal range at any given gestational age and so it is not possible to assess an individual baby's cortical maturity from one single EEG recording. A longitudinal study of the EEG will, however, allow the measurement electrophysiologically of the increasing maturity of the cerebral cortex in an individual baby [25].

## The significance of abnormality in the EEG of very preterm babies

The premature infant's brain is very vulnerable to a variety of stresses and insults. This is reflected in the high incidence of EEG abnormalities recorded from these infants in the NICU. It is beyond the scope of this review to discuss in detail every type of EEG abnormality associated with neurological illness or complications in the premature infant. This would not in any case be helpful because the abnormalities are non-specific and only rarely, if ever, can an aetiological diagnosis be assigned to a particular EEG pattern. Instead evidence is presented to support the proposal that abnormalities in the EEG provide a means of assessing acutely the severity of a brain injury even in these very preterm infants.

The value of the EEG in the prediction of the long-term neurological outcome of neonates who have sustained a variety of brain injuries has been assessed many times [24,26–28]. Although a statistical relationship between the EEG findings and the long-term outcome has been established in these studies, the EEG findings proved unreliable in correctly predicting the outcome for at least 25% of babies [24]. This unreliability has made the EEG an unsatisfactory method of assessing the prognosis of

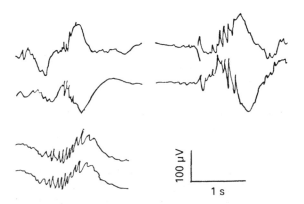

**Figure 18.17** Delta brush recorded from a 31-week gestation baby

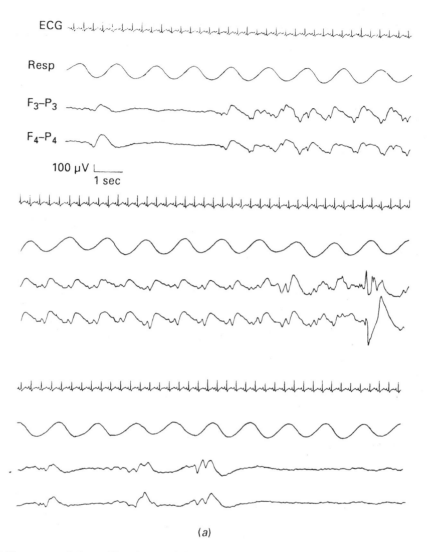

ECG

Resp

F₃–P₃

F₄–P₄

100 μV

1 sec

(a)

**Figure 18.18** *(a)* Electroencephalographic seizure activity recorded in a 26-week gestation infant showing rhythmical sharp and slow wave activity; *(b)* electroencephalographic seizure activity recorded in a 24-week gestation infant showing a burst of rhythmical activity of a single frequency

individual babies in the clinical situation. The majority of the studies, however, used intermittent and short recordings of the EEG. This made it impossible to determine in which babies the EEG abnormality was only present transiently and in which there was a much longer period of EEG abnormality. It is likely that transient abnormalities have less prognostic significance than similar abnormalities which persist for long periods. The use of intermittent EEG recordings is likely to introduce an error which interferes significantly with the prediction of outcome in individual babies.

We have recently completed a study to determine if data obtained prospectively from the continuous recording of the EEG during the period of acute illness and the intensive care could be predictive of the eventual outcome in babies of all gestational ages, including very preterm babies [21]. In this study the EEG of babies who required ventilation from within 5 hours after birth was recorded continuously while they received intensive care; 35 of these babies were less than 32 weeks in gestation (range 25–31 weeks) and their data are presented below. The EEG was analysed for

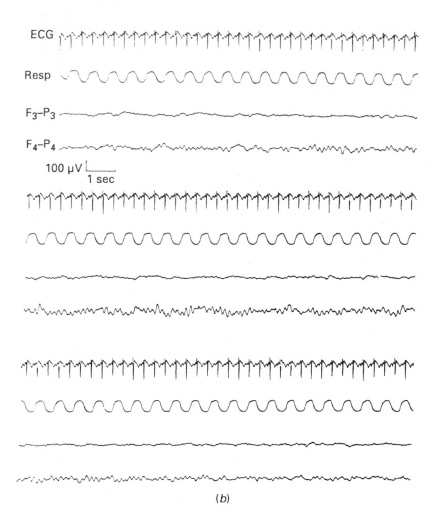

(b)

the presence and the total duration of electroencephalographic seizure activity and for the degree and duration of abnormalities in the background activity. The results of the EEG analyses were then correlated with the findings of an independent assessment of neuro-developmental outcome at 18 months.

### Seizures

Seizures in the newborn, particularly in the very preterm infant, may be very difficult to recognize from clinical signs alone. Subclinical seizures have frequently been reported in the newborn [18]. When there are clinical signs accompanying electrographic seizure activity, these are frequently atypical and subtle, e.g. eye movements, abnormal postures or apnoea. This makes diagnosis difficult. It has been proposed that seizures in the very preterm baby are much less common than in more mature babies because the preterm brain is too immature to sustain synchronized electrical activity. In addition, because of immature myelination, it has been proposed that the preterm baby rarely has generalized seizure activity.

In contrast to the clinical diagnosis, electrographic seizure activity in the newborn baby is easily recognized. There are two basic forms: the sudden onset of rhythmical sharp and slow waves (Figure 18.18a) or the paroxysmal appearance of rhythmic activity of a single frequency within the frequency range 5–13 Hz (Figure 18.18b). The spike and wave pattern typical of seizure activity in older children and adults is not seen in the neonate presumably because the immature myelination of pathways slows the conduction of spikes to scalp electrodes.

In the 35 babies of less than 32 weeks' gestation seizure activity was recorded in 13 (37%). The seizures began between 2 and 63 hours after birth with a median time of onset of 10 hours. Ten of the 13 babies began to have seizure activity within 24 hours after birth. The seizures persisted for between 1 and 5 days; however in 11 of the 13 babies (85%) the seizures were present for less than 72 hours. The total duration of seizure activity for each baby was greatest on the first day after seizure onset and decreased markedly over the subsequent days.

These results suggest that seizures represent an acute reaction to a perinatal insult. Discriminant analysis identified five perinatal factors strongly predictive of seizure onset:

(1)  The degree and duration of abnormal background EEG activity.
(2)  The Apgar scores at 1 and 5 min.
(3)  The maximum percentage of oxygen required.
(4)  The total number of pneumothoraces.
(5)  The lowest blood pH measured.

These data suggest that ischaemic hypoxic encephalopathy was the commonest cause of seizures during the period of intensive care of these very preterm babies. In total 755 separate episodes of seizure activity were recorded in these 13 babies; 36% of the seizures had a focal onset and remained confined to one hemisphere, 63% were primarily or became secondarily generalized. No significant differences could be found between these very preterm babies and the more mature babies in the study when the incidence, the predictive factors, the duration and the time course of seizure activity were considered.

A detailed assessment was made of the babies by an independent observer at 18 months. Nine had died, nine of the survivors

**Table 18.3. The incidence and duration of seizures in relation to outcome**

| Outcome | No. of patients with no seizures | No. of patients with seizures | Mean total duration of seizure activity (h) |
|---|---|---|---|
| Died | 1 | 8 | 3.70 |
| Abnormal | 5 | 4 | 1.31 |
| Normal | 16 | 1 | 0.49 |

had neuro-developmental abnormalities and 17 were normal. Both the occurrence and the duration of electrographic seizures were strongly related to outcome (Table 18.3). Seizures during the acute period of illness predicted death or abnormal survival with a sensitivity of 85%, a specificity of 94%, a positive predictive value of 92% and a negative predictive value of 72%.

The background EEG was classified into normal, mildly, moderately and severely abnormal activity and the total duration of each was measured during the recording period. These durations were then subsequently related to the neuro-developmental outcome (Table 18.4). The strong relationship between the degree and duration of abnormality in the EEG and the neuro-developmental outcome makes the quantitative analysis of an EEG recorded continuously during the period of acute illness useful for the assessment of the severity of the brain injury sustained.

## Conclusion

The recording of the EEG in newborn babies is relatively simple and non-invasive. The interpretation of the EEG is not, however, simple and requires considerable experience. The rapid development of the cortex in babies less than 32 weeks in gestation results in dramatic

**Table 18.4. The duration of normal and abnormal EEG in relation to outcome at 18 months**

| Outcome | Mean percentage of the EEG | | | |
|---|---|---|---|---|
| | Normal | Mildly abnormal | Moderately abnormal | Severely abnormal |
| Normal | 82 | 13 | 6 | 0 |
| Abnormal | 45 | 17 | 16 | 17 |
| Died | 0 | 3 | 34 | 67 |

changes in the pattern of the EEG with increasing gestational age. Longitudinal studies of the EEG in individual babies therefore will allow the process of cortical maturation and development to be followed electrophysiologically. In ill babies, acute abnormalities in the EEG are not usually diagnostic of the aetiology of the brain injury; the severity of the abnormality and its duration, however, are useful in the acute assessment of the severity of the injury sustained.

# References

1. Yudkin, P.L., Aboualfa, M., Eyre, J.A., Redman, C.W.G. and Wilkinson, A.R. (1987) Influence of elective delivery on birthweight and head circumference standards. *Arch. Dis. Childh.*, **62**, 24–29
2. Lemire, R.J., Loeser, J.D., Leech, R.W. and Alvord, E.C. Jr (1975) *Normal and Abnormal Development of the Human Nervous System*, Harper and Row, Hagerstown, Maryland
3. Yakovlev, P.I. (1959) Pathoarchitectonic studies of cerebral malformations. I. Arrhinencephalies (holoprosencephalies). *J. Neuropathol. Exp. Neurol.*, **18**, 22–35
4. Sidman, R.L., Miale, I.L. and Feder, N. (1959) Cell proliferation and migration in the primitive ependymal zone: an autoradiographic study of histogenesis in the nervous system. *Exp. Neurol.*, **1**, 322–326
5. Berry, M., Rogers, A.W. and Eayrs, J.F. (1964) Pattern of cell migration during cortical histogenesis. *Nature*, **203**, 591–593
6. Sidman, R.L. and Rakic, P. (1973) Neuronal migration with special reference to developing human brain: a review. *Brain Res.*, **62**, 1–15
7. Gruner, J.E. (1970) The maturation of human cerebral cortex in electron microscopy study of post-mortem punctures in preterm infants. *Biol. Neonate*, **16**, 243–247
8. Marin-Padilla, M. (1970) Prenatal and early postnatal ontogenesis of the human cortex: a Golgi study. 1. The sequential development of the cortical layers. *Brain Res.*, **23**, 167–169
9. Molliver, M.E., Kostovic, I. and Van Der Loos, H. (1973) The development of synapses in cerebral cortex of the human fetus. *Brain Res.*, **50**, 403–407
10. Purpura, D.P. (1959) Nature of electrocortical potentials and synaptic organisations in the cerebral and cerebellar cortex. *Int. Rev. Neurobiol.*, **1**, 47–163
11. Gibbs, F.A. and Gibbs, E.L. (1950) *Atlas of Encephalography*, Addison-Wesley, Reading, Massachusetts
12. Askerinsky, K.E. and Kleitman, N. (1953) Regularly occurring periods of eye motility and concomitant phenomena during sleep. *Science* **118**, 273–274
13. Askerinsky, K.E., Dement, W. and Klietman, N. (1957) Cyclical variations in EEG during sleep and their relation to eye movement, body motility, and dreaming. *Electroencephalogr. Clin. Neurophysiol.*, **9**, 680–690
14. Wolfe, P.H. (1959) State and neonatal activity. *Psychom. Med.*, **21**, 110–118
15. Prechtl, H.F.R. (1968) States of the infant. *Clin. Dev. Med.*, **28**, 27–41
16. Anders, T.F., Emde, R. and Parmelee, A.H. (1971) *A Manual of Standardized Terminology, Techniques and Criteria for Scoring States of Sleep and Wakefulness in Newborn Infants*, UCLA Brain Information Service, BRI Publications Office, Los Angeles, California, NNDS Neurological Information Network
17. Dreyfus-Brisac, C. (1968) Sleep ontogenesis in early human prematures from 24 to 27 weeks of conceptional age. *Dev. Psychol.*, **1**, 162–169
18. Dreyfus-Brisac, C. (1979) Neonatal electroencephalography. In *Reviews in Perinatal Medicine*, Vol. 3 (E.M. Scarpelli and E.V. Cosmi, eds), Raven Press, New York
19. Bergstrom, R.M. (1969) Electrical parameters of the brain during ontogeny. In *Brain and Early Behaviour* (R.J. Robinson, ed.), Academic Press, London, pp. 15–36
20. Eyre, J.A., Oozeer, R.C. and Wilkinson, A.R. (1983) Diagnosis of neonatal seizure by continuous recording and rapid analysis of the electroencephalogram. *Arch. Dis. Childh.*, **58**, 785–790
21. Eyre, J.A., Nanei, S. and Wilkinson, A.R. (1988) Quantification of changes of the normal neonatal electroencephalogram in relation to gestational age from continuous five day recordings. *Early Hum. Dev.*
22. Dreyfus-Brisac, C. (1970) Ontogenesis of sleep in human prematures after 32 weeks of conceptional age. *Dev. Psychol.*, **3**, 91–121
23. Anderson, C.M., Torres, F. and Faoro, A. (1985) The EEG of the early premature. *Electroencephalogr. Clin. Neurophysiol.*, **60**, 95–105
24. Watanabe, K. (1978) Neurophysiological approaches to the normal and abnormal development of CNS in early life. *Asian Med. J.*, **21**, 421–450
25. Lombroso, C.T. (1979) Quantified electrographic scales on 10 pre-term healthy newborns followed up to 40–43 weeks of conceptional age by serial polygraphic recording. *Electroencephalogr. Clin. Neurophysiol.*, **46**, 460–471
26. Monod, N. and Ducas, P. (1968) The prognostic value of the encephalogram in the first two years of life. In *Clinical Electroencephalography of Children* (P. Kellawat and Petersen, eds), Grune and Stratton, New York, pp. 61–76
27. Rose, A.L. and Lombroso, C.T. (1970) Neonatal seizure states. A study of clinical, pathological and electroencephalographic features in 137 full term babies with a long term followup. *Pediatrics*, **45**, 404–442
28. Engel, R.C.H. (1975) *Abnormal Electroencephalograms in the Neonatal Period*, C.C. Thomas, Springfield, Illinois

# IV. CRANIAL ULTRASONOGRAPHY

## Richard Cooke

Real-time ultrasound scanning of the cranium of newborn infants was introduced in 1979, and has become accepted as the best technique for imaging the brain in this age group. This is especially true when one considers the infant under 1000 g, because of their general fragility and their small size relative to the resolving power of equipment such as CT and MR scanners. The details of the techniques used to obtain suitable images of the brain with ultrasound in the neonates have been extensively described [1–3], and mention here will only be of points especially relevant to the ELBW infant.

## Technique

Although with a little experience information may be obtained on brain scan with almost any type of ultrasound imaging device, a real-time sector scanner with 5 and 7.5 MHz transducers is required to produce the best images in the tiniest infants. Most sector scanners are mechanical devices, although an increasing number of phased array devices are becoming available. The latter have the advantage of a steadier image and no moving parts, but may have fewer lines per sector and a lower lateral resolution. Linear resolution is higher with higher frequency transducers, although the actual resolution achieved depends on image processing factors and in practice the difference in resolution achieved for instance between a 5 and 7.5 MHz transducer may not be as great as theoretically expected.

The use of a sector format is essential in ELBW infants if more than the midline structures are to be seen. The transfontanellar approach produces the clearest images, and since most ELBW infants have a large anterior fontanelle this is not a problem [4]. By nature of the way in which the sector image is presented, structures very close to the transducer may be hidden in bright echoes from the scalp. The surface of the brain beneath the fontanelle may be more easily seen if a spacer device is used to provide an offset of 2–3 cm. A close focused 10 MHz transducer is also effective. Small superficial collections of blood are only visible by such means.

Images are best recorded on a digital image recorder, together with a written description of the examination. As a minimum, midcoronal, and right and left parasaggital cuts should be recorded.

## The purpose of scanning

Ultrasound scanning in ELBW infants can provide clinical diagnostic, management and prognostic information. Diagnostic information includes gestational age assessment [5], congenital malformations of the brain, periventricular and superficial haemorrhage [6,7], cerebral infarction and periventricular leucomalacia [8,9], hydrocephaly and ventriculitis. Evidence of haemorrhage or hydrocephalus may be an adequate explanation for convulsions or clinical deterioration at the bedside. The management of hydrocephaly is aided by having daily measurements of the ventricular size as a guide to the effectiveness of treatment [10], and the presence of extensive bilateral brain destruction may, together with clinical neurological signs, enable the discontinuation of intensive therapy in some cases. Long-term follow up from a number of centres now enables a reasonably accurate prognosis to be given with regard to neurological and cognitive development in ELBW survivors [8,9].

## Ultrasound diagnosis

When using cranial ultrasound in the very preterm infant, it is important to be aware of the differences that exist in anatomy between such infants and more mature ones. In the very preterm infant the brain itself is much less reflective of sound and appears consequently less detailed and darker. Structures such as the choroid plexus in comparison appear relatively more reflective and brighter, and may be confused with blood clot in the lateral ventricles. 'Side-lobe' artefacts produced by strong reflectors such as the choroid plexus are a particular problem with mechanical sector scanners, and may be mistaken for periventricular infarcts [11]. The lateral ventricles are

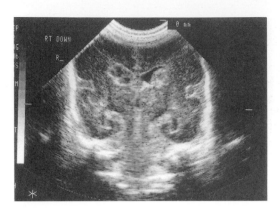

**Figure 18.19** Coronal scan showing blood clot in the lateral sulcus

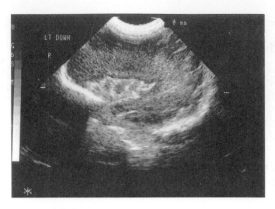

**Figure 18.20** Parasaggital scan showing blood clot in the lateral sulcus

relatively larger than in term infants, and are clearly seen, although the posterior horns of the lateral ventricles do not develop until after 30 weeks of gestation. The immature brain is smaller than the skull and so the subarachnoid space is relatively large and can be easily visualized. Blood clot from subarachnoid haemorrhage not normally visible in older infants can be seen if it is in the lateral sulcus or the interhemispheric fissure (Figures 18.19 and 18.20). Tangential views of the brain in a parasaggital direction used to show the surface of the parietal and temporal lobes appear almost featureless in infants of under 27 weeks' gestation, except for the lateral sulcus. Gyral development may be used as a guide to gestational age.

Several cerebral malformations are relatively easy to diagnose using ultrasound. In many cases the diagnosis may be made clinically. The presence and extent of hydrocephaly in conjunction with myelomeningocele is easily assessed. Holoprosencephaly is not uncommon in ELBW infants and not always immediately clinically apparent. The ultrasound appearances, however, are very striking. Porencephaly in ELBW infants is usually the result of perinatal events, although established cysts may be observed in newborn infants presumably from adverse events *in utero* (Figure 18.21).

Perinatal infections give rise to characteristic ultrasound appearances. Intrauterine viral infections such as cytomegalovirus (CMV) may produce hydrocephaly, but also periventricular calcification which may be obvious on ultrasound before it is visible on X-ray. Infants with

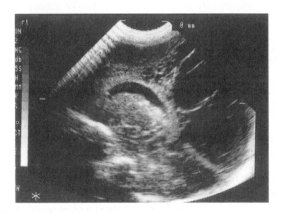

**Figure 18.21** Parasaggital scan showing extensive posterior cyst development, present at birth

hydrocephaly from malformations or as the result of intraventricular haemorrhage may develop ventriculitis. In the early stages a bright periventricular halo may be seen, and later either intraventricular strands of fibrin crossing the ventricles or debris resembling snowflakes when the infant's head is moved.

The various appearances of periventricular haemorrhage in preterm infants are well described and do not differ substantially in the ELBW infant (Figures 18.22 and 18.23). More recently interest has focused on periventricular leucomalacia which is very common in this group, and in particular its early precystic appearances (Figures 18.24 and 18.25). Small flare-like echoes are frequently seen extending from the lateral angles of the lateral ventricles on the first few days of life. Many of these disappear early and seem to be of little later consequence. Their aetiology is unclear. In

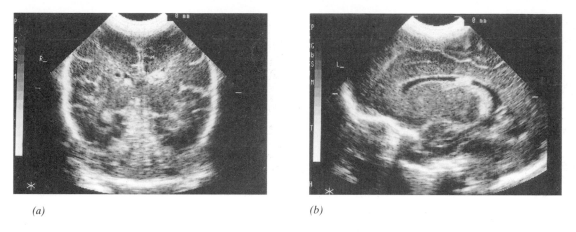

*(a)*             *(b)*

**Figure 18.22** Coronal and parasaggital scans showing small GLH/IVH

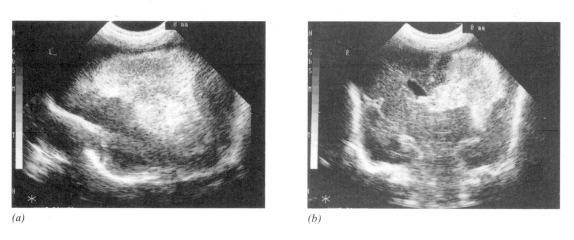

*(a)*             *(b)*

**Figure 18.23** Coronal and parasaggital scans showing major infarction

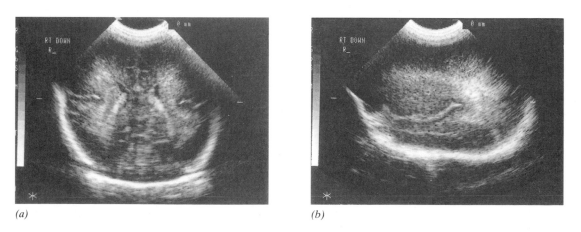

*(a)*             *(b)*

**Figure 18.24** Coronal and parasaggital scans showing 'flares', or early periventricular leucomalacia at 2 days after birth

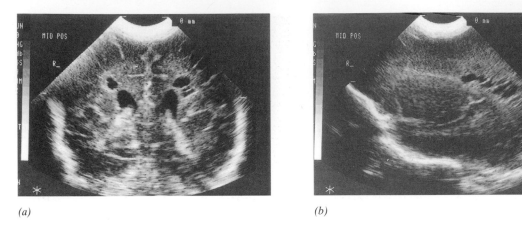

*(a)*                                                    *(b)*

**Figure 18.25** Coronal and parasaggital scans 3 weeks after birth showing periventricular cyst formation

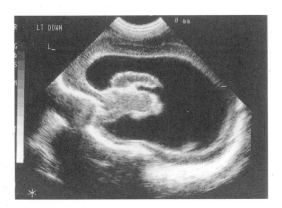

**Figure 18.26** Parasaggital scan showing progressive hydrocephaly

some cases these flares are brighter and persist for a week or more, frequently resulting in localized cyst formation at 2–3 weeks after birth [12,13]. These are the appearances of early periventricular leucomalacia. The areas most often affected as seen on a parasaggital scan are the frontal and occipital areas. Care should be taken to avoid confusion with 'side-lobe' artefacts. Cyst formation may be minimal and the cysts fill in after a month or two, or they may be much more extensive and even extend well into the cerebral subcortical areas [14]. When such major lesions are seen, and especially when they occur bilaterally, cortical blindness, spastic quadriplegia and severe developmental delay are usually seen. Gross ventricular enlargement is easily seen on ultra-

sound and may reflect hydrocephaly with a raised intraventricular pressure, or local periventricular atrophy with a normal pressure (Figures 18.26 and 18.27). In the case of hydrocephaly the enlargement is smooth and balloon-like, but it is irregular and 'craggy' in the case of atrophy [9]. Both states may coexist. Further evidence of periventricular atrophy may often be seen in the form of small periventricular cysts. These may not be evident when hydrocephaly is rapidly progressive, but may appear after it has been treated by drainage or shunting (Figure 18.28). Ultrasound may be useful in the monitoring of such procedures, showing their effectiveness or otherwise, and some of the complications that may result.

Cerebral ultrasound is of considerable value in neurodevelopmental prognosis. In the acute stages of neonatal management, ultrasound appearances usually only confirm a clinical diagnosis of extensive brain injury and may allow cessation of intensive care to be considered. In infants with normal ultrasound scans, most follow-up studies show the risk of major disability to be less than 5%, allowing the clinician to be confident in reassuring parents of good outcome in the majority of infants at discharge. Details of outcome relating to specific lesions seen on ultrasound have only been published for infants of under 32 weeks or 1500 g [15,9], although these are not likely to differ much from ELBW infants. Because of the higher mortality of ELBW infants with major parenchyma lesions, they are relatively under-represented in such series. While simple

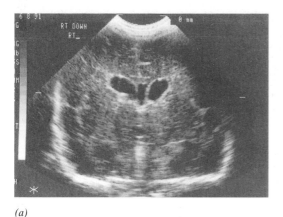

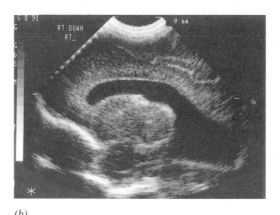

*(a)*                                          *(b)*

**Figure 18.27** Coronal and parasaggital scans showing persistent ventricular enlargement indicative of moderate cerebral atrophy

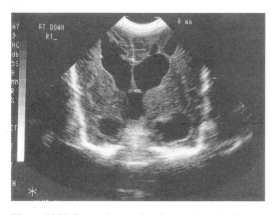

**Figure 18.28** Coronal scan showing periventricular cyst formation following treatment of hydrocephaly

**Practical points**

1. Transfontellar cranial ultrasound imaging effectively diagnoses cerebral malformations, haemorrhage, infarction and hydrocephaly in ELBW infants.
2. Serial examinations are needed to adequately interpret the signs of periventricular leucomalacia.
3. Infants without ultrasound scan evidence of cerebral lesions have a 95% chance of being free from major neurodevelopmental problems.

GLH/IVH has relatively benign outcome, later PVL may be associated with it which carries a poorer prognosis, emphasizing the value of repeated scans in the neonatal period.

Parenchyma unilateral cystic lesions are followed by major disabilities in over 60% of cases, mostly spastic hemiplegias. Bilateral cystic lesions are almost invariably followed by major disabilities and these are often multiple and severe. The results from cerebral ultrasound are proving valuable as a method of assessing the probable long-term effects of new procedures in neonatal care as well as a method for identifying high-risk groups for follow-up purposes. Future developments are likely to include more precise identification of more minor lesions, allowing prognoses to be more accurate.

## References

1. Rumack, C.M. and Johnson, M.L. (1984) *Perinatal and Infant Brain Imaging*. Yearbook Medical, Chicago
2. Levene, M.I., Williams, J.L. and Fawer, C.-L. (1985) Ultrasound of the infant brain. *Clin. Dev. Med.*, No. 92. SIMP, London
3. Naidich, T.P., Yousefzadeh, D.K. and Gusnard, D.A. (1987) Sonography of the normal neonatal head: state of the art imaging. In *Ultrasound of the Central Nervous System. Clinical Neurosonography*. (T.P. Naidich and R.M. Quencer, eds), Springer-Verlag, Berlin/New York, pp. 30–49
4. Cooke, R.W.I. (1979) Ultrasound examination of neonatal heads. *Lancet*, **ii**, 38
5. Murphy, N.P., Rennie, J.M. and Cooke, R.W.I. (1989) Cranial ultrasound assessment of gestational age in low birth weight infants. *Arch. Dis. Childh.*, **64**, 569–572

6. Cooke, R.W.I. (1981) Factors associated with periventricular haemorrhage in very low birthweight infants. *Arch. Dis. Childh.*, **56**, 425–431

7. Stewart, A.L., Thorburn, R.J., Hope, P.L., Goldsmith, M., Lipscomb, A.P. and Reynolds, E.O.R. (1983) Ultrasound appearances of the brain in very preterm infants and neurodevelopmental outcome at 18 months of age. *Arch. Dis. Childh.*, **58**, 598–604

8. DeVries, L.S., Dubowitz, L.M.S., Dubowitz, V. *et al.* (1985) Predictive value of cranial ultrasound in the newborn baby: a reappraisal. *Lancet*, **ii**, 137–140

9. Cooke, R.W.I. (1987) Early and late cranial ultrasonographic appearances and outcome in very low birthweight infants. *Arch. Dis. Childh.*, **62**, 931–937

10. Levene, M.I. (1981) Measurement of the growth of the lateral ventricles in preterm infants with real-time ultrasound. *Arch. Dis. Childh.*, **56**, 900–904

11. Farrell, E.E. and Birnholz, J.C. (1987) Neonatal neurosonography. *Pediatrics*, **79**, 1044–1048

12. DeVries, L.S., Pennock, J.M., Wigglesworth, J.S. and Dubowitz, L.M.S. (1988) Ultrasound evolution and later outcome of infants with periventricular echodensities. *Early Hum. Dev.*, **16**, 225–233

13. Appleton, R.E., Lee, R.E. and Hey, E.N. (1990) Neurodevelopmental outcome of transient neonatal intracerebral echodensities. *Arch. Dis. Childh.*, **65**, 27–29

14. DeVries, L.S., Eken, P., Groenendaal, F., van Haastert, I.C. and Meiners, L.C. (1993) Correlation between degree of periventricular leukomalacia diagnosed using cranial ultrasound and MRI later in infancy in children with cerebral palsy. *Neuropediatrics*, **24**, 263–268

15. Stewart, A.L., Hope, P.L., Hamilton, P.A. *et al.* (1987) Probability of neurodevelopmental disorders estimated from the ultrasound appearance of brains of very preterm infants. *Dev. Med. Child. Neurol.*, **29**, 3–11

# V. TREATMENT OF NEUROLOGICAL DISORDERS

## Andrew Whitelaw

The preceding chapters have described the major advances in our ability to diagnose and assess the severity of cerebral lesions in babies under 1000 g. The chapter on aetiology of neurological disorders refers to the extensive range of randomized trials to prevent periventricular haemorrhage. At the time of writing no treatment has been documented to prevent periventricular leukomalacia. Unfortunately, our ability to prevent cerebral lesions is still far from effective and clinical neonatologists are frequently faced with a baby under 1000 g with neurological damage that can be quite precisely defined using a combination of clinical examination, ultrasound and neurophysiological techniques. In this chapter we shall examine the evidence that treatment at this stage makes any difference to neurological outcome in: seizures, periventricular haemorrhage, or post-haemorrhagic ventricular dilatation.

## Treatment of seizures

### Diagnosis of seizure

The first essential is to define our diagnostic criteria for seizure in infants under 1000 g. Clonic movements which are rhythmic (1–3 per second), focal or generalized, have a high correlation with EEG seizure activity, as does tonic horizontal deviation of the eyes [1]. 'Subtle' activities such as eye opening, ocular movements, boxing or cycling, chewing and apnoea have a low correlation with EEG seizure activity. Tonic extension of both upper and lower extremities or flexion of the upper extremities and extension of the lower extremities correlate poorly with EEG seizures. However, focal tonic seizures have a high correlation with EEG seizure activity [1]. It has been postulated that tonic posturing and motor automatisms may be primitive brainstem and spinal motor patterns released from the tonic inhibition normally exerted by forebrain structures [2]. Such non-epileptic phenomena are usually provoked or exacerbated by sensory stimulation, are suppressed by passive restraint and are not accompanied by autonomic changes.

Confirmation of seizures has such importance for prognosis and treatment that we recommend that EEG be used whenever there is clinical suspicion of seizures. Even in the tiniest infants, it has been technically possible to record EEG using the Oxford Medilog System or Cerebral Function Monitor without interfering with intensive care. As all anticonvulsant drugs have potential problems, it is desirable that such drug treatment in infants below 1000 g be confined to EEG-confirmed seizures. In this group of infants, seizures are often the result of acute ischaemic, haemorrhagic, biochemical or infectious processes. After even one brief episode it is important to investigate and treat possible causes such as hypoglycaemia, hyponatraemia, hypocalcaemia and meningitis.

## Which seizures should be treated?

Clonic seizures and focal tonic seizures may be associated with a drop in $Po_2$ and changes in blood pressure. Thus it has been our practice to treat such seizures if they last over 3 minutes or if they are repeated. It is more difficult to know if seizures which do not disturb oxygenation or perfusion should be treated. This is particularly the case in infants receiving muscle-relaxant drugs such as pancuronium to facilitate mechanical ventilation.

## Seizures and retarded neonatal brain growth

Wasterlain and Plum administered 150 V shocks daily across the head of newborn rats [3]. Compared to control littermates, animals subjected to seizures between days 2 and 11 had a 14% reduction in brain weight and a 15% reduction in cell number. Rats having convulsions between days 9 and 18 subsequently had an 8% reduction in brain weight but no reduction in cell number. Animals who had convulsions after 18 days showed no reduction in brain weight or cell number. None of the brains showed any histological evidence of necrosis. The authors concluded that the brain still undergoing mitosis is more vulnerable to repeated seizures than the brain which is postmitotic. Considerable cell division takes place in the human brain after 28 weeks' gestation particularly in the cerebellum, brainstem and glial tissue.

## Can seizures produce cell death in the immature brain?

Seizures induced by bicuculline in newborn marmoset monkeys and lasting up to 4 hours did not result in any significant ultrastructural changes in the brain [4]. Energy metabolism has been studied during flurothyl or bicuculline induced seizures in mice, rats, dogs and monkeys [5–8]. A drop in glucose and phospho-

creatine was consistently found in the brain either by direct chemical analysis of brain biopsies or by magnetic resonance spectroscopy. However, ATP was not significantly decreased in mice, rats or dogs [5–7]. In the newborn monkeys, ATP was decreased by up to 40% and it was argued that immature primates (including humans) were especially prone to the brain damaging effects of status epilepticus [8]. However, a 40% reduction in ATP would not be expected to lead to necrosis by itself as levels of ATP in severe ischaemia are reduced by 60–99%.

There are grounds for suspicion, but not proof beyond reasonable doubt, that seizures themselves damage the preterm brain. At a consensus meeting in London in 1992 on management of neonatal seizures there was a majority vote for a randomized trial of anticonvulsant therapy to include a control group with no treatment for 24 hours. Many neonatologists feel that seizures are a symptom and that the outcome for the individual infant will be determined more by the nature of the underlying cerebral lesion than by anticonvulsant drugs.

## Phenobarbitone

Our practice is to treat seizures interfering with breathing or circulation and it is most important that the few available drugs are used to optimal effect with the minimum of adverse effects. Phenobarbitone is still the drug of first choice, more because of extensive experience than because of proven superiority over the alternatives. There is experimental evidence that phenobarbitone inhibits both the epileptic focus and the spread through cerebral tissue [9]. Phenobarbitone reacts with components of the GABA-A receptor in the brain and thereby enhances the efficacy of neurally released gamma-amino-butyric acid (GABA), the main inhibitory neurotransmitter [10].

### *Loading dose*

Older textbooks of neonatology tend to quote starting doses of $10 \text{ mg kg}^{-1}$ or less but there is good evidence that $20 \text{ mg kg}^{-1}$ is a better loading dose to achieve plasma levels that are in the range $15–30 \text{ mg l}^{-1}$ ($65–130 \text{ }\mu\text{mol l}^{-1}$). A single loading dose of $20 \text{ mg kg}^{-1}$ in infants with birth weights under $1500 \text{ g}$ gave mean phenobarbitone levels of $20.8 \text{ mg l}^{-1}$ ($89 \text{ }\mu\text{mol l}^{-1}$ at

24 hours, 19.2 mg l$^{-1}$ (83 $\mu$mol l$^{-1}$ at 48 hours and 18.1 mg$^{-1}$ (78 $\mu$mol l$^{-1}$) at 72 hours [11]. Lockman *et al.* studied the relationship between phenobarbitone loading dose, gestational age, blood level and seizure control in 39 neonates [12]. All twelve of the neonates who achieved seizure control had plasma levels of phenobarbitone above 16.9 mg kg$^{-1}$. A mean dose of 16.2 mg kg$^{-1}$ was required to achieve this plasma level. The 26 infants who continued to have seizures had plasma levels between 4 and 25 mg l$^{-1}$ (17–107 $\mu$mol l$^{-1}$). Gal *et al.* reported efficacy of 85% when the dose of phenobarbitone was increased to give a plasma level of up to 40 mg l$^{-1}$ (172 $\mu$mol l$^{-1}$) [13]. Studies using continuous EEG monitoring during phenobarbitone [14] have shown how the clinical seizures often stop but the electrical seizures continue. Absorption is unreliable from intramuscular injection and for babies under 1000 g; the intravenous route should be used for the loading dose.

### Adverse effects

Great care must be taken with the administration of phenobarbitone to non-ventilated infants below 1000 g as respiratory and circulatory depression may occur. In a randomized trial, babies under 1500 g who received 20 mg kg$^{-1}$ phenobarbitone were significantly more likely to develop respiratory failure and require ventilation than controls who received the placebo [11]. We have also observed that a rapid intravenous bolus injection of 20 mg kg$^{-1}$ phenobarbitone can lead to a significant drop in arterial blood pressure. We recommend that the rate of administration be 1 mg kg$^{-1}$ min$^{-1}$. Bradycardia has also been reported with serum levels in the range of 52 mg l$^{-1}$ (225 $\mu$mol l$^{-1}$) [15]. Untreated seizures may themselves cause hypoxia and acidosis. Oxygenation, acid–base balance, heart rate and blood pressure must be monitored effectively and hypotension, hypovolaemia, and hypoxaemia must be promptly corrected. If seizures continue after one loading dose, the dose can be repeated but careful physiological monitoring is even more essential.

### Are maintenance doses of phenobarbitone required?

Painter *et al.* found that maintenance doses of 5 mg kg$^{-1}$ day$^{-1}$ in neonates following a loading dose of 20 mg kg$^{-1}$ resulted in accumulation of the drug with plasma concentrations reaching about 40 mg l$^{-1}$ (172 $\mu$mol l$^{-1}$) after a week [16]. As the renal and hepatic elimination of virtually all drugs is slower in babies under 1000 g than in larger neonates, accumulation is likely to be even more of a problem. In this population of babies seizures are often the result of acute processes and the period during which anticonvulsant treatment is needed may be only a few days. Because of this, it is our practice not to routinely start maintenance therapy. Our approach is to try to achieve effective control with a loading dose(s) and observe without treatment for some days. If seizures which were initially controlled with phenobarbitone recur after a few days, maintenance phenobarbitone should be started at 4 mg kg$^{-1}$ day$^{-1}$. Monitoring of plasma levels is essential with the aim of maintaining a concentration of 15–30 mg l$^{-1}$ (65–130 $\mu$mol l$^{-1}$).

### What to use if phenobarbitone fails?

We favour intravenous diazepam or clonazepam as second choice because of the speed of action and the theoretical argument that the immature brain has a higher affinity for GABA and benzodiazepines than the mature brain.

### Benzodiazepines

*Diazepam* (in soya oil emulsion) can be given intravenously or rectally. The duration of action is unpredictable and the effective dose varies widely (0.1–0.5 mg kg$^{-1}$ i.v. bolus). Monitoring and support of respiration and circulation are essential. Respiratory depression is a common side-effect which may be of little significance if the infant is already mechanically ventilated and adequately monitored. The active metabolite, desmethyldiazepam, can persist for many days with long lasting hypotonia. Despite its drawbacks, diazepam is favoured by many because it often works faster than phenobarbitone or phenytoin [17]. Giving a continuous infusion of 0.7–2.75 mg kg$^{-1}$ hour$^{-1}$ has been reported to be 100% effective in neonatal seizures [18]. Diazepam crosses the blood–brain barrier rapidly and exerts its anticonvulsant effect by specific binding sites intimately linked to the GABA-A receptor in the brain, thus potentiating endogenously released GABA [19]. *Clonazepam* is also widely used and is thought to have a more predictable dose requirement 0.1–0.15 mg kg$^{-1}$ intravenously. *Lorazepam* is also gaining recognition as a neonatal anticonvulsant and has no active metabolite. A dose of 0.05 mg kg$^{-1}$ i.v. stopped seizures within 5 minutes in all seven infants studied [20].

### What to use if phenobarbitone and benzodiazepine fail?

Three different drugs have been advocated as the next line of treatment: phenytoin, paraldehyde, and lignocaine.

### Phenytoin

Concern has been expressed about adverse effects of phenytoin on cerebellar and cortical development but short-term use is still advocated [1]. Painter *et al.* reported that, of 49 infants unresponsive to phenobarbitone, 18 (41%) responded clinically to phenytoin [16]. We use phenytoin as third choice for neonatal seizures. A loading dose of 20 mg kg$^{-1}$ intravenously produced adequate plasma concentrations [16]; 5–14 mg l$^{-1}$ (20–56 µmol l$^{-1}$) is the preferred therapeutic range in preterm infants with decreased protein binding [16]. The intravenous loading dose must be given slowly (1 mg kg$^{-1}$ min$^{-1}$) as phenytoin can affect cardiac rhythm. Oral administration of phenytoin in ELBW infants is erratic and cannot be recommended.

### Paraldehyde

This traditional drug has the advantage of causing very little respiratory depression and we have found paraldehyde to be well tolerated by infants under 1000 g. Elimination is partly through the lungs. The original paraldehyde preparation has to be dissolved 1 in 20 to a 5% solution in 5% glucose and given as an intravenous infusion at 1–3 ml kg$^{-1}$ hour$^{-1}$. A bolus of 1 ml 5% paraldehyde can be given to initiate treatment. Paraldehyde dissolves rubber and some types of plastic (e.g. PVC) including three-way taps, but does not dissolve Teflon cannulae, polypropylene or polyethylene syringes and connecting tubes [21]. Undiluted intravenous paraldehyde solution is highly toxic. The plasma half-life of paraldehyde is considerably shorter (10.2 hour in term infants) than phenobarbitone

or phenytoin, but is probably longer in infants under 1000 g with lung disease [22]. Paraldehyde can be administered rectally by mixing 0.3 ml kg$^{-1}$ with an equal volume of mineral oil and injecting it through a Teflon, polypropylene or polyethylene tube passed a few centimetres into the rectum. This can be repeated every 4 hours but should be avoided if there is any suspicion of necrotizing enterocolitis [23].

### Lignocaine

Lignocaine can be used as an adjuvant anti-convulsant if previous treatment has failed. Continuous infusion at a rate of 4 mg kg$^{-1}$ hour$^{-1}$ was effective in 8 out of 10 neonates with refractory convulsions [24]. Effective blood levels of lignocaine appear to be in the range 0.5–4.0 mg l$^{-1}$ but lignocaine can itself be convulsant at plasma levels of 7.5 mg l$^{-1}$ and can cause bradycardia at levels of 8–12 mg l$^{-1}$. There is no information on half-life in babies under 1000 g.

## Treatment of periventricular haemorrhage (PVH)

### Acute consequences of blood loss

Large amounts of blood (half the circulating blood volume) may be lost in a massive PVH. Clinical observation of perfusion (capillary filling time should not exceed 3 seconds), blood pressure monitoring and regular acid–base and haematocrit measurements are the best guides to loss of blood in babies weighing less than 1000 g.

Mean arterial pressure (MAP) is used for decision making because it is less subject to damping than systolic or diastolic pressure. Infants with a gestation of 26 to 30 weeks who have no serious cerebral lesions on ultrasound and develop normally have usually maintained MAP over 30 mmHg [25]. A useful rule of thumb is that MAP in mmHg should not fall below the gestational age of the infant in weeks. Thus a 26-week infant may tolerate MAP as low as 26 mmHg as long as there is good peripheral perfusion, urine output and no metabolic acidosis.

In some neonatal intensive care units, an umbilical venous (in addition to an arterial) catheter is inserted into the inferior vena cava or right atrium of ill infants weighing less than 1000 g on admission to the unit. A secure route for fluids and drugs can thus be established and the risks of sepsis are much reduced if the catheter is inserted soon after birth rather than after the umbilicus has become heavily colonized. We do this on a selective basis and such a catheter provides a route for central venous pressure (CVP) measurement. Our immediate management plan for haemorrhagic hypovolaemia is:

(1) Transfuse 10 ml kg$^{-1}$ 5% albumin or heat treated plasma over 15 minutes. Repeat if necessary to raise MAP to 30 mmHg, improve perfusion and pH.

(2) If MAP has not risen to 30 mmHg, start dopamine 10 μg kg$^{-1}$ min$^{-1}$ intravenously while waiting for packed cells to arrive. Hypotensive infants under 1000 g usually fail to respond to dopamine infusions of 5 μg kg$^{-1}$ min$^{-1}$ [26]. The dopamine infusion can be increased to 15, 20 or 25 μg kg$^{-1}$ min$^{-1}$. Alternatively, noradrenaline can be started at 0.5 μg kg$^{-1}$ min$^{-1}$ increasing to 1.0 μg kg$^{-1}$ min$^{-1}$ as necessary.

(3) Transfuse packed red cells 15 ml kg$^{-1}$ if the haematocrit is below 0.36 or 20 ml kg$^{-1}$ of colloid has not normalized MAP.

(4) If there is a known or suspected coagulation abnormality, transfuse 15 ml kg$^{-1}$ fresh frozen plasma.

(5) If the platelet count is below 20 000 ml$^{-1}$, in the presence of haemorrhage, transfuse 10–15 ml kg$^{-1}$ platelet rich plasma.

## Post-haemorrhagic ventricular dilatation (PHVD)

Infants below 1000 g, who develop large IVH, are at risk of developing progressive ventricular dilatation leading to hydrocephalus. This type of hydrocephalus has a worse prognosis than congenital hydrocephalus. Epidemiological surveillance of neurological disabilities in South-West Sweden has shown a disturbing increase in the numbers of preterm infants surviving with post-haemorrhagic hydrocephalus and multiple severe disabilities: 78% of these infants subsequently developed cerebral palsy, 72% developmental or intelligence quotient below 70% and 56% had epilepsy [27]. In a group of 33 infants with PHVD followed to a mean age of 50 months,

58% had delayed motor development and 52% had delayed mental development [28].

## Mechanism of posthaemorrhagic ventricular dilatation

The mechanism of PHVD is thought to include initial obstruction of cerebrospinal fluid (CSF) pathways and the reabsorption channels, the arachnoid villi, by multiple small blood clots. Subsequently basal cistern arachnoiditis leads to obstruction of the foramina of the fourth ventricle and permanent hydrocephalus [29]. Animal models of hydrocephalus have demonstrated that ventricular dilatation driven by CSF pressure produces flattening and destruction of the ependymal lining, oedema and destruction of the periventricular white matter [30,31]. There is neuropathological evidence that a similar process can occur in the immature human brain [32]. Such periventricular damage would be likely to be neuromotor but if the effects of oedema and pressure were widespread in the preterm brain, mental and sensory functions of the brain might be damaged and epileptic foci established.

## Diagnostic criteria for PHVD

Diagnostic criteria for PHVD are:

(1) Intraventricular haemorrhage diagnosed with ultrasound or CT.

(2) Progressive increase in both ventricular widths reaching 4 mm over the 97th centile of Levene [33] (Figure 18.29). The ventricular width is measured in the transfontanelle midcoronal view just posterior to the interventricular foramina, taking the distance from the midline to the most lateral border of the ventricle. This means that for most babies weighing under 1000 g each ventricular width must be 15 mm.

In cerebral atrophy, the ventricles dilate, but this process can be distinguished from CSF-driven PHVD by the following features:

(1) In PHVD, the ventricles are usually rounded (ballooned), but in cerebral atrophy, the ventricles have an irregular outline.

(2) In PHVD, ventricular enlargement can be rapid with considerable growth within 24 hours, whereas cerebral atrophy is much slower in enlarging the ventricles.

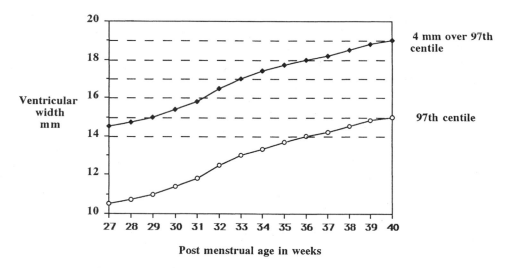

**Figure 18.29** The 97th centile for ventricular width according to postmenstrual age in weeks [33]: 4 mm over the 97th centile defines a group of infants with PHVD and a poor prognosis where intervention can be considered

(3)  Head circumference does not usually increase much in the early stages of PHVD but with progressive ventricular enlargement, head growth does eventually accelerate. In cerebral atrophy, head growth does not accelerate. There may be normal or subnormal growth.

(4)  In pure cerebral atrophy, intracranial pressure is not raised.

## CSF pressure in PHVD

Mean CSF pressure measured at lumbar puncture in normal infants, including those under 1000 g, is 2.8 mmHg with an upper limit of 6 mmHg [34]. We studied CSF pressure in 16 infants with PHVD [35]. Mean CSF pressure was 8.8 mmHg with a wide scatter from (standard deviation 4.6 mmHg). In babies under 1000 g ventricular enlargement can occur at very modest pressures because the immature brain and soft skull are very compliant. We cannot recommend non-invasive measurement of fontanelle pressure as the inaccuracy is too great for clinical decision making [36].

## Treatment of PHVD by CSF tapping

The experimental hydrocephalus findings and the moderately elevated CSF pressure suggested that early CSF tapping by lumbar puncture or ventricular puncture might benefit babies with PHVD by reducing pressure and so reducing periventricular tissue damage, and removing excess protein and blood in the CSF and so preventing permanent blockage of the CSF pathways.

Mantovani *et al.* [37] and Anwar *et al.* [38] carried out randomized trials of serial lumbar punctures in babies with large IVH. Both studies concluded that these measures did not reduce the progression to hydrocephalus and eventual surgical shunting. The hypothesis that early tapping by either lumbar or ventricular tapping might reduce neurodevelopmental impairment and disability was tested in a multi-centre trial which recruited 157 infants in England, Ireland and Switzerland from 1984 to 1987 [39]. Infants fulfilling the diagnostic criteria described above, were randomized to either early CSF tapping to prevent further ventricular enlargement or conservative management. The survivors were examined at 12 and 30 months past term by one developmental paediatrician. Mean CSF pressure was 9 mmHg in both treatment groups and early tapping did succeed in reducing the rate of ventricular and head expansion. Mean gestational age in the infants randomized was 28 weeks and many of them were under 1000 g birth weight; 62% of the survivors received ventriculoperitoneal shunts, the same percentage in each treatment group.

At 12 months past term, 85% of survivors had abnormal neuromotor signs and 77% had disability, with no difference between the treatment groups. The proportion of children with

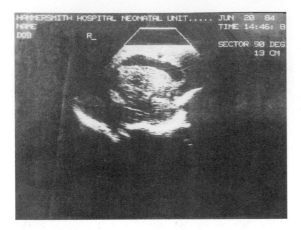

**Figure 18.30** Parasagittal cranial ultrasound scan of an infant with PHVD treated by ventricular tap. There is a needle track lesion extending upwards from the puncture site in the roof of the ventricle towards the fontanelle

neuromotor impairment plus other types of disability such as mental retardation, visual or hearing loss was not significantly different between the two treatment groups. There was a suggestion that infants who had already had a parenchymal cerebral lesion at the time of entry to the trial had a lower proportion of multisystem impairments at the 12-month follow-up examination but the level of significance was only 5% [39] and this finding was not confirmed at the 30-month examination (Ventriculomegaly Trial Group [40]). In this study 54% scored below 70 on the Griffiths Developmental Scales at 30 months; 90% had neuromotor impairment with 40% having severe disability. Vision was severely affected in 9% and 27% had a field defect; 6% had sensorineural hearing loss and 14% were taking regular convulsants. These findings were the same for both treatment groups. Repeated CSF tapping was followed by CSF infection (ventriculitis) in 11 infants, 7% [39]. An additional complication of repeated ventricular tapping is the production of needle track lesions through the cerebral hemisphere (Figure 18.30). Because of the lack of any consistent neurodevelopmental benefit, the absence of any reduction in surgical shunt dependence and because of the significant risk of serious infection, early treatment by CSF tapping cannot be recommended for PHVD.

We reserve CSF tapping for relief of symptoms associated with excessive pressure or excessive head expansion. We consider 12 mmHg to be an excessive CSF pressure. This is four times the normal mean and 100% over the upper limit of normal. This pressure is not necessarily associated with specific signs but we have often noted irritability and a tense fontanelle at this level. If tapping is carried out, then CSF should be allowed to drip out without suction. If pressure is measured (e.g. with an electronic pressure transducer) fluid can be removed until the normal mean of 3 mmHg is reached; 10–20 ml CSF $kg^{-1}$ is the volume we have found to be effective.

## Drugs to reduce CSF production

Because of the risks and lack of benefit from repeated tapping, non-invasive treatment to reduce the production of CSF has become an attractive alternative.

### *Acetazolamide*

Acetazolamide (Diamox) reduces CSF production by inhibiting carbonic anhydrase and has been used in many centres for treatment of PHVD. The most encouraging report was by Shinnar *et al.* [41]. They described a selected uncontrolled group of infants with hydrocephalus, some of whom were below 1000 g, in whom 100 mg $kg^{-1}$ $day^{-1}$ acetazolamide was combined with 1 mg $kg^{-1}$ $day^{-1}$ frusemide 1–3 mg $kg^{-1}$ $day^{-1}$. Frusemide has an inhibitory effect on CSF production in experimental animals. The authors concluded that they avoided shunt insertion in over 50% of the babies who would otherwise have been candidates for surgery. Our experience is that acetazolamide and frusemide can reduce ventricular and head expansion in cases where the process is relatively slow but are ineffective in rapidly progressive PHVD.

Acetazolamide has a number of effects on important physiological systems. Cerebral blood flow is increased substantially for several hours following 50 mg $kg^{-1}$. Blood pressure does not change but the cerebral vasodilatation can give a transient rise in intracranial pressure before the reduced production of CSF has time to reduce intracranial pressure [42]. These effects on the cerebral circulation are not thought to increase the risk of intraventricular haemorrhage in stable infants who are several weeks or months old.

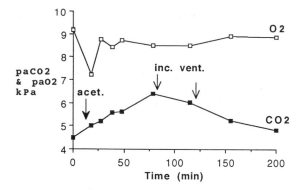

**Figure 18.31** Serial values for arterial $P_{O_2}$ and arterial $P_{CO_2}$ in a mechanically ventilated infant weighing <1000 g; 50 mg acetazolamide was given intravenously (acet). There was a progressive rise in $P_{a}CO_2$ from below 5.0 to 6.2 kPa. 'Inc vent' indicates where the ventilator rate was increased twice to correct the hypercapnea

The effects on $P_{CO_2}$ can be clinically significant. Carbonic anhydrase is necessary for the rapid conversion of circulating bicarbonate to $CO_2$ which can be eliminated as blood flows through the alveolar capillaries of the lungs. Acetazolamide inhibits pulmonary $CO_2$ elimination. In newborn piglets who had been tracheostomized, ventilated and paralysed to hold the $P_{CO_2}$ constant, intravenous acetazolamide produces an immediate reduction in end-tidal $CO_2$ measured by tracheal catheter and a rise in arterial $P_{CO_2}$ of 1.5 kPa within 10 minutes [43]. This inhibition of $CO_2$ elimination is not a clinical problem in infants with normal lungs as they can compensate by breathing faster, thus holding $P_{CO_2}$ constant. However, infants who are ventilator dependent or who have significant bronchopulmonary dysplasia cannot compensate [41]. In four such infants, acetazolamide produced a median increase of 2.0 kPa (range 0.6–3.4 kPa) with a corresponding reduction in pH such that acetazolamide had to be discontinued (Figure 18.31). Infants under 1000 g with PHVD are also likely to have chronic lung disease. Acetazolamide also has a mild diuretic effect and increases urinary excretion of bicarbonate. Thus it is normally necessary to give 4 mmol kg$^{-1}$ day$^{-1}$ sodium bicarbonate and, if frusemide is used as well, 1 mmol kg$^{-1}$ day$^{-1}$ potassium chloride, as replacement for urinary losses. A considerable proportion of infants under 1000 g with PHVD are also likely to have chronic lung disease and immature renal

function. Thus monitoring of blood gases, acid–base, fluid and electrolyte balance must be very carefully carried out and a few infants will not tolerate the treatment.

The preliminary results of a recent multi-centre randomized trial of acetazolamide and frusemide show no evidence of better outcome in infants who received drug therapy (Dr Peter Hope, personal communication).

### Isosorbide

Isosorbide reduces CSF production by an osmotic effect. Lorber described its use in infants with hydrocephalus [44] but his study did not involve babies under 1000 g and a high incidence of side-effects such as vomiting has been reported [45].

### Glycerol

Glycerol is another osmotic agent that has been used for control of hydrocephalus. There is no published experience with babies under 1000 g.

## Surgery for hydrocephalus

If there is persistent intracranial hypertension and excessive head growth despite attempts at medical management, surgical treatment becomes the only option.

### Ventricular reservoir

A ventricular catheter can be inserted through a burr hole in the parietal bone above and behind the right ear and connected to a subcutaneous reservoir (e.g. Rickham). Such a reservoir can be used to measure CSF pressure and remove CSF as often as is necessary to control pressure and head growth. This can be done even in the presence of blood stained, protein-rich or infected CSF. Such CSF tapping does require sterile technique and there is a small risk of introducing infection but it is considerably easier than ventricular or lumbar puncture. Another possible advantage is that fresh needle tracks are not made through the hemisphere every time CSF is removed. Thus a ventricular reservoir is an alternative to repeated ventricular punctures. The surgical procedure is shorter and simpler than a full shunt and many infants below 1000 g have been treated in this way [46]. A ventricular reservoir provides temporary control in hospital while waiting for: the PHVD to resolve spontaneously; protein and blood to clear from the CSF; growth and recovery of the infant from lung disease before insertion of a permanent shunt.

## Ventriculoperitoneal shunt (VPS)

If PHVD is relentlessly progressive despite the above measures, a permanent shunt is required. The ventricular catheter and Rickham reservoir described above are connected to a one way valve which may be Spitz–Holter, Pudenz, Hakim or any other type of small low pressure valve. Distal to the valve is connected a catheter which runs subcutaneously to the peritoneal cavity; 25–30 cm of tubing can be placed in the peritoneal cavity to allow for growth. Such a shunt may last several years before needing replacement. Because the ventricular pressure may be only 5–8 mmHg, the valve must be very compliant to allow flow at such pressures. There is evidence that blockage of the shunt is more likely if the CSF protein is elevated [47]. Despite the simple principles of the VPS, most centres experience a high rate of complications when operating on infants with birth weights under 1000 g [47]. Apart from blockage, infection is common with coagulase-negative staphylococci being the commonest organism. Ulceration of the thin skin over the reservoir can also occur in babies under 1000 g [48] and an immunological reaction to the silastic in the catheter has recently been described [49]. Siting the distal catheter in the right atrium necessitates repeated lengthening as the child grows and infection is much more dangerous because of the additional risks of emboli and glomerulonephritis [48]. For these reasons, it is advantageous to try to avoid, or delay as long as possible, shunt surgery in babies under 1000 g.

## Indications for shunting

Indications for shunting are:
(1)  Excessive head growth despite treatment. Excessive head growth is arbitrarily defined as an increase of 3 cm over 2 weeks or crossing from below the 50th to 2 cm over the 90th centile on the Gairdner growth chart [50].

(2)  If repeated tapping either by ventricular, spinal or reservoir puncture has been necessary (to control high pressure or excessive growth) for 4 weeks, shunting should be considered. If the infant's cardiorespiratory status is poor, or the CSF protein concentration is over 2 g dl$^{-1}$, non-surgical treatment should continue until these contraindications to shunting improve.

---

### Practical points

1.  The diagnosis of seizure requires clinical findings confirmed by EEG.
2.  Clinical seizures should be treated if they are repeated or are disturbing respiration or circulation. We have insufficient clinical trial data as to whether treatment of subtle or silent seizures benefits the infant.
3.  The drug of first choice is phenobarbitone 20 mg kg$^{-1}$. Assuming blood pressure and heart rate have not been depressed by the first dose, 20 mg kg$^{-1}$ can be repeated if seizures persist.
4.  Second choice drug is diazepam 0.3–0.5 mg kg$^{-1}$ followed by an infusion at 0.7–2.7 mg kg$^{-1}$ hour$^{-1}$ diazepam increasing the dose if seizures persist. Clonazepam 0.1–0.15 mg kg$^{-1}$ as a bolus is an alternative.
5.  Adverse effects of anticonvulsants on the circulation must be avoided. Oxygenation and acid–base balance must be adequately supported.
6.  Third line drugs include phenytoin, paraldehyde and lignocaine.
7.  Acute treatment of intraventricular haemorrhage involves correcting hypovolaemia and maintaining blood pressure.
8.  Treatment of progressive posthaemorrhagic ventricular dilatation (PHVD) by repeated early lumbar puncture or ventricular tap does not improve outcome.
9.  Current practice is to use CSF tapping via a reservoir only to prevent excessive intracranial pressure and to insert a ventriculoperitoneal shunt when the infant's size, general stability and the CSF protein are favourable.

## New approaches to PHVD

Because none of the existing treatment methods are free of serious complications and because of the unsatisfactory outcome of PHVD, an attempt is being made to treat the fundamental pathological process behind PHVD. Obstruction of the arachnoid villi and ventricular foramina by multiple small blood clots initiates PHVD and there is evidence of endogenous fibrinolysis in the CSF [51]. It seems logical to try to augment the natural fibrinolysis with a plasminogen activator in the CSF. In a pilot, non-randomized study, 9 infants with PHVD (same diagnostic criteria as above) received intraventricular infusions of streptokinase at 1000 units hour$^{-1}$ for about 48 hours. Secondary bleeding occurred in only one infant and the proportion of infants subsequently requiring shunt surgery was much lower than expected [52]. It has been shown that intraventricular streptokinase does produce the expected changes in the CSF, namely increased fibrin degradation products and consumption of plasminogen [53]. This approach is still purely investigational and is not appropriate for routine use.

# References

1. Volpe, J.J. (1989) Neonatal seizures: Current concepts and revised classification. *Pediatrics*, **89**, 422–428
2. Mizrahi, E.M. and Kellaway, P. (1987) Characterisation and classification of neonatal seizures. *Neurology*, **37**, 1837–1844
3. Wasterlain, C. and Plum, F. (1973) Vulnerability of the developing rat brain to electroconvulsive seizures. *Arch. Neurol.*, **29**, 38–45
4. Söderfeldt, B., Fujikawa, D.G. and Wasterlain, C. (1990) Neuropathology of status epilepticus in the neonatal marmoset monkey. In *Neonatal Seizures* (C. Wasterlain and P. Vert, eds), Raven Press, New York, 91–98
5. Sacktor, B., Wilson, J.E. and Tiekert, C.G. (1966) Regulation of glycolysis in brain, in situ, during convulsions. *J. Biol. Chem.*, **241**, 5071–5075
6. Wasterlain, C.G. and Duffy, T.E. (1976) Status epilepticus in immature rats: protective effects of glucose on survival and brain development. *Arch. Neurol.*, **33**, 821–827
7. Young, R.S.K., Osbakken, M.D., Briggs, R.W., Yagel, S.K., Rice, D.W. and Goldberg, S. (1985) NMR study of cerebral metabolism during prolonged seizures in the neonatal dog. *Ann. Neurol.*, **18**, 14–20
8. Fujikawa, D.G., Vanucci, R.C., Dwyer, B.E. and

9. Wasterlain, C.G. (1988) Generalised seizures deplete brain energy reserves in normoxemic newborn monkeys. *Brain Res.*, **454**, 51–9
9. Smith, M.C. and Riskin, B.J. (1991) The clinical use of barbiturates in neurological disorders. *Drugs*, **42**, 365–78
10. Roberts, E. (1984) GABA related phenomena, a model of nervous system function, and seizures. *Ann. Neurol.*, **16**, S77–S89
11. Whitelaw, A., Placzek, M., Dubowitz, L., Lary, S. and Levene, M. (1983) Phenobarbitone for prevention of periventricular haemorrhage in very low birth weight infants. A randomised double blind trial. *Lancet*, **ii**, 1168–70
12. Lockman, L.A., Kriel, R., Zaske, D., Thompson, T. and Virnig, N. (1979) Phenobarbital dosage for control of neonatal seizures. *Neurology*, **29**, 1445–9
13. Gal, P., Tobock, J., Boer, H. *et al.* (1988) Efficacy of phenobarbital monotherapy in treatment of neonatal seizures – relationship to blood levels. *Neurology*, **32**, 1017–8
14. Eyre, J., Oozeer, R.C. and Wilkinson, A. (1983) Continuous electroencephalographic recording to detect seizures in paralysed newborn babies. *Br. Med. J.*, **286**, 1017–1018
15. Svenningsen, N.W., Blennow, G., Landroth, M. *et al.* (1982) Brain oriented intensive care treatment in severe neonatal asphyxia. *Arch. Dis. Childh.*, **57**, 176–183
16. Painter, M.J., Pippinger, C., MacDonald, H. and Pitlick, W. (1978) Phenobarbital and diphenylhydantoin levels in neonates with seizures. *J. Pediatr.*, **92**, 315–319
17. Hakeem, V.F. and Wallace, S.J. (1990) EEG monitoring of therapy for neonatal seizures. *Dev. Med. Child Neurol.*, **32**, 858–864
18. Gamstorp, I. and Sedin, G. (1982) Neonatal convulsions treated with continuous intravenous diazepam. *Uppsala J. Med. Sci.*, **87**, 143–149
19. Gallager, D., Mallorga, P. and Thomas, J. (1980) GABA–benzodiazepine interactions: physiological, pharmacological and developmental aspects. *Fed. Proc.*, **39**, 3043–3049
20. Deshmukh, A., Witlert, W., Schnitzler, E. *et al.* (1986) Lorazepam in the treatment of refractory neonatal seizures. *Am. J. Dis. Child.*, **140**, 1042–1044
21. Johnson, C.E. and Vogoureaux, J.A. (1984) Compatibility of paraldehyde with plastic syringes and needle hubs. *Am. J. Hosp. Pharm.*, **41**, 306–308
22. Giacoia, G.P., Gessner, P.K., Zaleska, M.M. and Boutwell, W.C. (1984) Pharmokinetics of paraldehyde disposition in the neonate. *J. Pediatr.*, **104**, 291–295
23. Painter, M.J. and Alvin, J. (1990) Choice of anticonvulsants in the treatment of neonatal seizures. In *Neonatal Seizures* (C. Wasterlain and P. Vert, eds), Raven Press, New York, pp. 243–256
24. Norell, E. and Gamstorp, I. (1970) Neonatal seizures: effect of lidocaine. *Acta Paediatr. Scand.*, **206**, (Suppl.), 97–98

25. Miall-Allen, V.M., De Vries, L.S. and Whitelaw, A.G.L. (1987) Mean arterial blood pressure and neonatal cerebral lesions. *Arch. Dis. Childh.*, **62**, 1068–1069

26. Miall-Allen, V.M. and Whitelaw, A.G.L. (1989) Response to dopamine and dobutamine in the preterm infant less than 30 weeks' gestation. *Critical Care Med.*, **17**, 1166–1169

27. Fernell, E., Hagberg, G. and Hagberg, B. (1990) Infantile hydrocephalus – the impact of enhanced preterm survival. *Acta Paediatr. Scand.*, **79**, 1080–1086

28. Shankaran, S., Koepke, T., Woldte, E. *et al.* (1989) Outcome after posthaemorrhagic ventriculomegaly in comparison with mild haemorrhage without ventriculomegaly. *J. Pediatr.*, **114**, 109–114

29. Larroche, J.C. (1972) Posthaemorrhagic hydrocephalus in infancy. *Biol. Neonat.*, **20**, 287–299

30. Weller, R. and Wisnieski, H. (1969) Histological and ultrastructural changes with experimental hydrocephalus in adult rabbits. *Brain*, **92**, 819–828

31. Weller, R., Wisnieski, H., Shulman, K. and Terry R. (1971) Experimental hydrocephalus in young dogs: histological and ultrastructural study of the brain tissue damage. *Neuropath. Exp. Neurol.*, **30**, 613–627

32. Weller, R. and Shulman, K. (1972) Infantile hydrocephalus: clinical, histological, and ultrastructural study of brain damage. *J. Neurosurg.*, **36**, 255–265

33. Levene, M.I. (1981) Measurement of the growth of the lateral ventricles in preterm infants with real time ultrasound. *Arch. Dis. Childh.*, **56**, 999–904

34. Kaiser, A. and Whitelaw, A. (1986) Normal cerebrospinal fluid pressure in the newborn. *Neuropediatrics*, **17**, 100–102

35. Kaiser, A. and Whitelaw, A. (1985) Cerebrospinal fluid pressure in infants with post-haemorrhagic ventricular dilatation. *Arch. Dis. Childh.*, **60**, 920–924

36. Kaiser, A. and Whitelaw, A. (1987) Non-invasive measurement of intracranial pressure. Fact or fancy. *Dev. Med. Child. Neurol.*, **29**, 320–326

37. Mantovani, J.F., Pasternak, J.F., Mathew, O.P. *et al.* (1980) Failure of daily lumbar punctures to prevent the development of hydrocephalus following intraventricular haemorrhage. *J. Pediatr.*, **97**, 278–81

38. Anwar, M., Kadam, S., Hiatt, I.M. and Hegyi, T. (1985) Serial lumbar punctures in prevention of posthaemorrhagic hydrocephalus in preterm infants. *J. Pediatr.*, **107**, 446–449

39. Ventriculomegaly Trial Group (1990) Randomised trial of early tapping in neonatal posthaemorrhagic ventricular dilatation. *Arch. Dis. Child.*, **65**, 3–10

40. Ventriculomegaly Trial Group (1994) Randomised trial of early tapping in neonatal posthaemorrhagic ventricular dilatation. *Arch. Dis. Child.*, **70**, F129–136

41. Shinnar, S., Gammon, K., Bergman, E.W., Epstein, M. and Freedom, J.M. (1985) Management of hydrocephalus in infancy: use of acetazolamide and furosemide to avoid cerebrospinal fluid shunts. *J. Pediatr.*, **107**, 31–36

42. Thoresen, M. and Whitelaw, A. (1990) Effect of acetazolamide on cerebral blood flow velocity and $CO_2$ elimination in normotensive and hypotensive newborn piglets. *Biol. Neonate*, **58**, 200–207

43. Cowan, F. and Whitelaw, A. (1991) Acute effects of acetazolamide on cerebral blood flow velocity and $P_{CO_2}$ in the newborn infant. *Acta Paediatr. Scand.*, **80**, 22–27

44. Lorber, J. (1975) Isosorbide in treatment of infantile hydrocephalus. *Arch. Dis. Child.*, **50**, 431–436

45. Liptak, G.S., Gellerstedt, M.E. and Klionsky, N. (1992) Isosorbide in the medical management of hydrocephalus in children with myeodysplasia. *Dev. Med. Child. Neurol.*, **34**, 150–154

46. Anwar, M., Dolye, A.J., Kadam, S., Hiatt, I.M. and Hegyi, T. (1986) Management of post-haemorrhagic hydrocephalus in the preterm infant. *J. Pediatr. Surg.*, **21**, 334–337

47. Hislop, J., Dubowitz, L., Kaiser, A., Singh, P. and Whitelaw, A. (1988) Outcome of infants shunted for post-haemorrhagic ventricular dilatation. *Dev. Med. Child. Neurol.*, **30**, 451–456

48. Punt, J. (1988) Hydrocephalus. In *Fetal and Neonatal Neurology and Neurosurgery* (M. Levene, M. Bennett and J. Punt, eds), Churchill Livingstone, Edinburgh, pp. 586–591

49. Goldblum, R.M., Pelley, R.P., O'Donell, A.A., Pryon, D. and Heffers, J.P. (1992) Antibodies to silicone elastomers and reactions to ventriculoperitoneal shunts. *Lancet*, **340**, 510–513

50. Gairdner, D. and Pearson, J. (1971) A growth chart for premature and other infants. *Arch. Dis. Childh.*, **46**, 783–787

51. Whitelaw, A., Creighton, L. and Gaffney, P. (1991) Fibrinolytic activity in cerebrospinal fluid after intraventricular haemorrhage. *Arch. Dis. Childh.*, **66**, 808–809

52. Whitelaw, A., Rivers, R., Creighton, L. and Gaffney, P. (1992) Low dose intraventricular fibrinolytic therapy to prevent posthaemorrhagic hydrocephalus. *Arch. Dis. Childh.*, **67**, 12–14

53. Whitelaw, A., Mowinckel, M.C., Larsen, M. and Abildgaard, U. (1994) Intraventricular streptokinase increases cerebrospinal D dimer in preterm infants with posthaemorrhagic ventricular dilatation. *Acta Paediatrica*, **83**, 270–2

# 19

# Retinopathy of prematurity

## David Clark

Retinopathy of prematurity (ROP), previously known as retrolental fibroplasia, was first reported by Terry in 1942 [1]. The condition he described occurred in infants, mostly 8 weeks preterm, and consisted of a fibroblastic membrane behind the lens, thought to be due to persistence of the vascular supply to the developing lens and vitreous [2]. We now recognize these features as the cicatricial end-stage of the disease process.

In a retrospective study by Campbell in 1951 the link with oxygen therapy was made [3]. Thereafter animal model experiments and clinical trials seemed to confirm this hypothesis [4–8]. Guy *et al.* were confident enough to suggest that all ROP could be eliminated by the judicial curtailment of oxygen therapy [9]. Certainly the incidence of ROP fell dramatically but it never completely disappeared. Despite these predictions, Phelps estimated that the annual incidence of ROP-blindness in 1979 almost equalled that of the 1943–53 epidemic [10]. Gibson has since confirmed that this second epidemic is due to the increasing birth weight specific survival of infants born at <1000g [11,12].

## Normal vasculogenesis

The retinal vasculature develops from spindle cells which are probably of mesenchymal origin. They migrate from the area of the optic disc at 16 weeks' gestation and reach the ora serrata (anterior retina) at 29 weeks. The cells become canalized and gradually a network of capillaries develop. Through a process of selective atrophy and hypertrophy, dependent on the metabolic demands of the adjacent retina, the definitive vessel is formed. The retinal vessels reach the nasal ora at 36 weeks and the temporal ora at 40 weeks from conception. An incomplete and, therefore, vulnerable vasculature is fundamental to the development of ROP.

## Pathogenesis

In the 1950s it was naively thought that ROP was due solely to the unrestricted administration of oxygen. However, even in the clinical trials ROP occurred in the absence of oxygen therapy [13]. Numerous reports have since documented ROP in infants who never received supplemental oxygen [14], at birth [15], in cyanotic heart disease [16], and no retinopathy despite very high oxygen levels [17]. It is currently thought that the aetiology of ROP is multifactorial. Oxygen, though important, is but one of a number of factors, many of which are still poorly understood and under investigation.

The animal model experiments of Ashton [4–6] in the UK and Patz [7] in the USA demonstrated the effect of high oxygen concentrations on the blood vessels of newborn kittens. When the kittens were nursed in 60–80% oxygen environments marked vasoconstriction and often complete obliteration of the retinal circulation occurred. On reintroducing the kitten to normal atmospheric oxygen intense neovascular proliferation was found. This was postulated to be due to the secretion of a vasoformative substance by the now ischaemic peripheral retinal. The sensitivity to oxygen damage was directly proportional to the degree of immaturity of the retinal vessels, the duration of oxygen exposure and the concentration of oxygen. The initial vasoconstriction is probably a normal protective mechanism to reduce the damaging effect of a high blood oxygen level on the developing endothelial cells [18]. Flower found the protective mechanism was inhibited by manipulating prostaglandin synthesis using aspirin or by oxygen/carbon dioxide mixtures in the inspired air [19]. In both experiments the resultant retinopathy was more severe than in the control. These findings were consistent with the work of Ashton and Pedler on the cytotoxic effects of oxygen on endothelial cells [20].

The kitten has an incompletely vascularized retina similar to the premature infant and was thought to be a good model for experimental work. However, there are no spindle cells in the kittens' retinal vasculature and the cicatricial stages of ROP never develop. Hittner and Kretzer have shown that the spindle cell plays an important role in the pathogenesis of ROP [21]. They have found that the migrating spindle cells become gap-junction linked when they are 'stressed' thus preventing further migration. The cells then show an increase in rough endoplasmic reticulum implying protein synthesis, perhaps of an angiogenic factor that could stimulate abnormal fibrovascular proliferation. It is therefore the spindle cells peripheral to the ridge that induce stage 3 disease. Nissenkorn *et al.* have applied this theory clinically [22]. Rather than treating the whole avascular area with cryotherapy they confined treatment to the area just anterior to the ridge. Complete regression occurred in all cases confirming that the main stimulus for neovascularization comes from the avascular retina adjacent to the ridge.

Hyperoxia and hypoxia have been postulated to 'stress' spindle cells [23]. Hyperoxia and hypoxia are known to generate free radicals. The premature infant being deficient in antioxidants, notably vitamin E and the iron-associated antioxidants ceruloplasmin and apotransferrin, is therefore potentially susceptible to free radical damage. Light and iron are other sources of free radicals and alone or in combination with oxygen derived free radicals may be involved in the development of neovascularization [24–28].

## Classification

The International Classification of ROP divides the retina into three zones centred on the optic disc [29]. Zone I is a circle whose radius extends from the disc to twice the distance from the disc to the fovea. ROP located in Zone I is usually severe. Zone II extends from the nasal ora serrata to the temporal equator. Zone III consists of the retina peripheral to the edge of Zone II (Figure 19.1). ROP located in Zone III is usually mild.

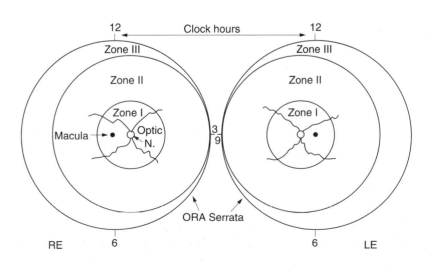

**Figure 19.1** Diagram showing the location of the zones and clock hours used to describe the position of ROP and extent of involved retina

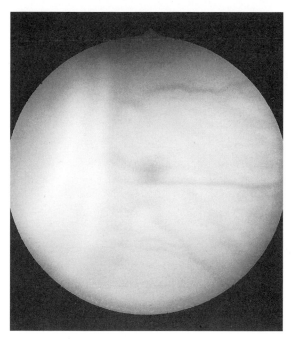

**Figure 19.2** Stage 2 (Ridge), with isolated shunts and small retinal haemorrhage. (Second white line is artefact from indentation)

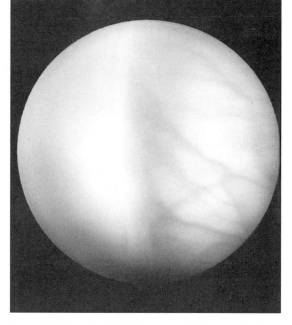

**Figure 19.3** Stage 3 – Mild (extraretinal fibrovascular proliferation)

The extent of the retina with ROP is specified by the number of clock hours involved, each clock hour being equivalent to a 30 degree sector. The severity of ROP is classified into 5 stages:

- Stage 1 (Demarcation Line) is a thin white line separating the avascular and vascular retina. Histologically it represents spindle cell proliferation [30].
- Stage 2 (Ridge) develops when the demarcation line has bulk and volume (Figure 19.2). It no longer lies in the plane of the retina but extends up out of it. It may be white or pink. Sometimes isolated tufts of new vessels posterior to the ridge may be found.
- Stage 3 (Extra-retinal Fibrovascular Proliferation) describes the ridge plus extra-retinal fibrovascular proliferative tissue (Figure 19.3 to 19.5). It may be further subdivided into mild, moderate or severe. It is characteristically located either continuous with the posterior aspect of the ridge, immediately posterior but not connected to the ridge or into the vitreous.
- Stage 4 (Sub-total Retinal Detachment) describes a sub-total retinal detachment

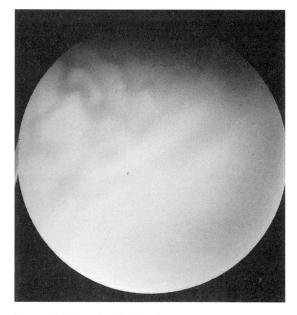

**Figure 19.4** Stage 3 – Moderate

that is nearly always tractional. Stage 4A if the fovea is not involved, stage 4B if it is.

- Stage 5 (Total Retinal Detachment) is a

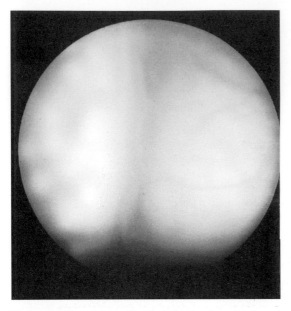

**Figure 19.5** Stage 3 immediately following laser treatment to avascular retina

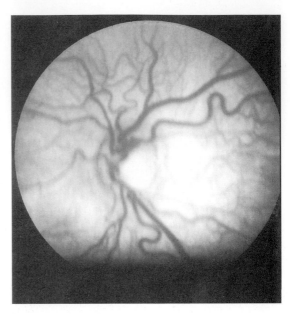

**Figure 19.6** 'Plus' disease

total retinal detachment and can be further classified according to its configuration.

- 'Plus' Disease. The designation 'plus' is added to the stage if the posterior vessels are dilated and tortuous (Figure 19.6). There may also be vitreous haze, iris vessel engorgement and pupil rigidity.

## Incidence and severity

Recent publications report the incidence of ROP in babies under 1000 g to be about 88% [31–33]. However, the incidence of severe disease, stage 3 or worse varies from 20% to 53%, probably differing because of different survival rates, referral patterns and screening methods.

**Table 19.1.** **Median and ranges of birth weight and gestational age for worst stage of ROP (either eye)**

| | No. of babies | Birth weight (g) | | Gestation (weeks) | |
|---|---|---|---|---|---|
| | | Median | Range | Median | Range |
| Stage 1 | 30 | 849 | 595–990 | 28 | 24–30 |
| 2 | 60 | 835 | 560–990 | 26 | 24–31 |
| 3 | 47 | 780 | 450–982 | 26 | 22–28 |
| 4/5 | 13 | 720 | 600–982 | 25 | 24–27 |

The worst stage of ROP (either eye) in 144 babies under 1000 g examined in Liverpool (1989–1992) was stage 1, 28 (19.4%); stage 2, 56 (39%); stage 3, 47 (32.6%) and stage 4–5, 13 (9%). The worst stages of ROP occur in the most premature and the smallest babies (Table 19.1 and Figure 19.7).

## Screening

The working party of the British Association of Perinatal Medicine and the College of Ophthalmologists recommend that all premature infants of 31 weeks' gestation or less and/or under 1500 g birth weight be screened for ROP [34].

The timing of screening is based on the gestation and postnatal age rather than birth weight. To keep the number of examinations to a minimum the infant should be seen at about 7 weeks postnatal age and thereafter fortnightly until there is no risk or the retinopathy is regressing [35]. However, in infants with a gestational age of 25 weeks or less the screening should begin earlier, at 5 weeks, as these babies are at risk of developing a more aggressive form of the disease. This is known as Rush Disease and carries a poor prognosis unless treated early.

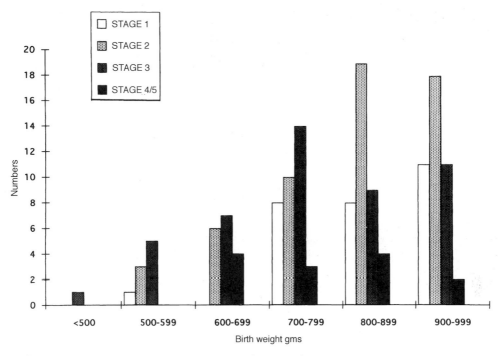

**Figure 19.7** Birth weight distribution of worst stage of ROP (either eye)

The eyes are dilated with cyclopentolate 0.5% one drop every 15 min for one hour and one drop of phenylephrine 2.5%, commencing about an hour before the examination. The adrenergic effect of phenylephrine causes blanching of the lids and surrounding skin. It may cause increased blood pressure and slowing of the heart rate even at this concentration, so must be used with caution.

Although not essential, the use of a lid speculum and scleral indentation facilitates the examination and is carried out using 0.4% oxybuprocaine, a topical anaesthetic. All infants should be monitored during the procedure because of the oculocardiac reflex and the general instability of these infants. Minor changes in heart rate and oxygen saturation occur frequently. Clarke *et al.* reported a 31% incidence of bradycardia (which they defined as a 10% decrease from base-line) in 54 infants examined. The bradycardia occurred most frequently during instillation of the drops and insertion of the lid speculum [36]. However, serious complications are rare. Clark *et al.* recorded three episodes of apnoea in over 600 examinations [32]. One case had recurrent apnoeic episodes before and after the screening procedure, a second had chronic lung

disease and the third was found to be anaemic (Hb 8 g dl$^{-1}$). A further examination a week later after a transfusion was uneventful. A prospective study by Laws *et al.* reported no clinically significant effects from the drops or from the eye examination [65].

## Natural history

### Age of onset

The age of onset of ROP occurs later in terms of postnatal age but earlier in relation to post-conceptional age for infants <28 weeks' gestation than for those of 28 weeks or above. Fielder *et al.* found a highly significant difference in median postnatal age at onset of 51 and 40 days respectively for these two groups [37]. They also noted that the ROP commenced 2 weeks earlier from conception (median 33.7 weeks) for infants <28 weeks compared to their older counterparts.

The onset is determined by the gestational age (and therefore the immaturity of the retina) and by the neonatal events. It is speculated that the very immature infant has less differentiation of the retina and therefore there is a greater time delay before metabolic demands provoke further vasogenesis [38].

## Location and severity

The extent of retinal vascularization is dependent on the gestational age and birth weight of the infant. The more premature infant having the least vascularized retina. Kretzer *et al.*, have shown that for an infant with the appropriate gestational age weighing 600 g or less at birth, ROP will develop in Zone I, those weighing 801 g or more will develop ROP in Zone II and those weighing 601–800 g may have ROP in either Zone I or II [39].

ROP that is located in Zone I is more likely to progress to severe disease than ROP in Zone III which only rarely develops to stage 3. The rate of progression from onset to stage 3 is also affected by the location, stage 3 developing more rapidly in zone I [40].

The disease often starts and is initially worse on the nasal side in babies under 1000 g [41,33]. The reason for this is unknown. However, the later cicatricial disease is usually worse temporally as the temporal retina has the larger area of unvascularized retina.

## Rush disease

This condition first described in the Japanese literature is a very severe and rapidly progressive form of ROP [42,43]. It is nearly always confined to the very premature baby of 26 weeks' gestation or less. The disease is located in Zone I and often associated with extensive preretinal haemorrhages. It has a rapid course, hence the name but does not progress in a step-by-step fashion through the stages. The terminal vessels arbourize and join, 'plus' disease develops and fibrovascular proliferation quickly follows with retinal, or sometimes vitreous, haemorrhages. Tasman says a ridge may be detected on indentation but this is often very difficult to visualize [44]. The success of treatment depends on its early detection. The presence of 'plus' disease even in the absence of the usual appearance of ROP may be the first sign this condition is developing.

## Treatment

If only stages 1 or 2 ROP are reached then spontaneous regression always occurs. Stage 3 however may regress or may progress to a retinal detachment. The American CryoROP study has demonstrated an initial 50% reduction in unfavourable outcome which they defined as a posterior retinal detachment, posterior retinal fold or retrolental tissue obscuring a view of the posterior retina [45]. The 12-month outcome confirmed these results [46]. The treatment involved ablation of the avascular retina using cryotherapy. The development of portable laser systems delivered through the indirect ophthalmoscope provides us with another modality of treatment, though a clear view of the retina must be present. Laser treatment is less traumatic for the infant and has the advantage that posteriorly located disease is more easily treated. It has been shown to be as effective as cryotherapy [47–49]. The response to laser may take a few days longer than cryotherapy but if there is no evidence of regression after 7 days for either modality of treatment, further laser or cryotherapy can be given to untreated areas.

Although the treatment can be carried out with the infant sedated under a local anaesthetic, we prefer a general anaesthetic. The infants are paralysed using pancuronium, intubated and ventilated. Fentanyl (15 µg kg$^{-1}$ induction dose; maintenance infusion 1–3 µg/kg/hour) is given for analgesia [32].

## Complications of treatment

### *Operative*

The main ocular complication encountered in the CryoROP trial was a 19% incidence of retinal or vitreous haemorrhage [45]. The risk of haemorrhage is increased if the vascular shunt is directly treated. As this is unnecessary it should be avoided.

Systemic complications include bradycardia (including asystole), cyanosis and respiratory arrest. Brown *et al.* reported three instances of respiratory arrest and one of cardiopulmonary arrest amongst 80 infants treated [50]. In each case a local anaesthetic was employed. Retrobulbar injections are not recommended because of the risk of globe perforation or inadvertent intracranial injection through the thin orbital bone.

### *Late complications*

Retinal detachments occurring more than a year after treatment have been described [51].

In each case the retinal tear occurred at the treated/untreated interface. The cause is speculated to be a consequence of the chorioretinal adhesion produced by cryotherapy. As the eye grows tension is exerted at this point.

Myopia has long been recognized to occur in regressed ROP before cryotherapy was routinely performed [52]. In a small series of 17 eyes treated with cryotherapy, myopia was increased in the treated cases but the amount was not statistically significant [53]. Further long-term follow up to determine the true incidence of side-effects of treatment is still needed.

### Results

The visual results of treating stage 3 ROP were significantly better than no treatment, 35% versus 56% unfavourable outcome respectively [46]. However, better visual outcomes have been reported, albeit in a smaller series of 79 infants, using 3 clock hours of stage 3 as the criteria for treatment [54]. Earlier intervention may therefore be beneficial, though some infants would undoubtedly be treated unnecessarily.

The threshold agreed by the CryoROP study was a 50% probability of blindness if untreated. However, the incidence of blindness in untreated Zone I disease at this threshold is 95% [55]. Perhaps treating these cases at a sub-threshold level will improve the successful outcome [56].

The visual acuity attained is not solely dependent on successful regression of the disease as defined in the CryoROP study. Mild traction on the retina sufficient to cause macula ectopia (dragging of the retina usually temporally) would be classified as a successful outcome in the trial. Macula ectopia can reduce the vision and substantially if the ectopia is severe [57,58].

Frequently there are associated cranial ultrasound abnormalities. Luna *et al.* used acuity cards to measure grating acuity in 17 infants with regressed stage 3 ROP (mean birth weight 910 g) [59]. Ten had grade 3 or 4 intraventricular haemorrhage (IVH) or periventricular leucomalacia (PVL). All ten had acuity scores below the seven with no neurological complications. Burgess *et al.* examined 49 out of 68 surviving children with a birth weigh <1000 g

or gestation ≤28 weeks [60]: 59% had ocular abnormalities, only two had cicatricial ROP, 25 had strabismus (squint), 10 were myopic, 10 had optic nerve abnormalities and one was cortically blind.

It is important, therefore, when counselling parents on the future visual outcome of their children, that these points are taken into account and not simply the success or otherwise of ROP treatment.

## Vitreoretinal surgery

The only controlled clinical trial of the outcome of vitreoretinal surgery for stage 5 ROP reported little improvement on vision even when the retina was anatomically reattached [61]. The results of surgery for stage 4B may be more promising but to date no prospective controlled trial has been published.

## Prevention

The strongest predictor of developing ROP is the degree of prematurity. Unfortunately the most premature is often the sickest infant, and despite all attempts at homeostasis, frequent fluctuations in cardiopulmonary status occur [62]. Flynn *et al.*, re-evaluating data from a previous trial, found a significant association between the amount of time the $tcPo_2$ was ≥80 mmHg and the incidence and severity of ROP [63]. The conclusion of the study was that it is not possible to prevent ROP with current methods of monitoring and oxygen delivery. Indeed fluctuations within the range 5–10 kPa in the first 2 weeks of life can increase the risk of developing severe ROP [66]. Research to develop a method of adjusting the oxygen to prevent fluctuations in arterial concentration may be the way forward.

Vitamin E therapy has not lived up to its expectations in preventing ROP in the <1000 g baby. Law *et al.* makes the point that only 0.1% of ELBW infants would avoid blindness from Vitamin E therapy, a figure too low to justify its use given the associated side-effects [64]. However, further research into free radical damage and the use of other antioxidants is still necessary.

Methods of reducing the incidence of premature birth should not be overlooked as the attention of research is focused on this disorder.

## Summary

The baby under 1000 g has a very high probability of developing ROP and in some this will progress to stage 3. The major advance in the management of ROP has been the demonstration that cryotherapy or laser therapy can reduce the frequency of unfavourable visual outcomes. The disappointing results of vitreoretinal surgery and the short time window when cryotherapy/laser can be given places the emphasis on an adequate screening (and treatment) programme in each NICU for these at-risk infants.

---

**Practical points**

1. The baby under 1000 g, especially if <750 g birth weight, is at risk of developing sight-threatening ROP for which a treatment modality is available.
2. Screening of these at-risk infants should commence at 6–7 weeks, but earlier at 5 weeks if the gestation is <26 weeks.
3. Treatment success depends upon early diagnosis and prompt treatment with either cryotherapy or laser.
4. Screening complications are rare, but monitoring of the infant during the procedure is recommended.
5. Parents should be informed early of the possibility of the condition occurring.
6. The aetiology of ROP is multifactorial. Free radical damage is thought to be the common pathway leading to its development.

---

## References

1. Terry, T.L. (1942) Extreme prematurity and fibroblastic overgrowth of persistent vascular sheath behind each crystalline lens. *Am. J. Ophthalmol.*, **25**, 203–204
2. Terry, T.L. (1942) Fibroblastic overgrowth of persistent tunica vasculosa lentis in infants born prematurely. *Am. J. Ophthalmol.*, **25**, 1409–1423
3. Campbell, K. (1951) Intensive oxygen therapy as a possible cause of retrolental fibroplasia: A clinical approach. *Med. J. Aust.*, **2**, 48–50
4. Ashton, N., Ward, B. and Serpell, G. (1953) Role of oxygen in the genesis of retrolental fibroplasia. *Br. J. Ophthalmol.*, **37**, 513–520
5. Ashton, N., Ward, B. and Serpell, G. (1954) Effect of oxygen on developing retinal vessels with particular reference to the problem of retrolental fibroplasia. *Br. J. Ophthalmol.*, **38**, 397–432
6. Ashton, N. (1954) Pathological basis of retrolental fibroplasia. *Br. J. Ophthalmol.*, **38**, 385–396
7. Patz, A., Eastham, A., Higgenbotham, D.H. and Kleh, T. (1953) Oxygen studies in retrolental fibroplasia II. The production of the microscopic changes of retrolental fibroplasia in experimental animals. *Am. J. Ophthalmol.*, **36**, 1511–1522
8. Kinsey, V.E. (1956) Retrolental fibroplasia. Cooperative study of retrolental fibroplasia and the use of oxygen. *Arch. Ophthalmol.*, **56**, 481–543
9. Guy, L.P., Lanman, J.T. and Dancis, J. (1956) The possibility of total elimination of retrolental fibroplasia by oxygen restriction. *Pediatrics*, **17**, 247–249
10. Phelps, D.L. (1979) Retinopathy of prematurity: an estimate of vision loss in the United States. *Pediatrics*, **67**, 924–926
11. Gibson, D.L., Sheps, S.B., Schechter, M.T., Wiggins, S. and McCormick, A.Q. (1989) Retinopathy of prematurity: A new epidemic? *Pediatrics*, **83**, 486–492
12. Gibson, D.L., Sheps, S.B., Uh, S.H., Schechter, M.T. and McCormick, A.Q. (1990) Retinopathy of prematurity-induced blindness: Birth weight-specific survival and the new epidemic. *Pediatrics*, **86**, 405–412
13. Lucey, J.F. and Dangman, B. (1984) A reexamination of the role of oxygen in retrolental fibroplasia. *Pediatrics*, **73**, 82–96
14. Adamkin, D.H., Shott, R.J., Cook, L.N. and Andrews, B.F. (1977) Nonhyperoxic retrolental fibroplasia. *Pediatrics*, **60**, 828–830
15. Addison, D.J., Font, R.L. and Manschot, W.A. (1972) Proliferative retinopathy in anencephalic babies. *Am. J. Ophthalmol.*, **74**, 967–976
16. Johns, J.J., Johns, J.A., Feman, S.S. and Dodd, D.A. (1991) Retinopathy of prematurity in infants with cyanotic congenital heart disease. *Am. J. Dis. Child.*, **145**, 200–203
17. Aranda, J.V. and Sweet, A.Y. (1974) Sustained hyperoxia without cicatricial retrolental fibroplasia. *Pediatrics*, **54**, 434–437
18. Flower, R.W. and Blake, D.A. (1981) Retrolental fibroplasia: Evidence for a role of the prostaglandin cascade in the pathogenesis of oxygen-induced retinopathy in the newborn beagle. *Pediatr. Res.*, **15**, 1293–1302
19. Flower, R.W. (1985) Perinatal retinal vascular physiology. In *Retinopathy of Prematurity* (W.A. Silverman and J.T. Flynn, eds), Blackwell Scientific, Oxford, pp. 97–120
20. Ashton, N. and Pedler, C. (1962) Studies on developing retinal vessels: IX Reaction of endothelial cells to oxygen. *Br. J. Ophthalmol.*, **46**, 257–276
21. Kretzer, F.L. and Hittner, H.M. (1985) Initiating

events in the development of retinopathy of prematurity. In *Retinopathy of Prematurity* (W.A. Silverman and J.T. Flynn, eds), Blackwell Scientific, Oxford, pp. 121–152

22. Nissenkorn, I., Axer-Siegel, R., Kremer, I. and Ben-Sira, I. (1991) Effect of partial cryoablation on retinopathy of prematurity. *Br. J. Ophthalmol.*, **75**, 160–162

23. Kretzer, F.L., Mehta, R.S., Johnson, A.T., Hunter, D.G., Brown, E.S. and Hittner, H.M. (1984) Vitamin E protects against retinopathy of prematurity through action on spindle cells. *Nature*, **309**, 793–795

24. Riley, P.A. and Slater, T.F. (1991) Retinopathy of prematurity. *Lancet*, **ii**, 492–493

25. Slater, T.F. and Riley, P.A. (1970) Free radical damage in retrolental fibroplasia. *Lancet*, **ii**, 467

26. Sullivan J.L. (1988) Iron, plasma antioxidants, and the 'oxygen radical disease of prematurity'. *Am. J. Dis. Child.*, **142**, 1341–1344

27. Slater, T.F. (1984) Free-radical mechanisms in tissue injury. *Biochem. J.*, **222**, 1–15

28. Cooke, R.W.I., Clark, D.I., Hickey-Dwyer, M. and Weindling, A.M. (1993) The apparent role of blood transfusions in the development of retinopathy of prematurity. *Eur. J. Pediatr.*, **152**, 833–836

29. The Committee for the Classification of Retinopathy of Prematurity (1984) An international classification of retinopathy of prematurity. *Arch. Ophthalmol.*, **102**, 1130–1134

30. Foos, R.Y. (1975) Acute retrolental fibroplasia. *Albrecht Von Graefes Arch. Klin. Exp. Ophthalmol.*, **195**, 87–100

31. Acheson, J.F. and Schulenburg, W.E. (1991) Surveillance for retinopathy of prematurity in practice: Experience from one neonatal intensive care unit. *Eye*, **5**, 80–85

32. Clark, D.I., O'Brien, C., Weindling, A.M. and Saeed, M. (1992) Initial experience of screening for retinopathy of prematurity. *Arch. Dis. Childh.*, **67**, 1233–1236

33. Fielder, A.R., Shaw, D.E., Robinson, J. and Ng, Y.K. (1992) Natural history of retinopathy of prematurity: A prospective study. *Eye*, **6**, 233–242

34. Anonymous (1990) College News: Retinopathy of Prematurity screening duty. *Q. Bull. Coll. Ophthalmol.* (**Autumn**), 6

35. Palmer, E.A. (1981) Optimal timing of examination for acute retrolental fibroplasia. *Ophthalmology*, **88**, 662–666

36. Clarke, W.N., Hodges, E., Noel, L.P., Roberts, D. and Coneys, M. (1985) The oculocardiac reflux during ophthalmoscopy in premature infants. *Am. J. Ophthalmol.*, **99**, 649–651

37. Fielder, A.R., Ng, Y.K. and Levene, M.I. (1986) Retinopathy of prematurity: Age of onset. *Arch. Dis. Childh.*, **61**, 774–778

38. Quinn, G.E., Johnson, L. and Abbasi, S. (1992) Onset of retinopathy of prematurity as related to postnatal and postconceptional age. *Br. J. Ophthalmol.*, **76**, 284–288

39. Kretzer, F.L. and Hittner, H.M. (1988) Retinopathy of prematurity: clinical implications of retinal development. *Arch. Dis. Childh.*, **63**, 1151–1167

40. Schulenburg, W.E., Prendiville, A. and Ohri, R. (1987) Natural history of retinopathy of prematurity. *Br. J. Ophthalmol.*, **71**, 837–843

41. Nissenkorn, I., Kremer, I., Cohen, S. and Ben-Sira, I. (1989) Nasal versus temporal preretinal vasoproliferation in retinopathy of prematurity. *Br. J. Ophthalmol.*, **73**, 747–749

42. Uemura, Y. (1977) Current status of retrolental fibroplasia: report of the joint committee for the study of retrolental fibroplasia in Japan. *Jpn. J. Ophthalmol.*, **21**, 366–378

43. Majima, A. (1977) Studies on retinopathy of prematurity 1. Statistical analysis of factors related to occurrence and progression in active phase. *Jpn. J. Ophthalmol.*, **21**, 404–420

44. Tasman, W. (1985) Zone I retinopathy of prematurity. *Arch. Ophthalmol.*, **103**, 1693–1694

45. Cryotherapy for Retinopathy of Prematurity Cooperative Group (1988) Multicenter trial of cryotherapy for retinopathy of prematurity: Preliminary results. *Arch. Ophthalmol.*, **106**, 471–477

46. Cryotherapy for Retinopathy of Prematurity Cooperative Group (1990) Multicenter trial of cryotherapy for retinopathy of prematurity: One year outcome – Structure and function. *Arch. Ophthalmol.*, **108**, 1408–1416

47. Landers, M.B., Toth, C.A., Semple, H.C. and Morse, L.S. (1992) Treatment of retinopathy of prematurity with argon laser photocoagulation. *Arch. Ophthalmol.*, **110**, 44–47

48. Clark, D.I. and Hero, M. (1994) Indirect diode laser treatment for stage 3 retinopathy of prematurity. *Eye*, **8**, 423–426

49. McNamara, J.A., Tasman, W., Brown, G.C. and Federman, J.A. (1991) Laser photocoagulation for stage 3+ retinopathy of prematurity. *Ophthalmology*, **98**, 576–580

50. Brown, G.C., Tasman, W., Naidoff, M., Schaffer, D.B., Quinn, G. and Bhutani, V.K. (1990) Systemic complications associated with retinal cryoablation for retinopathy of prematurity. *Ophthalmology*, **97**, 855–858

51. Greven, C.G. and Tasman, W. (1989) Rhegmatogenous retinal detachment following cryotherapy in retinopathy of prematurity. *Arch. Ophthalmol.*, **107**, 1017–1018

52. Birge, H.L. (1955) Myopia caused by prematurity. *Trans. Am. Ophthalmol. Soc.*, **53**, 219–230

53. Ben-Sira, I., Nissenkorn, I., Weinberger, D., Shohat, M., Kremer, I., Krikler, R. *et al.* (1986) Long-term results of cryotherapy for active stages of retinopathy of prematurity. *Ophthalmology*, **93**, 1423–1428

54. Nissenkorn, I., Ben-Sira, I., Kremer, I. *et al.* (1991) Eleven years experience with retinopathy of prematurity: visual results and contribution of cryoablation. *Br. J. Ophthalmol.*, **75**, 158–159

55. Sternberg, P., Lopez, P.F., Lambert, H.M., Aaberg, T.M. and Capone, A. (1992) Controversies in the management of retinopathy of prematurity. *Am. J. Ophthalmol.*, **113**, 198–202
56. Tasman, W. (1992) Threshold retinopathy of prematurity revisited. *Arch. Ophthalmol.*, **110**, 623–624
57. Katsumi, O., Mehta, M.C., Matsui, Y., Tetsuka, H. and Hirose, T. (1991) Development of vision in retinopathy of prematurity. *Arch. Ophthalmol.*, **109**, 1394–1398
58. Cryotherapy for Retinopathy of Prematurity Cooperative Group (1993) Multicenter trial of cryotherapy for retinopathy of prematurity: 3½ year outcome – structure and function. *Arch. Ophthalmol.*, **111**, 339–344
59. Luna, B., Dobson, V. and Biglan, A.W. (1990) Development of grating acuity in infants with regressed stage 3 retinopathy of prematurity. *Invest. Ophthalmol. Vis. Sci.*, **31**, 2082–2087
60. Burgess, P. and Johnson, A. (1991) Ocular defects in infants of extremely low birth weight and low gestational age. *Br. J. Ophthalmol.*, **75**, 84–87
61. Quinn, G.E., Dobson, V., Barr, C.C. *et al.* (1991) Visual acuity in infants after vitrectomy for severe retinopathy of prematurity. *Ophthalmology*, **98**, 5–13
62. Phelps, D. (1992) Retinopathy of prematurity. *N. Engl. J. Med.*, **326**, 1078–1080
63. Flynn, J.T., Bancalari, E., Snyder, E.S. *et al.* (1992) A cohort study of transcutaneous oxygen tension and the incidence and severity of retinopathy of prematurity. *N. Engl. J. Med.*, **326**, 1050–1054
64. Law, M.R., Wijewardene, K. and Wald, N.J. (1990) Is routine vitamin E administration justified in very low-birthweight infants? *Dev. Med. Child. Neurol.*, **32**, 442–450
65. Laws, D.E., Moreton, C., Weindling, M. and Clark, D. (1996) Systemic effects of screening for retinopathy of prematurity. *British J. Ophthalmology*, **80**, 425–428
66. Saito, Y., Omoto, T., Cho, Y., Hatsukawa, Y. *et al.* (1993) The progression of Retinopathy of Prematurity and fluctuation in blood gas tension. *Graefe's Arch. for Clinical and Experimental Ophthalmology*, **231**, 151–156

# 20

# Necrotizing enterocolitis

**Richard Cooke**

Necrotizing enterocolitis (NEC) is the most common gastroenterological complication of ELBW infants, occurring in about 10% of infants cared for in major centres [1], although very much higher rates have been described in some units. Early surgical description of the disorder date back to the last century [2], but the term 'necrotizing enterocolitis' was first used in 1961 [3], and a full clinical description published in 1963 [4]. The infants described in earlier papers tended to be relatively mature infants, and factors such as umbilical catheterization and exchange transfusions dominated the aetiological theories [5]. In more recent years the increased survival of ELBW infants in whom the condition was more common, meant that the majority of affected infants were in this group. The disorder is now regarded principally as a failure of adaptation of the immature gastrointestinal tract to the stresses of extrauterine life.

NEC presents as a range of clinical disorders, ranging from intolerance of oral feeds and ileus, to septic shock, gastrointestinal haemorrhage and bowel perforation [6]. In infants who survive, late complications include stricture formation and feed intolerance. Regarded initially as a surgical condition, the emphasis has now moved to medical management at least in the early phases of the condition, and a greater attention to prevention.

## Aetiology and pathogenesis

NEC is the pathological response of the immature gut to injury by a variety of insults.

The primary problems appears to be *ischaemic damage* to the mucosa, but the presence of *bacteria* and a nutrient *substrate* are also needed to produce the disease. The many factors associated with an increased risk of the development of NEC, each act through one or more of these three pathways [7]. The greater risk of developing NEC in the ELBW infants only reflects the higher prevalence of these conditions in the very immature [8].

### Ischaemic damage to the gut

Underperfusion of the gut may result from a range of insults. Abnormal patterns of flow velocity (absent or reversed end diastolic flow) in the fetal aorta have been detected *in utero* using Doppler ultrasound techniques in IUGR fetuses, and are associated with a high risk of NEC and other morbidities after birth [9,10]. During cardiorespiratory illness in the early neonatal period, poor cardiac output and systemic hypotension lead to poor peripheral perfusion [11,12]. In particular, the gut appears to lose blood flow to more immediately critical organs such as brain, heart, kidney and adrenals [13], in a process analogous to the diving reflex in some aquatic animals [14]. Persistence of the arterial duct may result in a marked left-to-right shunt giving rise to retrograde flow in the aorta during diastole, and compromising flow to the superior mesenteric artery [12]. Reduction of mesenteric perfusion may also be the reason that both umbilical arterial and venous catheters have been associated as risk factors in NEC [15]. Polycythaemia has also been associated with NEC, and if this is a causal relationship, a reduction in intestinal perfusion might be responsible [16].

In the very immature infant, the gut lacks much of the protection of mucus and secretory IgA present in older infants, and is also more permeable to molecules such as toxins and bacterial antigens [17–19]. Intestinal mucosal maturation has been shown to be promoted by corticosteroids, and it is known that antenatal steroids given to the mother reduce the risk of NEC in preterm infants [20].

### Bacterial infection

Although it is not widely believed that NEC occurs *primarily* as the result of bacterial infection, up to half of all infants with the fully developed condition have positive blood cultures, with the same organisms as are found in the bowel or peritoneum [21]. No one organism is consistently associated with NEC although Gram negative bacteria such as Klebsiella Sp. and *Escherichia coli* are commonly identified [22,23]. Changes in gut flora have been noted to occur in the 72 hours preceding clinically obvious NEC, and have been ascribed to changes in intraluminal conditions following gut ischaemia [24]. Various species of Clostridium have also been cultured from cases of NEC. Because they are known to produce toxins which damage the gut mucosa, and have been implicated in such enterocolitides as darmbrand [25] and pig-bel [26] and enterocolitis necroticans [27] in older individuals, Clostridia Sp. have been suggested as the primary insult in the NEC. Although found in infants during epidemics of NEC in a single nursery [28], they are not usually present in isolated cases [29], suggesting that their presence is fortuitous.

The gut organisms involved in NEC produce hydrogen and methane, which in turn are responsible for the intramural gas seen on abdominal radiographs in severe cases [30]. Endotoxins produced by these bacteria are absorbed readily into the circulation, and probably cause the picture of shock, and renal and hepatic failure which can occur.

### Enteral feeds

Milk in the gut provides an abundant substrate for bacterial proliferation. Most infants with florid NEC have been fed at some time after birth, and the timing of the onset of NEC relates strongly to the introduction of enteral feeds [21]. The volume and type of feed are also related to the risk. The use of hyperosmolar feeds and large volumes of milk in order to promote growth is associated with increased risk [32–34], and the use of human milk with reduced risk [35].

## Clinical presentation

The presentation of NEC varies greatly, and may initially be very non-specific, especially in the least mature. Classically, abdominal distension, bile stained gastric aspirates and blood and mucus in the stools are seen, together with pallor or a shock-like picture. In ELBW infants, a more gradual deterioration is usually seen, with recurrent apnoea, lethargy, and unstable vital signs, leading to pallor, mottling, jaundice and a generalized bleeding tendency. Bowel sounds are generally absent. Abdominal tenderness, crepitus, an abdominal mass or discoloration of the abdominal wall are ominous signs. A sudden increase in abdominal girth usually indicates acute perforation.

Laboratory investigations show a positive blood culture in up to one half of all cases. This is often accompanied by a relative neutropenia, a low platelet count, and an elevated C-reactive protein level. The last two investigations are useful for monitoring the course of the disease, and their early return to normal carries a good prognosis.

A plain abdominal radiograph may reveal an isolated distended loop of gut (fixed loop), usually on the right side, although it may only show ascites or thickened gut walls and fluid levels [36]. As many ELBW infants will not have been fed early, the pathognomonic appearance of intramural gas (pneumatosis intestinalis) is not seen as often as in larger babies. Gas in the portal venous system may occasionally be seen over the liver, and is regarded as a poor prognostic sign. Perforation leading to a pneumoperitoneum is not always very obvious on a plain anteroposterior film, and is usually more clearly evident on a film taken with the baby in the lateral decubitus position. Contrast radiographs are unnecessary during the acute illness, although may be invaluable for the assessment of stricture in the recovery period. Because of a risk of deterioration, probably

**Table 20.1. A staging system for necrotizing enterocolitis (after Bell *et al.* [6])**

**Stage 1** (suspected)
Unstable temperature, lethargy, apnoea, bradycardia.
Poor feeding, increased gastric aspirates, vomiting, mild abdominal distension, blood in stool.
Distended loops of gut on radiograph.

**Stage 2** (definite)
Above signs plus gross bleeding or abdominal distension.
Ileus, thickened bowel wall or intramural gas, portal vein gas on radiograph.

**Stage 3** (advanced)
Above signs plus deteriorating vital signs, septic shock, marked gastrointestinal haemorrhage.
Pneumoperitoneum.

related to sepsis, associated with contrast enemata in NEC, antibiotic prophylaxis has been advocated [37].

The clinical findings described above have been used by Bell *et al.* to stage the disease [6], and this system has been widely adopted (Table 20.1).

X-ray appearances of NEC in the ELBW infant are often less florid than in larger infants, and gross pneumatosis is rarely seen (Figures 20.1–20.4).

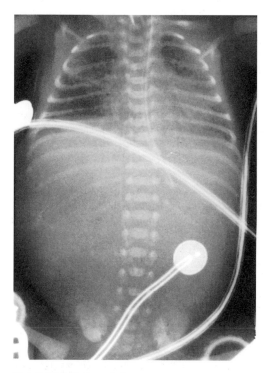

**Figure 20.1** Gasless abdomen

# Treatment

There have been no controlled trials of *treatment* of NEC that have shown benefit, and so management of the condition is essentially supportive and based on empirical interven-

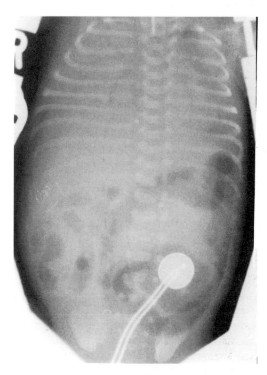

**Figure 20.2** Fixed (unchanging) bowel loops

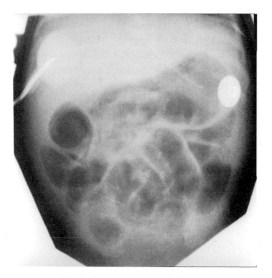

**Figure 20.3** Small bowel obstruction

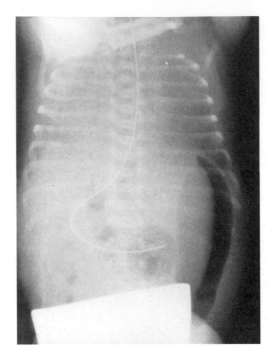

**Figure 20.4** Pneumoperitoneum

tions. Cessation of feeds for a variable period, intravenous antibiotics, transfusion of blood and other fluids, and total parenteral nutrition are all widely used as required. Emergency surgical intervention by laparotomy is now much less frequently resorted to, although about half of all more serious cases come to surgery. Initial medical treatment is given for 48 hours or so until the infant is stable and more likely to survive surgery. Such a policy has resulted in fewer infants undergoing very extensive gut resections [38]. Even perforation of the gut, once viewed as an absolute indicator for surgical intervention, may be treated initially by abdominal drainage by paracentesis, followed by interval laparotomy especially in frail ELBW infants [39]. The more conventional procedure is to do a limited laparotomy, pulling out a loop of bowel nearest to a perforation to form a double-barrelled ostomy, and allowing drainage of the upper gut and defunctioning of the lower bowel. Repair of the ostomy may often be postponed for 2 or 3 months, although excessive fluid loss from the ostomy may limit the infant's ability to thrive, forcing earlier closure [38].

Primary anastomosis of the gut ends may be attempted especially if the NEC is localized to a small part of the gut. It has been claimed that up to half of all patients are suitable for such a procedure and that it leads to a quicker recovery [40]. Surgery may often also be required later in infants managed initially entirely medically. Stricture formation may remain silent until refeeding occurs when obstruction becomes evident. Resection of the stenotic segment is then indicated. Contrast radiographic studies with a non-ionic contrast medium are helpful in identifying the site of the stricture.

Two randomized controlled trials of medical therapy have been carried out in infants with NEC. Hansen *et al.* gave gentamicin orally via the nasogastric tube after NEC had been diagnosed [41]. No differences in rate of resolution, mortality, or complications was observed. Faix *et al.* added clindamycin parenterally to the routine antibiotic therapy already being given, but was not able to demonstrate any clinical advantage [42].

## Prevention

In the light of relatively few proven treatment options in established NEC, prevention of the disease is a priority, and a number of strategies have been assessed in controlled clinical trials.

### Prenatal corticosteroids

Several controlled trials of antenatal corticosteroid prophylaxis for respiratory distress syndrome recorded the incidence of NEC as a secondary outcome variable [43–45]. In a meta-analysis of these studies, the event rate ratio (ERR) was 0.28 (95% CI 0.13–0.59) suggesting a strongly protective effect [46]. This could be mediated simply through a lower incidence of RDS, with which NEC is associated, or by a maturing effect on the gut itself [47].

There is also some limited evidence to suggest that steroids given postnatally may reduce NEC, although trial results were inconclusive [48].

### Antibiotics

Trial data have shown that antibiotics given to the mother prenatally do not prevent NEC [45,49,50]. Postnatally, however, there are five studies to date that show a reduction in NEC when oral aminoglycosides are given prophylactically to preterm infants at risk of developing NEC [51–55]. A meta-analysis of these studies, each of which is quite small, indicates a significant benefit with a likely ERR of 0.45 (95% CI 0.22–0.91) [46]. Although these studies were published some time ago, concern over the development of bacterial resistance has limited their acceptance. There is to date no evidence that this is actually a problem [56], but further studies are clearly needed.

## Immunoglobulins

Although a few early studies indicated that intravenous immunoglobulins may have a protective effect against infections in preterm infants, these early promises have not been borne out in larger subsequent trials. A protective effect for NEC was also anticipated, but generally no significant effects have been observed [57–59].

## Incidental outcomes of other treatments

In the course of controlled trials to prevent or treat other neonatal disorders in ELBW infants, NEC has often been recorded as a secondary or incidental outcome variable.

PDA is strongly associated with NEC, although whether this is a causal relationship is unclear. In seven controlled trials, use of *indomethacin* either prophylactially or as a treatment for PDA was not associated with a reduction in the incidence of NEC in treated infants [46]. The effects of closure of PDA with indomethacin and by *surgery* have also been compared, and again no significant differences in the incidence of NEC observed [60].

A significant reduction in NEC when PDA was ligated on day one in infants of less than 1000 g was observed by Cassady *et al.* [61], although it was noteworthy that the rate of NEC in the control group was exceptionally high at 30%. Cotton *et al.* found a higher rate of NEC in a group of low birth weight infants treated surgically for PDA, but there were no cases of NEC in the control group [62]. It remains uncertain as to whether treatment or prevention of PDA can alter the frequency of NEC. *Vitamin E* has been used for 30 years or more as a prophylactic measure against retinopathy, intraventricular haemorrhage and PDA. NEC has often been recorded as a

secondary outcome in controlled trials of vitamin E, and in a meta-analysis of seven such trials an increase in the frequency of NEC in the treated group was observed which did not reach statistical significance [46].

Because of the beneficial effect of antenatal steroid prophylaxis for RDS on the incidence of NEC, it had been assumed that the introduction of effective *exogenous surfactant therapy* would also produce a reduction in NEC, possibly through a reduction of hypoxia and ischaemia because of less severe lung disease. Neither individual controlled trials nor overviews have shown such an effect [46]. If such an effect does indeed exist, it is just possible that the increased survival of infants vulnerable to NEC in the surfactant treated group has masked it.

Although *mechanical ventilation* is the mainstay of neonatal therapy, NEC has not usually been an outcome variable in the few controlled trials of ventilation that have been carried out. In one recent trial comparing high frequency ventilation with conventional ventilation no differences in NEC rates were observed [63].

Early reports of NEC were of cases that had developed in infants following exchange transfusion through *umbilical catheters*. The association of umbilical catheterization with NEC has been observed in several epidemiological studies. Whether a causal relationship exists is uncertain. Mechanisms such as circulatory disturbance in the coeliac axis during exchange transfusion and leaching of plasticizers from polyvinyl chloride catheters have been proposed [63,64]. High catheter placement avoiding the coeliac axis does not appear to confer any advantage over low placement in the frequency of NEC [65,66]. Trials of partial exchange transfusion for polycythaemia have shown an increase in NEC in treated infants suggesting that the transfusion itself may have an aetiological role [67]. Reduced frequency of exchange transfusion in recent years makes this mechanism less important, particularly in the ELBW infant.

High rates of *fluid intake* have been associated with NEC. Bell *et al.* compared high and low fluid intakes, and showed a higher rate of NEC in those infants with an intake of more than 160 ml kg$^{-1}$ day$^{-1}$ [68,69]. Lorenz *et al.* [70] in a similar study did not show a significant excess of NEC cases in those on a high fluid regime, although they did take daily weight loss into account when calculating fluid intake. The two studies together tend to suggest an increased rate of NEC with high fluid intake, and that excess early fluid administration should be avoided.

NEC is rare prior to the onset of *oral feeding*, probably as the feed itself provides a substrate for bacterial proliferation, and secondary invasion of the bowel. Feeding precipitates the manifestation of a previous bowel insult which remains occult until demands are made on the bowel to function. Controlled trials of parenteral, compared to oral, feeding [71], and parenteral, compared to transpyloric, feeding [72] although small in size, both indicate the expected excess of NEC cases in the enterally fed groups. Anderson and Kliegman [73] in a retrospective study showed that the volume and rate of advancement of enteral feeding was all important.

It is probable that what the ELBW infant is fed as well as the rate of advancement of feed volume, relates to the incidence of NEC. Epidemiological studies and anecdotal reports have indicated for some time that *human milk* was likely to have a protective effect on the preterm gut when compared with artificial feeds. The mechanisms put forward included the presence of immunoglobulins and of live cells such as lymphocytes and macrophages. Eibl *et al.* were able to show that oral administration of a mixture of immunoglobulins A and G reduced the NEC rate to nil [74].

Intensive investigation of methods for feeding the preterm infant over the last 50 years, have concentrated mainly on short-term growth as an outcome measure. In the ELBW infant, consideration has also been given to morbidity such as NEC arising from attempts to emulate intrauterine growth rates. In large-scale studies, Lucas and Cole showed that preterm infants fed solely on human milk, from their mother or pooled donor milk, were the least likely to develop NEC [35]. Those fed a mixture of human milk supplemented with formula milk, were less likely to develop NEC than those fed formula alone. The groups in this study were not truly randomized as the infants' mothers preferences affected the choice of feeding method.

*Minimal enteral feeding* during parenteral feeding has been suggested to confer theoretical advantages such as better growth and earlier maturation of function as the gut obtains some of its nutrition directly from the contents of the lumen. Two small controlled trials have addressed this, and have shown an earlier full tolerance of enteral feeding [75,76]. This may have been because infants with complications such as NEC were excluded from the final analyses. NEC occurred more often in the minimally enterally fed groups although these differences were not statistically significant.

## Conclusions

The ELBW infant is particularly prone to NEC because of an immature gut, and exposure to hypoxic stresses often exacerbated by the effects of intrauterine growth retardation. Because of its multifactorial origins, NEC is unlikely to be prevented by a single intervention. Antenatal corticosteroid prophylaxis, human milk feeding after an initial short period of parenteral nutrition, and postnatal oral prophylaxis with non-absorbable antibiotics offer the best prospects of avoiding the condition.

Treatment is essentially supportive, and a conservative approach to surgical intervention carries fewer risks of extensive gut loss.

---

**Practical points**

1. Identify infants at highest risk, e.g. with IUGR and clinical signs of asphyxia or recurrent apnoea.
2. Reduce risk by use of human milk feeds and prophylactic oral non-absorbable antibiotics, and prenatal corticosteroid therapy where possible.
3. Conservative initial surgical management produces the best survival with fewest long-term sequelae.

---

## References

1. Palmer, S.R., Biffin, A. and Gamsu, H.R. (1989) Outcome of neonatal necrotising enterocolitis; results of a BAPM/CDSC surveillance study, 1981–4. *Arch. Dis. Childh.*, **64**, 388–394
2. Genersich, A. (1891) Banchfellenzundung beim

neugeboren in Folge von Perforation des Ileums. *Arch. Path. Anat.*, **126**, 484–494

3. Cruze, K. and Snyder, W.H. (1961) Acute perforation of the alimentary tract in infancy and childhood. *Ann. Surg.*, **154**, 93–99

4. Waldhausen, J.A., Herenden, J. and King, H. (1963) Necrotising enterocolitis of the newborn. *Surgery*, **54**, 365–372

5. Corkery, J.J., Dubowitz, V., Lister, J. and Moosa, A. (1968) Colonic perforation after exchange transfusions. *Br. Med. J.*, **4**, 345–349

6. Bell, M.J., Ternberg, J.L. and Feigin, R.D. (1978) Neonatal enterocolitis: Therapeutic decisions based on clinical staging. *Ann. Surg.*, **187**, 1–7

7. Palmer, S.R., Thomas, S.J., Cooke, R.W.I. *et al.* (1989) Birthweight specific risk factors for necrotising enterocolitis. *J. Epidemiol. Commun. Health*, **41**, 210–214

8. Beeby, P.J. and Jeffery, H. (1992) Risk factors for necrotising entero colitis: Influence of gestational age. *Arch. Dis. Childh.*, **67**, 432–435

9. Hackett, G.A., Campbell, S., Gamsu, H., Cohen-Overbeek, T and Pearce, J.M. (1987) Doppler studies in the growth retarded fetus and prediction of neonatal necrotising enterocolitis, haemorrhage and neonatal morbidity. *Br. Med. J., Clin. Res. Edn.*, **294**, 13–16

10. Malcolm, G., Ellwood, Devonald, K., Beilby, R. and Henderson Smart, D. (1991) Absent or reversed end diastolic flow velocity in the umbilical artery and necrotising entcrocolitis. *Arch. Dis. Childh.*, **66**, 805–807

11. Coombs, R.C., Morgan, M.E., Durbin, G.M., Booth, I.W. and McNeish, A.S. (1992) Abnormal gut blood flow velocities in neonates at risk of necrotising enterocolitis. *J. Pediatr. Gastroenterol Nutr.*, **15**, 13–19

12. Coombes, R.C., Morgan, M.E., Durbin, G.M., Booth, I.W. and McNeish, A.S. (1990) Gut blood flow velocities in the newborn: Effects of patent ductus arteriosus and parenteral indomethacin. *Arch. Dis. Childh.*, **65**, 1067–1071

13. Kempley, S.T., Gamsu, H.R., Vyas, S. and Nicholaides, K. (1991) Effects of intrauterine growth retardation on post natal visceral and cerebral blood flow velocities. *Arch. Dis. Childh.*, **66**, 1115–1118

14. Irving, L., Scholander, P.F. and Gormnel, S.W. (1942) The regulation of arterial blood pressure in the seal during diving. *Am. J. Physiol.*, **135**, 557

15. Touloukian, R.J., Posch, J.N. and Spencer, R. (1972) The pathogenesis of ischaemic gastroenterocolitis of the neonate: Selective gut mucosal ischaemia in asphyxiated neonatal piglets. *J. Pediat. Surg.*, **7**, 194–205

16. Le Blanc, M.H., D'Cruz, C. and Pate, K. (1984) Necrotising enterocolitis can be caused by polycythemic hyperviscosity in the newborn dog. *J. Pediat.*, **105**, 804–806

17. Bounous, G. and Hugon, J.S. (1983) Is neonatal necrotising enterocolitis a variant of acute necrosis of the intestinal mucosa in the adult. *Specul. Sci. Technol.*, **6**, 361–367

18. Walker, W.A. (1985) Absorbtion of protein and protein fragments in the developing intestine: Role of immunologic/allergic reactions. *Pediatrics*, **75**, 167–171

19. Weaver, L.T. and Walker, W.A. (1989) Uptake of macromolecules in the neonate. In *Human Gastroenterological Development* (E. Leenthal, ed.), Raven Press, New York, pp. 731–748

20. Bauer, C.R., Morrison, J.C. and Poole, K. (1984) A decreased incidence of necrotising enterocolitis after prenatal glucocorticoid therapy. *Pediatrics*, **73**, 682–688

21. Barnard, J., Greene, H. and Cotton, R. (1983) Necrotising enterocolitis. In *Nutritional Adaptation of the Gastrointestinal Tract of the Newborn* (N. Kretchmer and A. Minkowski, eds), Raven Press, New York, pp. 107–126

22. Brown, E.G. and Sweet, A.Y. (1982) Neonatal necrotising enterocolitis. *Pediatr. Clin. N. Am.*, **29**, 1149–1170

23. Millar, M.R., McKay, P., Levene, M., Langdale, V. and Martin, C. (1992) Enterobacteracae and neonatal necrotising enterocolitis. *Arch. Dis. Childh.*, **67**, 53–56

24. Hoy, C., Millar, M.R., McKay, P., Godwin, P.G., Langdale, V. and Levene, M.I. (1990) Quantitative changes in faecal microflora preceding necrotising enterocolitis in preterm infants. *Arch. Dis. Childh.*, **65**, 1057–1059

25. Zeissler, J. and Rassfeld-Sternberg, L. (1949) Enteritis necroticans due to *Clostridium welchii* type F. *Br. Med. J.*, **1**, 267–271

26. Lawrence, G. and Walker, P.D. (1976) Pathogenesis of enteritis necroticans in Papua New Guinea. *Lancet*, **i**, 125–139

27. Arseculeratne, S.N., Panabokke, R.G. and Navaratnam, C. (1980) Pathogenesis of necrotising enteritis with special reference to intestinal hypersensitivity reactions. *Gut*, **21**, 265–278

28. Han, V.K.M., Sayed, H., Chance, G.W., Braybyn, D.G. and Shaheed, W.A. (1983) An outbreak of Clostridium difficile necrotising enterocolitis: A case for oral vancomicin therapy. *Pediatrics*, **71**, 935–941

29. Thomas, D.F.M., Fernie, D.S., Bayston, R. and Spitz, L. (1984) Clostridial toxins in neonatal necrotising enterocolitis. *Arch. Dis. Childh.*, **59**, 270–272

30. Bell, M.J., Feigen, R.D., Ternberg, J.T. and Brotherton, T. (1978) Evaluation of gastrointestinal microflora in necrotising enterocolitis. *J. Pediatr.*, **92**, 589–591

31. Kliegman, R.M. and Fanaroff, A.A. (1984) Necrotising enterocolitis. *New Engl. J. Med.*, **17**, 1093–1103

32. Torma, J., DeLemos, R.A., Rogers, J.R. and Diserens, H.W. (1973) Necrotising enterocolitis in infants: Analysis of 45 consecutive cases. *Am. J. Surg.*, **126**, 758–761

33. Book, L.S., Herbst, J.J. and Jung, A.L. (1976) Comparison of fast- and slow-feeding rate schedules to the development of necrotising enterocolitis. *J. Paediatr.*, **89**, 463–466

34. Goldman, H.L. (1980) Feeding and necrotising enterocolitis. *Am. J. Dis. Child.*, **134**, 553–555

35. Lucas, A. and Cole, T.J. (1990) Breast milk and necrotising enterocolitis. *Lancet*, **336**, 1519–1523

36. Johnson, J.F., Robinson, L.H. (1984) Localised bowel distension in the newborn. A review of the plain film analysis and differential diagnosis. *Pediatrics*, **73**, 206–215

37. Brand, I.R. and Arthur, R.J. (1992) Contrast enemas after necrotising enterocolitis: A case for prophylaxis. *Pediatr. Radiol.*, **22**, 571–572

38. Lister, J. and Tam, P.K.H. (1990) Necrotising enterocolitis. Ch. 34 In *Neonatal Surgery. 3rd edn* (J. Lister and I.M. Irving, eds), Butterworths, London, pp. 485–498

39. Cheu, H.W., Sukarochana, K. and Lloyd, D.A. (1988) Peritoneal drainage for necrotising enterocolitis. *J. Pediatr. Surg.*, **23**, 557–561

40. Griffiths, D.M., Forbes, D.A., Pemberton, P.J. and Penn, I.A. (1989) Primary anastomosis for necrotizing enterocolitis: a 12 year study. *J. Pediatr. Surg.*, **24**, 515–518

41. Hansen, T.N., Ritter, D.A., Speer, M.E., Kenny, J.D. and Rudolph, A.J. (1980) A randomised, controlled study of oral gentamicin in the treatment of necrotising enterocolitis. *J. Pediatr.*, **97**, 836–839

42. Faix, R.G., Polley, T.Z. and Grasela, T.H. (1988) A randomised, controlled trial of parenteral clindamycin in neonatal necrotising enterocolitis. *J. Pediatr.*, **112**, 271–277

43. Bauer, C.R., Morrison, J.C., Poole, W.K. *et al.* (1984) A decreased incidence of necrotising enterocolitis after prenatal glucocorticoid therapy. *Pediatrics*, **73**, 682–688

44. Morales, W.J., Diebel, N.D., Lazar, A.J. and Zadrozny, D. (1986) The effect of antenatal dexamethasone administration on the prevention of respiratory distress syndrome in preterm gestations with premature rupture of the membranes. *Am. J. Obstet. Gynecol.*, **154**, 591–595

45. Morales, W.J., Angel, J.L., O'Brien, W.F. and Knuppel, R.A. (1989) Use of ampicillin and corticosteroids in premature rupture of membranes: A randomised study. *Obstet. Gynecol.*, **73**, 721–726

46. Bauer, C.R. (1992) Necrotising enterocolitis. Ch. 25 In *Effective Care of the Newborn Infant* (J.C. Sinclair and M.B. Bracken, eds), Oxford Medical Publication, pp. 602–616

47. Moog, F. (1962) Developmental adaptations of alkaline phosphatases in the small intestine. *Fed. Proc.*, **21**, 51–56

48. Halac, E., Halac, J., Begue, E.F., Casanas, J.M., Indiveri, D.R. and Petit J.F. (1990) Prenatal and postnatal corticosteroid therapy to prevent neonatal necrotising enterocolitis: A controlled trial. *J. Pediatr.*, **117**, 132–138

49. Amon, E., Lewis, S.V., Sibai, B.M., Villar, M.A. and Arheart, K.L. (1988) Ampicillin prophylaxis in preterm premature rupture of the membranes. *Am. J. Obstet. Gynecol.*, **159**, 539–543

50. Johnston, M.M., Sanchez-Ramos, L., Vaughn, A.J.,

Todd, M.W. and Benrubi, G.I. (1990) Antibiotic therapy in preterm premature rupture of the membranes: A randomised, prospective, double-blind trial. *Am. J. Obstet. Gynecol.*, **163**, 743–747

51. Egan, E.A., Mantilla, G., Nelson, R.M. and Eitzman, D.V. (1976) A prospective controlled trial of oral kanamycin in the prevention of neonatal necrotising enterocolitis. *J. Pediatr.*, **89**, 467–470

52. Rowley, M.P. and Dahlenburg, G.W. (1978) Gentamicin in prophylaxis of neonatal necrotising enterocolitis. *Lancet*, **ii**, 532

53. Grylac, L.J. and Scanlon, J.W. (1978) Oral gentamicin therapy in the prevention of neonatal necrotising enterocolitis. *Am. J. Dis. Child.*, **132**, 1192–1194

54. Boyle, R., Nelson, J.S., Stonestreet, B.S., Peter, G. and Oh, W. (1978) Alterations in stool flora resulting from kanamycin prophylaxis of necrotising enterocolitis. *J. Pediatr.*, **93**, 857–861

55. Brantley, V.E., Hiatt, I.M., Hegyi, T. (1980) The effectiveness of oral gentamicin in reducing the incidence of necrotising enterocolitis in treated and control infants. *Pediatr. Res.*, **14**, 592A

56. Grylack, L., Neugebauer, D. and Scanlon, J.W. (1982) Effects of oral antibiotics on stool flora and overall sensitivity patterns in an intensive care nursery. *Pediatr. Res.*, **16**, 509–511

57. Chirico, G., Rondini, G., Plebani, A., Chiara, A., Massa, M. and Ugazio, A.G. (1987) Intravenous gammaglobulin therapy for prophylaxis of infection in high-risk neonates. *J. Pediatr.*, **110**, 437–442

58. Clapp, D.W., Kliegman, R.M., Bayley, J.E., Shenker, N., Kyllonen, K., Fanaroff, A.A. and Berger, M. (1989) Use of intravenously administered immune globulin to prevent nosocomial sepsis in low birth weight infants. *J. Pediatr.*, **115**, 973–978

59. Baker, C.J. The Neonatal IVIG Collaborative Study Group. (1989) Multicenter trial of intravenous immunoglobulin (IVIG) to prevent late onset infection in preterm infants. Preliminary results. *Pediatr. Res.*, **25**, 275A

60. Gersony, W.M., Peckham, G.J., Ellison, R.C., Mietteinen, O.S. and Nadas, A.S. (1983) Effects of indomethacin in premature infants with patent ductus arteriosus: Results of a national collaborative study. *J. Pediatr.*, **102**, 859–906

61. Cassady, G., Crouse, D.T., Kirklin, J.W., Strange, M.J., Joiner, C.H. and Godoy, G. (1989) A randomised controlled trial of very early prophylactic ligation of the ductus arteriosus in babies who weighed 1000 g or less at birth. *New Engl. J. Med.*, **320**, 1511–1516

62. Cotton, R.B., Stahlman, M.T., Bender, H.W., Graham, T.P., Catterton, W.Z. and Kovar, I. (1978) Randomised trial of early closure of symptomatic patent ductus arteriosus in small preterm infants. *J. Pediatr.*, **93**, 647–651

63. Rogers, A.F. and Dunn, P.M. (1969) Intestinal perforation, exchange transfusion and PVC. *Lancet*, **ii**, 1246

64. The HIFI Study Group (1989) High frequency oscillatory ventilation compared with conventional mechanical ventilation in the treatment of respiratory failure in preterm infants. *New Engl. J. Med.*, **320**, 88–93

65. Mokrohisky, S.T., Levine, R.L., Blumhagen, J.D., Wesenberg, R.L. and Simmons, M.A. (1978) Low positioning of umbilical-artery catheters increases associated complications in newborn infants. *New Engl. J. Med.*, **299**, 561–564

66. Harris, M.S. and Little, G.A. (1985) Umbilical artery catheters: High, low or no. *J. Perinatol. Med.*, **6**, 15–21

67. Black, V.D., Rumack, C.M., Lubchenco, L.O. and Koops, B.L. (1985) Gastrointestinal injury in polycythaemic term infants. *Pediatrics*, **76**, 225–231

68. Bell, E.F., Warburton, D., Stonestreet, B.S. and Oh, W. (1979) High volume fluid intake predisposes premature infants to necrotising enterocolitis. *Lancet*, **ii**, 90

69. Bell, E.F., Warburton, D., Stonestreet, B.S. and Oh, W. (1980) Effect of fluid administration on the development of symptomatic patent ductus arteriosus and congestive heart failure in premature infants. *New Engl. J. Med.*, **302**, 598–604

70. Lorenz, J.M., Kleinman, L.I., Kotagal, U.R. and Reller, M.D. (1982) Water balance in very low birth weight infants: Relationship to water and sodium intake and effect on outcome. *J. Pediatr.*, **101**, 423–432

71. Yu, V.Y.H., James, B., Hendry, P. and MacMahon, R.A. (1979) Total parenteral nutrition in very low birth weight infants: A controlled trial. *Arch. Dis. Childh.*, **54**, 653–661

72. Glass, E.J., Hume, R., Lang, M.A. and Forfar, J.O. (1984) Parenteral nutrition compared with transpyloric feeding. *Arch. Dis. Childh.*, **59**, 131–135

73. Anderson, D.M. and Kliegman, R.M. (1991) The relationship of neonatal alimentation practices to the occurrence of endemic necrotising enterocolitis. *Am. J. Perinatol.*, **8**, 62–67

74. Eibl, M.M., Wolf, H.M., Furnkranz, H. and Rosenkranz, A. (1988) Prevention of necrotising enterocolitis in low birth weight infants by IgA-IgG feeding. *New Engl. J. Med.*, **319**, 1–7

75. Dunn, L., Hulman, S., Weiner, J. and Kliegman, R. (1988) Beneficial effects of early hypocaloric enteral feeding on neonatal gastrointestinal function: Preliminary report of a randomised trial. *J. Perinatol.*, **112**, 622–629

76. Slagle, T.A. and Gross, S.J. (1988) Effect of early low-volume enteral substrate on subsequent feeding tolerance in very low birth weight infants. *J. Pediatr.*, **113**, 526–531

# 21

# Iatrogenic disease

**Jean W. Keeling, Elizabeth M. Bryan and Janice M. Fearne**

The baby who weighs less than 1000 g at birth is unlikely to survive without active medical support and highly skilled nursing. ELBW infants are at increased risk of birth injury, many have respiratory problems and require ventilation, and they need assistance to achieve adequate nutrition. Treatment of infection, anaemia and jaundice is often necessary.

The introduction of intensive care of LBW newborn infants has been followed by the recognition of a range of complications of monitoring and of treatment. In very immature babies, the margins of safety between effective treatment and iatrogenic injury are often precariously narrow. Preterm delivery itself may be iatrogenic when it follows amniocentesis, undertaken either for prenatal diagnosis [1] or for the management of rhesus disease [2] or when premature operative delivery is undertaken because of severe maternal pre-eclampsia or intrauterine growth retardation.

Some complications are immediately apparent and may be life-threatening; others may not be recognized for several years. We here examine the complications of essential care of the ELBW neonate which are encountered at necropsy examination in the neonatal period and early infancy and look at the sequelae of intensive care amongst survivors during early childhood. Table 21.1 summarizes the most common iatrogenic lesions observed at necropsy examination in ELBW babies, grouped by age at death.

## Birth injury

The very immature baby is at risk of intracranial trauma during vaginal delivery. The cranium is easily deformed as skull bones are thin and poorly mineralized, connective tissue along suture lines is immature and cartilaginous junctions within the occipital bone are wide. Skull fractures and tears of falx and tentorium are uncommon, but cranial deformity is more likely to result in tearing of bridging veins as they cross the subdural space or direct compression of the brain. One form of cranial injury of which the very preterm infant is at risk is occipital osteodiastasis. This type of injury is more commonly found after breech delivery, a relatively frequent mode of presentation for the infant under 34 weeks' gestation. Furthermore, a smaller deforming force is probably required in the preterm infant.

Pressure between the internal aspect of the maternal pubic bones and the inferior part of the fetal occipital bone results in internal displacement of the latter and either compression or contusion of the cerebellum or tearing of the overlying sigmoid sinus causing subdural haemorrhage [3].

Vaginal breech delivery also predisposes to fractures of long bones, usually the femur, but fractures of the humerus are described when difficulties are encountered in bringing down the arms [4]. Bleeding into the muscles of legs and buttocks results from hypoxic capillary damage and increased hydrostatic pressure in fetal dependent parts whilst awaiting delivery

**Table 21.1.** **Iatrogenic pathology observed at necropsy amongst 131 babies of birth weight <1000 g by age at death. Necropsies were performed at John Radcliffe Hospital, Oxford between 1975 and 1986 and include babies treated in that intensive care nursery and those referred for postmortem examination**

| | 0–24 h | | | | 2–7 days | | | | 8–28 days | | | |
|---|---|---|---|---|---|---|---|---|---|---|---|---|
| | M | F | Total | Percentage of group (%) | M | F | Total | Percentage of group (%) | M | F | Total | Percentage of group (%) |
| Ventilation | | | | | | | | | | | | |
| Laryngeal injury | 3 | 8 | 11 | 16 | 7 | 9 | 16 | 36 | 7 | 2 | 9 | 45 |
| Tracheal injury | 5 | 5 | 10 | 15 | 4 | 3 | 7 | 16 | 5 | 1 | 6 | 30 |
| Interstitial emphysema | 11 | 10 | 21 | 31 | 4 | 9 | 13 | 30 | 3 | 1 | 4 | 20 |
| Pneumothorax | 12 | 4 | 16 | 24 | 5 | 8 | 13 | 30 | 4 | 2 | 6 | 30 |
| Lung perforation by chest drain | 2 | | 2 | 3 | 3 | | 3 | 7 | | 1 | 1 | 5 |
| Bronchopulmonary dysplasia | | | | | 1 | 1 | 2 | 5 | 11 | 5 | 16 | 75 |
| Large vessel cannulation | | | | | | | | | | | | |
| Aortic/iliac thrombosis | | 1 | 1 | 2 | 8 | 6 | 14 | 32 | 3 | 2 | 5 | 25 |
| Periumbilical a. haemorrhage | 1 | 2 | 3 | 5 | 2 | | 2 | 5 | | | | |
| Pulmonary thromboembolism | | | | | 2 | 1 | 3 | 7 | 2 | | 2 | 10 |
| Gangrene of extremities | | | | | | | | | 1 | 1 | 2 | 10 |
| Delivery or resuscitation trauma/hypoxia | | | | | | | | | | | | |
| Bruising | 13 | 5 | 18 | 27 | 5 | 7 | 12 | 27 | 4 | 1 | 5 | 25 |
| Subcapsular haematoma liver | 6 | 4 | 10 | 15 | 3 | 2 | 5 | 11 | 2 | | 2 | 10 |
| Haemoperitoneum | 2 | 2 | 4 | 6 | 5 | | 5 | 11 | 1 | | 1 | 5 |
| Skin excoriation | 3 | | 3 | 5 | 6 | 3 | 9 | 20 | 2 | 1 | 3 | 15 |
| Total in group | 43 | 24 | 67 | 100 | 22 | 22 | 44 | 100 | 14 | 6 | 20 | 100 |

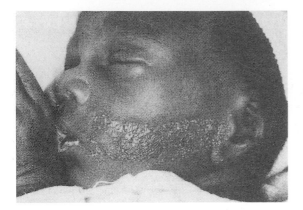

**Figure 21.1** Cutaneous excoriation caused by adhesive strapping

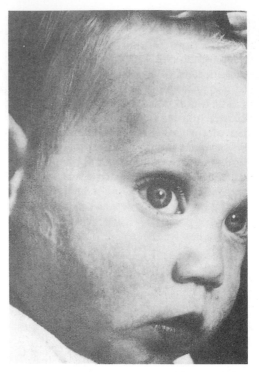

**Figure 21.2** Two-year-old with facial scarring from adhesive strapping

of the head [5]. The blood loss can be considerable and require replacement, and marked hyperbilirubinaemia may occur.

Visceral injuries result from manipulation of the fetal trunk. Hypoxia-induced hypotonia is a contributory factor. The most common injury is subcapsular haematoma of the liver, usually affecting the anterior surface of the right lobe. Postero-superior tears in the liver capsule close to the emergence of the inferior vena cava may result in severe haemorrhage; rupture of haematomata, producing a haemoperitoneum, is often rapidly fatal. More commonly the hepatic capsule remains intact and the extent of haemorrhage is restricted by increasing pressure within the haematoma. Injuries to the spleen, intestine and mesentery are less frequent.

## Ventilation

Complications of ventilation can be conveniently considered in relation to the apparatus and to the mode of administration and composition of ventilating gases.

### Apparatus

Orotracheal and nasotracheal tubes are kept in place by the use of adhesive strapping to the face. The epidermis of the preterm infant is thin and poorly keratinized, so cutaneous excoriation is easily produced by frequent changes of tube (Figure 21.1). This can cause lasting marks which are disfiguring in both light and dark skinned children (Figure 21.2).

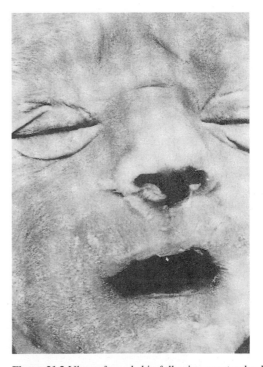

**Figure 21.3** Ulcer of nasal skin following nasotracheal intubation [40]

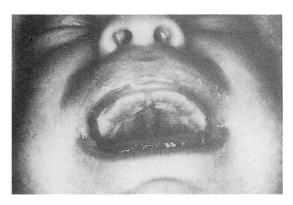

**Figure 21.4** Palatal groove following prolonged orotracheal intubation

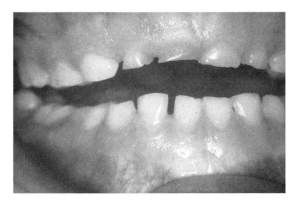

**Figure 21.5** Localized asymmetrical defects associated with neonatal oral intubation

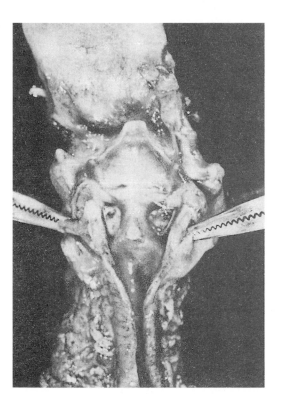

**Figure 21.6** Larynx opened posteriorly: ulceration in the midline and to either side below the vocal cords following chronic intubation [40]

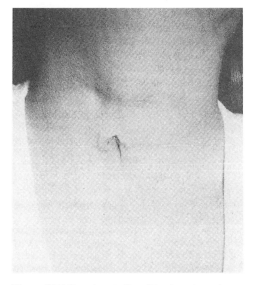

**Figure 21.7** Scarring at site of tracheostomy in a six-year-old girl

Pressure from the tube itself results in local injury at any point along its length. Nasotracheal tubes can cause ulceration at the external nares (Figure 21.3), and in some cases soft tissue injury is accompanied by pressure necrosis of the underlying cartilage which results in permanent disfigurement.

Palatal grooving and central clefts (Figure 21.4) have been reported following the long-term use of orotracheal tubes [6,7] and these can trap milk during feeding and encourage aspiration pneumonitis. The original reports suggested that direct pressure of tube on palate was responsible for the deformity, but Carillo [8] proposed that the continued presence of the tube prevents apposition of tongue and palate and so interferes with the normal spreading and reduction of the postalveolar ridges. Whilst this mechanism would accentuate any secondary palatal grooves, it is unlikely to produce clefts.

Localized asymmetrical defects of primary dentition are common in LBW children [9] (Figure 21.5) in association with oral intubation [10].

Laryngeal ulceration is a particularly serious side-effect of intubation. Ulceration occurs either along the free margin of the vocal cords or in the subglottic region (Figure 21.6). Superficial ulceration is repaired by rapid re-epithelialization following removal of the tube, but deeper ulcers result in necrosis of cartilage [11] or narrowing of the lumen during maturation and subsequent shrinkage of fibrous scars. Laryngeal or tracheal stenosis occurs in about 1.5% of chronically intubated infants [12]; intubation for 4 weeks or more predisposes to stenosis. Some children require tracheostomy for many years because of laryngeal stenosis and residual scarring is difficult to avoid (Figure 21.7).

Less severe damage to the vocal cords may go unrecorded, but persistent stridor causes anxiety to the parents and attracts distressing comments from outsiders; an abnormal speaking voice may be a grave social disadvantage. Some babies are not able to gain attention by crying, which must be frustrating as well as potentially dangerous.

Tracheal ulceration, usually manifest as focal anterior midline ulcers overlying consecutive cartilaginous rings, is sometimes seen. Squamous metaplasia of the tracheal epithelium is often extensive and involves the whole area of contact between tube and trachea, although epithelium overlying the posterior muscle is usually spared. This change seems to regress rapidly following extubation, but there may be interference with normal bronchial toilet in the period immediately after extubation and this predisposes to infection. Perforation of the trachea [13] or oesophagus [14] are infrequent complications of endotracheal intubation.

Oxygen is sometimes delivered by means of a face mask. This must fit tightly around the mouth and is usually secured by means of a broad (approximately 2 cm) Velcro band. Ischaemic necrosis and haemorrhage in the cerebellum have been observed following its use [15]; these are related to inward displacement of the occipital bone.

## Pressure of ventilating gases

Interstitial emphysema is a common complication of ventilation of immature lungs. Gas accumulates initially in the interstitial connective tissue around intrapulmonary bronchi and vessels and along interlobular septa. From this situation gas can collect beneath the pleura where it can be seen as small blebs.

Accumulation of gas also occurs in the interlobar fissures and at the hila. Rupture of the pleural surface produces pneumothorax. Eventually such defects close spontaneously. From hilar accumulations gas may track up into the mediastinum and thence to subcutaneous tissues over the head and neck, where

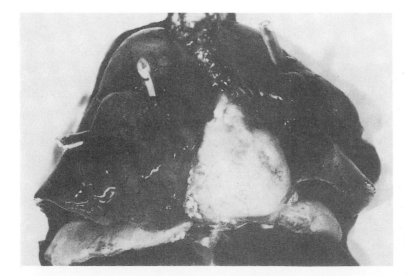

**Figure 21.8** Perforation of the lung by a chest drain

its crepitant quality is readily apparent. Gas may accumulate within the pericardial sac, occasionally giving rise to tamponade, or track downwards into retroperitoneal tissues where it may mimic pneumoperitoneum occurring in the course of necrotizing enterocolitis.

Pneumothorax is a common complication of ventilation in the very preterm infant. Estimates of its frequency vary widely and are closely related to both the admissions policy of a particular unit and the maximum ventilatory pressures used. Lindroth *et al.* [16] observed pneumothorax in 20% of babies receiving intermittent positive pressure ventilation in their unit. A frequent complication of management of this life-threatening event is perforation of the lung by a chest drain (Figure 21.8), particularly if a rigid introducer is used. Such perforation can provoke considerable haemorrhage without injury to large vessels because of the gross pulmonary congestion which is usually present. Injury to major vessels or other mediastinal structures is unusual. The authors have seen major haemothorax when an intercostal artery was torn during introduction of a chest drain. There was extensive retropleural and intramuscular haemorrhage as well.

An anterior chest drain scar is not only unsightly but may affect female breast development. Whenever possible the axilla is a preferable site as this ensures that the scar is hidden and the risk to the breast is removed.

### Composition and delivery of gas mixtures

Bronchopulmonary dysplasia (BPD) is a frequent and serious complication of ventilation. Its cause continues to be disputed. All of the histological features of BPD can be produced in animals by administration of increased oxygen concentrations at atmospheric pressures [17]. Edwards, Dyer and Northway [18] were able to induce pulmonary changes comparable to BPD by ventilating with air at the same pressure. In the human infant a relationship to gas pressures and length of ventilatory cycle has been described [19]. Interstitial oedema secondary to elevated pulmonary arterial pressure [20] may also be important.

The histological appearances of BPD were first described by Northway, Rosan and Porter [21]. Some of the features originally described are now rarely seen. Squamous metaplasia of intrapulmonary bronchi, for instance, is now uncommon. It was only seen in patients who died before 20 days of age.

## Oxygen monitoring

Recognition of an association between administration of oxygen-rich mixtures and retrolental fibroplasia in preterm infants (retinopathy of prematurity) [22] led to the introduction of methods of monitoring oxygen levels to maintain them within the confines of adequacy and safety. Intermittent sampling from peripheral arteries is less satisfactory than continuous monitoring because of limitation of the number of samples by availability of sampling sites and the inaccuracy of results obtained when a baby is disturbed by the procedure.

Temporal artery sampling was largely discontinued following reports of contralateral

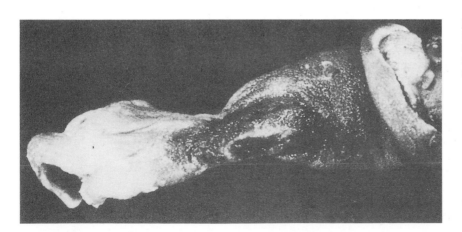

**Figure 21.9** Gangrene of forearm necessitating amputation following radial then brachial artery sampling [40]

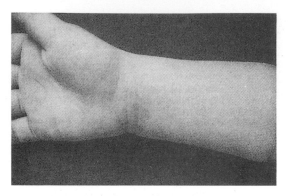

**Figure 21.10** Scarring and depigmentation of forearm following multiple radial artery sampling in the neonatal period at 6 years

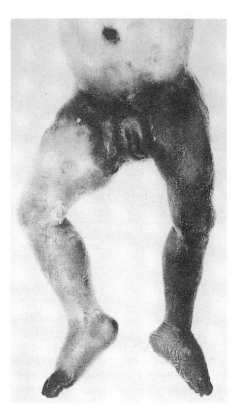

**Figure 21.11** Gangrene of the lower limbs and genitalia following massive aortic thrombosis

hemiplegia during the ensuing months due to cerebral infarction [23]. Radial artery sampling is sometimes followed by carpal tunnel syndrome due to haematoma [24], or gangrene of the forearm (Figure 21.9) but minor bruising is often the only sequel [25]. However, in the longer term extensive scarring and depigmentation of the forearm (Figure 21.10), particularly against a sun tan, may cause embarrassment.

Indwelling aortic cannulae which permit withdrawal of regular blood samples or have an oxygen detecting electrode incorporated into the tip have been used for systemic oxygen monitoring. Use of such cannulae in ELBW infants is always a cause of concern as their presence produces a marked reduction in the cross-sectional area of the vessel. In addition, intimal injury is common and predisposes to thrombosis. Minor thrombosis is a frequent complication of chronic aortic cannulation [26]; major thrombosis results in gangrene of lower limbs (Figure 21.11), ischaemic necrosis of the buttocks and external genitalia or visceral infarction. The risk and degree of thrombosis is related to the duration of cannulation, whether the cannula is used for intravenous alimentation, site of hole (side-hole cannulae have a dead space at the tip) and, finally, the position of the cannula. Aortic aneurysm is an uncommon complication and appears to be related to concomitant septicaemia [27,28]. Hypertension is an infrequent but serious late complication and is responsible for the majority of cases of hypertension seen in children in the UK and USA. Peripheral artery cannulation is now

being more often used thus reducing major complications, although serious local ischaemia can occur. The magnitude of the complications of invasive methods of oxygen monitoring has stimulated the development of non-invasive monitoring techniques. The use of transcutaneous oxygen electrodes has produced only minor, transient erythema.

## Umbilical venous cannulation

Umbilical vein cannulation was undertaken initially for exchange transfusions in the treatment of rhesus disease. Later it was used for blood sampling and intravenous alimentation as it is technically easier than umbilical arterial catheterization. The rate of complications resulting from thrombosis around or beyond the catheter is very high (Figure 21.12). Pulmonary thromboembolism and hepatic

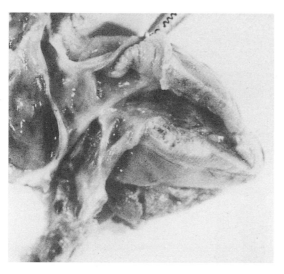

**Figure 21.12** Heart from right side: a cylindrical thrombus is present in the inferior vena cava and extends through the foramen ovale [40]

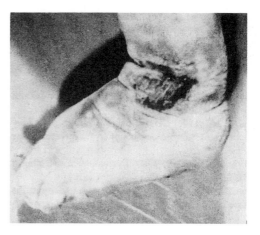

**Figure 21.13** Ulceration and dystrophic calcification around a venepuncture site following extravasation of calcium gluconate

vein or inferior vena cava thrombosis are frequent; massive hepatic necrosis is also recorded and portal hypertension is a late complication [29], and perforation of the heart has also been reported [30]. Necrotizing enterocolitis has been recognized as a complication of this procedure for many years [31,32].

## Drugs and their administration

Side-effects of drugs do not pose as great a problem in the neonatal period as they do in adults, perhaps because of the restricted range of drugs prescribed in the neonatal period. The side-effects of some drugs are predictable; tolazoline with its histamine-like structure, used in the neonate to reduce pulmonary hypertension, provokes gastric ulceration, sometimes accompanied by massive haemorrhage. Gentamicin is toxic to the auditory nerve.

The method of administering drugs may cause damage. Some antibiotics such as nafcillin give rise to soft tissue necrosis should extravasation of the infusion occur [33]. Extravasation of calcium gluconate has resulted in dystrophic calcification around the drip site (Figure 21.13). Quadriceps contrac-

ture is an unusual but well recognized complication of intramuscular injections in the thigh [34]. An abscess at the site of an intramuscular injection has led to osteomyelitis and deformity [35]. Intravenous alimentation is more hazardous in the ELBW baby than in mature infants and is in part related to immaturity of the reticuloendothelial system and liver. Pulmonary lipid thromboembolism has been reported following the administration of lipid emulsions as a bolus [36] and subsequently when administered continuously [37]. Pulmonary infarction was reported by the latter group. Lipid is present throughout the reticuloendothelial system and work in animals indicates compromised handling of microorganisms which might be an additional hazard in the ELBW infant whose immune competence is incompletely developed.

Amino acid infusions induce cholestasis and portal fibrosis [38]. This usually reverses after cessation of infusion but occasionally there is progression to cirrhosis. Cholelithiasis has been described when frusemide has been given at the same time as amino acid infusions: the drug enhances calcium secretion into the biliary tract [39].

## Topical applications

The skin of the ELBW infant is poorly keratinized and is thus readily permeable. This

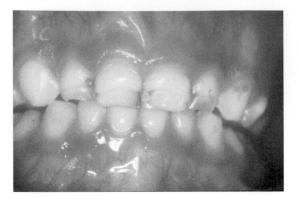

**Figure 21.14** Neonatal enamel hypoplia in primary incisors from LBW

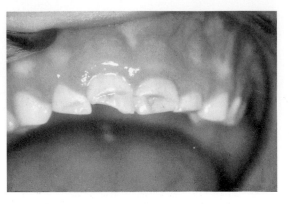

**Figure 21.15** Defects of the primary incisors

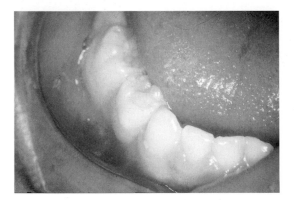

**Figure 21.16** Defective first primary molar

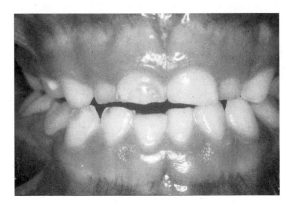

**Figure 21.17** Defects of upper incisors in orally intubated child

permeability allows absorption of constituents of topical applications (see Chapter 8).

## Dental problems

An increased prevalence of enamel defects (enamel hypoplasia) has been reported in the primary dentition of LBW children, particularly those who are sick, preterm infants, requiring ventilator support and/or intravenous alimentation [41].

Enamel hypoplasias are developmental in origin and are the result of a disturbance during enamel formation (amelogenesis). A systemic illness or upset occurring during amelogenesis may give rise to a generalized, symmetrical distribution of enamel hypoplasia affecting all the teeth mineralizing at the time. Such defects are often referred to as

'chronological hypoplasias' as it is possible to date approximately the time of the insult from the position of the defects on the teeth. Localized hypoplasia affecting one or a group of teeth (often asymmetrically) may be the result of a localized insult such as trauma or infection.

In LBW children systemic disturbances such as hypoxia [42], hypocalcaemia [43] and hyperbilirubinaemia [44] during the perinatal period have been associated with chronological enamel hypoplasia in the primary dentition. More defects are found in the very low birth weight (VLBW) and extremely low birth weight (ELBW) compared to the LBW children [45]. In a preterm infant the defects tend to be located on the incisal half of the incisors (Figures 21.14 & 21.15) and the occlusal surface of the first primary molar (Figure 21.16). In a full term infant, with more advanced dental development, the defects would tend to be in the gingival half of the primary incisors and also involve the second primary molars.

Localized, asymmetrical defects (Fig. 21.5) or defects only affecting upper incisors (Fig. 21.17) have been reported in association with neonatal oral intubation [9,10]. Traumatic forces either from the laryngoscope or from pressures exerted by the oral endotracheal tubes are thought to be transmitted through the alveolus to the underlying developing primary tooth germ which is lying close to the mucosa. Where the laryngoscope was applied to the left of the midline during intubation defects were found three times as often on the left side of the mouth [9]. The side affected may also reflect the side on which the oral tube was secured. It has been suggested that the defects occur as a result of trauma during intubation together with the systemic condition which makes the tooth germ more susceptible to injury. That is 'the adverse effect of systemic factors on amelogenesis in LBW infants may be confounded by traumatic forces from either the laryngoscope or the orotracheal tube'. This has been demonstrated in animal studies. Orthodontic forces on developing teeth produce hypoplasia in hypocalcaemic but not in normocalcaemic rats [46].

In a severe case of repeated orotracheal intubation during infancy the left primary incisor was rotated in its crypt and failed to erupt and the right primary incisor showed delayed eruption [47].

A histological study of exfoliated primary teeth from LBW children showed that in some cases the hypoplastic enamel is also hypomineralized with as much as a 10% reduction in mineral content [48].

The permanent teeth of LBW children do not appear to show the same increase in enamel hypoplasia [49]. The permanent teeth start to mineralize much later than the primary teeth. The first permanent molar commences around birth (40 weeks) and the incisors not until 2 to 3 months after birth. This suggests that the permanent teeth escape the effects of the neonatal upset, particularly in a child born preterm. However, an increase in the frequency of mild opacities of permanent enamel in LBW children compared to normal birth weight children has been suggested [49,50]. Illnesses in the first year of life might explain these findings.

## Conclusion

The price of intensive care of ELBW babies who survive may be iatrogenic damage which can, at worst, produce lasting physical or emotional handicap and at least a social embarrassment. Constant vigilance is essential if the long-term happiness of these ELBW survivors is not to be marred by some avoidable action on the part of the caretakers in the early weeks.

## References

1. Medical Research Council (1978) An assessment of the hazards of amniocentesis. *Br. J. Obstet. Gynaecol.*, **85** (Suppl. 2), 1–41
2. Brinsmead, M.W. (1976) Complications of amniocentesis. *Med. J. Aust.*, **1**, 379–385
3. Wigglesworth, J.S. and Husemeyer, R.P. (1977) Intracranial birth trauma in vaginal breech delivery: the continued importance of injury to the occipital bone. *Br. J. Obstet. Gynaecol.*, **84**, 684–691
4. Wigglesworth, J.S. (1984) Intrapartum and early neonatal death: the interaction of asphyxia and trauma. In *Perinatal Pathology*, W.B. Saunders, Philadelphia, pp. 93–112
5. Ralis, Z.A. (1975) Birth traumas to muscles in babies born by breech delivery and its possible fatal consequence. *Arch. Dis. Childh.*, **50**, 4–13
6. Duke, P.M., Coulson, J.D., Santos, J.I. and Johnson, J.D. (1976) Cleft palate associated with prolonged orotracheal intubation in infancy. *J. Pediatr.*, **89**, 990–991
7. Erenberg, A. and Nowak, A.J. (1984) Palatal groove formation in neonates and infants with orotracheal tubes. *Am. J. Dis. Child.*, **138**, 974–975
8. Carrillo, P. (1985) Palatal groove formation and oral endotracheal intubation. *Am. J. Dis. Child.*, **139**, 589–590
9. Seow, W.K., Brown, J.P., Tudehope, D.I. and O'Callaghan, M. (1984) Developmental defects in the primary dentition of low birthweight infants: Adverse effects of laryngoscopy and prolonged endotracheal intubation. *Pediatr. Dent.*, **6**, 28–31
10. Moylan, F.M.B., Seldin, E.B., Shannon, D.C. and Todres, I.D. (1980) Defective primary dentition in survivors of neonatal mechanical ventilation. *J. Pediatr.*, **96**, 106–108
11. Gould, S.J. and Howard, S. (1985) The histopathology of the larynx in the neonate following endotracheal intubation. *J. Pathol.*, **146**, 301–311
12. O'Neill, J.A. Jr (1984) Experience with iatrogenic laryngeal and tracheal stenoses. *J. Pediatr. Surg.*, **19**, 235–238
13. Reynolds, E.O.R. and Taghizadeh, A. (1974) Improved

prognosis of infants mechanically ventilated for hyaline membrane disease. *Arch. Dis. Childh.*, **49**, 505–515

14. Clarke, T.A., Coen, R.W., Feldman, B. and Papile, L. (1980) Esophageal perforations in premature infants and comments on the diagnosis. *Am. J. Dis. Child.*, **134**, 367–368

15. Pape, K.E., Armstrong, D.L. and Fitzhardinge, P.M. (1976) Central nervous system pathology associated with mask ventilation in the very low birth weight infant: a new aetiology for intracerebellar haemorrhages. *Pediatrics*, **58**, 473–483

16. Lindroth, M., Svenningsen, N.W., Ahlstrom, H. and Jonson, B. (1980) Evaluation of mechanical ventilation in newborn infants. *Acta Paediatr. Scand.*, **69**, 143–149

17. Bonikos, D.S., Bensch, K.G., Ludwin, S.K. and Northway, W.H. (1975) Oxygen toxicity in the newborn. The effect of prolonged 100% $O_2$ exposure on the lungs of newborn mice. *Lab. Invest.*, **32**, 619–635

18. Edwards, D.K., Dyer, W.M. and Northway, W.H. (1977) Twelve years' experience with bronchopulmonary dysplasia. *Pediatrics*, **59**, 839–845

19. Taghizadeh, A. and Reynolds, E.O.R. (1976) Pathogenesis of bronchopulmonary dysplasia following hyaline membrane disease. *Am. J. Pathol.*, **82**, 241–258

20. Brown, E.R., Stark, A., Sosenko, I., Lawson, E.E. and Avery, M.E. (1978) Bronchopulmonary dysplasia: possible relationship to pulmonary edema. *J. Pediatr.*, **92**, 982–984

21. Northway, W.H. Jr., Rosan, R.C. and Porter, D.Y. (1967) Pulmonary disease following respirator therapy of hyaline membrane disease. Bronchopulmonary dysplasia. *N. Engl. J. Med.*, **276**, 357–368

22. Ashton, N., Ward, B. and Serpell, G. (1954) Effect of oxygen on developing retinal vessels with particular reference to the problem of retrolental fibroplasia. *Br. J. Ophthalmol.*, **38**, 397–432

23. Simmons, M.A., Levine, R.V., Lubchenco, L.O. and Guggenheim, M.A. (1978) Warning: serious sequelae of temporal arterial catheterisation. *J. Pediatr.*, **92**, 284

24. Koenigsberger, M.R. and Moessinger, A.C. (1977) Iatrogenic carpal tunnel syndrome in the newborn infant. *J. Pediatr.*, **91**, 443–445

25. Adams, J.M. and Rudolph, A.J. (1975) The use of indwelling radial artery catheters in neonates. *Pediatrics*, **55**, 261–265

26. Wesstrom, G., Finnstrom, O. and Stenport, G. (1979) Umbilical artery catheterization in newborns. I. Thrombosis in relation to catheter type and position. *Acta Paediatr. Scand.*, **68**, 575–581

27. Rajs, J., Finnstrom, O. and Wesstrom, G. (1976) Case report. Aortic aneurysm developing after umbilical artery catheterization. *Acta Paediatr. Scand.*, **65**, 495–498

28. Colclough, A.B. and Barson, A.J. (1981) Infantile aortic aneurysm complicating umbilical arterial catheterisation. *Arch. Dis. Childh.*, **56**, 795–797

29. Lauridsen, U.B., Enk, B. and Gammeltoft, A. (1978) Oesophageal varices as a late complication to neonatal umbilical vein catheterization. *Acta Paediatr. Scand.*, **67**, 633–636

30. Purohit, D.M. and Levkoff, A.H. (1977) Pericardial effusion complicating umbilical venous catheterization. *Arch. Dis. Childh.*, **52**, 520

31. Corkery, J.J., Dubowitz, V., Lister, J. and Moosa, A. (1968) Colonic perforation after exchange transfusion. *Br. Med. J.*, **ii**, 345–349

32. Orme, R.L.E. and Eades, S.M. (1968) Perforation of the bowel in the newborn as a complication of exchange transfusion. *Br. Med. J.*, **iv**, 349–351

33. Tilden, S.J., Craft, C., Cano, R. and Daum, R.S. (1980) Cutaneous necrosis associated with intravenous nafcillin therapy. *Am. J. Dis. Child.*, **134**, 1046–1048

34. Lloyd-Roberts, G.C. and Thomas, T.G. (1964) The etiology of quadriceps contracture in children. *J. Bone Joint Surg.*, **46B**, 498–502

35. Elliman, A.M., Bryan, E.M. and Elliman, A.D. (1986) Low birth weight babies at three years of age. *Child Care, Health Dev.*, **12**, 287–311

36. Barson, A.J., Chiswick, M.L. and Doig, C.M. (1978) Fat emulsion in infancy after intravenous fat infusions. *Arch. Dis. Childh.*, **53**, 218–223

37. Levene, M.I., Wigglesworth, J.S. and Desai, R. (1980) Pulmonary fat accumulation after Intralipid infusion in the preterm infant. *Lancet*, **ii**, 815–818

38. Peden, V.H., Witzleben, C.L. and Skelton, M.A. (1971) Total parenteral nutrition. *J. Pediatr.*, **78**, 180

39. Whitington, P.F. and Black, D.D. (1980) Cholelithiasis in premature infants treated with parenteral nutrition and frusemide. *J. Pediatr.*, **97**, 647–649

40. Keeling, J.W. (1981) Iatrogenic disease in the Newborn. *Virchows Archiv. (Pathol. Anat.)*, **394**, 1–29

41. Fearne, J.M., Bryan, E.M., Elliman, A.M., Brook, A.H. and Williams, D.M. (1990) Enamel defects in the primary dentition of children born weighing less than 2000 g. *Br. Dent. J.*, **168**, 433–437

42. Johnsen, D., Krejci, C., Hack, M. and Fanaroff, A. (1984) Distribution of enamel defects and the association with respiratory distress in very low birthweight infants. *J. Dent. Res.*, **63**, 59–64

43. Seow, K.W., Brown, J.P., Tudehope, D.I. and O'Callaghan, M. (1984) Dental defects in the deciduous dentition of premature infants with low birthweight and neonatal rickets. *Pediatr. Dent.*, **6**, 88–92

44. Miller, J. and Forrester, R.M. (1959) Neonatal enamel hypoplasia associated with haemolytic disease and prematurity. *Br. Dent. J.*, **106**, 93–104

45. Seow, W.K., Humphreys, C. and Tudehope, D.I. (1987) Increased prevalence of developmental dental defects in low birthweight prematurely born children: a controlled study. *Pediatr. Dent.*, **9**, 221–225

46. Engstom, C. and Noren, J.G. (1985) Effects of orthodontic forces on enamel formation in normal and hypocalcaemic rats. *J. Oral. Pathol.*, **15**, 78–82

47. Mason, C., Odell, E.W. and Longhurst, P. (1994) Dental complications associated with repeat orotracheal intubation in infancy: a case report. *Int. J. Paed. Dent.*, **4**, 257–264

48. Fearne, J.M., Elliot, J.C., Wong, F.S.L., Davis, G.R., Boyde, A. and Jones, S.J. (1994) Deciduous enamel defects in low birthweight children: correlated X-ray microtomographic and backscattered electron imaging study of hypoplasia and hypomineralization. *Anat. Embryol. (Berlin)*, **189**, 375–381

49. Fearne, J.M. (1994) A longitudinal study of the teeth of low birthweight children: Variation in enamel structure and crown size. PhD Thesis, University of London

50. Pimlott, J.F., Nikiforuk, G., Thomas, P.H. and Fitzhardinge, P.M. (1985) Enamel defects in prematurely born low birthweight infants. *Pediatr. Dent.*, **7**, 218–223

# 22

# Nursing care

**Ann Maloy**

Over the last few years, neonatal care has developed rapidly in an attempt to meet the changing needs of the extremely low birth weight babies who now survive delivery.

Staff working within the NICU are highly trained and are required to respond quickly and effectively in situations which are often unpredictable and constantly changing.

The ability to work in such situations, dealing with families who are also in need of help and support, places huge demands on the nursing staff. The effects of stress and subsequent burnout are well documented in this group and mechanisms to recognize and address causes should be maximized in all SCBU and NICU.

## Handling

The promotion of a minimal handling approach to care is recognized as an effective method of reducing stress in these vulnerable patients. The continued assessment and planning of care to maximize periods of undisturbed rest by skilled neonatal nurses will help to minimize the harm that over stimulation can cause. Colour changes, tachycardia, tachypnoea, bradycardia and jitteriness are all responses that handling can precipitate. Sleep patterns are also disturbed, and it is important to remember that infants may only cope with one stimulus at a time. The infant may require time to recover from one procedure before another is performed, rather than all necessary tasks and tests being carried out in one sequence.

The baby's ability to cope will change constantly and needs to be continually assessed.

Many infants of low birth weight will be nursed on an open cot with a radiant heat source above. As these infants lose body fluids readily due to an increased skin permeability, various techniques and aids can be employed to minimize water loss.

The use of a plastic blanket to cover the naked infant reduces fluid loss and does not block out the heat delivered. Baumgart [1] also reported reductions in oxygen consumption in babies using a thermal blanket. Humidity delivered directly into closed incubators will help to minimize evaporative water loss. The early work of Silverman *et al* [2] will continue to be explored as equipment is further developed.

Many nurseries will use a combination of both open and closed incubators in maximizing the benefits that both have to offer [3].

Care must be taken, however, as high humidity could provide an ideal environment to host harmful organisms, although studies have been reassuring.

## Interventions

### Noise

Infants are exposed to high levels of noise continuously in NICUs. *In utero*, although exposed to noise, these sounds are muffled through amniotic fluid and often more comforting, such as the heart beat or the familiar sounds of the mother's voice. Studies have recorded sound levels in NICUs far exceeding those known to contribute to hearing loss in the adult population. Not only does this suggest that the potential for damage is ever present, but that other adverse effects are witnessed such as crying, reduced oxygenation, tachycardia and tachypnoea [4].

Strauch and colleagues [5] describe the use of a protocol where for a specified time on each shift, a designated quiet hour was established. The results showed that noise levels can be significantly decreased and that this has a positive impact on infant behaviour. This protocol has been adopted within our own nursery but is highly dependent upon the collaboration of all health care staff and families involved [6].

Sparshott [7] points out the need for every neonatal unit to design its own protocol for the use of beneficial aural stimulation such as cassette recordings of familiar family voices, womb sounds or music.

## Lighting

Many nurseries today have been designed with alternative methods of lighting control. The introduction of concealed lighting, dimmer facilities and better shades for natural light have reduced the impact that brightly lit nurseries used to have on the sick, immature infant. Glass *et al.* [8] suggested that continuous bright light had a contributory role in the aetiology of retinopathy of prematurity.

The adherence of nurseries to day and night routine for infants has been beneficial in the earlier organization of the infants' behaviour and sleep patterns.

Incubators, wherever possible, should also be adequately shaded for directional light, helping to maximize sleep quality. Parents often comment that after discharge, their infant is very restless in a quietened environment or more restful with the addition of a nightlight. This clearly demonstrates the impact the nursery environment has on the developing infant.

## Positioning

Neonatal staff can easily identify with the infant who appears restless and agitated in his cot, arms and legs outstretched in a startled action. *In utero*, flexor tone increases as the infant approaches term in his cramped environment. Immature infants never become large enough to develop this physiological flexion and tend to favour an extension preference. This is seen in the classic 'frog' positioning of the preterm infant. The early recognition and use of positioning techniques to minimize postural problems may improve the development of these infants.

Flexion can be increased when prone by tucking knees under the chest, arms held close to the body and the use of a small towel roll under the hips. This position has also been shown to improve oxygenation and lung compliance, reduce gastric reflux and risk of aspiration.

For side lying, infants need to be stabilized by using a small towel roll behind them and a wrap stretched across the pelvis to maintain flexion. These supports help to improve tone as they provide surfaces to flex against. The baby who is repeatedly found at the bottom of the incubator tray is searching to find boundaries. The careful 'nesting' of such infants with rolled towels will help to promote rest and reduce energy expenditure.

The positioning of hands in the midline or near the mouth will encourage hand-to-mouth orientation [9].

## Massage

The involvement of parents in the art of gentle massage has been very successful within our own department. An experienced neonatal nurse who has practised these techniques over many years will instruct and support both families and staff who wish to develop these skills.

Aracis oil is used to massage, initially localized areas such as the hand or upper arm are mastered, particularly in infants who have required splintage of the limb for i.v. fluid administration. This is particularly rewarding for parents who often feel that the splinted limb may cause discomfort for the infant. Parents will practise and extend the time and surfaces massaged with an appreciation of when to stop. Behavioural and biochemical [10] changes have been reported as beneficial, but further studies are required.

Improved attachment and confidence in caregiving have been demonstrated in this group within our own population.

## Skin integrity

Skin integrity is extremely important as breaches can lead to both localized and systemic infections. Correct positioning and the use of comfort aids such as bean bags, sheepskins or pressure mats will minimize injury.

Care must be taken in the choice and application of monitoring aids in this group.

Skin sites must be adequately prepared as skin breakdown, irritation and burns have all been reported. Frequent assessment and changing of sites will minimize trauma. Many of our practices such as heel pricks, venupuncture, adhesive strapping and removal of urine bags will breech the function of the skin as a barrier and should be used as little as is possible.

## Parent contact

Various studies since the early work of Klaus and Kennell [11] have looked at the effect of increased mother/infant contact. For the pregnancy which has terminated earlier than expected, the parental expectations of their full term infant are often exploded when faced with the very premature infant.

Attachment, due to their expectations and separation, may affect the subsequent relations within the family unit.

The opportunity to involve the parents actively, and as early as possible, is a challenge relished by NICU staff.

Early handling, stroking, breast feeding and contact with the parents should be supported to enhance attachment with the family unit.

### Skin-to-skin care

Skin-to-skin care as reported from Colombia [12] was undertaken to promote early discharge from overcrowded nurseries, promoting lactation and bonding, and impacted infant mortality rates.

Nursing the baby naked in a vertical position against the mother's skin, has been widely adopted and investigated since the discovery.

Acolet *et al.* [13] reported changes in oxygenation and the maintenance of skin temperature during the contact. Whitelaw *et al.* [14] continued to look at the effect this technique may have on a longer period.

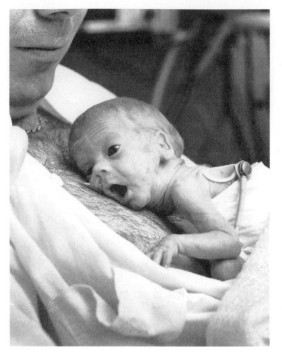

**Figure 22.1** Father and premature infant, skin-to-skin contact

Outcome measures such as duration of lactation and infant crying at 6 months showed that the group practising skin-to-skin contact lactates longer and had infants who cried significantly less at 6 months of age.

---

### Practical points

1. Neonatal nurses must be as pro-active as possible in supporting the whole family in the care of their sick newborn infant.
2. Neonatal Units need to have an awareness of their own unique environmental issues and their potentially harmful impact on the sick newborn.
3. A minimal handling approach which balances periods of rest with nursing and medical interventions is critical in this vulnerable group.
4. As technology races on, neonatal staff must not abandon the interventions that require minimal resources or cost little as their impact is often greatly underestimated.

This has also proved to be a particular care activity that fathers can actively participate in and achieve significant personal pleasure from (Figure 22.1).

Sadly, fathers have been largely seen as supports for mothers with their own needs often ignored. Vine [15] examines the changes in society and the expectations of men in the areas of childcare and how their roles can be fulfilled. Socioeconomic changes have resulted in fathers carrying out the childcare with mothers becoming the main breadwinners in some families. Their participation and involvement in the direct provision of care can only enhance the continued development of the family unit [16].

# References

1. Baumgart, S. (1984) Reduction of oxygen consumption, insensible water loss and radiant demand with the use of a plastic blanket for low birthweight infants under radiant warmers. *Pediatrics*, **75**, 89–95
2. Silverman, W., Agate, F. and Fertig, J. (1963) A sequential trial of non-thermal effect of atmospheric humidity on survival of newborn infants of low birthweight. *Pediatrics*, **31**, 719–724
3. Merenstein, G., Koziol, D.F., Brown, G.L. and Weisman, L.E. (1979) Radiant warmers vs. incubators for neonatal care. *Am. J. Dis. Child.*, **133**, 857–858
4. Long, G.J., Lucey, J.F. and Philip, A.G.S. (1980) Noise and hypoxaemia in the intensive care nursery. *Pediatrics*, **65**, 203–207
5. Strauch, C., Brandt, S. and Edwards-Beckett, J. (1993) Implementation of a quiet hour: effect of noise levels and infant sleep states. *Neonatal Network*, **12**(2), 31–35
6. Catlett, A.T. and Horditch-Davis, D. (1990) Environmental stimulation of the acutely ill premature infant; physiological effects and nursing implications. *Neonatal Network*, **8**(6), 19–26
7. Sparshott, M.M. (1995) 'The sound' – of neonatal intensive care: Effect of noise levels in the neonatal unit on the sleep patterns of sick preterm infants. *J. Neon. Nurs.*, **2**(1), 7–9
8. Glass, P., Avery, G.B., Subramanian, K.N. *et al.* (1985) Effect of bright light in the hospital nursery on the incidence of retinopathy of prematurity. *N. Engl. J. Med.*, **313**, 401–404
9. Jorgensen, K.M. (1993) *Developmental Care of the Pre-term Infant: A Concise Overview*. Children's Medical Ventures, Inc., South Weymouth, MA
10. Acolet, D., Modi, N., Giannakoulopoulos, X. *et al.* (1993) Changes in plasma cortisol and catecholamine concentrations in response to massage in pre-term infants. *Arch. Dis. Childh.*, **68**, 29–31
11. Klaus, M.H. and Kennell, J.H. (1976) *Parent–Infant Bonding*. Mosby, St Louis.
12. Whitelaw, A. and Sleath, K. (1985) Myth of the marsupial mother: home care of very low birthweight babies in Bogota, Columbia. *Lancet,* **ii**, 1206–1208
13. Acolet, D., Sleath, K. and Whitelaw, A. (1989) Oxygenation, heart rate and temperature in very low birthweight infants during skin-to-skin contact with their mothers. *Acta Paediatr. Scand.*, **78**, 189–193
14. Whitelaw, A., Sleath, K. and Acolet, D. (1988) Safety and effectiveness of skin-to-skin contact for very low birthweight infants. *Pediatric. Res.*, **3**, 430A
15. Vine, T. (1995) The father's role on the neonatal unit: the importance of the father as a full carer of his sick child as part of the family centred care on the N.I.C.U. *J. Neon. Nurs.,* **2**(1), 23–27
16. Gunderson, L.P. and Kenner, C. (1990) Care of the 24–25 week gestational age infant (small baby protocol). *Neonatal Network*, **1**, 160–163

# 23

# The social and emotional needs of the parents and baby

**Martin Richards and Janet Rennie**

While there is general agreement among clinicians and nursing staff that the birth and early months of life of an ELBW baby are often stressful for parents, the amount of research on the problem is very limited and most of what is available relates to very small samples. To add to our difficulties we need to be rather cautious in generalizing from findings from one centre to another as much may depend on the ways in which staff relate to parents, as well as such factors as attitudes in the community towards very small babies and their problems. It is tempting to fill in the gaps in our knowledge from the results of studies of larger preterm babies on the assumption that the issues and problems for the ELBW baby and parents will be much the same in kind, though more frequent and more serious. Up to a point, this strategy is probably not too misleading; however, it must be remembered that there are differences in the patterns of association with social and demographic variables for the larger and smaller preterm babies.

## The parents' perspective

Like many of the crises of parenting, one of the difficulties of the situation of the birth of an ELBW baby is that at a time when great emotional demands are likely to be made of parents, they are already in a stressed state. The early birth and the small baby are, in themselves, factors that often stress parents. Apart from the point that an earlier than expected birth may upset all sorts of practical arrangements, it may mean that parents are not psychologically ready for the birth.

For a mother there may be a sense of failure and inadequacy at being unable to carry a pregnancy to term and perhaps guilt at having done things which she feels may have caused the preterm delivery or a slow rate of fetal growth. For the father there could be a conflict of interest between his concern for his wife who is seriously ill and his new baby, also in a critical condition. A woman's capacity as a mother is often seen as a basic part of her nature and the ability to grow a fetus adequately may seem to a mother herself as the fundamental part of that capacity [1–3]. Reactions will vary widely, however, not only because of differing attitudes towards motherhood but also because in some situations a mother may have had some warning of the likelihood of an ELBW baby. While one might expect that warning and specific preparation for a preterm delivery are likely to ameliorate the stress of such birth, there appears to be no direct evidence for this.

Parents often have an image of the baby they would like to have and so part of what they have to face at the birth is the grief of the loss of that imaginary baby. This grief makes it hard to relate to the ELBW baby.

Among the feelings of any pregnancy for both mothers and fathers there is often anxiety that all may not go well. There are fears and fantasies of producing a damaged child. In recent years a growing number of screening and diagnostic techniques, such as amniocentesis and ultrasound, are being deployed as part of medical care in pregnancy. We know that in some situations their use increases anxiety [4–6].

The final point to be considered here is the birth itself. Caesarean section is commonly employed for the delivery of very preterm babies. There is accumulating evidence that some mothers are less responsive to their babies and feel more negative about the birth in general after a Caesarean section [7]. So, all is not likely to be equal at the birth of an ELBW baby; not only may the mother be recovering from a surgical delivery, but she and her partner will often have troubled feelings of failure, guilt and anxiety and perhaps a sense that their worst fears have been realized.

## The ELBW baby

An ELBW baby is likely to be moved straight from the delivery room to a neonatal unit. If the mother is conscious, she may have a chance to hold the baby briefly or at least have a glimpse before the baby is carried off. The baby she sees will not be the conventional image of the newborn child so prominent in the photographs in baby books and magazines. For some the first sight will be in the NICU with the baby in an incubator, attached to monitoring devices and perhaps on a ventilator, appearances matter. While the work does not specifically relate to ELBW babies, we know that parents of preterm and other babies receiving specialized neonatal care are very concerned about their baby's appearance [8,9]. It is easy to understand why this may be particularly important for parents of ELBW babies. These babies do not correspond to the expected image of a newborn son or daughter, but appearance is more or less all that parents have to go on. Dressing infants can help to make them appear more like the baby the parents were expecting. As excellent patterns exist for sewing and knitting tiny garments, the extended family can become involved in providing for their baby.

Because the baby cannot be freely held and is a poor partner in social interaction, appearance has a special importance. This also goes for the wider family whose members might expect to visit and hold a newborn full-term baby at home, but are likely to have to make do with a photograph and the parents' descrip-

tion of a baby who remains in the NICU: video recordings and photographs can help. In this connection, it is important to note that there may be negative images of preterm babies in the community. In one study in which mothers were given strange babies to hold, reactions were more guarded and negative when the mother was told (falsely) that the babies had been born prematurely [9].

The average length of stay for ELBW infants is of the order of 3 months. This can place a great strain on the parents' relationship and finances. Work patterns are disrupted and the time spent travelling and visiting the baby isolates the parents from family and friends and changes the tenor of the parents' lives. In one study it was found that 5% of a group of parents travelled more than 100 miles to visit their offspring [10] and the costs of visiting were more than £1000 for some parents. Siblings of the ELBW baby suffer more than is realized. It may be difficult for either parent to resume a demanding job effectively whilst the baby remains ill in a neonatal unit. Maternity leave is currently granted from the time that the baby is actually born rather than the due date, which can result in the mother having to resume her job just as the baby is discharged from hospital.

*Hospitalization* of parents is a well-recognized, if poorly documented, consequence of prolonged contact with a high-stress environment. Parents become dependent upon the unit's staff and regime for their social and emotional life, including celebrations such as Christmas, anniversaries and birthdays. They become *indispensable* members of the team. It is a tribute to most parents' good sense that they develop strategies of coping with this dramatic change in their lives and it is hardly surprising that observed responses amongst parents vary from an addiction to detail, including studying medical textbooks, to absenting themselves altogether from the neonatal unit. More research is needed on these kinds of response. We need to know the benefits of different coping strategies and how parents can be helped to develop those appropriate to their situation. It goes without saying that provision of accurate, consistent information about their baby of an appropriate level should be available to parents at all times and financial help for travel costs made easy to obtain. Support from employers can be excellent if the right letters are written in time, but this cannot be assumed and intervention may be needed. The luxury of a specific parent advocate and counsellor is probably of benefit, but is available to only a few units.

During the time that an ELBW baby is in a neonatal care unit, the parents have two crucial psychological issues to deal with: the containment of their anxiety about the baby's survival and prognosis, and the building of their relationship with him or her. Of course, the two issues may become linked as some parents may manage their fears and anxieties by remaining distant until they feel confident that their child will survive. This is an important point to bear in mind when discussing visiting with parents. The frequency of chronic lung disease in this group makes this a common problem, and many parents remark on the difficulty they have in conveying the uncertain prognosis to their friends and relations after the initial crisis period is over and the months of oxygen therapy begin. Lack of knowledge in the community, including among the medical and nursing profession about the prognosis, does not help. The parents may rapidly become more expert than their local advisers. As well as the obvious practical difficulties which may arise because of such things as travel costs and the need to care for older children at home, there may be psychological issues to resolve. Indeed, some regard regular visiting as a sign that these have been successfully worked through.

Parents (and some professionals) vary widely in their understanding of the complications of extremely low birth weight and the likely prognosis. Most will, at least at times, fear the worst: but what constitutes the worst is not the same for all. For some survival seems to be all that matters, but for others the thought of a severely damaged baby is worse than a death. These are very difficult issues for most parents (and, indeed, paediatricians and nurses) to confront openly even between themselves, let alone with those who have responsibility for the care of their child. Most parents have a great need to talk about their baby's problems and, not surprisingly, studies in neonatal units show that they are not always satisfied with the time available to see the paediatrician [11]. Despite the need to talk, they may find it very hard to ask for more time, not least because they may fear that such discussion time takes the staff away from caring for their baby. Some units have found it of great help to have someone with counselling or psychotherapy skills available to talk to parents (and to staff) [12]. Accurate information needs to be passed on to the family doctor, other caretakers, and community midwives to avoid the damage to confidence patiently built up by the neonatal unit staff which incorrect chance remarks from professionals subsequently encountered (ranging from anaesthetists to ENT surgeons) can cause.

Increasingly, the attitude amongst staff in neonatal units is that they should be straightforward and full in the explanations offered to parents, 'honest but not cruel' as one writer has put it [13]. Often parents will need to go over the same ground several times before they can accept and understand what is being said. Often the uncertainty of the developmental process may lead to difficulties. Not unnaturally, parents want to know about the longer-term prognosis – how will she do at school, will he be of normal height and so on – and they may find it hard to accept that precise answers cannot be given and may feel that the uncertainty is because something is being hidden from them.

But psychological work with parents suggests that for many, but not all, parents full information and the opportunity to talk are not enough. Some parents wish to be fully involved in all important decisions about the care of their child and, if the situation arises, about the withdrawal of some forms of treatment [14–16]. There has been some resistance to policies of this kind, not least on the grounds that most parents do not have sufficient knowledge and understanding of the relevant technical questions. The Dutch experience has been that the response to published guidelines regarding termination of neonatal life where the prognosis is poor has been widely accepted by the medical profession and parents but not by the lawyers [17]. There are indications that the grieving process is eased for parents who felt that they were involved in the important decisions [18].

While there is a growing body of data on the psychological development of low birth weight children [19] the great bulk of the psychological research carried out on the parent–child relationship of preterm babies has centred on the possible effects of early separation or, as it has come to be known, on the question of bonding. As specialized units for neonatal care grew up, there was growing disquiet among some parents and professionals about the possible consequences of the parent–infant separation. These concerns became focused on the concept of bonding, originally proposed by Klaus and Kennell [20]. Drawing on some research on animal species as well as on human data, these authors suggested that mothers enter a sensitive period after delivery during which they are particularly able to form a relationship with their baby. They further suggested that if mother and baby were separated during this sensitive period, which was hypothesized to last only 2 days, there might be long-term, if not permanent, difficulties in subsequently forming a satisfactory relationship. Many studies have been carried out to test these ideas and there have been several theoretical discussions of the concepts involved [21–24]. The general consensus is that while there may be some short-term effects of early separation, there are powerful recuperative processes so that separation *per se* does not seem to have long-term effects. Nevertheless, most parents dislike enforced separation; this and the short-term effects that have been demonstrated make the avoidance of separation a high priority in neonatal care. Indeed, the evidence goes further than this and indicates that more is required than the avoidance of separation and that active steps should be taken to engage parents in as much caretaking of their baby as they may feel comfortable with. This involvement appears to reduce the short-term effects of separation that have been described, such as a feeling of lack of confidence in being able to cope with the baby and a distance and strangeness in the relationship. In recent years, units have gained considerable experience with a wide range of techniques and practices designed to foster good relationships and reduce the inevitable stresses created by an admission to a neonatal unit [25]. These range from skin-to-skin contact [26] to massage, which has been shown to reduce the levels of cortisol and catecholamine levels in the blood of preterm infants [27]. The dangers of touching and disturbing these fragile babies may have been overstated in the past, and there may well be a place for gentle handling in the convalescent phase. Parents rapidly learn how to tube feed and care for the baby. This new approach not only includes parents but also siblings and grandparents.

As these kinds of programmes have developed, research interest and accompanying practice have focused on a somewhat different issue: the behaviour of preterm babies and the difficulties of building satisfactory relationships with them. The analysis of the growth of social relationships of full term infants and their caretakers has demonstrated the importance of mutuality in interactions. Even from the first days after birth, the normal full-term infant's behaviour has a structure that is relatively predictable so that the caretaker can mould his or her behaviour around what the infant is doing. This, in turn, provides a predictable social world for the infant. For the caretaker, the sense that the infant can respond in some way to what she is doing seems to be a crucial step in the early formation of their relationship.

The extent to which an infant's behaviour is structured (and there is a possibility of interactive behaviour) is related to gestational age. So, quite simply, preterm babies make very poor social partners. Their behaviour is unpredictable and disorganized and it is very difficult for the parent to get any sense of being engaged in a social relationship. Direct observation of preterm babies with their parents demonstrates differences in interaction which may persist for some weeks, if not months, after birth [28]. While it is important not to overstress differences of this kind, parents often need support and the reassurance that, with time, satisfactory relationships will develop. Especially in the USA, various home visiting programmes have been developed, some of which have specifically set out to enhance parent–infant interaction. Some of these programmes have demonstrated beneficial effects on mothers; initial adjustment to their infants and a positive longer-term (4 years) effect on the child's cognitive development [29]. However, though it is somewhat difficult to generalize, the more broadly based programmes of support, such as are offered by health visitors in the UK and elsewhere, seem as effective as those with more specific aims [30–32]. Given the relatively high rates of problems indexed by such measures as hospital re-admissions that ELBW babies and their parents experience at least for the first couple of years, there is a case for follow-up studies which would investigate more fully the psychological problems that might arise in this period [33].

An issue that has been the subject of a good deal of research is the extent to which maternal interactions with ELBW infants may differ from those of full term infants. Most studies are reassuring in that they demonstrate few if any differences in the attachment pattern of low birth weight singleton or twins over the first months of life [34,35]. Some, however, have reported that mothers of preterm infants left them alone more, and talked and interacted with them less, at least in the early weeks [36]. Interestingly, there are indications that while the development of preterm and full term children may be broadly similar after the first few weeks or months, they may reach this status in rather different ways [37]. Quality of input from a caretaker may be more crucial for the preterm infants. Satisfactory catch up is achieved where there are positive maternal attitudes, again underlining the need for support and help for the roles of parents. The wider kin network, especially grandmothers, is likely to be of special importance here. However, there is evidence from a USA study [38] that the birth of an ELBW baby does not evoke the same degree of positive support from the kinship network as that of a full term baby. Like parents, perhaps grandparents need to grieve over the loss of the idealized grandchild.

## The emotional needs of the ELBW baby

Despite the considerable interest among psychologists in bonding and the early parent–infant relationship of preterm and LBW babies, there has been little interest in the emotional needs of the babies themselves in the neonatal period. While it is possible to point to a whole number of features of this early environment which set it apart from that of a full term baby, it is another matter to assess the significance of these differences.

An incubator seems to operate as a psychological, as well as physical, barrier for parents and caretakers [10]. The baby's crying is difficult to hear and this, together with features of the way in which nursing care is usually organized, means that there is a lack of correlation between the infant's behaviour and that of the caretakers [39]. Again, compared with the normal situation, a very large number of different caretakers are likely to be involved

and any one of them is unlikely to learn in detail about a baby's individual characteristics. There are also aspects of the physical environment such as the general noise level and the repeated sharp sounds that are heard when a hard object is placed on an incubator. Light levels may be high and vary little by day or night. There may be a very high rate of medical intervention, including procedures that are painful [40], and this may permanently blunt pain responses. For tube-fed babies there is the lack of sucking experience. Here there is evidence that the provision of a teat to suck on during a tube feed may be associated with higher rates of weight gain [41]. However, this study, like the many others that have tested a wide range of interventions from stroking through rocking water beds to the provision of piped music, did not involve ELBW babies.

Studies are required of the physical and social environment of these babies and of ways in which these may be enhanced. In particular, it needs to be established if the use of potentially stressful and painful procedures can be reduced or their effect ameliorated. The issue of pain in immature babies is a controversial one. However, there is sufficient evidence from infant studies to suggest that we cannot continue to assume that babies lack pain perception and the use of pain relieving techniques may improve the medical prognosis [42].

## Multiple births

A final issue that requires brief mention is that of multiple births which figure prominently among ELBW babies. While the evidence, such as it is, about the social relationships of LBW twins is relatively reassuring [43], the same may not be true for higher multiples. The birth of three or more infants, even in relatively ideal situations, may cause extreme stress for parents. When the babies are all of VLBW it is likely that these problems are multiplied [44,45] and it should be remembered that such births are to become more frequent with the deployment of techniques for assisted conception.

## Conclusion

It is disappointing that with the great strides that have been made in the medical care of the

ELBW baby, there has not been a corresponding growth of our knowledge of social and psychological matters. Most of what can be said has still to be based on extrapolations from studies of heavier babies. While these do provide a general understanding, much more work is needed to see what specific problems may accompany the birth of a baby weighing less than 1000 g.

---

**Practical points**

1. A photograph of the baby (dressed if possible) given to the mother immediately after birth is a simple and effective way to encourage the development of a social relationship and overcome anxiety about the baby's appearance in the early days. Further prints may be required for grandparents and other relatives.

2. Written information about the equipment and common complications of prematurity should be available to back up what is said in interviews. Translation into foreign languages through an interpreter, and sign language interpreters for the deaf, should be available with an on-call system.

3. A separate, quiet, suitably furnished area off the intensive care unit should be created for counselling parents. It is difficult for parents to concentrate with all the distractions of the intensive care area and information is not retained well.

4. Accurate, up-to-date information related to gestational age regarding the prognosis of preterm infants needs to be widely disseminated amongst midwives and obstetric junior and senior staff in a maternity hospital to avoid false information being given in the labour ward in an emergency.

5. Post-discharge support by a community special care sister and a telephone help line needs to be available to parents after they take their small baby home for the first time. Here, too, accurate and up-to-date information is needed by all professionals who may have contact with these babies.

---

# References

1. Silcock, A. (1984) Crises in parents of prematures: an Australian study. *Br. J. Dev. Psychol.*, **2**, 257–268
2. Yu, V.Y.H. (1977) Caring for parents of high-risk infants. *Med. J. Aust.*, **2**, 532–537
3. Richards, M.P.M. (1992) Psychological aspects of neonatal care. In *Textbook of Neonatology* (N.R.C. Roberton, ed.) 2nd edition, Churchill Livingstone, Edinburgh, pp. 29–42
4. Green, J., Statham, H. and Snowdon, C. (1992) Screening for fetal abnormalities: attitudes and experiences. In *Obstetrics in the 1990s: current controversies* (T. Chard and M.P.M. Richards, eds), *Clin. Dev. Med.*, **123–124**, pp. 65–89, Mac Keith Press, London.
5. Rothman, B.K. (1986) *The Tentative Pregnancy: Prenatal Diagnosis and the Future of Motherhood.* Viking, New York
6. Richards, M.P.M. (1989) Social and ethical problems of fetal diagnosis and screening. *J. Reprod. Infant Psychol.*, **71**, 671–685
7. Marut, J.S. and Mercer, R.T. (1979) The Caesarian birth experience: implications for nursing. *Nurs. Res.*, **28**, 260–266
8. Goodman, J.R. and Sauve, R.S. (1985) High risk infant: concerns of the mother after discharge. *Birth*, **12**, 235–242
9. Stern, M. and Hildebrandt, A. (1986) Prematurity stereotyping: effects on mother–infant interaction. *Child Dev.*, **57**, 308–315
10. McLoughlin, A., Hillier, V.F. and Robinson, M.J. (1993) Parental costs of neonatal visiting. *Arch. Dis. Childh.*, **68**, 597–599
11. Jacques, N.C.S., Hawthorne-Amick, J.T. and Richards, M.P.M. (1983) Parents and the support they need. In *Parent–Baby Attachment in Premature Infants* (J.A. Davis, M.P.M. Richards and N.R.C. Roberton, eds), Croom Helm, London, 100–128
12. Bender, H. and Swan-Parente, A. (1983) Psychological and psychotherapeutic support of staff and parents in an intensive care baby unit. In *Parent-Baby Attachment in Premature Infants* (J.A. Davis, M.P.M. Richards and N.R.C. Roberton, eds), Croom Helm, London, 165–178
13. Bogdan, R., Brown, M.A. and Foster, S.B. (1982) Be honest but not cruel: staff parent communications on a neonatal unit. *Hum. Org.*, **41**, 6–16
14. Whitelaw, A. (1986) Death as an option in neonatal intensive care. *Lancet*, **ii**, 328–331
15. Harrison, H. (1986) Neonatal intensive care: parents' role in ethical decision making. *Birth*, **13**, 165–175
16. Richards, M.P.M. (1989) The withdrawal of treatment from newborn infants. *Early Hum. Dev.*, **18**, 263–272
17. Versulys, C. (1993) Ethics of neonatal care. *Lancet*, **341**, 193–195
18. Stinson, R. and Stinson, P. (1983) *The Long Dying of Baby Andrew*. Little Brown, Boston
19. Freidman, S.L. and Sigman, M.D. (1992) *The Psychological Development of Low Birthweight Children.* Ablex, New York

20. Klaus, M.H. and Kennell, J.H. (1982) *Parent–Infant Bonding.* Mosby, St Louis

21. Campbell, S.B.G. and Taylor, P.M. (1980) Bonding and attachment: theoretical issues. In *Parent–Infant Relationships* (P.M. Taylor, ed.), Grune and Stratton, New York, 3–25

22. Herbert, M., Sluckin, W. and Sluckin, A. (1982) Mother-to-infant 'bonding'. *J. Child. Psychol. and Psychiatr.*, **23**, 205–217

23. Richards, M.P.M. (1983) The myth of bonding. In *Progress in Child Health* (J.A. Macfarlane, ed.), Churchill Livingstone, Edinburgh, pp. 113–120

24. Goldberg, S. (1983) Parent–infant bonding, another look. *Child. Dev.*, **54**, 1355–1382

25. Davis, J.A., Richards, M.P.M. and Roberton, N.R.C. (1983) *Parent–Baby Attachment in Premature Infants.* Croom Helm, London

26. Acolet, D., Sleath, K. and Whitelaw, A. (1989) Oxygenation, heart rate and temperature in very low birthweight infants during skin-to-skin contact with their mothers. *Acta Paediatr. Scand.*, **78**, 189–193

27. Acolet, D., Modi, N., Ginnakoulopoulos, X. *et al.* (1993) Changes in plasma cortisol and catecholamine concentrations in response to massage in preterm infants. *Arch. Dis. Childh.*, **68**, 29–31

28. Goldberg, S. and Divitto, B.A. (1992) *Born Too Soon.* Freeman, San Francisco

29. Raul, V.A., Achenbach, T.M., Nurcombe, B., Howell, C.T. and Teti, D.M. (1988) Minimizing adverse effects of low birthweight: four-year results of an early intervention program. *Child Dev.*, **59**, 544–553

30. Barrera, M.E., Rosenbaum, P.L. and Cunningham, C.E. (1986) Early home intervention with low birth-weight infants and their parents. *Child Dev.*, **57**, 20–33

31. McCormick, M., Bernbaum, S., Stemmlet, M. and Farran, A. (1984) The LBW infant goes home: impact on the family. *Paediatr. Res.*, **18**, 109

32. Ferrari, L., Pelafigue, A. and Salbreux, R. (1988) Early and continuous action to prevent breakdown in the care of infants and their families after serious neonatal episodes. *Inf. Ment. Health J.*, **9**, 82–92

33. Ford, G., Rickards, A., Kitcher, W.H., Ryan, M.M. and Lissenden, J.V. (1986) Relationship of growth and psychoneurologic status of 2 year old children of birth-weight 500–999 g. *Early Hum. Dev.*, **13**, 329–337

34. Goldberg, S., Perrotta, M. and Munde, K. (1986) Maternal behaviour and attachment in low-birth-weight twins and singletons. *Child Dev.*, **57**, 34–46

35. Easterbrooks, M.A. (1989) Quality of attachment to mother and to father: effects of perinatal risk status. *Child Dev.*, **60**, 825–830

36. Davis, D.H. and Thomas, E.B. (1989) The early social environment of premature and full term infants. *Early Hum. Dev.*, **17**, 221–232

37. Greenberg, M.T. and Crnic, K.A. (1988) Longitudinal predictors of developmental status, and social interaction in premature and full-term infants at age two. *Child Dev.*, **59**, 554–570

38. Zarling, C.L., Hirsch, B.J. and Landry, S. (1988) Maternal social networks and mother-infant interaction in full-term and very low birthweight, preterm infants. *Child Dev..*, **59**, 178–185

39. Prince, J., Firlej, M. and Harvey, D. (1978) Contact between babies in incubators and their caretakers. In *Separation and Special Care Baby Units* (F.S.W. Brimblecombe, M.P.M. Richards and N.R.C. Roberton, eds), *Clin. Dev. Med.*, **68**, Heinemann Medical Books, 55–63

40. Murdock, D.R. and Darlow, B.A. (1984) Handling during neonatal care. *Arch. Dis. Childh.*, **59**, 957–961

41. Ignatoft, E. and Field, T. (1982) Effects of non-nutritive sucking during tube-feeding on the behaviour and clinical course of ICU preterm neonates. In *Infant Behavior and Development: Perinatal Risk and Newborn Behaviour* (L.P. Lipsitt and T.M. Field, eds), Albex, New York, pp. 107–115

42. Anand, K.J.S., Sippell, W.G. and Aynsley-Green, A. (1987) Randomised trial of fentanyl anaesthesia on preterm babies undergoing surgery: effects on the stress response. *Lancet*, **i**, 62–65

43. Goldberg, S., Perrotta, M., Minde, K. and Corter, C. (1986) Maternal behaviour and attachment in low-birth-weight twins and singletons. *Child Dev.*, **57**, 34–46

44. Botting, B., MacFarlane, A. and Price, F. (1990) *Three Four and More: a National Study of Triplets and Higher Order Births* (Price Report). HMSO, London

45. Harvey, D. (1992) *The Stress of Multiple Births.* Multiple Birth Foundation, London

# 24

# Pain

**Nicholas Rutter**

Pain is the sensation one feels when hurt. As such it is subjective, easily perceived but difficult to describe or to measure objectively. The human infant is born at a stage of cortical immaturity, and this has led in the past to the view that because consciousness is poorly developed, so too is pain. Philosophical arguments about what an infant perceives, interprets and perhaps later remembers as pain are a distraction. What is important is whether a newborn baby, in particular one born prematurely, is able to recognize a painful stimulus and to react to it. There is evidence that even the most immature infant is able to recognize and react to painful stimuli. A number of manoeuvres including the administration of anaesthesia and analgesia will modify the pain responses of the newborn infant, supporting the view that pain relief in the newborn should be considered in a similar way to that in children or adults. Anand and Hickey [1] and Anand and Carr [2] have reviewed the subject of pain and its effect in the human fetus, neonate, infant, and child. Evidence that the immature newborn baby feels and reacts to pain is taken from their reviews.

## Are pain pathways developed?

Pain pathways travel from sensory receptors in the skin, mucous membranes and internal organs to the sensory cortex.

## Pain receptors

The density of pain receptor nerve endings in the skin of the newborn baby is similar to, or greater than in adult skin. These sense receptors first appear around the mouth at 7 weeks of gestation, and by 20 weeks have spread to all cutaneous and mucous surfaces.

## Peripheral nerve fibres

Pain fibres in the peripheral nerve are either myelinated (fast pain) or poorly or non-myelinated (slow pain) in the adult. Fast pain is rapid in onset, sharp and well localized. Slow pain is slower in onset, prolonged, dull and aching. Myelination of the fast pain fibres is incomplete in preterm infants but slower conduction is compensated for by the much shorter distance the impulses need to travel. Slow pain fibres are poorly myelinated anyhow. Thus, lack of myelination of pain fibres in immature infants does not support that argument that such infants cannot feel pain.

## Spinal cord

Pain fibres in peripheral nerves synapse with spinal neurones in the dorsal horn of the spinal cord grey matter. Differentiation of the dorsal horn neurones begins at 13 weeks. By 30 weeks the synaptic connection and specific neurotransmitter vesicles have matured. Pain impulses are carried along spinal and brainstem tracts to the thalamus. These tracts are fully myelinated by 30 weeks.

### Cortex

Connections between the thalamus and the sensory cortex are established by 20 to 24 weeks' gestation. Myelination is complete by 37 weeks' gestation. By 20 weeks' gestation the cortical neurone complement is complete. EEG activity, somatosensory evoked responses, and sleep/wake cycles are developing between 24 and 28 weeks' gestation.

The newborn baby, even if born very early, has well defined and functioning pain pathways. Much less is known about maturation of the neurochemical systems associated with the perception of pain. However, substance p, a tachykinin, well established as a transmitter and controller of pain impulses, can be demonstrated within the central nervous system of human fetuses early in their development. Endogenous opioids, particularly β-endorphin, can be found in high levels in plasma and cerebrospinal fluid of premature babies.

## Reactions of the immature infant to a painful stimulus

The reaction of a newborn infant to pain is clearly less sophisticated than that of an adult. However, a reaction is well developed even in the most immature baby. Reaction to a painful stimulus takes three forms: physiological, hormonal and behavioural.

### Physiological reactions to pain

#### Cardiovascular

Cardiovascular reactions are well recognized. Heart rate and blood pressure increase acutely in response to a painful stimulus such as heelprick blood sampling or circumcision, in both term and preterm infants [3–7]. The magnitude of the response is in part related to the length and intensity of the stimulus and can be modified by analgesia or local anaesthesia. Fluctuations, particularly falls, in transcutaneous arterial $Po_2$ or oxygen saturations occur in preterm infants following a painful stimulus and again this can be modified by drugs.

Tracheal intubation and suction are manoeuvres which produce marked cardiovascular and oxygenation changes in preterm infants [8–10], and they too can be reduced or abolished by drugs [11].

### Intracranial pressure

Intracranial pressure increases in response to tracheal intubation in preterm infants, a combination of arterial and venous hypertension associated with struggling [12,13]. The increase can be abolished by anaesthetic.

### Palmar sweating

Palmar sweating is a response to emotional rather than thermal stimulation and relates well in the term infant to state of arousal [14]. In response, for example, to heelprick blood sampling, there is an abrupt sustained increase in palmar water loss which continues until the stimulus is removed. This is a useful objective tool for measuring response to a painful stimulus and its modification but only in mature infants [15]. Palmar sweating does not develop before 37 weeks' gestation and its development is not hastened by premature delivery.

### Hormonal reactions to pain

The production of hormones in response to stress has been well studied in preterm and term infants subjected to the stress of surgery. There is a marked release of catecholamines, growth hormone, glucagon, cortisol, aldosterone and other steroids. This leads to the breakdown of fat and carbohydrate stores, protracted hyperglycaemia and increases in lactate, pyruvate, ketone bodies and non-esterified fatty acids. Older infants and children show similar hormonal changes. Although their catecholamine and glucagon responses are smaller, their corticol responses are greater and more prolonged. Effective anaesthesia combined with analgesia will abolish these responses. Although these very marked hormonal changes could be regarded as having positive benefit in the acute phase of stabilization following injury and in promoting wound healing, in a hospital setting they serve no useful function. The hypermetabolic state may well lead to increased morbidity and mortality.

## Behavioural reactions to pain

These have been studied in preterm and term infants. Clearly they may be limited in a preterm infant because of illness, endotracheal intubation and restraint of the head and limbs. The more immature the infant, the more these behavioural responses are likely to be limited. However, a healthy 24-week gestation infant will respond in a similar way to a full term infant when subjected to painful stimuli.

### *Simple motor responses*

Simple motor responses are demonstrated when a limb is painfully stimulated, as in a heelprick. There is flexion and adduction of all four limbs as well as crying and facial movements [16,17]. Such responses are seen in the most immature infants [18]. The same movements are described in the midtrimester fetus in response to an amniocentesis needle.

### *Crying*

Crying is the major mode of communication in the newborn baby and is elicited by pain as well as hunger or discomfort. The cry of pain has characteristics which can be recognized by the mother and distinguished from crying for other reasons. It is possible to analyse crying by spectrographic means and this is used as a measure of pain in research [1]. Even extremely immature infants are able to cry if they are in good health and not intubated.

### *Facial expression*

Facial expression changes according to the mood of the newborn infant. Pleasure, pain, sadness and surprise elicit distinct expression. Pain is associated with intense grimacing as well as crying and body movement.

### *Complex behaviours*

Complex behaviour changes in response to pain are also reported in the newborn baby, although not in the most immature infant. For example, circumcision without analgesia disturbs the normal sleep/wake cycle and results in more non-rapid eye movement sleep [19]. There is increased wakefulness and irritability. Similar changes occur after blood sampling. It is possible to assess and score behaviour so that it can be used as a research tool in measuring pain and its relief. In one study, for example, 90% of newborn infants showed prolonged alteration in behaviour after circumcision, although such behaviour was only recorded in 16% of non-circumcised controls [20]. There is evidence that altered behaviour occurs in response to a variety of measures in neonatal intensive care, and that this is complex, subtle and capable of being recognized and modified to the benefit of the infant.

In summary, newborn infants, even those who are born extremely prematurely, show physiological, hormonal and behavioural responses to painful stimuli. There is much evidence that these responses can be modified by drug therapy.

## Pain and discomfort in neonatal intensive care

Most pain and discomfort which preterm infants experience is caused by procedures or treatment rather than directly by their illness. It is inflicted. Since the smallest, most immature infants are also the sickest, their need for intensive care will be greater and longer. They are therefore subjected to more painful stimuli than larger infants [21] and thus the need to avoid, modify or relieve their pain is greater.

### Trauma

Most trauma is inflicted in the intensive care unit after delivery. Trauma during delivery is less common in the most immature infants because of their small size. Much trauma is caused by needles. This takes the form of heel or finger stabs, venepuncture, the insertion of intravenous and intra-arterial cannulae, and lumbar puncture. Extravasation of fluid from a cannula into the subcutaneous tissue, a common occurrence with intravenous infusions in small infants, is particularly painful. The insertion of drains into the chest or abdomen usually involves a small skin incision and is likely to be more painful than venepuncture. Surgery is sometimes necessary in immature infants, particularly laparotomy, thoracotomy and hernia repair. Adhesive skin trauma, such as the removal of sticking plaster or an ECG electrode, is common. The behavioural changes which a small infant shows when the plaster or electrode is removed suggests that it is as painful as it would be to a child.

### Intubation

Insertion of a laryngoscope into the pharynx and of a tube into the trachea in an awake patient may not be traumatic (although it often is in very small sick infants) but it is, however, intensely unpleasant and elicits very marked behavioural and physiological responses in all but the sickest, most depressed infants. Pharyngeal and tracheal suctioning elicits similar if milder responses in intubated babies.

### Inflammation

Peritonitis is clearly painful to small infants, as judged by the behavioural and physiological response to abdominal palpation. Meningitis may be similarly painful, and the irritability which is often seen may be due in part to headache rather than direct cerebral irritation.

### Discomfort

The distinction between pain and discomfort is difficult to define and perhaps unnecessary. However, adults who have experienced major surgery or intensive care are often distressed by factors which compound any pain they feel. Constant disturbance as a result of bright light, noise, repeated handling by staff, or being too warm or too cool, results in poor sleep, a lack of feeling rested, lowering of morale and delayed recovery. Although there may be a large cerebral element to these feelings which might be lacking in a very immature infant, discomfort in the newborn intensive care unit is worth examining.

The sick preterm infant is usually nursed in constant bright light, is subjected to constant background noise with frequent peaks of loud sound, and is unlikely to experience periods of quiet and low light intensity until the need for intensive care is over. The infant nursed in a closed incubator may feel cold because of thermal stress. The infant under an overhead radiant heater may feel alternately hot and cold as the heater cycles on and off, with a variable draught coming from the room. Most sick immature infants are nursed naked and therefore lack the comfort as well as warmth which clothing provides. Furthermore, they usually lie on a firm and unyielding mattress. Handling by staff is frequent, especially if the infant is sick, which results in disturbed sleep and causes restlessness, instability of heart rate, blood pressure and oxygenation, and cold stress. It is possible to address some of these environmental factors and modify them, using the principle that what would be considered beneficial for a child or adult is likely to be good for a newborn baby too.

## Prevention of pain

This is difficult, since those procedures which cause pain are usually necessary for the monitoring and treatment of the infant's illness. Arterial cannulae once inserted provide a painless method of blood sampling and blood pressure monitoring. Intravenous central lines provide long-term venous access and avoid the need for constant re-insertion of tissued drips. Clearly though, there is a price to be paid for this convenience.

Heel blood sampling can be effectively performed using a spring-loaded automated device, either a lance (e.g. Autolet, Owen Mumford, UK) or a blade (e.g. Tenderfoot, International Technidyne Corporation, USA) [22]. This is less painful than manual lancing of the heel [15,23], a distressing and unacceptable way of taking blood from a small infant. The use of Karaya gum ECG electrodes is more practical and less painful than the standard adhesive electrode [24]. Powerful adhesive tape which is sometimes used to fix endotracheal tubes or chest drains should be avoided, particularly in the very immature infant with a thin, weak epidermis.

## Improvement of comfort

Thought needs to be given to the provision of a period of uninterrupted rest for sick preterm infants. Nursing cares, medical examination and investigation can often be concentrated into a short spell, then to be followed by a period of unbroken rest which is only interrupted in an emergency. Reduction, either periodically or constantly, of noise and light levels is possible and unlikely to be harmful. Provision of clothing and a soft yielding surface to lie on may well have a calming effect on the infant.

# Relief of pain

## Analgesia and sedation

Pure sedatives are rarely used in neonatal care, although their use in paediatric and adult intensive care units is common. Opiates, however, with varying analgesic and sedative properties, are widely used in neonatal intensive care in the UK [25]. Non-opiate analgesia is less commonly used and little is known about properties of such drugs in the preterm newborn.

### Opiates

Opiates are used for pain relief during and after surgery, for intubation and to provide sedation of infants who are being ventilated. In the latter case they provide constant analgesia which reduces the pain and discomfort of intensive care. Morphine is the most widely used, particularly in ventilated infants where its respiratory depressant effect may be beneficial. Its use is associated with a significant reduction in the hormonal stress response in ventilated preterm infants [26]. Metabolism and excretion is delayed in the preterm compared with term infants [27,28]. Elimination half-life and clearance are reduced. Diamorphine is similarly effective. It has been shown to reduce the hormonal stress response in ventilated preterm infants [29]. It appears to be safe if given as a constant infusion ($15 \mu g \, kg^{-1} \, hour^{-1}$) following a small loading dose ($50 \mu g \, kg^{-1}$ over 30 min) [29,30]. It is rapidly metabolized to morphine in even the most immature infant [31] and both elimination and clearance are reduced in the more immature infants. Fentanyl and its close relatives alfentanil and sufentanil are short-acting and more popular for use during and after surgery. Pharmacokinetic studies in the preterm infant are limited but suggest that half-life and clearance are prolonged [32]. Efficacy of the opiates is difficult to quantify, although the blunting of the massive hormonal response to surgery is well documented. Reduction in the hormonal stress response during neonatal intensive care has been demonstrated in research work [26,29] but cannot be used in clinical practice to demonstrate efficacy. Use of opiates is largely based on clinical impression of pain relief and ease of ventilation, as judged by behavioural and physiological effects [29,33,34]. Side-effects include hypotension, respiratory depression, urine retention and constipation. It is thought that hypotension and respiratory depression are more likely to occur with bolus injections. Opiates are best given intravenously as a slow loading dose over 30 minutes or so, followed by a low dose constant infusion [26,30,29]. It is an impression that opiates are as effective and safe in the very immature infant below 1000 g birthweight, as in less preterm infants, although information in this group is understandably limited.

### Non-opiates

Non-opiates are sometimes used, particularly paracetamol as an analgesic and chloral hydrate as a sedative. Little is known about their metabolism and elimination in very immature infants, and less is known about their efficacy.

## Anaesthesia

### General and regional anaesthesia

There is evidence that aggressive anaesthesia decreases the stress responses of newborn infants undergoing surgery and reduces their morbidity and mortality. In a randomized controlled trial, preterm infants undergoing duct ligation received either paralysis and nitrous oxide alone or with additional intravenous fentanyl [35]. There were eight infants in each treatment group, of mean gestation 28 weeks and mean birth weight 1000 g. The marked hormonal stress responses were significantly decreased in the babies who received fentanyl. Increases in blood glucose, lactate and pyruvate were prevented in the fentanyl group and there was less breakdown of endogenous protein and fewer postoperative complications. In another randomized controlled trial, term infants undergoing surgery were either paralysed and received nitrous oxide alone, or received additional halothane [36]. Halothane and nitrous oxide together results in significant reduction in the hormonal responses to surgery, less metabolic disturbance and a better outcome. In a further randomized trial carried out in newborn babies undergoing cardiac surgery, one group were given halothane and low-dose morphine, the other received halothane and high-dose sufentanil [37,38]. Hormonal stress responses were very marked in the low-dose morphine group, with marked metabolic responses. Both hormonal and metabolic responses were substantially reduced in the high-dose sufentanil group. Furthermore, postoperative complications and mortality were significantly lower in the sufentanil group. Aggressive anaesthesia therefore decreases stress response of neonatal surgery and improves postoperative outcome. Little information is available on the very immature infants but there is no reason to suppose that their need for adequate anaesthesia and analgesia is any less. Regional anaesthesia, spinal epidural, is useful for minor surgery such as inguinal hernia repair in an immature, non-ventilated infant with chronic lung disease.

### *Local anaesthesia*

Local anaesthesia is not commonly used in neonatal care. It is argued that the injection required to give the local anaesthetic is as painful as the venepuncture or lumbar puncture itself. The use of topical local anaesthesia, though, needs exploring. The lignocaine prilocaine cream (EMLA) which is used so effectively in children has potential dangers in the very immature infant. Local anaesthetics are poorly absorbed through mature skin but are likely to be rapidly absorbed through the poor epidermal barrier of the immature infant. The prilocaine component of the EMLA cream causes methaemoglobinaemia in older infants and is likely to have a more marked effect in preterm infants.

Lignocaine alone has been shown *in vitro* to be absorbed through the skin of preterm infants in amounts which have been estimated to provide local anaesthesia without systemic toxicity [39]. *In vivo*, however, topical lignocaine does not appear to have a local anaesthetic effect in preterm infants [40,41], either because it is not sufficiently absorbed or because it is not pharmacologically active. There is a need for further research to find an effective safe topical agent to provide local anaesthesia for practical procedures in the preterm infant.

**Practical points**

1. Neural pathways for nociception are well developed in even the most immature infants.
2. Immature infants respond to pain and stress with physiological, behavioural and hormonal changes.
3. Opiate analgesics will blunt the hormonal stress responses during surgery and intensive care. They appear to be safe if given as a continuous, low dose infusion.
4. Painful procedures are commonly carried out in babies of less than 1000 g and should, where possible, be reduced or modified.
5. There is a need for an effective and safe topical local anaesthetic for use in the premature newborn.

## References

1. Anand, K.J.S. and Hickey, P.R. (1987) Pain and its effects in the human neonate and fetus. *N. Engl. J. Med.*, **317**, 1321–1329
2. Anand, K.J.S. and Carr, D.B. (1989) The neuroanatomy, neurophysiology, and neurochemistry of pain, stress, and analgesia in newborns and children. *Ped. Clin. N. Am.*, **36**, 795–822
3. Williamson, P.S. and Williamson, M.L. (1983) Physiologic stress reduction by a local anesthetic during newborn circumcision. *Pediatrics*, **71**, 36–40
4. Holve, R.L., Bromberger, B.J., Groverman, H.D., Klauber, M.R., Dixon, S.D. and Snyder, J.M. (1983) Regional anesthesia during newborn circumcision: effect on infant pain response. *Clin. Pediatr. (Phila.)*, **22**, 813–818
5. Owens, M.E. and Todt, E.H. (1984) Pain in infancy: neonatal reaction to a heel lance. *Pain*, **20**, 77–86
6. Johnson, C.C. and Strada, M.E. (1986) Acute pain response in infants: a multidimensional description. *Pain*, **24**, 373–382
7. Field, T. and Goldson, E. (1984) Pacifying effects of non-nutritive sucking on term and preterm neonates during heelstick procedures. *Pediatrics*, **74**, 1012–1015
8. Kelly, M.A. and Finer, N.N. (1984) Nasotracheal intubation in the neonate: physiologic responses and effects of atropine and pancuronium. *J. Pediatr.*, **105**, 303–309
9. Marshall, T.A., Deeder, R., Pai, S., Berkowitz, G.P. and Austin, T.L. (1984) Physiologic changes associated with endotracheal intubation in preterm infants. *Crit. Care Med.*, **12**, 501–503

10. Gibbons, P.A. and Swedlow, D.B. (1986) Changes in oxygen saturation during elective tracheal intubation in infants. (Abstract) *Anesth. Analg.*, **65**, 558

11. Hickey, P.R., Hansen, D.D., Wessel, D.L., Lang, P., Jonas, R.A. and Elixson, E.M. (1985) Blunting of stress responses in the pulmonary circulation of infants by fentanyl. *Anesth. Analg.*, **64**, 1137–1142

12. Raju, T.N.K., Vidyasagar, D., Torres, C., Grundy, D. and Bennett, E.J. (1980) Intracranial pressure during intubation and anesthesia in infants. *J. Pediatr.*, **96**, 860–862

13. Friesen, R.H., Honda, A.T. and Thieme, R.E. (1987) Changes in anterior fontanel pressure in preterm neonates during tracheal intubation. *Anesth. Analg.*, **66**, 874–878

14. Harpin, V.A. and Rutter, N. (1982) Development of emotional sweating in the newborn infant. *Arch. Dis. Childh.*, **57**, 691–695

15. Harpin, V.A. and Rutter, N. (1983) Making heel pricks less painful. *Arch. Dis. Childh.*, **58**, 226–228

16. Rich, E.C., Marshall, R.E. and Volpe, J.J. (1974) The normal neonatal response to pin-prick. *Dev. Med. Child Neurol.*, **16**, 432–434

17. Franck, L.S. (1986) A new method to quantitatively describe pain behavior in infants. *Nurse Res.*, **35**, 28–31

18. Fitzgerald, M., Shaw, A. and MacIntosh, N. (1988) The postnatal development of the cutaneous flexor reflex: a comparative study in premature infants and newborn rat pups. *Dev. Med. Child. Neurol.*, **30**, 520–526

19. Emde, R.N., Harmon, R.J., Metcalf, D., Koenig, K.L. and Wagonfeld, S. (1971) Stress and neonatal sleep. *Psychosom. Med.*, **33**, 491–497

20. Marshall, R.E., Stratton, W.C., Moore, J.A. and Boxerman, S.B. (1980) Circumcision. I. Effects upon newborn behaviour. *Infant Behav. Dev.*, **3**, 1–14

21. Barker, D.P. and Rutter, N. (1995) Exposure to invasive procedures in neonatal intensive care unit admissions. *Arch. Dis. Childh.*, **72**, 47–48

22. Barker, D.P., Latty, B.W. and Rutter, N. (1994) Heel blood sampling in preterm infants – which technique? *Arch. Dis. Childh.*, **71**, 206–208

23. McIntosh, N., van Veen, L. and Brameyer, H. (1994) Alleviation of the pain of heel prick in preterm infants. *Arch. Dis. Childh.*, **70**, F177–181

24. Cartlidge, P.H.T. and Rutter, N. (1987) Karaya gum E.C.G. electrodes for the preterm infant. *Arch. Dis. Childh.*, **62**, 1281–1282

25. Rutter, N. and Richardson, J. (1992) A survey of the use of analgesia in newborn intensive care. *Int. J. Pharm. Pract.*, **1**, 220–222

26. Quinn, M.W., Wild, J., Dean, H.G. *et al.* (1993) Randomised double-blind controlled trial of effect of morphine on catecholamine concentrations in ventilated preterm babies. *Lancet*, **342**, 324–327

27. Choonara, I.A., McKay, P., Hain, R. and Rane, A. (1989) Morphine metabolism in children. *Br. J. Clin. Pharmacol.*, **28**, 599–604

28. Mercurio, M., Nelli, C., Gettner, P., Sherwonit, E., Williams, Jl. and Ehrenkranz, R. (1989) Morphine pharmacokinetics in premature newborns. *Paediatr. Res.*, **25 (71A)**, A408

29. Barker, D.P., Simpson, J., Pawula, M. *et al.* (1996) A randomised, double-blind trial of two loading dose regimens of diamorphine in ventilated newborn infants. *Arch. Dis. Childh.*, **73**, F22–26

30. Elias-Jones, A.C., Barrett, D.A., Rutter, N., Shaw, P.N. and Davis, S.S. (1991) Diamorphine infusion in the preterm infant. *Arch. Dis. Child.*, **66**, 1155–1157

31. Barrett, D.A., Elias-Jones, A.C., Rutter, N., Shaw, P.N. and Davis, S.S. (1991) Morphine kinetics after diamorphine infusion in premature neonates. *Br. J. Clin. Pharmacol.*, **32**, 31–37

32. Marlow, N., Weindling, A.M., Van Peer, A. and Heykants, J. (1990) Alfentanil pharmacokinetics in preterm infants. *Arch. Dis. Childh.*, **65**, 349–351

33. Chay, P.C.W., Duffy, B.J. and Walker, J.S. (1992) Pharmacokinetic-pharmacodynamic relationship of morphine in neonates. *Clin. Pharmacol. Ther.*, **51**, 334–342

34. Quinn, M.W., Otoo, F., Rushforth, J.A. *et al.* (1992) Effect of morphine and pancuronium on the stress response in ventilated preterm infants. *Early Hum. Dev.*, **30**, 241–248

35. Anand, K.J.S., Sippell, W.G. and Aynsley-Green, A. (1987) Randomised trial of fentanyl anaesthesia in preterm babies undergoing surgery: Effects on the stress response. *Lancet*, **1**, 243

36. Anand, K.J.S., Sippell, W.G., Schofield, N.M. *et al.* (1988) Does halothane anaesthesia decrease the stress response of newborn infants undergoing operation? *Br. Med. J.*, **296**, 668

37. Anand, K.J.S., Carr, D.B. and Hickey, P.R. (1987) Randomised trial of high-dose sufentanil anesthesia in neonates undergoing cardiac surgery: hormonal and hemodynamic stress responses. *Anesthesiology*, **64**, A501

38. Anand, K.J.S. and Hickey, P.R. (1987) Randomised trial of high-dose sufentanil anesthesia in neonates undergoing cardiac surgery: effects on the metabolic stress response. *Anesthesiology*, **67**, A502

39. Barrett, D.A. and Rutter, N. (1994) Percutaneous lignocaine absorption in the newborn. *Arch. Dis. Childh.*, **71**, 122–124

40. Rushforth, J.A., Griffiths, G., Thorpe, H. *et al.* (1995) Can topical lignocaine reduce behavioural response to heel prick? *Arch. Dis. Childh.*, **72**, F49–51

41. Barker, D.P. and Rutter, N. (1995) Topical lignocaine as a local anaesthetic in the preterm newborn. *Arch. Dis. Childh.*, **72**, F203–204

# 25

# Outcome

Ann Stewart

As more and more extremely low birth weight (ELBW) infants survive, demands for information about their long-term outcome increase. Society questions the ethics of the survival of such tiny infants and financial constraints mean that cost effectiveness should be examined. In the early 1960s, similar questions were asked about infants who weighed less than 1500 g. Since then the lower limit of survival has moved down until now it is realistically quoted as 500 g in specialist centres in Europe, North America and Australasia; and attention is focused on infants who weigh less than 1000 g.

The first published report devoted exclusively to these tiny infants was made in 1972 [1]. There were few more reports until the 1980s, by which time survival had improved dramatically, as illustrated by results from England and Wales shown in Table 25.1 [2]. By the early 1990s, reports of studies of school-age ELBW infants began to emerge. This chapter will review the literature with the specific intention of providing answers to the questions which parents and society ask about the quality of life to be expected if such tiny infants survive, namely:

(1) What sort of citizens do ELBW infants grow into?
(2) Can good and bad outcomes be predicted; and how soon?
(3) What impact do these infants have on health care and educational resources?

Parents have an immediate need for reassurance; and society is concerned that scarce resources should be spent wisely. Both have to accept that there is rarely a simple choice between intact survival and death; survival with brain damage leading to life-long disabilities has to be considered also, and it should be remembered that it is the most costly option in both emotional and financial terms.

## Source material

Forty-two reports were reviewed [1,3–43], including ten [34–43] which exclusively concerned infants who weighed less than 800 g, recently described in North America as 'Micropremies'. All of these reports were published after 1972 and referred to infants born after 1965. They were chosen because they were the only ones which gave information about both neonatal (28-day) and long-term mortality as well as morbidity, including the number of infants

Table 25.1. Mortality at 7 and 28 days of ELBW infants born in England and Wales, 1981–1989 [2]

| Year | Mortality (%) | |
|------|---------|---------|
| | 7 days | 28 days |
| 1981 | 55 | 62 |
| 1982 | 54 | 60 |
| 1983 | 49 | 54 |
| 1984 | 45 | 51 |
| 1985 | 47 | 52 |
| 1986 | 42 | 48 |
| 1987/8 | 41 | 48 |

**Table 25.2.** First-year mortality and morbidity (disabling neurodevelopmental impairments) of ELBW infants aged less than 3 years, born 1965–1989, calculated as proportions of total admissions from pooled data from reports in the world literature

| Year | Studies (n) | Infants (n) | Died (%) | Disabled (%) | No disability (%) |
|---|---|---|---|---|---|
| **<1000 g** | | | | | |
| 1965–74 | 4 | 416 | 75 | 5 | 20 |
| 1975–79 | 8 | 623 | 68 | 6 | 26 |
| 1980–84 | 11 | 1593 | 63 | 7 | 30 |
| 1985–89 | 2 | 782 | 58 | 7 | 35 |
| **<800 g** | | | | | |
| 1974–80 | 9 | 704 | 68 | 8 | 24 |
| 1981–84 | 2 | 81 | 79 | 7 | 14 |
| 1985–89 | 2 | 241 | 76 | 5 | 19 |

followed up, the methods of ascertainment used and details of the impairments included when defining an adverse outcome. Follow up had been continued until the end of the first year of life in all the studies. The median value for the minimum age at final assessment was 2 years, but final assessments were made at ages ranging from ten months to 8 years, including three reporting the results of assessment at 8 years [30,31,33] and reporting results at least 6 years [32,40]. Confirmation of these reports was also sought in research abstracts presented at meetings of the American Pediatric Society and the Society for Pediatric Research [eg. 42].

Adverse outcome was clearly and consistently defined in all of the reports. Affected infants had neurodevelopmental impairments which caused disability and required specific interventions or management (analogous to 'special needs' as defined in the UK Education Act, 1981) [44]; and they were usually serious and permanently disabling. They included neuromotor disabilities, deafness due to sensory neural hearing loss severe enough to require aiding, partial or total blindness usually due to retinopathy of prematurity, overall developmental delay in the younger children and cognitive deficits (IQ two or more standard deviations below the test mean) in those over the age of about 4 years. In addition, in 14 reports [6,11–14,19,20,27,29–31, 33,38,40] infants were described as having *minor* neurodevelopmental abnormalities which had been defined as deviations from normal development, according to age-specific standards, without disability requiring intervention at the age of assessment. In these studies it was possible to calculate the total

number of infants whose development was in any way abnormal; and by contrast, the numbers of infants whose development could be regarded as completely normal – at least at the age of assessment. Unfortunately, these 14 reports were in the minority, so it was only possible to examine all the data for trends in the proportions of mortality, disabling impairments and survival without disability. The results have been tabulated with long-term mortality, disability and survival without disability calculated as proportions of the total number of ELBW live births enrolled in the study (Table 25.2), and survival with and without disability calculated as proportions of the total number of ELBW long-term survivors (Table 25.3). The results for the tiniest infants weighing less than 800 g are shown separately (Tables 25.2 and 25.3). Table 25.4 shows the results of the school-age studies, including IQ and educational needs.

**Table 25.3.** Morbidity (disabling neurodevelopmental impairments) of ELBW infants aged less than 3 years, born 1965–1989, calculated as a proportion of survivors from pooled data from reports in the world literature

| Years | Studies (n) | Survivors (n) | Impaired (%) |
|---|---|---|---|
| **<1000 g** | | | |
| 1965–74 | 4 | 102 | 21 |
| 1975–79 | 8 | 207 | 18 |
| 1980–84 | 11 | 594 | 20 |
| 1985–89 | 2 | 323 | 16 |
| **<800 g** | | | |
| 1974–80 | 9 | 223 | 24 |
| 1981–84 | 3 | 89 | 26 |
| 1985–89 | 2 | 50 | 26 |

**Table 25.4.    Outcome of ELBW infants at school age (6–8 years), including impairments with moderate or severe disability, disabling neuromotor impairments, mean IQ and proportions in special schools and receiving extra educational provision. Values for infants of birth weight 1000–1499 g from one study are also shown for comparison**

| Study and dates | n | Disabling impairment (%) | Disabling neuromotor impairment (%) | IQ | Extra educational provision | |
|---|---|---|---|---|---|---|
| | | | | | Special school (%) | All extras (%) |
| **<1000 g** | | | | | | |
| Victoria, Australia [30] | | | | | | |
| 1977–80 | 88 | 36 | | 97[a] | 11 | ? |
| Hamilton, Ontario [31] | | | | | | |
| 1977–81 | 129 | >15 | | 91[a] | 14 | ? |
| North Carolina[c] [32] | | | | | | |
| 1980 | 28 | 54 | | 86[b] | ? | ? |
| UCH, London [60,62] | | | | | | |
| 1979–83 | 56 | 23 | 7 | 92[a] | 11 | 30 |
| **<800 g** | | | | | | |
| Ohio[c] [40] | | | | | | |
| 1982–86 | 67 | ? | 12 | 84[b] | ? | 45 |
| **1000–1499 g** | | | | | | |
| UCH, London [60,62] | | | | | | |
| 1979–83 | 259 | 10 | 7 | 102[a] | 8 | 15 |

[a]WISC (R) IQ
[b]K-ABC mean processing composite
[c]6 years of age

## Quality of the source material

Although 42 fully documented reports were found for review, only 11 [13,14,16,21,22,25, 27–31] were population-based. The remainder were from specialist centres where selection for admission was likely to have occurred. Almost all of the studies were small, reflecting the low proportion of ELBW infants among live births. According to one relatively recent UK regional study [21], these infants represented approximately 3 per 1000 live births in the region under consideration who were born in the years 1979–81. Comparable figures for England and Wales in 1982 were 2.6 per 1000 [2], but more recent birth weight-specific data for England and Wales [2,41] indicated that the proportion had increased to 3 per 1000 live births by 1987. These may represent true population differences over time or between an individual region in the UK and the country as a whole. However, they could be the result of variations in reporting policies throughout the country. For example, Dunn [45] showed that the numbers of ELBW notifications in one UK Health District (Avon) increased more than four-fold in 3 years following the adoption of a policy of offering full intensive care to all ELBW infants without congenital malformations. During the same period in England and Wales, the rate of registration remained constant and comparable to the initial rate in Avon.

Variation in notification policy, both in the official guidelines issued and in their implementation, is probably the most important factor accounting for differences in ELBW studies. It is extremely difficult to document for ethical reasons as the lower legal limit of viability rarely corresponds with the biological limit in current practice at any time, yet it affects the interpretation of all data concerning ELBW or extremely short gestation infants. For example, it could be argued that ELBW infants will only be referred to specialist centres for care when they are in good condition, thus producing a bias in the notification of these infants towards under-reporting and favourable results. In contrast, specialist centres themselves will regard as potentially viable even the tiniest infants born within their own units, regardless of condition, which will bias notification in the opposite direction. Confirmation of such differing attitudes between units comes from three studies, including two regional ones in the UK.

In 1987–88, Fenton *et al.* [46] examined how local attitudes to management of extremely preterm labour may influence data on perinatal mortality. They found large variations in the proportion of infants regarded as viable among infants born at or before 27 weeks of gestation in the 17 perinatal units in their region (Trent, UK). Rates ranged from 7.2 to 0 per 1000 live births. By contrast, differences were not noted among births from 28–32 weeks. They concluded that local attitudes have the potential to affect perinatal mortality rates and made a plea for a standard recording scheme for all infants weighing more than 500 g. Similar results were reported by the National Institute of Child Health and Human Developmental Neonatal Network, USA [28] who found inter-centre variability of mortality rates for infants weighing less than 1000 g of about 35% whereas the variability for heavier infants (1000–1500 g) was under 10%. Wariyar *et al.* [47] investigated the outcome of all pregnancies, registered for antenatal care in their region, that ended between 24 and 31 weeks. They were confident that they had full ascertainment and showed small but significant differences from formally collected regional statistics.

A lowering of the limit of legal viability from 28 to 24 weeks of gestation, introduced in the UK in October 1992 [48], should result in a more consistent notification policy in the UK in the future. Meanwhile, data concerning ELBW infants born before the end of 1992 in the UK, or elsewhere if the 24-week limit has not been observed, will still be subject to the variations and biases described above which must be considered when interpreting results. These considerations, however, must not be used as an excuse to disregard the results of all studies of ELBW infants.

Data from England and Wales have drawn attention to another interpretation problem. The national figures for ELBW neonatal mortality in England and Wales, UK are similar to the pooled data (Table 25.1), year for year [2]. The most recent value of 48% is in keeping with 55% in the pooled data derived from published reports and with figures of 50% usually now quoted from specialist centres; and these data indicate a similar acceleration in the downward trend noted in the pooled data, resulting in almost 50% more ELBW survivors in England and Wales in the 5-year period

1983–87 [2,41]. However, there was an even greater reduction in first week deaths that was not sustained in the neonatal figures, providing good evidence of postponement of death from the first week, rather than an absolute fall in mortality. Workers in specialist units have increasingly expressed concern about this effect in recent years and cautioned that age of death must be remembered and considered carefully when interpreting mortality figures, especially changes over time.

The results of the reports reviewed here indicated in general that the proportions of dead, disabled and surviving pre-school ELBW infants without serious impairments were consistent between specialist centres at any one time; and the results of the population-based studies were similar to those from specialist centres for the same years. This finding was noted previously among VLBW infants and was interpreted as meaning that the outcome for such infants depends predominantly upon expertise available at the time [49]. In the case of the ELBW infant, it may also be argued that the results apply to infants registered as livebirths at the time [50]; this at least gives an indication of what can be achieved, given the notification policy prevailing at the time and place under consideration.

## Outcome

During the 25 years under review, infant mortality (total deaths from birth to the end of the follow-up period) fell consistently and significantly ($P<0.001$) among the ELBW subjects of the reports (Tables 25.1 and 25.2). The proportion of infants surviving without disabilities in the preschool period rose correspondingly ($P<0.01$), but the proportion of disabled survivors calculated as a proportion of the total livebirths remained constant or possibly even rose. Until the early eighties, this trend was accounted for by changes in the outcome of the larger infants who weighed 751–1000 g [see references 10,13–15,17,18,27, 29]. Among infants born since about 1986, the trend has also been reported among the smallest infants weighing 501–800 g [41].

Three groups [27,29,43] have reported improvements in morbidity up to 3 years of age as well as in mortality during the past 10 years, based on regional data. Considering the studies independently, the changes in neurodevelopmental morbidity are impressive; 51% down to 30% [27], 24% down to 17% [29] and 16% down to 9% [43]. However, these figures refer only to neurological impairments in very young children, and in one study [27], only to major impairments causing serious disability. In the most recent study [43], change was attributed to a reduction in blindness resulting from retinopathy of prematurity, believed to be due to improved control of homeostasis after birth. As the authors point out, these trends must be interpreted with great caution as the children were too young for assessments of cognitive or fine motor functioning, of visual-motor integration or for evaluation of learning ability and school performance. Hence the values, as for all values derived from studies of such young children, are likely to under-estimate the eventual neurodevelopmental morbidity of ELBW children.

Because, in general, there were no changes in the proportion of disabled survivors, reductions in mortality resulted in significantly more survivors without disabilities detected in the preschool period, but the actual numbers of disabled ELBW children also must have risen. It is this aspect which has caused particular concern among those responsible for health and educational services. Although the proportion of disabled children is small when considered as a percentage of total ELBW live births, it averages 20% in the preschool period when calculated as a percentage of all ELBW survivors and 25% of those who weighed less than 800 g (Table 25.3) in the years covered by this review, and confirmed in several short reports in 1993 [42]. These values support the observation originally made by Orgill *et al.* [13] that among ELBW infants only mortality increases as birth weight decreases; the outcome for ELBW survivors is the same, no matter how low the birth weight. However, the proportions of impaired ELBW children are always larger than those (10%) reported in the heavier infants who weigh up to 1500 g (VLBW) (Table 25.5).

Since 1990, reports have been made concerning the school performance of ELBW survivors born since modern neonatal intensive care became generally available. Two regional case–control studies made at 8 years indicated that on all aspects studied, ELBW children performed appreciably worse than age-

**Table 25.5.** Neurodevelopmental impairments from reports of studies giving data according to birth weights 500–749 g, 750–999 g and 1000–1499 g for children born 1979–1989 and aged 3 years or less.

| | Birth weight (g) | | | | | |
|---|---|---|---|---|---|---|
| | 500–749 (n) | (%) | 750–999 (n) | (%) | 1000–1499 (n) | (%) |
| **With serious disability** | | | | | | |
| Netherlands [25] | | | | | | |
| 1983 | 18 | 0 | 112 | 9 | 640 | 6 |
| **With moderate/serious disability** | | | | | | |
| Merseyside [21] | | | | | | |
| 1979–81 | | | 46 | 15[a] | 276 | 11 |
| Northern, UK [50] | | | | | | |
| 1983 | | | 49 | 16[a] | 171 | 10 |
| USA ICU[b] [23] | | | | | | |
| 1979–84 | 66 | 27 | 114 | 27 | 641 | 10 |
| UCH, London | | | | | | |
| 1981–89[c] | 36 | 19 | 148 | 24 | 373 | 8 |

[a]500–999 g
[b]Pooled data from USA centres offering full level-three care;
[c]Stewart *et al.* 1993, unpublished data

matched classmates whose birth weight was normal [30,31]. Although within the normal range, the mean IQs (91 and 97 respectively) of the groups were significantly lower both than their controls and the test mean (100). More than 10% were in special schools. In a report of a smaller study of slightly younger infants weighing less than 750 g [40], almost half were receiving extra educational provision of some kind. This proportion was compared with 16% of normal birth weight controls, implying that three times as many ELBW infants weighing less than 750 g needed extra help. Results from 56 ELBW infants born in the years 1979–1983 and included in a cohort study of very preterm infants carried out at University College Hospital, London, were similar in many respects [33] (Table 25.4). However, the proportion receiving extra educational provision was smaller, at 30%. Nevertheless, this was approximately double the proportion found among the infants weighing 1000 g or more in the same cohort and, likewise, the proportion estimated for the school-age population in England and Wales [51].

The number of ELBW children born since the introduction of full intensive care who have been studied at school age is very small and justifies only the most tentative conclusions. However, the five studies quoted (Table 25.4)

**Table 25.6.** Probability estimates and 95% confidence intervals of neurodevelopmental impairments at 1 year for neonatal ultrasound brain scan findings at discharge from hospital in ELBW infants and in infants born before 33 weeks of gestation. Values calculated from Stewart *et al.* 1987 [55] plus additional data for infants born and enrolled in the study 1984–89

| | *n, % probability and 95% confidence interval* | | | | | |
| | *ELBW (<1000 g)* | | | *Very preterm (<33 weeks)* | | |
| | *n* | *Disabled** | *Total+* | *n* | *Disabled** | *Total+* |
|---|---|---|---|---|---|---|
| Normal scan or uncomplicated PVH[a] | 117 | 9   8% (3–14) | 39   33% (24–42) | 592 | 23   4% (2–6) | 76   13% (11–16) |
| Ventricular dilatation[b] | 46 | 17   37% (23–52) | 24   52% (37–67) | 91 | 13   14% (7–23) | 28   31% (22–41) |
| Hydrocephalus[c] | 4 | 1   25% (1–81) | 3   75% (19–99) | 14 | 5   36% (13–65) | 10   71% (42–92) |
| Cerebral atrophy[d] | 27 | 15   56% (35–75) | 22   81% (62–94) | 48 | 23   48% (33–63) | 33   69% (54–81) |
| Total | 194 | 42   22% (16–29) | 88   45% (39–54) | 745 | 64   9% (7–11) | 147   20% (17–23) |

*Neurodevelopmental impairments with disability
+Total of neurodevelopmental impairments with and without disability
Ultrasound definitions [55]:
[a]Uncomplicated periventricular haemorrhage (PVH): haemorrhage into the germinal layer or ventricles not associated with ventricular dilatation or marked periventricular echodensities indicating intraparenchymal haemorrhage.
[b]Ventricular dilatation: obvious dilatation of one or both lateral ventricles with cerebrospinal fluid, but insufficient to meet the criteria for a diagnosis of hydrocephalus.
[c]Posthaemorrhagic hydrocephalus: severe dilatation of a lateral ventricle with cerebrospinal fluid such that its width was 5 mm or more above the 97th centile for this dimension.
[d]Cerebral atrophy: loss of brain tissue from any cause, including cysts or irregular enlargement of the ventricular system consistent with periventricular leucomalacia or generalized atrophy of the brain.

gave similar results; mean IQ in the low normal range, more than 10% in special schools and proportions in excess of 25% of children needing some kind of extra educational provisions, usually because of cognitive deficits and learning difficulties. Indeed, the main problem experienced by ELBW children seems to be difficulty with various aspects of learning; and this cannot be diagnosed with certainty until the children have been in school for 2 or 3 years. Hence, preschool assessments probably underestimate the true prevalence of disabling impairments in ELBW children.

## Impact of ELBW infants on the community

Because VLBW births account for a small proportion of all live births, it has been calculated that disabled VLBW survivors contribute not more than 2% of disabled children entering the community in any one year [52]. As ELBW births account for an even smaller proportion of all live births, it is unlikely that they will contribute as much as 1% of the disabled children, in spite of the larger prevalence of

disability. For the same reason, the contribution made by ELBW children to the total who need extra educational provision in school is likely to be small although the available evidence suggests that the proportion needing help may be two or three times greater than that of their full term peers (approximately 15%) [33,40].

## Prediction of outcome in survivors

Early measures or observations which predict long-term outcome in survivors are needed for the rational management of all vulnerable children. Early prediction is particularly important in ELBW infants in whom the full impact of any impairment may not be recognized until at least 8 years of age. Objective measures of brain structure and function in the perinatal period have been developed for predictive purposes. Several have been shown to predict early outcome in VLBW or very preterm infants and in those who suffered birth asphyxia [53,54]. Ultrasound brain scanning is the best researched, and predictive indices have been reported for very preterm infants at 1 [55], 4 [56] and 8 years [33] on the basis of scan

**Table 25.7.**   **Probability estimates and 95% confidence limits of outcomes at 8 years according to neonatal ultrasound brain scan findings at discharge from hospital in ELBW infants and in very preterm infants born before 33 weeks of gestation. Calculated from data included in Roth *et al.* 1993 [33] and 1994 [60], with additional data from Kirkbride *et al.* 1994 [62]**

| | | *Outcome at 8 years* (n % probability and 95% confidence intervals) | | | | | |
|---|---|---|---|---|---|---|---|
| | | *Impairment* | | | *IQ* | | |
| | | *Disabled neuromotor*[a] | *Disabled all*[b] | *Total impaired*[c] | *<80* | *<70* | *Special educational provision* |
| **Extremely low birth weight, <1000 g** | | | | | | | |
| Normal scan or uncomplicated PVH | n=36 | 0 | 5  14% (5–30) | 17  47% (30–65) | 5  14% (5–30) | 4  11% (3–26) | 9  25% (12–42) |
| Ventricular dilatation | n=17 | 3  18% (4–43) | 6  35% (14–62) | 12  71% (44–90) | 7  41% (18–67) | 3  18% (4–43) | 4  24% (7–50) |
| Cerebral atrophy | n=3 | 1  3% (1–91) | 2  67% (9–99) | 3  100% (29–100) | 1  33% (1–91) | 2  67% (9–99) | 3  100% (29–100) |
| Total 'unfavourable'[d] | n=20 | 4  25% (6–44) | 8  40% (19–64) | 15  75% (51–91) | 8  40% (19–64) | 5  25% (9–49) | 7  35% (15–59) |
| Total | n=56 | 4  7% (2–17) | 13  23% (13–36) | 32  57% (43–70) | 13  23% (13–36) | 9  16% (8–28) | 16  29% (17–42) |
| **Very preterm, gestation <33 weeks** | | | | | | | |
| Normal scan or uncomplicated PVH | n=253 | 6  2% (1–5) | 16  6% (4–10) | 81  32% (26–38) | 19  8% (5–12) | 10  4% (2–7) | 31  12% (9–17) |
| Ventricular dilatation | n=37 | 6  16% (6–32) | 12  32% (18–50) | 22  59% (42–75) | 11  30% (16–47) | 6  16% (6–32) | 9  24% (12–41) |
| Hydrocephalus | n=8 | 2  25% (3–65) | 2  25% (3–65) | 6  75% (35–97) | 2  25% (3–65) | 1  13% (1–53) | 2  25% (3–65) |
| Cerebral atrophy | n=17 | 7  41% (18–67) | 10  59% (33–82) | 14  82% (57–96) | 6  35% (14–62) | 5  29% (10–56) | 8  47% (23–72) |
| Total 'unfavourable'[d] | n=62 | 15  24% (14–37) | 24  39% (27–52) | 42  68% (55–79) | 19  31% (20–44) | 12  19% (10–31) | 19  31% (20–44) |
| Total | n=315 | 21  7% (4–11) | 40  13% (10–18) | 123  39% (34–46) | 38  12% (9–17) | 22  7% (5–11) | 50  16% (13–21) |

[a]Neuromotor impairments with disability
[b]All neurodevelopmental impairments with disability
[c]Total of neurodevelopmental impairments with and without disability
[d]Ventricular dilatation, hydrocephalus or cerebral atrophy
For definitions of ultrasound diagnoses, see footnote to Table 25.6.

findings at discharge from hospital. Analysis in one study at 4 years indicated that birth weight did not affect the accuracy of prediction, although the absolute values of the probability estimates for the total of major and minor impairments changed with decreasing birth weight [56]. Probability estimates and 95% confidence limits for outcomes at 1 and 8 years are shown in Tables 25.6 and 25.7 with values for the whole cohort of infants born before 33 weeks of gestation for comparison.

Numbers in the group of ELBW infants were very small, consequently the 95% confidence intervals were wide. Nevertheless, the probability estimate values of disabling impairments for ELBW were similar at the two ages to those for the larger group of very preterm infants. By contrast, the probability estimates of minor impairments without disability, and hence of total impairments for normal scans or uncomplicated periventricular haemorrhage at 1 year were a little larger in the ELBW infants (Table 25.6). A similar effect was noted at 8 years; and at 8 years the differences were noted also in estimates of an IQ less than 80 and of the need for extra educational provision (Table 25.7). Ventricular dilatation, hydrocephalus and cerebral atrophy carried large probabilities for all adverse outcomes at 1 and 8 years in ELBW infants; and the values were similar to those reported for these lesions in very preterm infants, suggesting that scan findings at discharge from hospital can also be used to predict adverse outcomes in ELBW infants as

**Table 25.8.** Probability estimates and 95% confidence intervals of outcome at 8 years for neurodevelopmental impairments diagnosed at 1 year in ELBW infants and in very preterm infants born before 33 weeks of gestation. Calculated from data included in Roth *et al.* 1993 [60] and 1994 [60] with additional data from Kirkbride *et al.* 1994 [62]

| | | *Outcome at eight years*<br>*(n, % probability and 95% confidence intervals)* | | | | | |
|---|---|---|---|---|---|---|---|
| | | *Impairment* | | | *IQ* | | *Special educational provision* |
| | | *Disabled neuromotor*[a] | *Disabled all*[b] | *Total impaired*[c] | *<80* | *<70* | |
| **Extremely low birth weight, <1000 g** | | | | | | | |
| None | n=33 | 0 | 3   9% (2–24) | 12   36% (20–55) | 4   12% (3–28) | 1   3% (1–16) | 6   18% (7–35) |
| Without disability | n=12 | 0 | 2   17% (2–48) | 9   75% (43–95) | 2   17% (2–48) | 2   17% (2–48) | 4   33% (10–65) |
| With disability | n=11 | 4   36% (11–69) | 8   73% (39–94) | 11   100% (72–100) | 7   64% (31–89) | 5   45% (17–77) | 7   64% (31–89) |
| Total | n=56 | 4   7% (2–17) | 13   23% (13–36) | 32   57% (43–70) | 13   23% (13–36) | 8   14% (6–26) | 17   30% (19–44) |
| **Very preterm, gestation <33 weeks** | | | | | | | |
| None | n=21 | 1   <1% (0–2) | 8   3% (1–6) | 73   29% (23–34) | 16   6% (4–10) | 5   2% (1–5) | 25   10% (7–14) |
| Without disability | n=31 | 1   3% (<1–17) | 4   13% (4–30) | 19   61% (42–78) | 3   10% (2–26) | 2   6% (1–21) | 7   23% (10–41) |
| With disability | n=33 | 19   58% (39–75) | 28   85% (68–95) | 32   97% (84–99) | 19   58% (39–75) | 14   42% (25–61) | 24   73% (54–87) |
| Total | n=315 | 21   7% (4–11) | 40   13% (10–18) | 124   39% (34–46) | 38   12% (9–17) | 21   7% (4–11) | 56   18% (15–24) |

[a]Neuromotor impairments with disability
[b]All neurodevelopmental impairments with disability
[c]Total of neurodevelopmental impairments with and without disability

they grow older. For example, the sensitivity of prediction of 'unfavourable' scans for disabling neurodevelopmental impairments at 1 and 8 years was high (Tables 25.6 and 25.7), with values ranging from 100% for disabling neuromotor impairments at 8 years to 79% for all disabling impairments at 1 year and 62% at 8 years. The values for all impairments (56% at 1 year and 47% at 8 years), IQ below 80 (62%) and for extra educational provision (44%) were less good.

The results of structured neurological examination at one year have also been reported to be good predictors of neurological and cognitive outcomes and of school performance in both term [57,58] and preterm infants [59,60]. As for ultrasound, results have not been reported specifically for ELBW infants so recent data relating neurodevelopmental impairment identified at 1 year to outcome at 8 years have also been analysed for ELBW infants [60] and are shown in Table 25.8. These data confirmed that the relation between neurological impairments identified at 1 year

and long-term outcome at 8 years in very preterm infants born before 33 weeks also existed in ELBW infants (Table 25.8). Because neurological impairments at 1 year appear to predict school performance, prediction on this basis is potentially very valuable in the management of ELBW children.

## Can the prognosis of ELBW infants be improved?

Two pieces of information derived from the results of the investigations discussed above into the prediction of long-term outcome of ELBW infants, may provide clues to the aetiology of the poor school performance which appears to be an important cause of disability. They also provide reasons why the outcome of ELBW children is generally worse than that of their heavier peers weighing 1000 g or more (Table 25.4). For example, although the proportion of disabling neuromotor impairments was similar in the two groups studied, the numbers with cognitive deficits and those requiring extra educational provision were significantly larger in the ELBW children [33,60].

Considering first the neonatal ultrasound brain scan findings in ELBW and the infants weighing 1000 g or more in the University College study [33], a significantly larger proportion (30% versus 8%, $P = <0.005$) of the ELBW infants had ventricular dilatation (Table 25.7). In both groups, these lesions carried a large probability of impairment at 8 years [33] (Table 25.7) and affected children had lower cognitive scores and were more likely to be receiving extra educational provision than those with normal scans. By contrast, the proportions of infants with parenchymal lesions that also carried a large probability of disabling impairments were similar (5% versus 8%, NS), as were the proportions with disabling neuromotor impairments (Tables 25.4 and 25.7).

Considering the neurodevelopmental status of the infants at 1 year of age, the proportion of ELBW children in the study who had minor impairments was larger than that in the heavier infants (21% versus 10%, $P<0.025$) (Table 25.8). Like those with a diagnosis of ventricular dilatation, children with minor neurological impairments at 1 year had lower cognitive scores ($P<0.01$) [56] and were more likely to be receiving extra educational provision by the age of 8 years than children without detectable impairments at 1 year [60].

These observations concern very small numbers of children. However, first, they imply that ELBW infants are particularly vulnerable to the type of brain lesions (ventricular dilatation) often associated with periventricular leucomalacia and presumed to be due to hypoxic–ischaemic injury which carry a large probability of cognitive deficits and the need for extra educational provisions. Second, as an appreciable proportion of these children exhibit abnormal neurological signs at 1 year, signs of early neurological damage appear to persist. Thus, it may be inferred that the poor school performance reported in ELBW children is often a consequence of hypoxic–ischaemic insult. Prevention or avoidance of this type of insult should improve the prognosis of these children. Meanwhile, all ELBW infants, and particularly those who have ventricular dilatation diagnosed in the neonatal period with cerebral ultrasound and those who exhibit minor neurological impairments at 1 year, should be regarded as particularly vulnerable to later problems with learning, and receive close surveillance through infancy and their early school years.

## Appendix: follow-up protocol for ELBW infants

As ELBW infants are the highest risk infants to be cared for in neonatal intensive care units, careful follow-up by experienced personnel should be mandatory. Surveillance should continue until the children are established in school and have proved their ability to learn and make satisfactory progress. The following protocol suggests the minimum necessary to identify the abnormalities to which ELBW infants appear to be particularly prone. It assumes that 'normal' surveillance is available, including routine measurements, developmental checks and immunizations.

### In the Neonatal Unit

1. Serial ultrasound brain scans, including a scan at the gestational-equivalent age of term (40 weeks)
2. Other objective measures (magnetic resonance, near infrared, EEG) according to indication.
3. Auditory brainstem (ABR) testing before discharge.
4. Ophthalmological opinion after oxygen therapy discontinued to exclude retinopathy.

*If* a) the term ultrasound brain scan shows ventricular dilatation, hydrocephalus or cerebral atrophy, or definite lesions were identified on another objective measure, the infants should have three-monthly neurological examinations.

b) ABR is abnormal, appropriate referral should be made.

### At gestational-equivalent age of term (40 weeks)

1. Structured neurological examination [61].
2. Measurement of occipitofrontal head circumference (OFC) and weight.
3. Ultrasound brain scan.
4. Confirm ABR done or planned.

5. If visual behaviour is abnormal [62] in course of 1., arrange ophthalmological opinion immediately and visual testing at 3 months [63].

### At corrected age of 12 months

1. Developmental testing with, for example, the Griffiths Developmental Scales.
2. Structured neurological examination [64].
3. Measurement of OFC, weight and height.
4. Clinical examination.
5. Confirm ABR testing done *and* check for conductive loss (distraction testing and evidence of 'pre-language' on developmental testing).
6. Confirm ophthalmological appointments kept and visual testing done as indicated; check for squint.

*If*  a) abnormality diagnosed, refer for appropriate management and on-going surveillance.

    b) abnormal neurological signs without functional consequences noted, ensure child *cannot* be lost to follow-up, or arrange annual review.

    *NB* A. *To exclude spastic diplegia*: if not walking solo at 12 months:

      a) if any passive tone measurement in either leg outwith standard-for-age, and especially if ankle dorsiflexion >70°, review at 15 months (corrected).

      b) if passive tone within standards-for-age, review if not walking solo by 15 months – parents to report.

    B. *To confirm language development is starting*: if no pre-language noted at developmental assessment;

      a) if ABR and distraction testing indicate normal hearing, review at 18 months – or tell parents to return if the child is not talking in phrases.

      b) if any doubt about hearing, refer for oto-audiological opinion; if hearing normal, review at 18 months.

### Pre-school, 4–4½ years:

1. Assessment of cognitive functioning, for example, the McCarthy Scale of Children's Abilities which includes a motor scale [65].
2. Structured neurological examination [64].
3. Pure-tone audiogram.
4. Test of vision.
5. Clinical examination and measurement of OFC, weight and height.
6. Interval history, paying particular attention to seizures, CNS infections or head injuries.

### In-school, aged at least 8 years:

1. Assessments of:
   a) cognitive functioning, for example, the WISC-R [66].
   b) learning processes and achievement, for example the Kaufman Assessment Battery for Children (K-ABC) [67].
   c) visual–motor integration, Beery VMI test [68].
   d) motor impairment, for example the Henderson–Stott test (TOMI) [69].
   e) vision.
2. Neurological examination.
3. Pure-tone audiogram.
4. Clinical examination, including measurement of OFC, weight and height.
5. Standardized behavioural rating.
6. Interval history (as at four years).
7. School report.

## References

1. Alden, E.R., Mandelkorn, T., Woodrum, D.E., Wennberg, R.P., Parks, C.R. and Hodson, W.A. (1972) Morbidity and mortality of infants weighing less than 1000 grams in an intensive care nursery. *Pediatrics*, **50**, 49–49
2. Alberman, E. and Botting, B. (1991) Trends in prevalence and survival of very low birthweight infants, England and Wales: 1983–7. *Arch. Dis. Childh.*, **66**, 1304–1308
3. Stewart, A.L., Turcan, D.M., Rawlings, G. and Reynolds, E.O.R. (1977) Prognosis for infants weighing 1000 g or less at birth. *Arch. Dis. Childh.*, **52**, 97–104
4. Grassy, R.G., Hubbard, C., Graven, S.N. and Zachman, R.D. (1976) The growth and development of low birth weight infants receiving intensive neonatal care. *Clin. Pediatr.*, **15**, 549–553
5. Pape, K.E., Buncic, R.J., Ashby, S. and Fitzhardinge, P.M. (1978) The status at two years of low-birthweight infants born in 1978 with birth weights of less than 1001 g. *J. Pediatr.*, **92**, 253–260

6. Rothberg, A.D., Maisels, M.J., Bagnato, S., Murphy, J., Gifford, K. and McKinley, K. (1983) Infants weighing 1000 grams or less at birth: developmental outcome for ventilated and non-ventilated infants. *Pediatrics*, **71**, 599–602

7. Bhat, R., Raju, T.K.N. and Vidyasagar, D. (1978) Immediate and long-term outcome of infants less than 1000 grams. *Crit. Care Med.*, **6**, 147–150

8. Kumar, S.P., Anday, E.K., Sacks, L.M., Ting, R.Y. and Delivoria-Papadopoulus, M. (1980) Follow-up studies of very low birth weight infants (1250 grams or less) born and treated within a perinatal center. *Pediatrics*, **66**, 438–444

9. Picece Bucci, S., Colarizi, P., Di Tullio, F. *et al.* (1979) Prognosi a distanza di bambini con peso alla nascita di 1500 g o meno. *J. Ital. Pediatr.*, **5**, 583–591

10. Stewart, A.L., Reynolds, E.O.R. and Lipscomb, A.P.L. (1981) Outcome for infants of very low birth weight: survey of world literature. *Lancet*, **i**, 1038–1041

11. Ruiz, M.P.D., LeFever, J.A., Hakanson, D.O., Clark, D.A. and Williams, M.L. (1981) Early development of infants of birth weight less than 1000 grams with reference to mechanical ventilation in newborn period. *Pediatrics*, **68**, 330–335

12. Driscoll, J.M., Driscoll, Y.T., Steir, M.E. *et al.* (1982) Mortality and morbidity in infants less than 1001 grams birth weight. *Pediatrics*, **69**, 21–26

13. Orgill, A.A., Astbury, J., Bajuk, B. and Yu, V.Y.H. (1982) Early development of infants 1000 g or less at birth. *Arch. Dis. Childh.*, **57**, 823–827

14. Saigal, S., Rosenbaum, P., Stoskopf, B. and Sinclair, J.C. (1984) Outcome in infants 501 to 1000 g birth weight delivered to residents of the McMaster Health Region. *J. Pediatr.*, **105**, 969–976

15. Stewart, A.L. (1987) Unpublished data

16. Kitchen, W., Ford, G., Orgill, A. *et al.* (1984) Outcome in infants with birth weight 500 to 999 g: a regional study of 1979 and 1980 births. *J. Pediatr.*, **104**, 921–927

17. Hoskins, E.M., Elliot, E., Shennan, A.T., Skidmore, M.B. and Keith, E. (1983) Outcome of very low-birth weight infants born at a perinatal center. *Am. J. Obstet. Gynecol.*, **145**, 135–139

18. Kraybill, E.N., Kennedy, C.A., Teplin, S.W. and Campbell, S.K. (1984) Infants with birth weights less than 1000 g. *Am. J. Dis. Child.*, **138**, 837–842

19. Walker, D.-J.B., Feldman, A., Vohr, B.R. and Oh, W. (1984) Cost-benefit analysis of neonatal intensive care for infants weighing less than 1000 grams at birth. *Pediatrics*, **74**, 20–25

20. Skouteli, H.N., Dubowitz, L.M.S., Levene, M.I. and Miller, G. (1985) Predictors for survival and normal neurodevelopmental outcome of infants weighing less than 1001 grams at birth. *Dev. Med. Child Neurol.*, **27**, 588–595

21. Powell, T.G., Pharoah, P.O.D. and Cooke, R.W.I. (1986) Survival and morbidity in a geographically defined population of low birthweight infants. *Lancet*, **i**, 539–543

22. Yu, V.Y.H., Wong, P.Y., Bajuk, B., Orgill, A.A. and Astbury, J. (1986) Outcome of extremely low birth-weight infants. *Br. J. Obstet. Gynaecol.*, **93**, 162–170

23. United States Congress, Office of Technology Assessment (1987) Neonatal intensive care for low birth-weight infants: costs and effectiveness. (Health Technology Case Study 38). OTA-HCS-38 US Government Printing Office, Washington, DC, 20402-9325

24. Portnoy, S., Callias, M., Wolke, D. and Gamsu, H. (1988) Five-year follow-up study of extremely low-birthweight infants. *Dev. Med. Child. Neurol.*, **30**, 590–598

25. van Zeban-van der Aa, T.M., Verloove-Vanhorick, S.P., Brand, R. and Ruys, J.H. (1989) Morbidity of very low birthweight infants at corrected age of two years in a geographically defined population. *Lancet*, **i**, 253–255

26. Hack, M. and Fanaroff, A. (1989) Outcomes of extremely-low-birth-weight infants between 1982 and 1988. *N. Engl. J. Med.*, **321**, 1642–1647

27. Saigal, S., Rosenbaum, P., Hattersley, B. and Milner, R. (1989) Decreased disability rate among 3-year-old survivors weighing 501 to 1000 grams at birth and born to residents of a geographically defined region from 1981 to 1984 compared with 1977 to 1980. *J. Pediatr.*, **114**, 839–846

28. Hack, M., Horbar, J.D., Malloy, M.H., Tyson, J.E., Wright, E. and Wright, L. (1991) Very low birth weight outcomes of the National Institute of Child Health and Human Development Neonatal Network. *Pediatrics*, **87**, 587–597

29. Victorian Infant Collaborative Study Group (1991) Improvement of outcome for infants of birth weight under 1000 g. *Arch. Dis. Childh.*, **66**, 765–769

30. Victorian Infant Collaborative Study Group (1991) Eight-year outcome in infants with birth weight of 500 to 999 grams: continuing regional study of 1979 and 1980 births. *J. Pediatr.*, **118**, 761–767

31. Saigal, S., Szatmari, P., Rosenbaum, P., Campbell, D. and King, S. (1991) Cognitive abilities and school performance of extremely low birth weight children and matched term control children at age 8 years: a regional study. *J. Pediatr.*, **118**, 751–760

32. Teplin, S.W., Burchinal, M., Johnson-Martin, N., Humphry R.A. and Kraybill, E.N. (1991) Neurodevelopmental, health, and growth status at age 6 years of children with birth weights less than 1001 grams. *J. Pediatr.*, **118**, 768–777

33. Roth, S.C., Baudin, J., McCormick, D.C. *et al.* (1993) Relation between ultrasound appearance of the brain in very preterm infants and neurodevelopmental impairment at eight years. *Dev. Med. Child. Neurol.*, **35**, 755–768

34. Bennett Britton, S., Fitzhardinge, P.M. and Ashby, S. (1981) Is intensive care justified for infants weighing less than 801 g at birth? *J. Pediatr.*, **99**, 937–943

35. Buckwald, S., Zorn, W.A. and Egan, E.A. (1984) Mortality and follow-up data for neonates weighing 500 to 800 g at birth. *Am. J. Dis. Child.*, **138**, 779–782

36. Hirata, T., Epcar, J.T., Walsh, A. *et al.* (1983) Survival and outcome of infants 501 to 750 g: a six-year experience. *J. Pediatr.*, **102**, 741–748

37. Bennett, F.C., Robinson, N.M. and Sells, C.J. (1983) Growth and development of infants weighing less than 800 g at birth. *Pediatrics*, **71**, 319–323

38. Hack, M. and Fanaroff, A.A. (1986) Changes in the delivery room care of the extremely small infant (<750 g): effects on morbidity and outcome. *N. Engl. J. Med.*, **314**, 660–664

39. Hoffman, E.L. and Bennett, F.C. (1990) Birth weight less than 800 grams: changing outcomes and influences of gender and gestation number. *Pediatrics*, **86**, 27–34

40. Hack, M., Taylor, G., Klein, N. and Eiben, R. (1993) Outcome of <750gm birthweight children at school age. A regional study. *Pediatr. Res.*, **33**, 262A

41. Roberton, N.R.C. (1993) Should we look after babies less than 800 g?. *Arch. Dis. Childh.*, **68**, 326–329

42. American Pediatric Society and the Society for Pediatric Research (1993) Proceedings of 1993 Spring Meetings. *Pediatr. Res.*, **33**, 264A–279A

43. Perlman, M., Claris, O., Hao, Y. *et al.* (1995) Secular changes in the outcomes to eighteen to twenty-four months of age of extremely low birth weight infants, with adjustment for changes in risk factors and severity of illness. *J. Pediatr.*, **126**, 75–87

44. UK Education Act, 1981

45. Dunn, P.M. (1985) Fetal viability: a perinatal viewpoint. In *Preterm Labour and its Consequences* (R. Beard and F. Sharp, eds), Royal College of Obstetricians and Gynaecologists, London, pp. 295–301

46. Fenton, A.C., Field, D.J., Mason, E. and Clarke, M. (1990) Attitudes to viability of preterm infants and their effect on figures for perinatal mortality. *Br. Med. J.*, **300**, 434–436

47. Wariyar, U., Richmond, S. and Hey, E. (1989) Pregnancy outcome at 24–31 weeks' gestation: mortality. *Arch. Dis. Childh.*, **64**, 670–677

48. The UK Still-birth (Definition) Act, 1992

49. Koops, B.L., Morgan, L.J. and Battaglia, F.C. (1982) Neonatal mortality risk in relation to birth weight and gestational age: update. *J. Pediatr.*, **101**, 969–977

50. Wariyar, U., Richmond, S. and Hey, E. (1989) Pregnancy outcome at 24–31 weeks' gestation: neonatal survivors. *Arch. Dis. Childh.*, **64**, 678–686

51. Polnay, L. and Hull, D. (1993) *Community paediatrics* (2nd edn). Churchill Livingstone, Edinburgh

52. Alberman, E. (1982) The epidemiology of congenital defects: a pragmatic approach. In *Paediatric Research: A Genetic Approach* (M. Adinolfi, P. Benson, F. Giannelli and M. Seller, eds), Heinemann, London, pp. 1–12

53. Stewart, A.L. (1988) Prediction of long-term outcome in high-risk infants: the use of objective measures of brain structure and function in the neonatal intensive care unit. In *Baillière's Clinical Obstetrics and Gynaecology; Antenatal and Perinatal Causes of Handicap* (N. Patel, ed.), Baillière Tindall/WB Saunders, London, **2**, pp. 221–236

54. Stewart, A.L. (1993) Measures of outcome in the newborn. *Br. J. Obstet. Gynaecol.*, **100**, 711–713

55. Stewart, A.L., Reynolds, E.O.R., Hope, P.L. *et al.* (1987) Probability of neurodevelopmental disorders estimated from ultrasound appearance of brain in very preterm infants. *Dev. Med. Child. Neurol.*, **20**, 3–11

56. Costello, A.M. de L., Hamilton, P.A., Baudin, J. *et al.* (1988) Prediction of neurodevelopmental impairment at four years from beam ultrasound appearance of very preterm infants. *Dev. Med. Child. Neurol.*, **30**, 711–722

57. Amiel-Tison, C., Dube, R., Garel, M. and Jequier, J.C. (1984) Outcome at age 5 years of full term infants with transient neurologic abnormalities in the first year of life. In *Intensive Care in the Newborn*, Volume IV (L. Stern, ed.), Masson, New York, pp. 247–257

58. Pe Benito, R., Santello, M.D., Faxas, T.A., Ferretti, C. and Fisch, C.B. (1989) Residual developmental disabilities in children with transient hypertonicity in infants. *Pediatr. Neurol.*, **5**, 154–160

59. Stewart, A.L., Costello, A.M. de L., Hamilton, P.A., Baudin, J., Bradford, B.C. and Reynolds, E.O.R. (1989) Relation between neurodevelopmental status at one and four years in very preterm infants. *Dev. Med. Child. Neurol.*, **33**, 756–765

60. Roth, S.C., Baudin, J., Pezzani-Goldsmith, M., Townsend, J., Reynolds, E.O.R. and Stewart, A.L. (1994) Relation between neurodevelopmental status of very preterm infants at one and eight years. *Dev. Med. Child. Neurol.*, **36**, 1049–1062

61. Amiel-Tison, C. (1995) Clinical assessment of the infant nervous system. In: *Fetal and Neonatal Neurology and Neurosurgery* (2nd edn), (M.I. Levene and R.J. Lilford, eds), Churchill Livingstone, London, pp. 83–104

62. Kirkbride, V., Baudin, J., Townsend, J. *et al.* (1994) Neonatal visual responses and neurodevelopmental outcomes at 8 years in very preterm infants. (Abstract) *Pediatr. Res.*, **35**, 274

63. Atkinson, J. (1993) Cambridge assessment and screening of vision in high risk infants and young children. In *At Risk Infants: Intervention, Families and Research* (N.J. Anastasiow, S. Harel, eds) Paul H. Brooks Publishing, Baltimore, pp. 35–36

64. Amiel-Tison, C. and Stewart, A. (1989) Follow-up studies during the first five years of life: a pervasive assessment of neurological function. *Arch. Dis. Childh.*, **64**, 496–502

65. McCarthy, P. (1972) *McCarthy Scale of Children's Abilities*. The Psychological Corporation, New York

66. *Weschler Intelligence Scale for Children (WISC-III)* (1994) Psychological Corporation, New York and London

67. *Kaufman Assessment Battery for Children* (1983) American Guidance Inc, Circle Pines

68. Beery, K.E. (1989) *Developmental test of visual-motor integration*. Modern Curriculum Press, Cleveland

69. Henderson, E.H., Stott, H.D. and Moyes, F.A. (1987) *Test of Motor Impairment*. Harecourt Brace Jovanovich, London

# 26

# Ethical issues

## David Harvey

The birth of a baby is a major event for any family, but it is a crisis when the baby is born very prematurely, particularly when there are severe illnesses or congenital malformations. The care of such babies requires great medical and nursing skill and raises major financial and ethical issues [1,2]. It has been said that the care of the newborn baby is a minefield for those concerned with ethics in medicine; there are certainly many problems for the carers – there are even more for the parents. Even if the baby is relatively well, the equipment in the intensive care unit and the worry that the baby might die suddenly puts a great strain on most parents.

Some of the issues raised in this chapter are also discussed in other parts of the book, but they demonstrate the complexity of day-to-day work in a neonatal unit. This chapter could be used to suggest topics for discussion during seminars on ethics in perinatal care.

## Survival and prematurity

The strain on parents must always be recognized when we assess the remarkable medical and nursing advances in the last 2 decades which allow many babies to survive today who would have died in the past [3]. Several decades ago, the mortality of small babies was very high, as it is still today in many parts of the world. In the nationwide British survey of 1946, no baby under 1000 g survived, whereas it is now an everyday experience to see the care of such babies in modern neonatal units; 1000 g is the median birth weight at 28 weeks' gestation and the chance of survival of such a baby in a developed country today is 90% or more. Babies born at 23 weeks' gestation now survive and there is an occasional survivor at a presumed gestation of 22 weeks. At present one might expect a survival of 90% at 28 weeks, about 60% at 26–27 weeks, 20–40% at 24–25 weeks, but only about 5% at 23 weeks. Mortality rates are constantly improving because of the use of ventilation and other techniques of intensive care, but there must be doubt about the future because of the prolonged intensive care needed at 23 weeks' gestation. Everyone must weigh the benefits gained from neonatal care against the risk of later death or survival with serious disability.

In the past, major advances in neonatal care were made with very simple measures. Such techniques are still critical today: babies need adequate warmth particularly at birth; they must be dried quickly; and resuscitation must be available instantly with the use of endotracheal intubation and ventilation. All this means that doctors and nurses must take an active part in resuscitation, rather than waiting to see whether survival looks possible before proceeding. The study by Drew showed a significantly improved mortality in babies under 1500 g if they were intubated electively rather than selectively at birth [4]. This implies that some thought must be given before delivery to the likelihood of survival and whether the baby will be neurologically normal as a result. Most neonatal doctors and nurses have seen disasters when resuscitation was not undertaken at birth, but was attempted an hour later because the baby was still breathing. It is important for the professional team and the parents to have come to a clear decision beforehand and not to change their minds too readily. The ethical issues involved in the decisions about undertaking resuscitation are complex [5], but it is interesting that many people find it easier to withhold resuscitation of a very premature baby than to withdraw treatment some time later when the outlook appears bleak.

The shorter the gestational age, the longer the period of intensive care which is needed to keep the baby alive and in good health. A baby of 23 weeks' gestation may require many weeks, or even months, of ventilation and oxygen therapy before leaving hospital. In addition, there are still concerns about whether there is an increased risk of neurological impairment in babies of very short gestational age. Follow-up figures suggest that 5% of babies born at 28 weeks' gestation are liable to have a major disability as a result of an impairment in the brain occurring during the perinatal period [6]. Many feel that disability is still rather loosely defined, but for most people, professional or lay, a major neurological impairment would include at least the following: cerebral palsy, severe neural deafness, severe visual impairment, or severe mental handicap. These problems may be somewhat more common under 26 weeks' gestation where they are thought to occur in 10% of babies. Some authors have found that the risk of neurological impairment does not increase with decreasing birth weight or gestational age [7], but others have suggested a high risk of impairment at very short gestational ages, such as 23 weeks. The small number of survivors at this gestational age makes prognosis doubtful and larger studies are essential.

One disability has definitely returned – blindness due to retinopathy of prematurity [8], which used to be called retrolental fibroplasia. This was recognized as a major hazard of oxygen therapy in preterm infants in the late 1940s and the 1950s. The incidence of visual impairment from retinopathy decreased when oxygen therapy was restricted in the 1950s and 1960s, although this may have caused the death of a number of preterm babies from hypox-

aemia. In the 1970s and 1980s, it became usual to manage oxygen therapy by measuring the inspired oxygen concentration carefully and monitoring the arterial oxygen by a variety of techniques. These include direct sampling of arterial blood, measurement of oxygen tension through the skin ($tcPO_2$), or the more recent technique of measuring the saturation of haemoglobin with oxygen by shining a light through a peripheral part of the baby's body ($SaO_2$). None of these techniques is perfect, but they do allow closer control of oxygen therapy than in the past. Whereas blindness from retinopathy has largely disappeared in babies over 1000 g, it is now increasing in the babies under that birth weight. It is certainly not clear what is the cause of this increase, as blindness can occur in a baby whose oxygen therapy has been impeccably controlled. The most striking increase in the condition has occurred in the very tiny babies, under 750 g. Now that it is known that retinopathy can be treated by cryotherapy if the retinopathy is recognized early, babies' eyes should be examined at about the equivalent of 32 weeks' gestation and every 2 weeks until discharge from hospital. This can preserve vision in many babies who would otherwise become blind.

The use of ultrasound to produce a bedside image of the baby's brain has been a major advance, but there is a danger that the images may cause professionals to advise on outcome. Cerebral ultrasound was discovered to be a practical diagnostic tool in the late 1970s and is now commonplace in neonatal units [9]. Intraventricular haemorrhage is easily recognized; such bleeding into the cavities of the brain is characteristic of preterm babies. When it was first recognized on ultrasound, many parents were given a very gloomy prognosis and it was thought that such bleeding would inevitably damage the brain. It is very common under 30 weeks' gestation and occurs in the majority of babies under 26 weeks' gestation. There is some evidence that it occurs less often today than a few years ago. Interestingly, the blood is frequently absorbed completely, and brain damage only occurs in two instances: if blood ploughs through the wall of the ventricle into the brain substance itself, like some types of stroke in adults; or where the blood causes a blockage in the circulation of the cerebrospinal fluid so causing hydrocephalus, with gross enlargement of the ventricles and brain damage from stretching the cerebrum. These two complications of haemorrhage are relatively uncommon but have a much worse prognosis [10].

A lesion which has become much more clearly recognized recently is periventricular leucomalacia (PVL). This appears in the brain substance alongside the ventricles, although it can occur in any part of the brain. As a result, lack of blood supply causes infarction with areas of brain death. The damaged areas become cysts which can be recognized on ultrasound after a week or two before they disappear. These lesions now have a sinister reputation as many of the affected babies suffer from cerebral palsy and mental handicap. Ultrasound is thus very useful in making a prognosis about neurological development. Where only a tiny haemorrhage occurs or the brain scan is normal, 10% or less of babies have subsequent problems. Those with mild dilatation of the ventricles have an intermediate prognosis: around 40–50% of babies have problems. The most severe outcome occurs in those who have cerebral cysts as a result of haemorrhage into the brain substance, or where there is PVL: in such cases, 70–100% of the babies are left with clinical brain damage. We are therefore nearer the accurate detection of those babies with a poor prognosis, which would allow a discussion with the parents about whether further intensive care is indicated or not.

In addition to serious disability, many small preterm babies are found at school to have minor problems. They have difficulties with movement, so that they cannot skip or hop as effectively as other children, may be clumsy with their hands, or have difficulties with reading and writing [11]. Such problems, which may be regarded as minor by medical authors, are a source of great anxiety to families. However, it is difficult to know whether such future problems should be considered in ethical decisions about whether babies should receive intensive care or not. Most professionals and families seem to regard cerebral palsy, mental handicap, blindness and deafness as being in a different category compared to relatively minor problems which also commonly occur in many children who were born at term.

Advances in neonatal medicine are continuing; the use of surfactant to treat respiratory failure in the preterm baby has greatly improved survival. This therapy is expensive, but could become cheaper if the substance is produced artificially in large quantities. Methods of ensuring the survival of babies born earlier than 23 weeks, such as by the use of an artificial placenta, have not yet proved possible. It would be more important to prevent premature labour.

## Other consequences of neonatal care

Authors and professionals concentrate on neurological disorders when discussing the outcome of neonatal care, but many other problems may result. At the simplest, there are scars on the skin: it is easy to recognize a child who was a preterm baby by looking at the backs of the hands and wrists. There are tiny, white, pin-prick scars from venous infusions or puncture marks where blood samples were taken from radial arteries. Such scars may seem very minor, but they do show up clearly on pigmented skin. In other circumstances, scars may be much more severe – it is unfortunately common for infusion fluid to escape from a vein into the subcutaneous tissues. In most cases this presents no problem apart from a little bruising, but the skin can become necrotic producing an ugly scar. Children will not remember the intensive care which saved their lives, but may be embarrassed by ugly scars on the backs of their hands; the scars are with them for life, even if they are improved by plastic surgery.

A more serious consequence is chronic oxygen dependency. Such babies today are sometimes sent home on oxygen provided by a concentrator; the families become adept at managing the oxygen therapy and can recognize when the baby is hypoxaemic. Saturation monitors are provided, as well as small cylinders of oxygen, so that the baby can go out on a shopping expedition or to the park.

## Cost of neonatal care

Much more attention is now paid to the economic consequences of neonatal care. Every country has recognized that the demand for medical treatment outstrips the wealth of the community to provide it. This is as true in a developing country, where babies die because there is insufficient money to give them even a bare minimum of medical care, as it is in an industrialized country whose population demands sophisticated investigation and treatment. Even a rich country may deliver such care for most of the population without providing resources for the mentally handicapped, the mentally ill, or the poor.

Neonatal intensive care is, of course, relatively expensive because it is both labour intensive and requires expensive equipment. A number of studies have been done to estimate the costs of neonatal intensive care, and whether the balance of benefits and expenditure is worthwhile. It has been suggested that the care of babies over 1000 g is relatively cost-effective in producing healthy normal children who have required only a short period of intensive care. Intensive care for babies under 1000 g, particularly those under 750 g, is much more expensive and the risk of neurological and other damage is higher [12]. The cost in financial terms is increasingly expensive for these very premature babies because of the prolonged periods of ventilation and other technical support needed. However, the normal survivors in this group of very small babies are very important for their parents.

Added sophistication has been given to analyses by the use of estimations as quality-adjusted life years (QALYs). The principle behind these is that, in order to provide a proper economic comparison, it is important to recognize the financial benefits for a society of keeping a baby alive. A healthy survivor who lives for 70 years will contribute money to society which must be remembered when considering the expenditure of saving that individual's life when very young. Such an analysis is popular with paediatricians, because healthy survivors of infant disorders are likely to live a long time and return wealth to our communities. There might not be such enthusiasm for QALYs by geriatricians whose patients wanted treatment but were not so likely to pay society back because they had passed their years of employment.

By using QALYs and other analyses, it has been suggested that neonatal intensive care s not such a bad bargain. Many relatively common procedures in industrialized countries are more expensive than neonatal care; these include coronary by-pass surgery and haemodialysis for renal disorders [13].

There are, however, other costs in neonatal care – those which fall on the parents, both financially and emotionally. The increasing tendency to concentrate medical care in larger departments can produce great hardship for parents. It seems reasonable that large centres would be used for highly technical care; this produces better and cheaper results because of improved teamwork and expertise. The problem is that the centre providing this expert care may be at a great distance from the parents' home and from the hospital where the birth was originally booked. When such rationalization occurs in medical treatment, the costs to the parents are rarely considered and very little compensation is given. In many countries only certain parents, such as the unemployed, receive financial support for travel to visit their sick babies. Initially, the mother will be admitted for her own medical care to the hospital where the baby is receiving treatment. Soon, she will be discharged from hospital because she no longer needs medical care and she may prefer to be at home, particularly if she has other children. The financial costs of travel may be reimbursed or paid in advance for the very poor – those who are unemployed or are receiving some form of income support. The wealthy can manage to pay fares or use their own transport, even though this is a strain, but families who are employed on low income may be very hard hit. This needs careful attention in public policy, as it is likely to become an increasing problem. National publicity campaigns have so far failed to produce much help for these families, but it is essential that pressure should continue. Many charities have sprung up to support medical care; amongst these are some which provide specialized support for families who have to visit their children in hospital. However, one should not rely on charitable support, but expect travel to be part of the costs of providing highly technical and centralized medical care for infants.

Sometimes, improvements in access to hospitals may make things worse for some parents in monetary terms. For instance, many car parks in hospitals have been permanently blocked by the volume of cars from members of staff and visitors, so that it is very difficult for a parent to park a car for a short period for an outpatient appointment. The increasing tendency to charge for car-parking in hospitals has gone some way to resolve this problem as there are now spaces available during the day for outpatients and the cost is relatively modest for each hour. It is, however, very different for families who need to spend the whole day, and every day, at the hospital to be with their baby. The car-parking charges on an hourly basis can make a large hole in the parents' pocket.

Monetary costs are not the only ones. There is an enormous emotional cost of having a severely ill baby requiring many weeks of intensive care. Many parents speak of their distress and the prolonged tension which results from not knowing whether their baby is going to survive or not. They describe the desperate wait for the results of tests or for an improvement in the baby's condition. Although parents usually say that the stress was worthwhile and they appreciate the attempts that are made by the nursing and medical staff to save their baby, it can produce a huge strain on the marriage or the mental health of the parents.

## Involvement of parents in decisions

It is critically important that parents should be involved in decisions about the care of their children. In the past, parents were often not consulted about whether their children should be resuscitated when they were born very prematurely; it has even been said that it would be worrying for parents to be involved in such a decision when they are facing the anxiety of premature labour. It is important that parents should not be asked to bear the burden of making decisions on their own, but it is understandable that they would expect to be asked for their views so that a decision can be made.

There is a problem about how one regards decisions concerning the care of individual babies. It is common to say that all babies must be treated alike, but many people feel that this is not realistic, and that there are relative indications for different babies. To give one example, some people might agree that there is a difference between a baby born at 23 weeks who had been thought to be a miscarriage by an unmarried 19 year old who had not planned the pregnancy, and the baby of a mother of 40 years who had had nine previous pregnancies none of which had produced a live child. We still find it difficult to discuss the subtleties of the decision-making needed in such situations.

There are special difficulties in obtaining consent for research projects. Whereas a parent may be happy with an explanation that a standard drug is being used, they may be very unhappy if the same substance is being used in a careful research comparison with another standard therapy, and may be unnerved by having to sign a written consent form. These difficulties can only be overcome by longer discussions between the staff and the parents.

## Ethical decisions on the neonatal unit

Most ethical decisions involve questions about whether treatment is justified or not. A decision concerning the start of treatment may face a member of the junior medical staff when more senior help is not instantly available; the proper course is then to start therapy and consider later whether it should be discontinued.

It is a constant anxiety for medical and nursing staff, and of course for the parents, that too much treatment is being done and that the baby's life is being prolonged unnecessarily and causing the baby great distress. In some countries, the law unfortunately does not allow a doctor to withdraw life support. In our practice, we face such decisions frequently and treatment is not continued if it is judged to be useless or the outlook for the baby, particularly the neurological prognosis, is very bad indeed. First, the professionals need to discuss the case and reach a consensus about whether stopping life support is justified. The parents can then be approached by a senior member of staff to explain the situation and gently invite their views. This procedure must not be rushed and may require several interviews. The burden of decision making must not be put on the parents, but some have very strong views about the course of action which should be taken. In most cases, the parents are undecided and the doctor may need to suggest that ventilation should be stopped and ask if they will go along with such a plan. Such discussions usually concern very preterm infants, those with serious congenital abnormalities incompatible with a normal life, and babies damaged by severe birth asphyxia [14]. It is often difficult to judge the seriousness of the future for the baby; this will need widespread public discussion in the future, but the parents' views should not be overridden unless they are well outside what society would accept [15].

## Bereavement

Special attention should be paid to the parents when a baby dies. Quite simple measures for providing support have been shown to reduce the risk of mental symptoms in the mother 6 months later [16]. This care involves a sensitive, kind and sympathetic approach from the staff to the problems which the parents face when their baby is dying. It is important to allow them to be with the baby in private when death occurs. This is not always possible when desperate attempts are being made to save the baby's life; but when a decision has been made to withdraw life support, because of a hopeless prognosis, the parents can be given the baby to hold, after the endotracheal tube and monitoring devices have been removed. When the baby has died, two sets of photographs should be taken, of the baby naked and clothed; as parents sometimes do not know at the moment of death whether they want to keep photographs or not. An instant camera is very useful in a neonatal unit, but it should be of the type that allows very close-up pictures to be taken of the baby's face, so that the features are recognizable. The baby can be made to look very attractive when dressed and every hospital should have a place where the baby's body can be viewed by the parents and relatives. Some parents wish to go back many times to see the baby; although this is sometimes regarded as a morbid attachment to the baby by the staff, it is very important for some parents. Every culture and ethnic group has particular requirements for the funeral and disposal of the body. These should be respected carefully; the hospital must have efficient arrangements for advice from religious leaders and with undertakers for the funeral. It is easy to be insensitive and not recognize that what are apparently trivial matters are offensive to some people. For example, christian symbols should be removed from the chapel for those families who have a different religion.

The registration of the death of the baby can be relatively complicated, so the necessary bureaucratic procedures should be explained carefully. Written material can be very helpful and should be available in the common languages which are used by the population served by the hospital.

Many parents find the request for a postmortem examination very distressing, but it is often necessary in order to explain the baby's death fully. Parents sometimes say that they do not like the idea of their baby's body being 'cut up' or that 'the baby has already suffered enough'. The importance of a postmortem examination must be carefully explained: we often say that 'we strongly recommend a postmortem examination to explain your baby's death'.

Follow-up visits are critical. Many parents feel that they do not want a formal consultation with the obstetrician or paediatrician until all the results have been obtained, but they may want to keep in close contact with the staff on the neonatal unit, because they were the people with whom they talked during the distressing time of their baby's illness. Other parents find visits or calls to the hospital where their baby died overwhelmingly distressing. It is common to meet mothers who will avoid passing the hospital and will take a different route on a bus. For such parents, follow-up visits may need to take place at a different hospital.

The interview is best held when the baby's death has been discussed at one of the regular perinatal mortality conferences which are held in all obstetric units. This allows the paediatrician to give as much information as possible and report the conclusions from the multidisciplinary conference. Special appointments may need to be made, such as a consultation with a clinical geneticist to give advice about an inherited disorder and, of course, with the obstetrician to discuss the next pregnancy. It is common practice to recommend a wait of at least 6 months before starting a new pregnancy, so as to allow the mother's physical health to recover and for the family to have sufficient emotional stability for another birth; but all families are different and 6 months may be too long for some.

## Conclusions

The birth of a small baby is very difficult for the parents and for the professional staff. The parents' many questions must be answered honestly and plenty of time is needed for discussion. Full access must be encouraged for parents to visit and stay with their baby. Good facilities, including a bedroom, sitting room, television, and small kitchen are very important. Partnership in care should be encouraged.

# References

1. Campbell, A.G.M. (1988) Ethical issues in child health and disease. In *Child Health in a Changing Society* (J.O. Forfar, ed.), OUP, Oxford, pp. 215–253
2. Griffin, J. (1993) *Born Too Soon*. Office of Health Economics, London
3. Roberton, N.R.C., ed. (1992) *Textbook of Neonatology*. 2nd edn. Churchill Livingstone, Edinburgh, pp. 43–47
4. Drew, J.H. (1982) Immediate intubation at birth of the very-low-birth-weight infant: effect on survival. *Am. J. Dis. Child.*, **136**, 207–210
5. Campbell, A.G.M. (1992) Ethical problems in neonatal care. In *Textbook of Neonatology*. 2nd edn (N.R.C. Roberton, ed.), Churchill Livingstone, Edinburgh
6. Stewart, A.L., Reynolds, E.O.R. and Lipscomb, A.P. (1981) Outcome for infants of very low birthweight: survey of world literature. *Lancet*, **i**, 1038–1041
7. Yu, V.Y.H., Loke, H.L., Bajuk, B., Szymonowicz, W., Orgill, A.A. and Astbury, J. (1986) Prognosis for infants born at 23 to 28 weeks' gestation. *Br. Med. J.*, **293**, 1200–1203
8. Lucey, J.L. and Dangman, B. A re-examination of the role of oxygen in retrolental fibroplasia. *Pediatrics*, **73**, 82–96
9. Pape, K.E., Blackwell, R.J., Cusick, G. *et al.* (1979) Ultrasound detection of brain damage in pre-term infants. *Lancet*, **ii**, 1261–1264
10. Stewart, A.L., Reynolds, E.O.R., Hope, P.L. *et al.* (1987) Probability of neurodevelopmental disorders estimated from ultrasound appearance of brains of very preterm infants. *Dev. Med. Child. Neurol.*, **29**, 3–11
11. Elliman, A.M., Bryan, E.M., Elliman, A.D., Walker, J. and Harvey, D.R. (1991) Coordination in low-birth-weight seven-year-olds. *Acta Paediatr. Scand.*, **80**, 316–322
12. Boyle, M.H., Torrance, G.W., Sinclair, J.C. and Horwood, S.P. (1983) Economic evaluation of neonatal intensive care of very low birthweight infants. *N. Engl. J. Med.*, **308**, 1330–1337
13. Torrance, G.W. and Zipursky, A. (1984) Cost effectiveness of antepartum prevention of Rh immunisation. *Clin. Perinatol.*, **11**, 267–281
14. Whitelaw, A. (1986) Death as an option in neonatal intensive care. *Lancet*, **ii**, 328–331
15. Royal College of Pediatrics and Child Health (1997) *Witholding or Withdrawing Life Saving Treatments in Children: a Framework for Practice.* RCPCH, London
16. Forrest, G.C., Standish, E. and Baum, J.D. (1982) Support after perinatal death. *Br. Med. J.*, **285**, 1475–1479

# 27

# The cost of intensive care

**Richard Cooke**

In an ideal world there would be infinite resources available for health care and it would not be necessary to consider the cost of caring for sick and ELBW infants; but in reality we are forced to do this. In making decisions about resource allocations we reveal something of our attitudes toward our patients, their parents, and our own feelings about disability in later life. In this chapter we will discuss the methods by which the costs of care have been examined, how they compare with the costs of other forms of medical care, and to what extent we are able to and are justified in containing them.

In the earliest days of intensive care for LBW babies, intensive treatment for the infant under 1000 g was rarely attempted. The very high mortality with the techniques which were then available, and the generally low expectations of parents and doctors, meant that no real dilemma existed. Gradually as results improved there was an enthusiasm to extend attempts at intensive care further down the birth weight scale until the first gloomy follow-up reports caused a reappraisal. At about the same time units undertaking intensive care for the ELBW infant became all too aware of the very extended periods of care required by some survivors, particularly those who had developed chronically disabling disorders such as bronchopulmonary dysplasia and post-haemorrhagic hydrocephalus. In countries without a free health service the costs of this care had to be borne mainly by the hospital or university, as the parents could rarely meet the enormous bills generated. Intense interest in the actual costs of care and the factors influencing them has developed as a result.

## Costs

In 1959 Baumgartener, Jacobziner and Pakter [1] reported that the cost of neonatal care for US hospitals was about $25 per day, but it is unlikely that this included many ELBW infants or represented a level of intensive care that we would recognize today. In comparison, a study of costs of intensive care for LBW infants in Calcutta between 1980 and 1983, using 'low cost indigenous human and material resources', showed average daily costs of $7.75 and an improved survival in infants under 1250 g of from 5.6% before the programme was instituted to 23.1% afterwards [2].

By 1978 escalating costs in the US, and in particular the inability of hospitals to collect these from parents of very premature infants, caused a reappraisal of the attitude that 'no cost is too great' when caring for the ELBW infant. Pomerance *et al.* [3] showed that the costs (adjusted for a 94% collection rate) were $450 per day for survivors and $825 per day for non-survivors. Total costs were lower for non-survivors at $14,236 compared to $40,287 for survivors. The high rate of later disability in these infants was recognized in that the authors also quote a cost per 'normal' survivor of $88,058. They conclude: 'It is our belief that the cost of living for infants weighing less than

1000 g at birth is justifiable. Society, however, must be the ultimate judge, for society must pay the bill and reap the benefits and the heartaches as well'. The approach to costs in this paper did not try to take into account any of the long-term costs of care for the disabled, their loss of income and increased use of medical resources in later years, and so an economic appraisal of the value of neonatal intensive care was not possible.

In the same year, however, Marsh, Coleman and Jung [4] drew attention to the serious stress being placed on families who had to meet medical costs of ELBW infants admitted to intensive care. In the following year there was a report of the costs of neonatal intensive care which included the extra considerable transport costs experienced in Denver, Colorado [5]. Day costs for ELBW survivors were $340 and average total costs $24,150. They noted large debts written off by the hospital, and some parents were sued by debt collection agencies. Costs compared favourably with those for adult intensive care, although survival rates were three times higher. Nevertheless, the highest charges were paid by the parents of the babies with the worst outcomes who were usually the smallest.

Phibbs, Williams and Phibbs [6] in 1981, when using a multiple regression analysis to investigate the sources of the high costs in neonatal intensive care, found that three measures of risk – low birth weight, mechanical ventilation and surgical intervention – explained a significant proportion of the variation in individual costs. Variations between institutions in costs were due to differences in case mix. Stevenson *et al.* determined actual costs of care for a geographical cohort of VLBW infants during their first 4 years, and estimated lifetime costs of care for disabled survivors. Birth weight was a poor predictor of lifetime costs, although clinical factors explained 60% of the variance in initial hospital costs, and 30% of the variance of life-time costs and the cost of quality-adjusted lives produced [7,8]. Shankaran *et al.* [9] similarly studied ongoing costs of care following discharge from an NICU in three groups of infants with increasing degrees of impairment. Greater degrees of impairment were associated with higher costs, although some of these costs were due to costs of occupational and physical therapy which the authors pointed out

was of unproven efficacy to date. Even 'normal' survivors had higher costs after discharge than those estimated for rearing ordinary children. More recently McCormick *et al.* showed an average first-year post-discharge cost of medical care for VLBW infants to be nine times that for term infants [10].

In looking for ways in which to contain hospital costs, Pomerance, Schifrin and Meredith [11] examined the theoretical reduction in costs that might be produced by the extension of gestation by admission of mothers in premature labour and the use of tocolysis. By identifying hospital costs for preterm infants they noted a linear relationship between cost of survival and gestational age. Between 29 and 34 weeks this cost an average of $772 per day. Since the cost of admitting the mother to hospital was $310 per day the difference represented a saving of $462 per day ('womb-rent') if that admission resulted in a prolongation of gestation. It was also pointed out, however, that if such an admission resulted in a 24-week gestation fetus being born at 25 weeks the effect would be in the opposite direction. The former would almost certainly die within a short time, but the latter would live expensively with a high chance of long-term sequelae. Although this argument has been repeated elsewhere, evidence that effective tocolysis of preterm labour is possible or even desirable from a fetal point of view in the ELBW is lacking.

Hack and Fanaroff [12] have recorded their anxieties about morbidity costs and outcome of infants under 750 g in Cleveland, Ohio. They noted increasing numbers of very immature infants whose prolonged and extremely complex courses resulted in many poor outcomes and an average cost of care of $158,800 (range $72,110–$524,110). Many of the mothers were socio-economically disadvantaged, young, unsupported and black. Some did not wish to or were unable to care for their infants after discharge and there were late deaths. The authors conclude that 'the implications and cost–benefit ratios of extending the trend whereby intensive care is applied to progressively smaller immature infants must be seriously considered in order for definitive guidelines to be devised'. A recent attempt to offer such guidelines has been made by the Canadian Paediatric Society and others [13].

They recommended no exceptional treatment for ELBW fetuses and infants of 22 weeks and less, but full care for those of 25 weeks and above. Infants with a gestational age of 23 or 24 completed weeks deserved 'careful consideration' before intensive care was undertaken.

In Europe and elsewhere, interest in the costs of neonatal intensive care was not apparent until nearly ten years after discussions had begun in the US. This was probably due in part to the slower development of such units in Europe, and to the effects of socialized health care making costs less immediately evident. In Paris in 1984, a study [14] showed costs to be mainly related to duration of stay which averaged 71 days for ELBW infants. These costs were increased most by the development of bronchopulmonary dysplasia or necrotizing enterocolitis in survivors. In the same year in the UK, Newns *et al.* published a costing study which gave day costs as £235 for intensive care, £122 for high dependency care and £43 for special care [15]. The average cost for an ELBW survivor was £10,000, but for a non-survivor £800, reflecting the short duration of care for the latter also seen in previous US costings. More enthusiastic efforts with very immature babies have resulted in increased costs for those who eventually die in the UK in a way similar to the Cleveland experience with infants under 750 g.

A similar study to that of Newns *et al.* was published in 1986 from Liverpool, UK [16]. It showed very similar day costs when corrected for inflation, but markedly dissimilar costs for non-survivors. They cost nearly as much as survivors, presumably as they survived longer as the result of more energetic care. It is clear that medical policies concerning the approach to the tiniest babies may radically alter the overall costs of a service without necessarily substantially altering outcome. Such factors need to be taken into account when comparing costings. In the same study the relationship between cost and birth weight was examined, as almost all similar studies have shown a negative correlation between the two. A significant correlation was seen but this was found to be largely an artefact produced by grouping the data in 100 g groups before calculating the correlation. When a correlation was sought using data from individual patients, the correlation, whilst still statistically significant, was very weak ($r^2 = 0.04$). This indicates that most of the variance in costs was due to factors other

than birth weight. All other studies had previously calculated correlations with grouped data thus exaggerating the effect of weight on cost and outcome. Further similar attempts at local costing studies have been made in Australia [17–19], Ireland [20], South Africa [21] and Leeds, UK [22] with broadly similar results. Different methodologies, time-periods and currencies make further comparisons difficult.

In a detailed review in 1981, Sinclair *et al.* [23] pointed out that although some of the individual interventions in neonatal intensive care programmes had been evaluated scientifically, their overall effectiveness had not. Such non-experimental evidence that existed derived from referral units and did not describe the effect on the actual population served. They believed that the greatest priority for a full economic evaluation was the care of the VLBW infant because of the very high financial outlay involved and the ethical issues this raised. They also pointed out that 'there was no firm evidence that measures of the use of neonatal intensive care adequately reflect the desire, need, or demand for these services. Indeed it is possible that the supply of neonatal intensive care determines its use, rather than the converse'.

Walker *et al.* [24] performed a cost–benefit analysis on the care of 247 ELBW infants admitted to a single unit over a 5-year period. Using follow-up data in conjunction with hospital and estimated future therapeutic care required by disabled children, total life-time costs were estimated. An inverse correlation between cost and weight was obtained ranging from $362,992 per survivor at 600–699 g to $40,647 at 900–999 g. Estimates were then made at current rates of life-time earnings and these ranged from $0 for the lowest weight group to $77,084 for the highest. Only in the 900–999 g group did life-time earnings exceed life-time costs of care. In a subsequent publication [25], the authors point out the many limitations of their study, and that they have not considered any intangible benefits or what alternatives might reasonably be followed. To answer some of these questions they produced a further cost–benefit analysis for all infants less than 1500 g born in a geographically defined area (Rhode Island) during two periods, 1974–75 and 1979–80. In the former period intensive care was in its initial stages but it was considered to be established in the later period. Costs per survivor over the two periods remained essentially the same, but life-time earnings increased largely as the result of an increase in normal survivors. When costs and benefits were compared an excess of benefit over cost of $1,390,000 in the former period and $3,706,000 in the latter was observed although this was not a statistically significant difference. When ELBW infants were examined as a subgroup, the benefits to costs were –$74,310 in the former period and –$378,774 in the latter period. Increased intensive care for ELBW infants produced an increased life-time deficit for the region.

These findings reflect those of the most detailed study to date by Boyle *et al.* [26] from Ontario in Canada, of the economic aspects of neonatal intensive care. They used outcomes and costs of care before and after the introduction of a regional neonatal intensive care programme in Hamilton-Wentworth County. Two periods 1964–69 and 1973–77 were compared. Health outcomes were expressed in terms of both life years gained and quality-adjusted life years (QALY) gained. The latter were produced using a range of utility values for different health states derived by interviewing parents of school children in the area. These ranged from 1 for perfect health to 0 for dead. As some states were perceived as worse than death by some parents, the range of values extended to –0.39. Hospital costs and long-term costs and estimated life-time earnings were obtained. Cost-effectiveness, cost–utility, and cost–benefit analyses were performed. A 5% discount rate to allow for inflation was used. For infants weighing less than 1000 g each additional survivor produced by intensive care cost $102,500 and $9,300 per life year gained. When utility values were included a cost of $22,400 per QALY was derived. For ELBW infants the net economic loss produced by intensive care was $16,100 per live birth. When subgroups by weight below 1000 g were examined, the results were even worse with a net economic loss of $25,500 for infants between 750 and 999 g (smaller infants still were less costly as they lived for a shorter time and the few survivors did better). The authors suggested that similar methodologies to theirs be used to evaluate other therapeutic interventions so that direct comparisons could be made which would allow more rational use of health care resources. They have published

some approximate comparisons in terms of cost ($US 1983) per QALY: antepartum anti-D prophylaxis, $1220; screening for congenital hypothyroidism, $6,300; post-menopausal oestrogen therapy, $27,000; coronary single vessel graft for angina, $36,000; hospital haemodialysis, $54,000. Using data from their 1983 study, and comparing it with a period 10 years earlier, Sandhu *et al.* [16] were able to produce similar QALY costs for neonatal care of VLBW infants in the UK. The costs were $1500 as compared with similarly estimated UK costs per QALY of £750 for hip replacement and £3000 for renal transplantation.

Further studies on the economic impact of neonatal intensive care become more difficult as its widespread implementation precludes suitable control groups. The biggest step change in survival was produced by the introduction of mechanical ventilation, although the more recent widespread adoption of antenatal steroid prophylaxis and postnatal exogenous surfactant therapy have dramatically improved survival further, and rendered most costing studies published to date obsolete. Because of the apparently high cost of commercially available surfactants, numerous studies have looked at the economic impact of their introduction. Maniscalco *et al.* showed that mortality in preterm infants with RDS was reduced with a concurrent reduction in daily hospital charges of nearly $2000 per week. Hospital charges to produce a surviving infant were $18,500 less in the surfactant-treated group [27]. Mugford *et al.* estimated the economic effects of using both antenatal steroids and surfactant, using data from controlled trials and costs on a regional neonatal unit [28]. Used in all babies below 35 weeks' gestation the cost per survivor was estimated to be reduced by 16%. In infants below 31 weeks, reduction in costs per survivor was lower, and increased survival would lead to increased costs of care of up to 32%. Other authors have reached similar conclusions [29–31]. Similar cost–benefit analyses have been done for other interventions such as the use of erythropoietin for anaemia of prematurity [32]. Despite demonstrable efficacy, the incurred costs of the therapy exceeded the averted costs by $300 per infant.

Many perinatologists writing on the subject of extreme prematurity and its medical and economic costs, preface their comments by saying that the most effective way of producing improvement would be to change the life-style or habits of the pregnant mother. Economic studies clearly show the association between maternal smoking habit [33,34] and cocaine use [35–37] and increased costs of neonatal and subsequent care. Poor antenatal care has also been linked with increased subsequent neonatal care costs [38] and intervention by means of a targeted preterm birth prevention project claimed to reduce the costs of neonatal care [39].

Although in recent years we have learned a lot about costs of care for preterm infants in the neonatal unit, it does not necessarily help the clinician to make daily decisions. While we may recognize that care for infants of less than 900 g birth weight as a group may not pay long-term economic dividends, we are all aware that the majority of those surviving will be normal adults. If a patient's future earning power was the key to decision making for health care in our society there would be no care after retirement. If we use the QALY as a tool for decision making, this will inevitably discriminate between patient groups. It is a useful tool to determine cost-effectiveness, but a relatively poor one for cost–benefit. The health economist feels the need for a mechanism in health care provision whereby the planners may be assisted in improving value for money in the face of an increasing demand for health care with limited resources. The QALY may provide this. It is very important that the methodology is the same when comparisons are made, and so far this has not often proved to be the case.

The clinician's responsibility is not so much the provision of resources, but the effects at an individual level of their restriction. There is a fear that excessive expenditure on the tiny infant with a poor prognosis may deflect funds from the care of the more numerous larger infants who stand a better chance of a good outcome if treated well. The clinician seeks a set of rules that might guide in making non-treatment or selective treatment decisions. Such rules should make meaningful distinctions between classes of patients to be treated or not, but with complex and multiple diagnoses, rules based on a single characteristic such as weight or gestational age will never be adequate or fair. It is necessary to balance equity with efficiency in resource allocation. Clinical decision making involves these bal-

ances, and knowledge of costs can help a clinician in assessment of the efficiency side of the equation.

---

**Practical points**

1. Cost–benefit analyses have not shown positive gains when infants of less than 900 g as a group have been studied. Such analyses cannot be applied to individuals.
2. Economic studies are most useful in examining the merits of competing therapies or strategies.
3. Costs of care for an infant relate well to duration and intensity of care, but poorly to weight or gestational age.

---

# References

1. Baumgartner, L., Jacobziner, H. and Pakter, J. (1959) A critical survey of the New York program for the care of premature infants. *J. Pediatr.*, **54**, 725–729
2. Subramanian, C., Clark-Prakash, C., Dadina, Z.K., Ferrara, B. and Johnson, D.E. (1986) Intensive care for high-risk infants in Calcutta. Efficacy and cost. *Am. J. Dis. Child.*, **140**, 885–888
3. Pomerance, J.J., Ukrainski, C.T., Ukra, T., Henderson, D.H., Nash, A.H. and Meredith, J.L. (1978) Cost of living for infants weighing 1000 g or less at birth. *Pediatrics*, **61**, 908–910
4. Marsh, L.A., Coleman, T.D. and Jung, A.L. (1978) Financial impact to families of less than 1000 g babies admitted to an NICU. *Pediatr. Res.*, **12**, 374–376
5. McCarthy, J.T., Koops, B.L., Honeyfield, P.R. and Butterfield, L.J. (1979) Who pays for neonatal intensive care? *J. Pediatr.*, **95**, 755–762
6. Phibbs, C.S., Williams, R.L. and Phibbs, R.H. (1981) Newborn risk factors and costs of neonatal intensive care. *Pediatrics*, **68**, 313–321
7. Stevenson, R.C., Pharoah, P.O.D., Cooke, R.W.I. and Sandhu, B. (1991) Predicting costs and outcomes of neonatal intensive care for very low birthweight infants. *Public Health*, **105**, 121–126
8. Pharoah, P.O.D., Stevenson, R.C., Cooke, R.W.I. and Sandhu, B. (1988) Costs and benefits of neonatal intensive care. *Arch. Dis. Childh.*, **63**, 715–718
9. Shankaran, S., Cohen, S.N., Linver, M. and Zonia, S. (1988) Medical care costs of high-risk infants after neonatal intensive care: a controlled study. *Pediatrics*, **81**, 372–378
10. McCormick, M.C., Bernbaum, J.C., Eisenberg, J.M.,

Kustra, S.L. and Finnegan, E. (1991) Costs incurred by parents of very low birthweight infants after the initial neonatal hospitalisation. *Pediatrics*, **88**, 533–541

11. Pomerance, J.J., Schifrin, B.S. and Meredith, J.L. (1980) Womb rent. *Am. J. Obstet. Gynecol.*, **137**, 486–490

12. Hack, M. and Fanaroff, A.A. (1986) Changes in the delivery room care of the extremely small infant (<750 g): effects on morbidity and outcome. *N. Engl. J. Med.*, **314**, 660–664

13. Fetus and Newborn Committee, Canadian Paediatric Society, Maternal–Fetus Medicine Committee, Society of Obstetricians and Gynaecologists of Canada (1994) *Can. Med. Assoc. J.*, **151**, 547–553

14. Monset-Couchard, M., Jaspar, M.L., Bethmann, O. and Relier, J.P. (1984) Cout de la prise en charge initiale des enfants de poids de naissance inferieur ou egal a 1500 g en 1981. *Arch. Fr. Pediatr.*, **41**, 579–585

15. Newns, B., Drummond, M.F., Durbin, G.M. and Culley, P. (1984) Costs and outcomes in a regional neonatal intensive care unit. *Arch. Dis. Childh.*, **59**, 1064–1067

16. Sandhu, B., Stevenson, R.C., Cooke, R.W.I. and Pharoah, P.O.D. (1986) Cost of neonatal intensive care for very low birthweight infants. *Lancet*, **i**, 600–603

17. Tudehope, D.I., Lee, W., Harris, F. and Addison, C. (1989) Cost-analysis of neonatal intensive and special care. *Aust. Paediatr. J.*, **25**, 61–65

18. Marshall, P.B., Halls, H.J., James, S.L., Grivell, A.R., Goldstein, A. and Berry, M.N. (1989) The cost of intensive care and special care of the newborn. *Med. J. Aust.*, **150**, 568–569, 572–574

19. Doyle, L.W., Murton, L.J. and Kitchen, W.H. (1989) Increasing the survival of extremely immature (24–28 week gestation) infants – at what cost? *Med. J. Aust.*, **150**, 558–563, 567–568

20. Connolly, M., Fox, G., O'Connor, G., Clarke, T.A. and Mathews, T.G. (1989) Cost of neonatal intensive and special care. *Ir. Med. J.*, **82**, 34–36

21. Malan, A.F., Ryan, E., van-der-Elst, C.W. and Pelteret, R. (1992) The cost of neonatal care. *S. Afr. Med. J.*, **82**, 417–419

22. Ryan, S., Sics, A. and Congdon, P. (1988) Cost of neonatal care. *Arch. Dis. Childh.*, **63**, 303–306

23. Sinclair, J.C., Torrance, G.W., Boyle, M.H., Horwood, S.P., Saigal, S. and Sackett, D.L. (1981) Evaluation of neonatal intensive care programs. *N. Engl. J. Med.*, **305**, 489–493

24. Walker, D.J.B., Feldman, A., Vohr, B.R. and Oh, W. (1984) Cost–benefit analysis of neonatal intensive care for infants weighing less than 1000 g at birth. *Pediatrics*, **74**, 20–25

25. Walker, D.J.B., Vohr, B.R. and Oh, W. (1985) Economic analysis of regionalised neonatal care for very low birthweight infants in the State of Rhode Island. *Pediatrics*, **76**, 69–74

26. Boyle, M.H., Torrance, G.W., Sinclair, J.C. and Horwood, S.P. (1983) Economic evaluation of neonatal intensive care of very low birthweight infants. *N. Engl. J. Med.*, **308**, 1330–1337

27. Maniscalco, W.M., Kendig, J.W. and Shapiro, D.L. (1989) Surfactant replacement therapy: impact on hospital charges for premature infants with respiratory distress syndrome. *Pediatrics*, **83**, 1–6

28. Mugford, M., Piercy, J. and Chalmers, I. (1991) Cost implications of different approaches to the prevention of respiratory distress syndrome. *Arch. Dis. Childh.*, **66**, 757–764

29. Phibbs, C.S., Phibbs, R.H., Wakeley, A., Schlueter, M.A., Sniderman, S. and Tooley, W.H. (1993) Cost effects of surfactant therapy for neonatal respiratory distress syndrome. *J. Pediatr.*, **123**, 953–962

30. Diwaker, K., Roberts, S. and John, E. (1993) Surfactant replacement therapy in neonates less than 32 weeks' gestation: effect on neonatal intensive care resource utilization. *J. Pediatr. Child. Health.*, **29**, 434–437

31. Wach, R., Darlow, B., Bourchier, D., Broadbent, R., Knight, D. and Selby, R. (1994) Respiratory distress syndrome in New Zealand: evidence from the OSIRIS trial of exogenous surfactant (Exosurf). *N.Z. Med. J.*, **107**, 234–237

32. Shireman, T.I., Hilsenrath, P.E., Strauss, R.G., Widness, J.A. and Mutnick, A.H. (1994) Recombinant human erythropoietin vs transfusions in the treatment of anaemia of prematurity. A cost–benefit analysis. *Arch. Pediatr. Adolesc. Med.*, **148**, 582–588

33. Marks, J.S., Koplan, J.P., Hogue, C.J. and Dalmat, M.E. (1990) A cost–benefit/cost-effectiveness analysis of smoking cessation for pregnant women. *Am. J. Prevent. Med.*, **6**, 282–289

34. Oster, G., Delea, T.E. and Colditz, G.A. (1988) Maternal smoking during pregnancy and expenditures on neonatal health care. *Am. J. Prevent. Med.*, **4**, 216–219

35. Phibbs, C.S., Bateman, D.A. and Schwartz, R.M. (1991) The neonatal costs of maternal cocaine use. *J. Am. Med. Assoc.*, **266**, 1521–1526

36. Calhoun, B.C. and Watson, P.T. (1991) The cost of maternal cocaine abuse: 1. Perinatal cost. *Obstet. Gynecol.*, **78**, 731–734

37. Chiu, T.T., Vaughn, A.J. and Carzoli, R.P. (1990) Hospital costs for cocaine-exposed infants. *J. Fla. Med. Assoc.*, **77**, 897–900

38. Wilson, A.L., Munson, D.P., Schubot, D.B., Leonardson, G. and Stevens, D.C. (1992) Does prenatal care decrease the incidence and cost of neonatal intensive care admissions? *Am. J. Perinatol.*, **9**, 281–284

39. Ross, M.G., Sandhu, M., Bemis, R., Nessim, S., Bragonier, J.R. and Hobel, C. (1994) The West Los Angeles Preterm Birth Prevention Project: II. Cost-effectiveness analysis of high-risk pregnancy interventions. *Obstet. Gynecol.*, **83**, 506–511

# 28

# Respiratory audit and the CRIB score

William Tarnow-Mordi, Gareth Parry and Ashley Buckner

*'Clinical audit provides the basis for determining whether cost-effective methods are in use and whether they are being used appropriately. Quality of treatment is influenced by severity of illness, professional skills, staffing, and facilities, and to assess it we require reproducible measures of health that can be applied before and after treatment. Since the lead time between research and practical development is shorter than it used to be, we need to think in advance about the possible impact of new discoveries and techniques upon organisation of care, the workforce, the design of treatment facilities and so on.'*
*Professor Michael Peckham, Director of NHS Research and Development [1]*

The increasing survival of ELBW infants owes much to the efforts and enthusiasm of those who treat them. Without systematic audit of the outcome of care however, these efforts may do more harm than good. ELBW infants with respiratory illness are at much greater risk of death, lung damage, poor nutrition and neurodevelopmental impairment than those without, so audit of respiratory care is particularly important. This chapter outlines a simple system of respiratory audit. It is designed to help busy clinicians improve the quality of perinatal care and its major respiratory outcomes by maximizing the use of effective treatments.

The system is also compatible with studies being conducted within the International Neonatal Network, which is a worldwide collaborative group of over 125 neonatal units. The International Neonatal Network aims to develop accurate predictive models for mortality and major morbidity in preterm infants, to allow more reliable comparisons of the risk-adjusted performance of neonatal units.

## Substantive or surrogate measures of outcome?

Substantive outcomes are important clinical events like death or major morbidity. Surrogate outcomes are physiological measurements or intermediate end points. Although surrogate outcomes can serve as convenient proxies for substantive outcomes, they provide a less reliable basis for clinical policy. For example, acute improvements in gas exchange are sometimes used as a surrogate outcome in trials of surfactant therapy. In the Curosurf 4 trial comparing surfactant regimens in high versus low dose, high doses led to faster improvements in oxygenation at 48 hours and fewer infants requiring $FiO_2$ >40% after 3 days, but there were no differences in death, chronic lung disease or major cerebral abnormality. Based on these substantive measures of outcome, the low-dose regimen was therefore more cost-effective [2]. The system of audit proposed here includes only substantive clinical outcomes.

## Which outcomes and treatments should we audit?

The Concise Oxford Dictionary defines an outcome as a 'result or visible effect'. Not all important adverse events in ELBW infants are a result of poor perinatal care. For example, cases of cystic leucomalacia can originate before birth through unavoidable insults for which no effective treatment exists. If such cases were typical, postnatally detected brain damage would be neither an outcome of antenatal or postnatal care nor a measure of its quality. The system of audit outlined here therefore only classifies clinical events as outcomes if there is good evidence that they can be modified by perinatal or respiratory care. Lethal congenital anomlies are therefore excluded.

By the same token, there is little point in auditing the many treatments which have not yet been shown to be effective in improving substantive clinical outcomes. We have therefore only included treatments if there is convincing evidence that they reduce mortality or major morbidity. Wherever possible, this evidence is based on overviews of well-designed randomized controlled trials (RCTs). Where controlled trials are not available, the evidence is based on observational studies.

Surprisingly few outcomes or treatments satisfy these simple criteria for audit. They are summarized in Tables 28.1 and 28.2.

A major problem in auditing outcomes in individual or small groups of neonatal units is that these events are often infrequent, giving widely overlapping confidence intervals and inconclusive comparisons [3,4]. A more reliable approach is to audit pre-specified outcomes in large groups of neonatal units [5] or in single units over long periods [6–8]. Auditing the use of effective treatments [9] in individual units is statistically more reliable than auditing outcomes, as the number of patients eligible for treatment are much larger than the numbers of outcomes [5–10].

## Evidence that each of the major clinical outcomes selected in Table 28.1 can be modified by perinatal or respiratory care

Overviews and individual RCTs confirm that hospital mortality and cerebral haemorrhage in

**Table 28.1. Suggested outcomes for respiratory audit in ELBW (or any high-risk) infants**

**Short-term outcomes**
1. Death in any hospital before discharge
2. Pneumothorax
3. Chronic lung disease of prematurity with oxygen dependency at 36 weeks post-conceptional age
4. Major cerebral abnormality on any ultrasound scan before discharge[a], defined as:
   - Intraventricular haemorrhage with ventricular dilatation >97th centile but less than 4 mm above 97th centile for gestation [11] OR
   - Any parenchymal haemorrhagic lesion OR
   - Hydrocephalus, defined as ventricular dilatation >4 mm above the 97th centile for gestation [11] OR
   - Porencephalic cyst or cystic leucomalacia
5. Retinopathy of prematurity
   - Prethreshold ROP, according to the International Classification [12,13]

Intraventricular haemorrhage in the first 12 hours after birth may often reflect antenatal or intrapartum rather than postnatal events. The same is true of cystic lesions in the first 10 days after birth [14].

**Longer term outcome**
1. Health status and functional ability at 2 years:
   - This should be assessed by an observer independent of those who provided neonatal care.
   - A minimum dataset for assessment which could be adopted nationally has recently been proposed [15].
   - So far there is little firm evidence that health status at 2 years reflects the quality of perinatal care (see Table 28.4, Figure 28.7 and text).

preterm infants at risk of respiratory illness are reduced by antenatal corticosteroids [16,17], that deaths, chronic lung disease and pneumothorax are reduced by prophylactic surfactant therapy [18–20] and that natural surfactant is more effective than synthetic surfactant [21]. RCTs also suggest that certain methods of mechanical ventilation can increase the risk of pneumothorax [22,23]. Observational studies suggest that pneumothorax may predispose to abnormal cerebral haemodynamics and intraventricular haemorrhage [24,25] and that hypocarbia caused by overventilation may lead to cystic periventricular leucomalacia [26], perhaps because of ischaemia associated with cerebral vasoconstriction. RCTs confirm that hyperoxia is a causal factor in retinopathy of prematurity [27,28] and a recent observational study [29] suggested that incidence and severity of ROP was related to the duration of time that transcutaneous $Po_2$ exceeded 80 mmHg (10.6 kPa). Recently the Multicenter Trial of Cryotherapy for Retinopathy of Prematurity has

**Table 28.2. Suggested treatments for respiratory audit in ELBW (or any high-risk) infants**

| Treatment | Scientific status | Questions for audit in your hospital district or region (Italics indicate suggested measures of good practice) |
|---|---|---|
| Antenatal steroids | ◆ Proven effective in RCTs in over 3000 infants [16,17]<br>◆ Reduce mortality and major morbidity in infants born before 31 weeks' gestation by 60–70% [16,17]<br>◆ Recommended even with ruptured membranes, if there is no chorioamnionitis or other contraindication [16,17,35]. | 1. How many women delivered before 34 weeks' gestation?<br>2. *How many of these received antenatal steroids?*<br>3. How many women delivered before 34 weeks' gestation were admitted <48 hours before birth without contraindication to steroids?<br>4. *What proportion of these received antenatal steroids for over 24 hours?* [36]<br>5. *Are these figures published in your hospital's perinatal report?* |
| Resuscitation with IPPV at birth | ◆ Accepted as mandatory in infants with respiratory failure at birth. This is supported by RCTs [37] and observational data [38].<br>◆ Exact indications are undefined. | 1. *Was there a written protocol for resuscitation in the neonatal unit and labour ward?*<br>2. Were all new SHOs given a formal training course in resuscitation?<br>3. *Are these figures published in your annual perinatal report?* |
| Exogenous surfactant | ◆ Compared with no treatment, surfactant reduced mortality and major morbidity by 40–50% in RCTs in over 4000 infants at all gestations [18].<br>◆ Early or prophylactic treatment was more effective than rescue treatment in infants at high risk of RDS [19,20].<br>◆ Compared with rescue treatment, prophylaxis reduced mortality by 40% in infants <750 g or <27 weeks' gestation but long-term morbidity in the most immature infants is unknown [19,20]. | 1. How many infants born before 32 weeks' gestation were intubated (a) before admission and within 72 hours of birth?<br>2. *What proportion of each group had surfactant within 15 minutes of intubation?,*<br>3. *What proportion received more than the maximum number of recommended doses?*<br>4. *Are these figures published in your annual perinatal report?* |
| Screening and retinal ablation for threshold ROP | ◆ In an RCT of 291 infants of <1251 g birthweight, systematic screening and cryotherapy reduced severe visual impairment by 50% [30]. | 1. *What proportion of infants had screening performed at the appropriate time [13]?*<br>2. *What proportion of infants with threshold ROP had retinal ablation performed at the appropriate time [13,30]?*<br>3. *Are these figures published in your annual perinatal report?* |

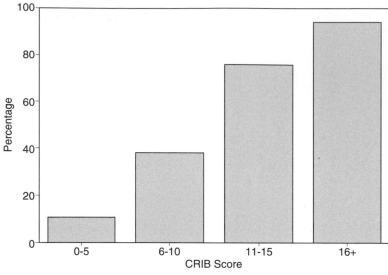

**Figure 28.1** Hospital mortality in 676 ELBW infants by CRIB score, International Neonatal Network, 1992–3

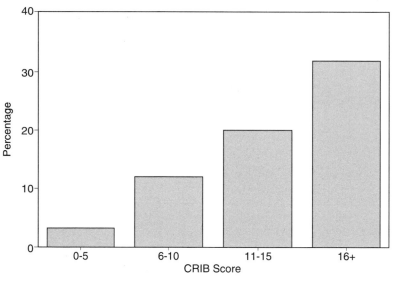

**Figure 28.2** Pneumothorax in ELBW infants by CRIB score. International Neonatal Network, 1992–3

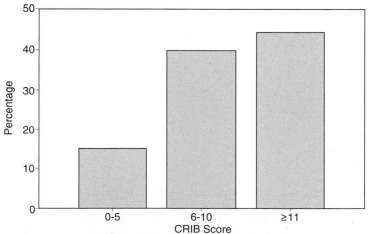

**Figure 28.3** Oxygen dependency at 36 weeks post-conceptional age in ELBW survivors, International Neonatal Network, 1992–3

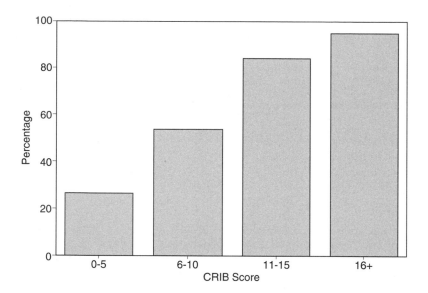

**Figure 28.4** Death or major brain damage in ELBW infants. International Neonatal Network, 1992–3

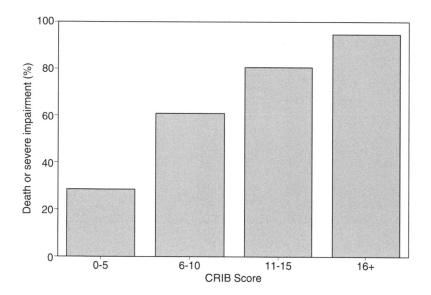

**Figure 28.5** Death or severe neurodevelopmental impairment at 2 years (corrected for gestation) by CRIB score in 271 ELBW infants treated in eight Scottish hospitals in 1988–90

shown that screening and retinal ablative treatment during the appropriate 'window of opportunity' reduce severe visual impairment by 50% [30].

Unpublished observational data from the International Neonatal Network and from Richardson's group in Boston, and a recent publication from Manchester, UK, show that each of the outcomes listed in Table 28.1 is also directly associated with the degree of initial neonatal risk and severity of illness as measured by the CRIB (clinical risk index for babies) or SNAP (score for acute neonatal physiology) scoring systems (Figures 28.1–28.5) [31–34]. These data indicate that illness severity is a major prognostic variable which can be accurately quantified. This is an important finding. It raises the possibility that many interventions which reduce initial severity of illness may improve short- and long-term outcome. It may also allow more reliable comparison of outcome between different types of neonatal unit after stratification of outcomes by differences in initial risk and illness severity – an issue discussed in more detail below.

## Promising treatments which may merit audit in the future

It is important to stress that several other treatments not listed in Table 28.2 appear promising, but have not yet been shown unequivocally to improve substantive clinical outcomes in RCTs. Examples are:

(1)  Effects of surfactant treatment in extremely low birth weight on survival and long-term morbidity [19,20].
(2)  Antenatal treatment in women at high risk of preterm delivery with antibiotics [39,40].
(3)  Delayed clamping of the cord in preterm infants [41].
(4)  Postnatal corticosteroids [18,42–44].
(5)  Inositol supplementation [18,45] in infants with, or at risk of, respiratory illness.
(6)  Neonatal immunoglobulin therapy as prophylaxis or treatment for sepsis [46, 47].

Clinicians are encouraged to participate in well designed controlled trials of these interventions and to keep their status under regular review. The Cochrane Library provides an excellent and inexpensive means of doing this, and is updated every 3 months [48].

## Interpreting differences in outcome between neonatal units

Differences in major outcomes between neonatal units could reflect variations in quality of care, including the use of effective treatments, and differences in the case mix, or degree of clinical risk and illness severity, of each hospital population. Neonatal units which treat many immature or sick infants may easily have higher rates of death and morbidity, despite providing better care than neonatal units which treat infants of low risk. Unless these differences in risk are measured and accounted for, attempts to compare the performance of neonatal units may be misleading [42]. The

CRIB score has been developed as a simple method of adjusting for differences in risk and illness severity between neonatal units, using routine data [31].

## The CRIB score

CRIB was developed using methods similar to those employed in developing the PRISM (Pediatric Risk of Mortality) score in paediatric intensive care [49]. CRIB is based on a logistic regression equation for death in hospital which was derived in a development cohort of 812 infants of >1500 g birth weight of <31 weeks' gestation admitted to four UK teaching hospitals in 1988–90. More than 40 variables, including obstetric and neonatal factors, were screened for their strength of association with death before discharge. Those which were significantly associated with death on univariate analysis were then entered into a multiple logistic model for hospital death. The process yielded only six variables which remained independently associated with hospital death; three clinical variables: birth weight, gestation, and non-lethal congenital malformations, and three physiological variables: the maximum and minimum appropriate oxygen requirements and the worst base deficit recorded in the first 12 hours of life. Obstetric

**Table 28.3.  The CRIB (Clinical Risk Index for Babies) Score**

| | | |
|---|---|---|
| 1. Birth weight (g) | >1350 | 0 |
| | >850 ~ 1350 | 1 |
| | >700 ~ 850 | 4 |
| | ≤ 700 | 7 |
| 2. Gestation (weeks) | >24 | 0 |
| | ≤ 24 | 1 |
| 3. Non-lethal congenital malformations | None | 0 |
| | Not life threatening | 1 |
| | Life threatening | 3 |
| 4. Minimum (worst) base excess in first 12 h (mmol l$^{-1}$) | >−7.0 | 0 |
| | −7.1 ~ −10.0 | 1 |
| | −10.1 ~ −15.0 | 2 |
| | ≤−15.0 | 3 |
| 5. Minimum appropriate $F_{IO_2}$ in first 12 h | ≤0.4 | 0 |
| | 0.41 ~ 0.6 | 2 |
| | 0.61 ~ 0.9 | 3 |
| | 0.91 ~ 1.0 | 4 |
| 6. Maximum appropriate $F_{IO_2}$ in first 12 h | ≤0.4 | 0 |
| | 0.41 ~ 0.8 | 1 |
| | 0.81 ~ 0.9 | 3 |
| | 0.91 ~ 1.0 | 5 |

variables, such as use of antenatal steroids, did not increase the predictive power of the model. This suggests that the effect of steroids on major respiratory outcomes is expressed through a reduction in initial severity of respiratory illness. The six independently predictive variables were subdivided into categories which were themselves independently associated with death. The regression coefficients of each of these categories in the resulting expanded regression equation were calculated. These regression coefficients were rounded up to whole integers, in order to create a more user-friendly score to reflect the risk of death in relation to the degree of clinical risk and illness severity at 12 hours of age (Table 28.3). The higher this score, the greater the risk of subsequent death and major morbidity (Figures 28.1–28.5). CRIB was tested by demonstrating that it accurately predicted death in an independent validation cohort of 488 similar infants admitted concurrently to four different UK teaching hospitals [31]. CRIB performed nearly as accurately as PRISM and SNAP, both of which use considerably more variables, scored over the first 24 hours of admission [32,49].

## Limitations of the CRIB score

One problem common to all scoring systems is that poor early treatment may increase the initial severity of disease. Paradoxically, as this also makes the prognosis worse the predictive value of the score may not greatly alter. Nevertheless this could confound comparisons of the quality of care between neonatal units, by blunting the difference between poorly performing hospitals, where mildly ill patients die because of inappropriate early treatment, and better performing hospitals, where severely ill patients die despite appropriate early treatment. This might systematically bias risk-adjusted comparisons of mortality or adverse outcome *in favour* of hospitals which gave worse care, but only if they consistently did so solely in the first few hours after admission. One effect of inappropriate early treatment may therefore be to *underestimate true differences in performance* between well and poorly performing hospitals. The CRIB score was designed to reduce this postulated 'inappropriate early treatment bias' by reducing

the initial sampling period from 24 to 12 hours. As a result, CRIB may provide a more sensitive comparator for hospital performance than clinical and physiological scoring systems which sample initial disease severity up to 24 hours after admission like the PRISM [49], SNAP [32] and APACHE (Active Physiology and Chronic Health Evaluation) scores [50,51]. The issue requires further investigation.

A further limitation is that CRIB was developed and validated in high-risk preterm infants before the widespread introduction of surfactant therapy. Preliminary data indicate that CRIB remains a robust index of the risk of death in infants treated with surfactant [31]. This suggests that the effect of surfactant in improving major clinical outcomes is linked with its effect on the initial severity of respiratory illness. However, another version of CRIB is now being developed and it is likely that the variables incorporated into the new score and their associated regression coefficients will change (see author's note at the end of chapter).

## Using the CRIB score to compare the performance of neonatal units

Since CRIB is designed to compare the performance of neonatal units, it requires hospital-based rather than population-based cohorts of infants. In epidemiological terms the correct denominator for comparisons is those index infants treated in each neonatal unit rather than all those liveborn to residents of the area it serves. The outcomes of infants transferred from one neonatal unit to another after birth are assigned to the neonatal unit which provided the longer duration of the care between 12 and 72 hours of age. CRIB provides a quantitative estimate of an infant's early clinical risk and illness severity which can be used to compare the effectiveness of care after the initial sampling period of up to 12 hours of age. CRIB is therefore only suitable for risk-adjusted comparisons of the outcome of *neonatal care after the baseline sampling period*, and not of the obstetric or neonatal care which preceded it. A risk-adjusted comparison of the outcome of total perinatal care between different hospitals would require an accurate measure of total risk at the time of antenatal booking.

Preliminary comparisons of the performance of neonatal units using CRIB have suggested a

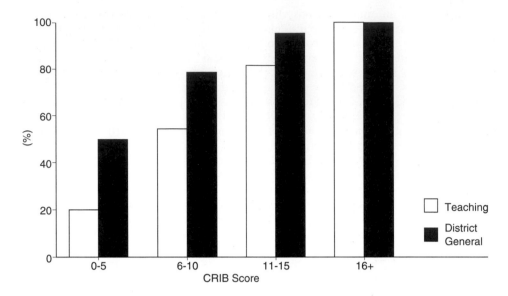

**Figure 28.6** Hospital mortality in ELBW infants by CRIB score: 271 infants treated in eight Scottish hospitals in 1988–90

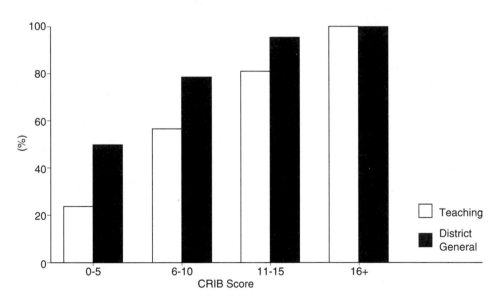

**Figure 28.7** Death or severe neurodevelopmental impairment by CRIB score: 271 infants treated in eight Scottish hospitals in 1988–90

difference in risk-adjusted hospital mortality for preterm infants between nine teaching and four district general hospitals [31] in the UK, in parallel with earlier findings from Trent region [52]. This difference in risk adjusted mortality persisted when outborn infants and the minority of infants (less than 10%) who died in the first 12 hours of age were excluded [31,53,54].

However in a cohort of 271 ELBW infants treated in five teaching and three district general hospitals in Scotland and followed up to the age of 2 years corrected for gestation, there was a significant excess in mortality between district general versus teaching hospitals but no statistically significant differences in death and severe neurodevelopmental

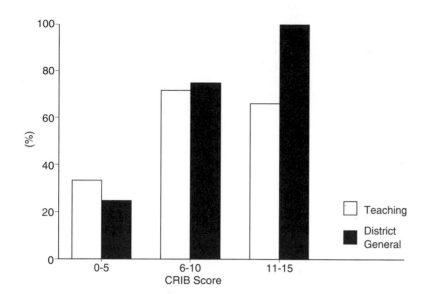

**Figure 28.8** Oxygen dependence at 36 weeks post-conceptional age in ELBW survivors by CRIB score: 271 infants treated in eight Scottish hospitals in 1988–90

impairment, or in severe chronic lung disease (defined as requiring oxygen at 36 weeks corrected for gestation) in survivors (Figures 28.6–28.8, Table 28.4). There were losses to follow up after 18 months, emphasizing the need for systematic assessment of all survivors of neonatal intensive care [15],

It must be stressed that these preliminary findings must not be taken as representative or typical of the UK. Nevertheless, they raise many questions.

Could the apparent differences between certain hospitals reflect differences in important prognostic variables which CRIB does not measure, such as social or obstetric risk factors, which might be more common amongst some populations? Are the differences in risk-adjusted mortality due to disparities in staffing levels, or other aspects of policy, resources or organization? Do certain hospitals achieve higher rates of

risk-adjusted survival at the cost of increased numbers of chronically disabled survivors? These questions cannot be reliably studied using annual league tables [55]. Several of these issues are being addressed in the UK Neonatal Staffing Study, a prospective cohort study of over 6,000 infants in a random sample of 54 neonatal units [56], which will relate outcomes to specific, alterable characteristics of organization, such as patient volume, staffing anbd workload. Research would be much enhanced by the establishment of coordinated national programmes to follow up the health status of high risk infants at 2 years of age or more [15].

One of the pitfalls of comparative audit is to fail to account for the effects of reporting bias, or selection bias between hospitals. For example, among infants born before 31 weeks' gestation in nine Scottish hospitals between 1988 and 1993, fewer of those delivered in

**Table 28.4.** Comparisons of major outcomes up to 2 years of age in 271 ELBW infants treated in three district general hospitals versus five teaching hospitals in Scotland between 1988 and 1990 after risk-adjustment using CRIB

| Outcome | Teaching hospital | District general hospital | Odds ratio adjusted for CRIB | 95% confidence intervals | P |
|---|---|---|---|---|---|
| Death in hospital | 94/203 | 40/68 | 2.54 | 1.31–4.92 | 0.006 |
| Death or chronic oxygen dependency at 36 weeks gestational age | 142/198 | 51/67 | 1.53 | 0.73–3.20 | 0.258 |
| Severe neurodevelopmental impairment in survivors | 14/108 | 1/17 | | | |
| Death or severe neurodevelopmental impairment | 109/203 | 41/68 | 1.70 | 0.90–3.20 | 0.099 |

**Practical points**

1. Outcomes are adverse events which can be prevented or reduced by perinatal or postnatal care.
2. Substantive outcomes, e.g. death, brain damage, chronic lung disease and retinopathy are more important than surrogate outcomes, e.g. acute changes in blood gases.
3. This system of respiratory audit concentrates on these four substantive adverse outcomes and the few treatments which have been proved effective in reducing them
   - antenatal steroids
   - resuscitation at birth
   - early surfactant replacement therapy
   - screening for retinopathy
4. Neonatologists should audit trends in the use of antenatal steroids, but obstetricians are better placed to make reliable comparisons of inter-hospital performance as they can measure the correct numerator and denominator, i.e. the women who received them and those who could have done.
5. The earlier surfactant replacement therapy is given to infants at high risk of respiratory distress syndrome, the more effective it is. This system audits the proportion of infants receiving surfactant replacement therapy within 15 minutes of intubation.

Authors' note: An up-to-date predictive equation for mortality using CRIB is available from Dr Parry at Medical Care Research Unit, School for Health and Related Research, University of Sheffield, 30 Regent Street, Sheffield SD 14A, UK. Email: g.parry@ sheffield.ac.uk. Further information on the Cochrane Library is available from Update Software, Summertown Pavilion, Oxford OX2 7LG.

# References

1. Peckham, M. (1991) Research and development for the National Health Service. *Lancet*, **338**, 367–371
2. Halliday, H., Tarnow-Mordi, W.O., Corcoran, J.D. and Patterson, C.C. (1993) Multicentre randomised trial comparing high and low dose surfactant regimens for the treatment of respiratory distress syndrome (the Curosurf 4 trial). *Arch. Dis. Childh.*, **69**, 276–280
3. de Courcy-Wheeler, R.H.B., Wolfe, C.D.A., Fitzgerald, A. *et al.* (1995) Use of the CRIB (clinical risk index for babies) score in prediction of neonatal mortality and morbidity. *Arch. Dis. Childh.*, **73**, F32–F36
4. Tarnow-Mordi, W.O., Parry, G.J., Gould, C. and Fowlie, P.W. (1996) CRIB and performance indicators for neonatal intensive care units (NICUs). *Arch. Dis. Childh.*, **70**, F79–F80
5. Richardson, D.K., Tarnow-Mordi, W.O. and Lee, S.K. (1999) Risk adjustment in quality improvement. *Pediatrics*, **103**, 255–265
6. Baumer, J.H., Wright, D. and Mill, T. (1997) Illness severity measured by CRIB score: A product of changes in perinatal care? *Arch. Dis. Childh.*, **77**, F211–F215
7. Kaaresen, P.I., Dohlen, G., Fundingsrud, H.P. *et al.* (1998) The use of CRIB (clinical risk index for babies) score in auditing the performance of one neonatal intensive care unit. *Acta Paediatrica*, **87**, 195–200
8. Richardson, D.K. and Tarnow-Mordi, W.O. (1998) Neonatal illness severity and new insights into perinatal audit. *Acta Paediatrica*, **87**, 134–135
9. Tarnow-Mordi, W.O. (1994) Comparing performance of hospitals. *Lancet*, **343**, 1162–1163
10. Mant, J. and Hicks, N. (1995) Detecting differences in quality of care: the sensitivity of measures of process and outcome in treating acute myocardial infarction. *BMJ*, **311**, 793–6
11. Levene, M.I. (1981) Measurement of the growth of the lateral ventricles in preterm infants with real time ultrasound. *Arch. Dis. Childh.*, **56**, 900–904
12. Committee for the Classification of Retinopathy of Prematurity (1984) An international classification of retinopathy of prematurity. *Br. J. OphthalmoL.*, **68**, 690–697
13. Fielder, A.R. and Levene, M.I. (1992) Screening for

district general hospitals received antenatal steroids than those delivered in teaching hospitals [36]. However, this does not prove that district general hospitals prescribed this highly effective treatment less frequently, as it may have reflected incomplete reporting by district general hospitals or the transfer of infants who had already started treatment in district general hospitals to delivery in teaching hospitals. A more reliable denominator population for comparisons of hospital performance would therefore be all premature births, including stillbirths, to women who were admitted to the hospital of birth at least 48 hours before delivery [36] (Table 28.2). As in all epidemiological comparisons, strict definition and ascertainment of denominators is essential.

retinopathy of prematurity. *Arch. Dis. Childh.*, **67**, 860–867

14. Murphy, D.J., Hope, P.L. and Johnson, A. (1996) Ultrasound findings and clinical antecedents of cerebral palsy in very preterm infants. *Arch. Dis. Childh.*, **74**, 105–109

15. National Perinatal Epidemiology Unit and Oxford Regional Health Authority (1994) Disability and perinatal care: measurement of health status at 2 years. NPEU, Oxford

16. Crowley, P., Chalmers, I. and Keirse, M.J.N.C. (1990) The effects of corticosteroid administration before preterm delivery: an overview of the evidence. *Br. J. Obstet. Gynaecol.*, **97**, 11–25

17. Crowley, P. (1998) Corticosteroids prior to preterm delivery (Cochrane Review). In: The Cochrane Library, Issue 4, Oxford, Update Software

18. Soll, R.F. and McQueen, M.C. (1992) Respiratory distress syndrome. In *Effective Care of the Newborn Infant* (J.C. Sinclair and M.B. Bracken, eds), Oxford University Press, pp. 329–355

19. Morley, C.J. (1997) Systematic review of prophylactic vs rescue surfactant. *Arch. Dis. Childh.*, **77**, F70–F74.

20. Soll, R.F. and Morley, C.J. (1998) Prophylactant surfactant vs treatment with surfactant (Cochrane Review). In: The Cochrane Library, Issue 4, Oxford, Update Software

21. Soll, R.F. (1998) Natural surfactant extract vs synthetic surfactant in the treatment of established respiratory distress syndrome (Cochrane Review). In: The Cochrane Library, Issue 4, Oxford, Update Software

22. Bancalari, E. and Sinclair, J.C. (1992) Mechanical ventilation. In *Effective Care of the Newborn Infant* (J.C. Sinclair and M.B. Bracken, eds), Oxford University Press, pp. 200–220

23. OCTAVE Study Group (1991) Multicentre randomised controlled trial of high against low frequency positive pressure ventilation. *Arch. Dis. Childh.*, **66**, 770–775

24. Lipscomb, A.P., Thorburn, R.J., Reynolds, E.O.R. *et al.* (1981) Pneumothorax and cerebral haemorrhage in preterm infants. *Lancet*, **1**, 414–416

25. Hill, A., Perlman, J.M. and Volpe, J.J. (1982) Relationship of pneumothorax to occurrence of intraventricular haemorrhage in the premature newborn. *Pediatrics*, **69**, 144–149

26. Calvert, S.A., Hoskins, E.M., Fong, K.W. *et al.* (1987) Etiological factors associated with the development of periventricular leucomalacia. *Acta Paediatrica Scandinavica.*, **76**, 254–259

27. Kinsey, V.E. (1956) Retrolental fibroplasia: cooperative study of retrolental fibroplasia and the use of oxygen. *Arch. Ophthalmol.*, **56**, 481–543

28. Flynn, J.T., Bancalari, E., Bawol, R. *et al.* (1987) Retinopathy of prematurity: a randomised, prospective trial of transcutaneous oxygen monitoring. *Ophthalmology*, **94**, 630–638

29. Flynn, J.T., Bancalari, E., Snyder, E.S. *et al.* (1992) A cohort study of transcutaneous oxygen tension and the incidence and severity of retinopathy of prematurity. *N. Engl. J. Med.*, **326**, 1050–1054

30. Cryotherapy for Retinopathy of Prematurity Cooperative Group (1990) Multicenter trial of cryotherapy for retinopathy of prematurity: one year outcome. *Arch. Ophthalmol.*, **108**, 1408–1416

31. International Neonatal Network (1993) The CRIB (clinical risk index for babies) score: a tool for assessing neonatal risk and comparing performance of neonatal intensive care units. *Lancet*, **342**, 193–198

32. Richardson, D.K., Gray, J.E., McCormick, M.C. *et al.* (1993) Score for Neonatal Acute Physiology: A physiology severity index for Neonatal Intensive Care. *Pediatrics*, **91**, 617–623

33. Richardson, D.K., Tarnow-Mordi, W.O. and Escobar, G.J. (1998) Neonatal risk scoring systems. Can they predict mortality and morbidity? *Clinics in Perinataology*, **25**, 591–611

34. Emsley, H.C.A., Wardle, S.P., Sims, D.G. *et al.* (1998) Increased survival and deteriorating developmental outcome in 23 to 25 week old gestation infants, 1990–4 compared with 1984–9. *Arch. Dis. Child.*, **78**, F99–F104

35. Royal College of Obstetricians and Gynaecologists. Medical Audit Committee (1993) *Effective Procedures in Obstetrics Suitable for Audit.* RCOG Medical Audit Unit, London

36. Scottish Neonatal Consultants Collaborative Study Group, International Neonatal Network (1996) Trends and variations in use of antenatal corticosteroids to prevent neonatal respiratory distress syndrome. Recommendations for national and international comparative audit. *British Journal of Obstetrics and Gynaecology,* **103**, 534–540

37. Tyson, J.E. (1992) Immediate care of the newborn infant. In *Effective Care of the Newborn Infant* (J.C. Sinclair and M.B. Bracken, eds), Oxford University Press, 28–39

38. Stilwell, J., Szczepura, A. and Mugford, M. (1988) Factors affecting the outcome of maternity care. 1. Relationship between staffing and perinatal deaths at the hospital of birth. *J. Epidemiol. Commun. Health*, **42**, 157–169

39. Mercer, B. and Arheart, K. (1995) Antimicrobial therapy in expectant management of preterm premature rupture of membranes. *Lancet*, **346**, 1271–1279

40. Kenyon, S. and Boulvain, M. (1998) Antibiotics for pretrm premature rupture of membranes (Cochrane Review). In: The Cochrane Library, Issue 4, Oxford, Update Software

41. Kinmond, S., Aitchison, T.C. Holland, B.M. *et al.* (1993) Umbilical cord clamping and preterm infants: a randomised trial. *Br. Med. J.*, **306**, 172–4

42. Halliday, H.L. (1998) Postnatal corticosteroids for prevention of chronic lung disease in the preterm infant. Early treatment (<96 hours) (Cochrane Review). In: The Cochrane Library, Issue 4, Oxford, Update Software

43. Halliday, H.L. (1998) Postnatal corticosteroids for

prevention of chronic lung disease in the preterm infant. Moderately early treatment (7–14 days) (Cochrane Review). In: The Cochrane Library, Issue 4, Oxford, Update Software

44. Halliday, H.L. (1998) Postnatal corticosteroids in preterm infants with chronic lung disease:: Late treatment (>3 weeks) (Cochrane Review). In: The Cochrane Library, Issue 4, Oxford, Update Software

45. Howlett, A. and Ohlsson, A. (1998) Inositol in preterm infants with RDS (Cochrane Review). In: The Cochrane Library, Issue 4, Oxford, Update Software

46. Ohlsson, A. and Lacy, J.B. (1998) Prophylactic intravenous immunoglobulin (IVIG) in preterm and/or low-birth-weight neonates (Cochrane Review). In: The Cochrane Library, Issue 4, Oxford, Update Software

47. Ohlsson, A. and Lacy, J.B. (1998) Intravenous immunoglobulin in suspected or subsequently proved neonatal infection (Cochrane Review). In: The Cochrane Library, Issue 4, Oxford, Update Software

48. The Cochrane Library. http://www.cochrane.co.uk

49. Pollack, M.M., Ruttimann, U.R. and Getson, P.R. (1988) Pediatric risk of mortality (PRISM) score. *Crit. Care Med.*, **16**, 1110–1116

50. Knaus, W.A., Draper, E.A., Wagner, D.P. *et al.* (1985) APACHE II: A severity of disease classification system. *Crit. Care Med.*, **13**, 818–828

51. Knaus, W.A., D.P. Wagner, Draper, E.A. *et al.* (1991) The APACHE III prognostic system: risk prediction of hospital mortality for critically ill hospitalised adults. *Chest*, **100**, 1619–1636

52. Field, D., Hodges, S., Mason, E. and Burton, P. (1991) Survival and place of treatment after premature delivery. *Arch. Dis. Childh.*, **66**, 408–11.55

53. Tarnow-Mordi, W.O. and Parry, G. (1993) The CRIB score. *Lancet*, **342**, 1365

54. Scottish Neonatal Consultants Collaborative Study Group and International Neonatal Network. (1995) CRIB (clinical risk index for babies) mortality and impairment after neonatal intensive care. *Lancet*, **345**, 1020–1022

55. Parry, G.J., Gould, C.R., McCabe, C.J. and Tarnow-Mordi, W.O. (1998) Annual league tables of hospital mortality in neonatal intensive care: longitudinal study. *BMJ*, **316**, 1931–35

56. Tarnow-Mordi, W.O., Tucker, J.S., McCabe, C.J., Nicolson, P., Parry, G.J. on behalf of the UK Neonatal Staffing Study Collaborative Group (1997) The UK Neonatal Staffing Study: a prospective evaluation of neonatal intensive care in the UK. *Semin. Neonatol.*, **2**, 171–179

# 29

# Practical procedures

**Richard Mupanemunda**

The premature infant has a thin skin with little or no subcutaneous fat. However, even the most immature infant has well defined pathways for the sensation of pain [1]. One should attempt therefore to treat pain in neonates adequately during procedures. The preterm infant's skin is also more vulnerable to irritants. Even apparently simple skin preparation for procedures must be undertaken with care. Excess 70% isopropyl alcohol can cause chemical burns if a neonate is allowed to lie in it for any length of time. Gloves should be worn for all procedures at birth and thereafter when contamination with blood is possible.

## Intubation

Extremely low birth weight infants usually require intubation and ventilation at birth (see Chapter 4). Often a brief period of bag and mask ventilation may be required first if the infant is hypoxic or apnoeic. An appropriately sized face mask (e.g. 00 Laerdal Infant Mask) is required and the neck should be slightly extended with the jaw held forward.

For intubation, the baby's neck is slightly extended and the blade of the laryngoscope (7.5 cm straight blade) carefully advanced through the right-hand side of the mouth deflecting the tongue to the left. Advance the blade into the vallecula and pull the epiglottis forward to reveal the larynx. If the vocal cords are not easily seen, the laryngoscope should not be rotated but gently lifted upwards in the direction of the handle. The vocal cords should then come into view and this may be further aided by slight pressure on the cricoid cartilage. With the cords in clear view, a 2.0 or 2.5 mm internal diameter endotracheal tube may then be gently inserted through the vocal cords (Figure 29.1). Withdraw the laryngoscope while the orotracheal tube is held against the roof of the mouth. Connect the tube to an oxygen supply and using a resuscitation bag or by a T-piece occlusion method administer positive pressure ventilation. An effective pressure-release system should be used with the pressure set at 20 cmH$_2$O (1.9 kPa). Adjust the flow and pressure until good chest movement can be observed. Ascertain equal air entry on both sides of the chest by auscul-

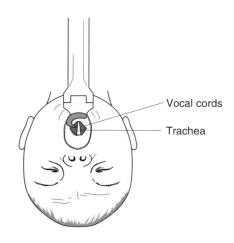

**Figure 29.1** Idealized view of the larynx at laryngoscopy

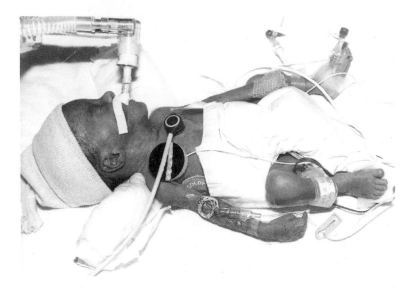

**Figure 29.2** Securing the endotracheal tube

tation. When breath sounds are reduced on the left the tube may have been pushed too far down the right main bronchus.

For nasal intubation a paediatric Magill forceps and a straight-walled tube are required. Lubricate the tip of the tube with K-Y jelly. Insert the tube into one of the nostrils aiming the tip anteriorly. Once the tip of the tube appears in the pharynx, use the Magill forceps to guide the tip through the vocal cords. While holding the nasotracheal tube in place, withdraw the Magill forceps and laryngoscope. Connect to a pressure-limited oxygen supply as described above.

The Cole (shouldered) tube is easier to insert and more suitable for resuscitation and emergencies. The straight-walled tubes (Portex or Vygon) may be more appropriate for long-term ventilation whether placed orally or nasally.

There are various ways of securing the endotracheal tube. One method not requiring special equipment is described. Clean and dry the upper lip and cheeks. Coat the upper lip and cheeks with tincture of benzoin and allow to dry. An H-shaped piece of white tape (e.g. Leukoplast™, Beiersdorf AG, Germany) previously prepared is then held up horizontally and the superior two limbs of the H applied to the upper lip and cheeks. The inferior limbs are wrapped around the orotracheal tube (Figure 29.2). For a nasotracheal tube the inferior limbs of the H-shaped tape are applied to the upper lip and cheeks and the

superior limbs wrapped around the tube. The tube is trimmed to an appropriate size and placement checked radiographically.

## Continuous positive airway pressure

Continuous positive airway pressure (CPAP) may be administered by a nasopharyngeal tube or prongs. For nasal prong CPAP, insert the prongs (Figure 29.3) into the nostrils and secure the prongs to the infant's hat. Connect to a source of positive pressure and adjust the pressure to 5 cmH$_2$O.

For nasopharyngeal CPAP, the procedure is the same as that for nasopharyngeal intubation. Using a laryngoscope to view the pharynx, advance the tube until the tip is just

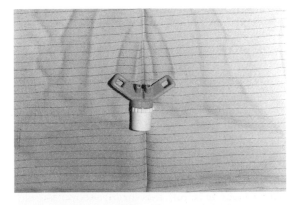

**Figure 29.3** CPAP nasopharyngeal prongs

visible at the margin of the soft palate. The tube is then secured as for nasotracheal intubation, and connected to a source of positive pressure. To prevent the tube from blocking with secretions, it should be suctioned regularly and the oxygen–air mixture humidified.

# Blood sampling

## Capillary sampling

Unless there is oedema of the extremities or poor perfusion, capillary blood obtained by the heel prick method is an extremely efficient method of obtaining small amounts of blood with minimal trauma. Such samples can be used for most biochemical and haematological evaluations. Warming the heel by wrapping the foot in a small towel pre-soaked in warm water improves the capillary free flow. The medial or lateral plantar aspects of the heel may be used (Figure 29.4). Clean the heel with an alcohol swab. The foot is held dorsiflexed between the fingers and the thumb and a clean lancet or stylet used to stab the heel on the medial or lateral aspects. The protruding spike on the stylet or lancet should not be longer than 2 mm or there may be a risk of causing puncture of the calcaneus with attendant infection [2]. A thin layer of soft paraffin wax may be applied just below the stab site to aid blood collection by preventing smearing. The blood should flow freely and should not be squeezed from the

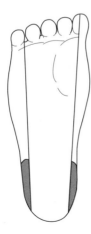

**Figure 29.4** The shaded areas represent sites where heel punctures should be performed for capillary samples, i.e. beyond lateral and medial limits of the calcaneus

heel or scraped from the heel into the containers as excessive haemolysis will occur.

## Venous blood

### *Venepuncture*

Blood may be obtained from any fair sized peripheral vein from scalp veins to the veins of the antecubital fossa. The largest veins are best reserved for percutaneously inserted central lines. The femoral veins should be avoided as they carry a higher risk of complications. The hip joint may be accidentally entered and infected and the adjoining artery and nerve traumatized with the risk of thrombosis of the vessels.

Clean the skin over the vein with an alcohol swab. Apply an occluding pressure to obstruct the venous drainage of the chosen area in order to distend the veins. Holding the skin taut around the vessel to be entered, puncture the skin 2 mm proximal to the vein with an FG 23 butterfly needle attached to a 2 ml syringe. Blood will readily flow into the tubing of the butterfly as soon as the vein is entered. Maintaining gentle venous occlusion while applying gentle suction on the syringe allows blood to flow back into the syringe. Excessive suction will collapse the vein and impede blood flow. A relatively large needle should be used as narrow needles produce a slow flow which predisposes to clot formation in the tubing.

### *Broken needle approach*

This is a very efficient way of obtaining blood for most purposes, except blood cultures. Clean the skin with an alcohol swab and distend the targeted vein by gentle distal occlusion of the regional venous drainage. An FG 21 or FG 23 needle with the hub broken off is then inserted into the distended vein with an immediate flow of blood from the broken end of the needle. The blood is collected in the appropriate containers (Figure 29.5). With continued gentle venous occlusion enough blood for all routine investigations can be obtained. It is not necessary to *milk* the blood out as this causes bruising to the site and produces haemolysed samples. When enough blood has been collected, remove the needle and apply constant pressure to the site until all bleeding has stopped.

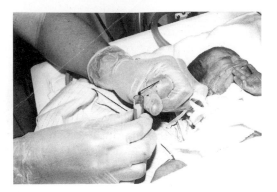

**Figure 29.5** Collecting venous blood by the broken needle method

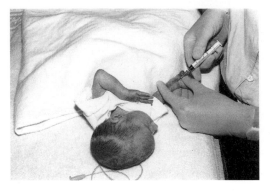

**Figure 29.6** Position for radial artery puncture

## Arterial blood

### Arterial puncture

In the immediate postnatal period only one artery should be used when performing blood gas analysis while sparing the other arteries for an indwelling arterial catheter. Suitable arteries are the temporal, radial, ulnar, posterior tibial and dorsalis pedis arteries. Thrombosis of the femoral or brachial arteries, which may follow arterial puncture, has serious consequences. These two arteries should therefore be avoided especially where repeated sampling is required. The artery to be punctured may be located by palpation or illuminating the limb from behind with a fibreoptic cold light source. The artery will be clearly visible in tiny infants particularly if the site has not been previously bruised.

### Temporal artery

The temporal artery is an end artery which runs just in front of the ear with its branches covering the lateral aspect of the skull. A heparinized FG 25 butterfly needle attached to a heparinized 1 ml syringe is used. Directing the needle towards the neck, the artery or its branches, may be entered at any point. On removing the needle, constant pressure should be applied to the site to ensure complete haemostasis.

### Radial artery

The radial artery may be readily identified by palpation in the lateral third of the flexor aspect of the wrist or visualized with a cold light source. In very small preterm infants the artery may be easily identified as a pulsating hump on the flexor aspect of the wrist. The right radial artery provides preductal samples. First confirm there is a patent ulnar artery by palpation or by showing that the hand remains pink when the radial artery is occluded. Clean the skin with an alcohol swab then slightly extend the wrist (Figure 29.6). The artery is entered at the wrist just proximal to the transverse creases at an angle of 30–45° to the skin. An FG 25 needle attached to a 1–2 ml heparinized syringe, or a heparinized FG 25 butterfly needle also attached to a heparinized syringe may be used. The latter has the advantage of being less easily dislodged from the artery when applying suction on the syringe. Syringes may also be changed over with ease to prevent blood clotting during collection when using a butterfly needle.

### Ulnar artery

The ulnar artery should not be used if the adjoining radial artery has been cannulated or punctured. The procedure for cannulation of the ulnar artery is the same as that for the radial artery.

### Posterior tibial artery

The technique for sampling of the posterior tibial artery is much the same as that already described for the radial artery. This may be more difficult to sample as it is not as easily identified. As a guide, aim for the midpoint between the posterior end of the calcaneus and the posterior border of the medial malleolus.

### *Dorsalis pedis artery*

While holding the foot slightly plantar flexed, the artery may be entered in the midpoint of the foot between the first and second metatarsals. The technique is the same as that described for sampling other arteries.

## Intravascular access

### Intravenous infusion

Peripheral veins initially suffice for the administration of fluid therapy and intravenous drugs. For long-term parenteral nutrition however, percutaneously inserted central venous lines are preferred. There is a significant morbidity associated with all peripheral or central lines. Extravasation of medications, parenteral nutrition solutions or blood from peripheral venous sites can result in extensive tissue damage and permanent scars. Infusion sites must therefore be regularly checked and suspect infusion lines replaced.

Any superficial vein may be used. The most commonly used are veins on the scalp, antecubital fossa, dorsa of the hand and foot, and the long saphenous vein. For fine scalp veins FG 23 or FG 25 butterfly needles may be used. For all other veins Teflon cannulae FG 24 or FG 26 (Jelco, Quick-Cath or Abbocath) are preferable as they last longer. Prepare strips of adhesive tape to be used for securing the cannula. A T-piece extension is attached to a 2 ml syringe filled with heparinized 0.45% sodium chloride. A well padded splint at least 8 cm long will be required (except when scalp veins are used). Wooden tongue depressors must not be used as they are often contaminated with fungi. Having chosen a good size straight vein, clean the overlying skin with an alcohol swab. Occlude the regional venous drainage at a distance from the site to be cannulated in order to distend the veins. Draw the skin taut to prevent the vein from sliding away during cannulation. Excessive pressure will collapse the vein making it difficult to visualize. Puncture the skin 2–3 mm proximal to the vein with the needle bevel facing up and advance the needle slowly towards the vein. With experience a *give* may be felt as the needle enters the vein and blood immediately flows back into the cannula. The cannula should be gently advanced another millimetre

to ensure that the Teflon catheter tip has also entered the vein. With some of the very fine vessels, there may be a very sluggish blood flow back when the vein is entered. Flushing the cannula with a small amount of heparinized saline will confirm whether the vessel has been cannulated. The needle trocar is withdrawn, the T-piece connected to the cannula and then slowly injected with heparinized saline while being advanced further into the vein. Where a butterfly needle is employed, the needle must be advanced as far as possible into the vein. The cannula or butterfly is secured with adhesive tape and finally the limb splinted. For scalp veins, a cushion of cotton wool is prepared with adhesive tape to protect the site. In all cases, the site of entry of the needle into the skin should be left visible to facilitate detection of early extravasation.

### Insertion of a central venous catheter

Full sterile precautions must be taken for this procedure. Specially prepared packs are now commercially available (Vygon, UK). These consist of an FG 23 graduated silicone catheter the proximal end of which is connected to a Luer lock compression hub, which in turn is connected to the infusion set via a Luer lock and an FG 19 butterfly needle. In addition, a sterile pair of fine non-toothed forceps and a 5 ml syringe filled with heparinized 0.45% sodium chloride are required.

The most suitable veins are the superficial temporal vein, external jugular vein, medial antecubital veins, or long saphenous vein on the medial aspect of the ankle. Measure the distance from the target site to the midpoint of the sternum. Clean the entire limb or a large area surrounding the temporal vein with iodine and cover with drapes. Flush the catheter with heparinized 0.45% sodium chloride. Using the fine toothed forceps thread the tip of the catheter 2–3 cm into the FG 19 butterfly needle. The catheter tip should not protrude from the sharp end of the needle. Distend the targeted vein by occluding it distally then approach the vein at a very acute angle (<30°) with the bevel of the needle upward. Once in the vein, blood immediately flows back into the needle and catheter with some blood seeping between the needle and the pre-threaded catheter. Pre-threading the catheter avoids unnecessary blood loss from the brisk bleeding which may occur once the FG 19 needle has entered the vein. Thread the catheter through the needle until a catheter length equal to the measured distance plus 2 cm has been threaded up the vein. Disconnect the catheter from the compression hub by loosening the blue hub. The blue hub should not be separated from its coupling clear hub as the interlinking washer may be lost. Remove the needle, re-insert the catheter into the compression hub and tighten it. Blood should rapidly flow back into the catheter if gentle suction is applied. If this does not occur the catheter may have been advanced too far and should be pulled back while applying gentle suction. Once a good blood flow back is obtained re-flush the system. Coil any excess catheter tubing besides the puncture site and cover with a neatly cut 1 cm square sterile gauze before covering the entire assembly with an occlusive transparent dressing (e.g. Tegaderm™, 3M, USA) (Figure 29.2).

The position of the catheter tip must be checked radiographically. Some 0.2–0.4 ml of contrast media (e.g. Omnipaque™, Nycomed, UK) may be injected into the catheter during radiography. The ideal position for the catheter tip is at the junction of the right atrium with the superior or inferior vena cava. Upon removal, the tip should be sent for culture. Catheter-related complications include septicaemia, venous thrombosis, hydrothorax and cardiac tamponade [3].

### Peripheral arterial catheterization

It is preferable to cannulate an artery with an indwelling catheter when repeated sampling is required. An FG 24 or FG 26 cannula may be used. A T-piece extension is attached to a 2 ml syringe with 0.45% heparinized sodium chloride and flushed. Locate the arteries as previously described under arterial puncture. Suitable arteries are the radial, dorsalis pedis or posterior tibial. Avoid the brachial, femoral or temporal arteries which carry a high risk of complications as they are end arteries.

Clean the skin over the artery with an alcohol swab then puncture the artery at an acute angle (<30°). On entering the artery an immediately blood flush back is observed. The trocar is partially retracted and the Teflon cannula gently advanced along the artery. The trocar is then completely withdrawn and the cannula connected to the T-piece extension.

The whole system is then gently flushed with correct siting of the cannula being confirmed by a transient blanching of the immediate area. The cannula is secured with adhesive tapes and the limb splinted. The cannula should be continuously perfused with heparinized 0.45% sodium chloride (1 unit ml$^{-1}$) at a rate of 1 ml hour$^{-1}$. This may be connected to a blood pressure transducer for continuous blood pressure monitoring. Luer lock connections should always be used to prevent potentially serious haemorrhage from accidental disconnections which may go undetected. For early detection of catheter-related complications, the tips of the fingers or toes (as appropriate) must be left exposed. Remove the catheter if digits spontaneously become discoloured or the limb is persistently cool. On removing the cannula, apply firm pressure over the puncture site until complete haemostasis is achieved.

### Umbilical vessel catheterization

Catheterization of the umbilical vessels is usually a necessity rather than an option in very premature infants. This is most easily done soon after birth but can be performed up to a week later. The procedure should be carried out with full aseptic precautions using either a plain end-hole type catheter (Argyle™ FG 3.5, Sherwood Medical, UK) or a side-hole catheter with an oxygen-sensing electrode (Neocath FG 4, Biomedical Sensors, UK). The infant should be carefully monitored during the procedure.

### Umbilical artery catheterization

The infant is gently restrained. Clean the umbilical stump with an iodine solution taking care to avoid the solution running down the flanks of the infant as prolonged contact of the solution with the skin under the infant can damage the skin. Drape the infant. Cut the cord obliquely with a scalpel some 2 cm from the base. An oblique cut exposes a greater surface area of the vessel improving the chances of a successful cannulation. Grasp the most superior edge of the cord with an artery clip. The umbilical vein is the largest vessel lying superiorly with the two thick walled arteries being inferiorly placed. The umbilical artery catheter is primed with heparinized 5% dextrose in preparation for catheterization.

Stabilize the cord stump with the artery clip and gently tease the lumen of one of the arteries open with a fine non-toothed forceps then further dilate with a probe to a depth of 1 cm. The already primed catheter (with an attached syringe) is then gently introduced into the open mouth of the dilated artery and gently advanced while the cord stump is pulled towards the infant's chest. It is worthwhile spending time gently dilating the mouth of the artery as the tiny vessels of small infants may be otherwise difficult to catheterize successfully and false passages are easily created. Resistance is often experienced as the artery turns caudally just below the umbilicus and at its junction with the internal iliac artery. Once the latter is traversed, an arterial pulsation becomes evident. If the catheter is advanced a distance equal to twice the distance between the groin and the base of the cord, its tip will be positioned at the L3/L4 level (low position). A high position at T8 can be achieved by advancing the catheter a further 5 cm. Either the high or low positions may be chosen, although the high position is reported to be associated with fewer complications and lasts longer [4].

The catheter is secured with a purse string around the base with further loops tied around the catheter. The catheter is further secured by a bridge tape (Figure 29.7). A constant infusion of heparinized 5% dextrose (1 unit ml$^{-1}$) is set up to run at 1 ml hour$^{-1}$, and connected to a blood pressure transducer as required. Infusing dextrose solutions avoids inappropriate sodium supplementation. The catheter position should be checked radiographically and adjusted as required. The radiograph has a

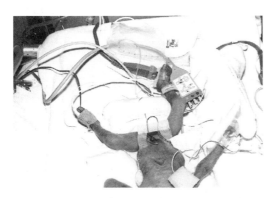

**Figure 29.7** Securing the umbilical artery catheter by a bridge tape

characteristic acute angle defining the internal iliac artery junction. Among the possible complications of umbilical artery catheterization are sepsis, arterial thrombosis and lower limb ischaemia. Should one or both lower limbs become persistently discoloured, the catheter should be removed.

## Umbilical vein catheterization

Umbilical vein catheterization is considerably easier than arterial catheterization as the vein is a large vessel readily cannulated with an FG 5 catheter. In the very small infant, umbilical vein catheterization soon after birth provides an alternative route for administering intravenous fluids during the first 48–72 hours of life. This avoids excessive handling of the infant when it is most unstable and peripheral vascular access difficult. When the infant's condition has stabilized, a percutaneous central line may then be inserted and the umbilical venous catheter removed. On the first day of life it is usually possible to advance the catheter through the ductus venosus into the right atrium.

Steady the cord by gripping the edge with an artery clamp. The primed catheter with an attached 5 ml syringe filled with heparinized 5% dextrose is advanced into the vein and aimed towards the chest. If the catheter impacts in the portal system a resistance will be felt with the catheter recoiling once the advancing pressure is released. Attempts to aspirate the catheter will not be successful. The catheter is pulled back 2 cm, twisted and re-threaded. When 6–7 cm of catheter has been advanced, the catheter does not spring back when released and there is free flow of blood on aspiration, the tip has most likely entered the inferior vena cava. Advance a further 1 cm to ensure the tip has entered the right atrium. The catheter is secured as described for the umbilical artery catheter, and continuously infused with heparinized 5% dextrose (1 unit ml$^{-1}$), [5].

The position of the catheter tip must be checked radiographically and adjusted as required. Umbilical venous catheters should not be used for infusions if the tip is in the liver as there is a risk of thrombotic complications and hepatic necrosis. Venous catheters do carry the risk of air embolism if the catheter is left open to the atmosphere.

### Catheter removal

Prior to removing the catheter, the stump is cleaned and dried Wharton's jelly removed. The catheter is drawn back slowly particularly the last 1–2 cm. Bleeding may be controlled by applying firm digital pressure with a sterile dressing. An additional suture is usually not required. The tip should always be sent for culture.

## Thoracentesis

### Chest transillumination

Transillumination of the chest with a fibre-optic cold-light source is a useful and rapid way of detecting a significant pneumothorax particularly in a ventilated infant whose condition suddenly deteriorates. With the cold-light closely applied to the chest, the affected side will appear hyperlucent. In very small preterm infants, however, the chest will be generally hyperlucent and unilateral pulmonary interstitial emphysema may be confused with a pneumothorax. Unless urgent measures are required, the suspicion of a pneumothorax must be confirmed radiographically, [5].

### Drainage of pneumothoraces

A ventilated infant who suddenly becomes hypoxaemic, bradycardic and hypotensive has probably developed a tension pneumothorax which requires immediate drainage. If the suspected diagnosis is supported by transillumination, an FG 25 or FG 23 butterfly needle attached to a three-way tap and 20 ml syringe is inserted anteriorly into the second intercostal space in a midclavicular line. The needle should not be advanced too far as it will puncture the lung as it re-inflates. The three-way tap allows drainage of air without disconnecting the syringe. A standard chest drain should be inserted as a sterile procedure following this emergency procedure.

After determining the most appropriate site for the drain, administer some intravenous analgesia (e.g. 1 mg pethidine). Rotate the infant slightly to expose the inferolateral chest wall with an assistant restraining the upper limbs. Clean the area with iodine and apply sterile drapes. Infiltrate the area with local anaesthetic, then make a small skin incision just above a rib using a straight-blade scalpel. Avoid the nipple and areolar area. Advance the blade 1–2 mm into the intercostal muscle then using an artery forceps continue teasing the muscles apart until the pleural space is entered – confirmed by a gush of air. An FG 12 chest drain with the trocar removed (to prevent lung puncture) is inserted 2 cm into the chest wall and directed towards the neck. Connect the drain to an underwater seal drain and secure the chest drain with a suture. The underwater seal should bubble or oscillate when correctly positioned. Cover the site with a transparent dressing (e.g. Tegaderm™, 3M, USA), further securing the chest drain to the chest wall. A low suction system (–5 cmH$_2$O) facilitates drainage. The position of the chest drain is checked radiographically [5,6].

When clamping the drain no longer leads to reaccumulation of air, the drain may be removed. After removing the tapes and dressing, the area is cleansed with iodine solution and a purse string suture placed around the drain. This is pulled tight as the drain is removed to prevent air entering the chest. Cover the site with a plastic dressing aerosol spray and a small adhesive plaster. The drain tip should be cultured.

### Drainage of pleural effusions

Pleural effusions merit drainage when causing respiratory compromise. A suitable drainage site is the fourth intercostal space on the posterior axillary line. Clean the site with iodine solution. Infiltrate the skin with local anaesthetic then gently insert an FG 19 cannula above the rib and advance slowly. Once the pleural space is entered, completely withdraw the trocar and attach a three-way tap and 10-ml syringe. Slowly aspirate the fluid into the syringe. Closely monitor the infant during the procedure. When the effusion has been completely drained, remove the cannula, spray the site with a plastic dressing and cover a small adhesive dressing.

### Pericardiocentesis

This is often a matter of urgency following a pneumopericardium or a pericardial effusion which leads to cardiac tamponade. Significant effusions are readily identified by echocardiography. An FG 19 or FG 21 cannula is required. Clean the skin of the anterior chest wall with iodine. Enter the left xiphocostal angle at an angle of 45° aiming the cannula at the left shoulder. At a depth of 5–10 mm the pericardium will be entered, the trocar completely withdrawn, a three-way tap attached and gentle suction applied. If fresh blood is withdrawn, the heart has been entered and the cannula should be withdrawn. A large pericardial fluid collection should be gradually drained to avoid sudden hypotension. Thick effusions may require insertion of an FG 10 pleural drain which may be left *in situ* and connected to an underwater seal drain [5,6].

### Abdominal paracentesis

This is most commonly done for marked ascites or pneumoperitoneum causing respiratory compromise, or for diagnostic purposes. It is prudent to perform an abdominal ultrasound scan prior to the procedure to determine the most appropriate drainage site. Otherwise the puncture should be in the left or right iliac fossae. Express the bladder. Clean the skin with iodine and infiltrate the site with 1% lignocaine. A large bore cannula (e.g. FG 18) is inserted through the skin and the trocar immediately withdrawn as soon as resistance gives way to prevent perforation of viscera. Advance the cannula a further 5–10 mm and attach a three-way tap and slowly aspirate the fluid. Large quantities of fluid should not be drained over a short period. Drains left *in situ* carry a risk of peritonitis. Upon removal cover the site with a plastic dressing aerosol spray (e.g. OpSite™ Smith & Nephew, UK) and a small adhesive dressing [5,6].

### Suprapubic bladder puncture

When confirmation of a possible urinary tract infection or urgent urine culture is required, suprapubic aspiration of urine is the method of choice for obtaining clean urine samples. This should be attempted at least 45 minutes after the last wet nappy. With the infant lying supine and the legs restrained, clean the skin above the symphysis pubis with iodine. Insert an FG 23 needle attached to a 5-ml syringe 1 cm above the symphysis pubis and in midline angling the needle into the pelvis. Apply constant gentle suction as the needle is advanced. The bladder will be entered at a

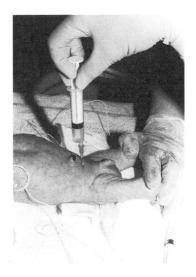

**Figure 29.8** Position for suprapubic bladder puncture

depth of approximately 1 cm and urine aspirated (Figure 29.8). The needle is then withdrawn and the site covered with a small adhesive dressing. The urine should immediately be forwarded for analysis.

### Lumbar puncture

Close monitoring is required during the procedure. The infant is placed in a lateral decubitus position and the spine gently flexed. The lumbar area is cleaned with iodine and sterile drapes applied. Identify the superior iliac crest and move down in a perpendicular line to the lumbar spine (spine of L4). A 3.6 cm FG 22 spinal needle is slowly inserted into the L3/L4 intervertebral space and advanced perpendicularly being pointed towards the umbilicus. As one commonly does not feel the needle entering the dural space and the subarachnoid space is only 5 mm from the surface, the stylet should be withdrawn frequently while advancing the needle. A common mistake is advancing the needle too far and puncturing the anterior vertebral venous plexus, testified by uniformly blood-stained fluid. Collect CSF for biochemical, bacteriological and viral analysis (7–10 drops per container). Re-introduce the stylet, gently remove the needle and spray the site with a plastic dressing. Finally cover with a small adhesive dressing.

## Ventricular tap

Ventricular taps may be required when managing progressive non-communicating hydrocephalus, confirming a diagnosis of suspected ventriculitis or rarely for administering intraventricular antibiotics. The procedure should only be performed when the ventricles are clearly dilated (confirmed ultrasonically) and with full sterile precautions. Place the infant supine with an assistant firmly holding the head. Shave and clean the skin overlying the anterior fontanelle. Insert a 5 cm long spinal needle through the lateral angle of the anterior fontanelle and slowly advance anteromedially towards the inner canthus of the eye. The dilated lateral ventricle is entered 1–2 cm from the surface. Allow the cerebrospinal fluid to drip from the needle (do not aspirate!). The needle should be advanced and retracted along the same track. Changing the direction of insertion *after* the brain is entered damages brain tissue. On removing the needle, cover the puncture site with a plastic aerosol dressing and apply a small adhesive dressing [5,6].

## Subdural tap

This procedure is rarely indicated because most subdural collections are small and do not require intervention. Subdural effusions can be diagnosed by ultrasound, magnetic resonance imaging or by computed tomography scanning. The procedure is similar to that described for ventricular puncture. The infant is similarly positioned and the scalp cleaned as already described. Using a subdural needle enter the subdural space from the lateral margin of the anterior fontanelle aiming towards the ipsilateral foot. The needle is often felt puncturing the dura at a depth of 2–3 mm. Withdraw the stylet and allow the fluid (if any) to drain. Congealed collections may not readily drip out and blood may require very gentle suction. If fluid is encountered on one side, the contralateral side should also be tapped. If no fluid is encountered on entering the dura, do not persist. The needle should not be pointed in different directions seeking a collection. A

successful tap makes repeat taps a necessity as subdural effusions commonly recur. On removing the needle cover the site with a plastic aerosol dressing and a small adhesive plaster.

---

### Practical points

1. Always administer analgesia before performing painful procedures.
2. Do not undertake procedures you have not been trained to perform.
3. Do not persist in any procedure(s) if repeatedly unsuccessfully, ask for assistance.
4. Only perform essential procedures in the critically ill infants as they may deteriorate significantly during procedures.
5. Monitor infants continuously during procedures and avoid hypothermia.
6. Make an accurate and legible record of all procedures (apart from the most minor ones) in the patient's medical records and record any adverse events.

---

# References

1. Anand, K.J.S. and Hickey, P.R. (1987) Pain and its effects in the human neonate and fetus. *N. Engl. J. Med.*, **317**, 1321–1329
2. Blumenfeld, T.A., Turi, G.K. and Blanc, W.A. (1979) Recommended site and depth of newborn heel skin punctures based on anatomical measurements and histopathology. *Lancet*, **1**, 230–233
3. Mupanemunda, R.H. and Mackanjee, H.R. (1992) A life-threatening complication of percutaneous central venous catheters in neonates. *Am. J. Dis. Child.*, **146**, 1414–1415
4. Kempley, S.T., Bennett, S., Loftus, B.G. and Gamsu, H.R. (1993) Randomized trial of umbilical arterial catheter position: clinical outcome. *Acta Paediatr.*, **82**, 173–176
5. Fletcher, M.A. and MacDonald, M.D. (eds). (1993) *Atlas of Procedures in Neonatology*. JB Lippincott Company, Philadelphia
6. Walsh-Sakys, M.C. and Krug, S.E. (1997) *Procedures in Infants and Children*. WB Saunders, Philadelphia, 1997

# Index

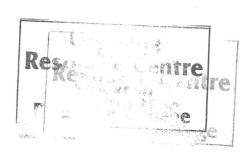